Biopsy interpretation of bone and bone marrow

Biopsy interpretation
of
bone and
bone marrow

Histology and immunohistology in paraffin and plastic

Prof. Bertha Frisch
Institutes of Pathology and Hematology
Diagnostic and Research Cancer Center
University of Tel-Aviv
TEL-AVIV
ISRAEL

Prof. Dr. med. Reiner Bartl
Medizinische Klinik III
Klinikum Großhadern
Ludwig-Maximilians-Universität
81377 MUNICH
GERMANY

Cytogenetics in collaboration with R. Rothman MSc

A member of the Hodder Headline Group
LONDON • SYDNEY • AUCKLAND
Copublished in the USA by
Oxford University Press, Inc., New York

First published in Great Britain in 1999 by
Arnold, a member of the Hodder Headline Group,
338 Euston Road, London NW1 3BH

http://www.arnoldpublishers.com

Co-published in the United States of America by
Oxford University Press Inc.,
198 Madison Avenue, New York, NY10016
Oxford is a registered trademark of Oxford University Press

Whilst the advice and information in this book are believed to be true and
accurate at the date of going to press, neither the authors nor the publisher
can accept any legal responsibility or liability for any errors or omissions
that may be made. In particular (but without limiting the generality of the
preceding disclaimer) every effort has been made to check drug dosages;
however it is still possible that errors have been missed. Futhermore,
dosage schedules are constantly being revised and new side-effects
recognized. For these reasons the reader is strongly urged to consult the
drug companies' printed instructions before administering any of the drugs
recommended in this book.

British Library Cataloguing in Publication Data
A catalogue record for this book is available from the British Library

Library of Congress Cataloging-in-Publication Data
A catalog record for this book is available from the Library of Congress

ISBN 0 340 74089 2

1 2 3 4 5 6 7 8 9 10

Typeset in 9.5/12.5 Stone serif by Best-set Typesetter Ltd., Hong Kong
Printed in Hong Kong

WITH THE INTRODUCTION, CONSTANT DEVELOPMENT AND RAPIDLY INCREASING APPLICATION OF THE TECHNIQUES OF MOLECULAR GENETICS, HISTOPATHOLOGY IS ON THE BRINK, OR RATHER, IS ALREADY IN THE THROES OF THE GREATEST REVOLUTION AND METAMORPHOSIS SINCE THE INITIAL OBSERVATION OF STAINED TISSUE SECTIONS IN THE LIGHT MICROSCOPE. THE EXAMPLES GIVEN IN THIS TEXT ARE ONLY THE TIP OF THE ICEBERG.

Contents

Preface

In recent years there has been a great increase in the number of bone marrow biopsies (BMB) taken because the indications have broadened in direct proportion to improvements in (1) biopsy needles, (2) methods of processing and therefore diagnostic reliability and (3) the number and range of additional investigative techniques available and applicable to bone biopsy sections. Consequently, the indications for taking biopsies have increased (see below) especially in internal medicine, oncology and osteology as well as in hematology. This is shown by the large number of articles and texts that have appeared over the past decade since the publication of the first edition in 1985.

This book deals with the diagnosis of bone and bone marrow histology and histopathology, with the emphasis on iliac crest biopsies, as these are clinically the most widely used. However, due to limitation of space and because this is intended principally to be a diagnostic text for bone and bone marrow biopsy histopathology, conditions in which a bone biopsy is unlikely to be performed have been omitted. As a result, emphasis has been placed on conditions in which biopsies are routinely taken as well as the disorders in which a bone biopsy can be expected to provide diagnostic and supplementary information. The length of the chapters consequently varies considerably and this also depends on whether a single disease entity or a group of disorders is dealt with. The first edition of this book was based on results of plastic-embedded bone biopsies because of the excellent preservation of the undecalcified bone and bone cells and the cytologic details of the bone marrow provided by this method. In this second edition have been added paraffin embedding and immunohistology as they are routinely employed and, in certain cases, provide additional information; for example, immunological characteristics for leukemia and lymphoma classification, and specific antibodies for identification of organ of origin in metastatic involvement of the bone marrow.

To increase the practical value of this edition, a biopsy check list has been added as well as characteristic clinical correlations at the end of many chapters, when appropriate. It should, however, also be borne in mind that an aspirate and smears or imprints are always taken and evaluated together with the histologic sections. Therefore, a working knowledge of the possibilities offered by application of the latest techniques for analysis of cell structure and function widens the scope for interpretation of bone biopsy histopathology. On tissue sections this is achieved by immunohistology, on aspirates by cytochemistry, immunology, flow cytometry (fluorescent-activated cell sorting, FACS) and cytogenetics, that is, characteristic clonal karyotypes. FACS is today an indispensible tool in the identification of the hematologic malignancies, as well as in the clarification of their origin and evolution. FACS is generally used for the flow cytometric analysis, though strictly speaking it is incorrect as in the examples given the results refer to the flow cytometry itself and a subsequent sorting was not carried out.

Cytogenetics today also constitutes an integral part of the initial investigation in hematologic (as well as other) malignancies, mainly because of the impressive advances made over the past decade which have transformed cytogenetic analysis into an investigative parameter contributing to diagnosis, classification and prognostic evaluation of hematologic malignancies, and thereby to therapeutic decisions. Since specific cytogenetic changes have been recognised and associated with distinct types of leukemias and malignant lymphomas, their detection is now considered an essential component not only of the initial diagnosis but also in follow-up, monitoring and determination of remission, residual disease and relapse. Chromosome analysis and molecular biology of the genes involved in chromosomal anomalies (the molecular basis of leukemia) have shown that the resulting encoded proteins participate in the process of malignant transformation. The genes resulting from chromosome alterations so far analysed encode: (1) tyrosine protein kinases, (2) serine protein kinases, (3) cell surface receptors, (4) growth factors and (5) mitochondrial membrane proteins. The largest group encodes transcriptional regulatory factors, which are crucial to cellular development, differentiation and function. Moreover, translocations in the lymphoid malignancies involving the immunoglobulin genes in B cell neoplasias and the T cell receptor genes in T cell neoplasias stimulate inappropriate expression of the other gene in the translocation. These and other far-reaching advances have provided new insights into the pathogenesis of the clinical manifestations of the leukemias and lymphomas, and the findings in bone marrow biopsies are one aspect of these manifestations. For example, the translocation t(14;18)(q32;q21) is a common chromosomal translocation in lymphoid malignancies, especially follicular lymphoma. BCL2 was discovered at the breakpoint of this translocation and is now known to be much more widely distributed. It is localised to mitochondria and blocks apoptosis – programmed cell death (PCD) – without affecting cellular proliferation. PCD is characterised morphologically by blebbing of nuclear and cell membranes, cell shrinkage and pyknosis. Many factors have been implicated in the regulation and modulation of apoptosis, and different cell types use different factors for the control of their own survival, proliferation, differentiation or death. Where appropriate and informative, results of FACS analysis have been given together with the bone biopsy findings. Only a few typical ones have been included, selected from over a thousand cases of biopsies and FACS analysis taken and done together. All these aspects are now considered (and will be, to ever greater degrees, as more and more antibodies are developed) in histopathological interpretation and consequent clinical implications for therapeutic decisions. The same applies to cytogenetics. The karyotypes given are derived from our own results and a survey of the literature; however, only the characteristic clonal karyotypes are listed. For a comprehensive coverage of clonal chromosomal aberrations, many characterised at the molecular level, see Mitelman *et al.* (1997) who provide an up-to-date map of each chromosome and the conditions that have been localised to it, as well as the genes involved.

Bibliography

Abstracts of 1st European Cytogenetics Conference (1991) *Cytogenetics and Cell Genetics*. Basel: Karger.

Ackerman (1966) *Surgical Pathology*, vol. 2, 8th edn. St Louis: Mosby.

Bain B., Clark D., Lampert E. (1992) *Bone Marrow Pathology*. Oxford: Blackwell.

Barbanti-Brodano G., Bendinelli M., Friedman H. (eds) (1995) *DNA Tumor Viruses: Oncogenic Mechanisms*. New York: Plenum.

Bartl R., Frisch B. (1993) *Biopsy of Bone in Internal Medicine: An Atlas and Sourcebook*, vol. 21. Dordrecht: Kluwer Academic.

Bernstein I. (1996) Hematologic malignancies. *Current Opinion in Hematol.*, **3 (4)**.

Beutler E., Lichtman M.A., Coller B.S., Kipps T.J. (eds) (1995) *Williams Hematology*, vol. 5. McGraw-Hill.

Bilezikian J.P., Raisz L.G., Rodau G.A. (1996) *Principles of Bone Biology*. San Diego: Academic.

Brunning R., McKenna R. (1994) *Tumors of the Bone Marrow*. Washington: AFIP.

Catovsky D. (ed.) (1991) *The Leukemic Cell*, 2nd edn. Edinburgh: Churchill Livingstone.

Clarkson B. (ed.) (1994) *Current Opinion in Hematology: Hematologic Malignancies*, **1 (4)**.

Cline M.J. (1994) The molecular basis of leukemia. *New Engl J Med.*, **330 (5)**, 328–36.

Connor M., Ferguson-Smith M. (1997) *Essential Medical Genetics*, 5th edn. London: Blackwell.

Cotran, Kumar, Robbins (1994) *Pathologic Basis of Disease*, 5th edn. Philadelphia: W.B. Saunders.

Fielding A.K., Ager S., Russell S.J. (1997) ABC of clinical hematology: the future of hematology, molecular biology, and gene therapy. *BMJ*, **314**, 1396.

Foucar K. (1995) *Bone Marrow Pathology*. Chicago: ASCP.

Frisch B., Bartl R. (1990) *Atlas of Bone Marrow Pathology*, vol. 15. Dordrecht: Kluwer Academic.

Ganser, A., Hoelzer D. (1994) Acute leukemia. *Current Opinion in Hematology*, **1**, 248–55.

Hoffbrand A.V., Pettit J.E. (eds) (1995) *Essential Hematology*, 3rd edn. Oxford: Blackwell Science.

Hoffman R., Benz E.J. Jr., Shattil S.J. *et al.* (1995) *Hematology: Basic Principles and Practice*, 2nd edn. Edinburgh: Churchill Livingstone.

Knowles D.M. (ed.) (1996) *Neoplastic Hematopathology*. Baltimore: Williams & Wilkins.

Korsmeyer S.J. (1992) Bcl-2 initiates a new category of oncogenes: regulators of cell death. *Blood*, **4**, 879–86.

Mitleman F., Mertens F., Johansson B. (1997) A breakpoint map of recurrent chromosomal rearrangements in human neoplasia. *Nature Genetics*, **15**, 417–19.

Mufti G.J., Flandrin G., Schaefer H.E. *et al.* (1996) *An Atlas of Malignant Hematology*. Martin Dunitz.

Odero M.D., Calasanz M.J., Marin J., *et al.* (1997) Cytogenetic analysis of neoplastic hematological disorders. A survey of 2,500 samples from a single institution. *Cytogenet Cell Genet.*, **77**, 129.

Rasko I., Downes C.S. (1995) *Genes in Medicine: Molecular Biology and Human Genetic Disorders*. London: Chapman &Hall.

Robinson J.P. (ed.) (1993) *Handbook of Flow Cytometry Methods*. Chichester: John Wiley.

Rodak B.F. (1995) *Diagnostic Hematology*. Philadelphia: W.B. Saunders.

Rozman C., Woessner S., Feliu E. *et al.* (1993) *Cell Ultrastructure for Hematologists*. Doyma.

Savill J. (1997) Role of molecular cell biology in understanding disease. *BMJ*, **314**, 203–8.

Strauchen Y. (1996) *Diagnostic Histopathology of the Bone Marrow*. New York: Oxford University Press.

Tang D.G., Porter A.T. (1996) Apoptosis: a current molecular analysis. *Pathol Oncol Res.*, **2 (3)**.

Testoni N., Martinelli G., Farabegoli P. *et al.* (1996) A new method of 'in-cell reverse transcriptase-polymerase chain reaction' for the detection of BCR/ABL transcript in chronic myeloid leukemia patients. *Blood*, **87 (9)**, 3822–7.

Veldman T., Vignon C., Schröck E. *et al.* (1997) Hidden chromosome abnormalities in hematological malignancies detected by multicolour spectral karyotyping. *Nature Genetics*, **15**, 406–10.

Weed L.L. (1997) New connections between medical knowledge and patient care. *BMJ*, **315**, 231–5.

Yates J.R.W. (1996) Medical genetics. *BMJ*, **312**, 2021–5.

Yawata Y. (1996) *Atlas of Blood Diseases: Cytology and Histology*. Martin Dunitz.

Acknowledgements

We wish to thank all doctors who referred patients or sent biopsies, as well as the staff of the histopathology and photographic departments. Special appreciation goes to our personal technical assistants Ms S. Choivenitsky and Ms J. Sturm; to Ms S Bar-On for performing the flow cytometry, and to Dr E. Berger, Head of the Immunology Laboratory. We are greatly indebted to Ms E. Asher for expert secretarial help and typing the manuscript. We thank Dr Lifshitz-Mercer for reading the manuscript, and Dr Baratz for scientific discussions.

1 Biopsy of bone and bone marrow

Indications for bone and bone marrow biopsies

Patients

Biopsies can be obtained from patients of all ages (1–96 years is the range in our institutes to date). Consequently, the differences in skeletal structure and bone marrow in different bones, as well as the age-related alterations in both osseous and hematopoietic components, must be taken into account, particularly with respect to histomorphometric measurements.

Indications

A long list of indications has now been established in osteology, hematology, internal medicine and oncology, and can be summarised as follows:

1. In all conditions that might affect the bone, either primarily or secondarily; when the diagnosis is in doubt; or when confirmation is sought of a specific process, e.g. metastases, multiple myeloma and systemic mastocytosis.

2. In all cases where aspiration of the bone marrow is considered as a diagnostic procedure, there are advantages in taking a biopsy at the same time. The patient is psychologically prepared, the local anesthetic will have been administered, and the mental and physical stress of another procedure at a later date will be avoided. Moreover, since aspiration and biopsy are complementary procedures, if the biopsy is omitted, the physician will not obtain maximum information and the patient will not have the full benefit of the investigation.

3. Clarification of numerous other disorders, such as infections, including AIDS, toxo- and histoplasmosis, granulomatous conditions, amyloidosis, vascular disease, pyrexia of unknown origin, and the effects of metabolic disturbances, and storage diseases.

4. Whenever a dry tap or insufficient material is obtained on aspiration.

5. Staging and classification in malignant lymphomas (ML), multiple myeloma (MM) and Hodgkin's disease (HD), and pattern of involvement and quantitation of the tumor cell burden in the bone marrow.

6. Diagnosis and evaluation of the bone marrow in myeloproliferative disorders (MPD), and in myelodysplastic syndromes (MDS).

7. Suspected minimal lesions and/or hypocellular variants of hematologic malignancies and other conditions (e.g. aplastic anemias).

8. Evaluation of fibrosis and other stromal reactions and manifestations, e.g. iron depletion or overload, serous (gelatinous) atrophy and inflammatory reactions.

9. Evaluation of residual normal hematopoiesis in involved bone marrows (e.g., in patients with ML and thrombocytopenia or anemia, are megakaryocytes present and is there red cell aplasia respectively?).

10. Monitoring of therapy, remission, relapse, disease progression or transformation (as in ML, MPD and MDS), and recognition of concomitant diseases in the bone marrow in any myelo- or lymphoproliferative disorder.

11. Evaluation of the bone marrow before bone marrow transplantation, and before harvesting of bone marrow of patients in remission for possible future autotransplantation in relapse.

1

12. There are many other indications in oncology, osteology and internal medicine, for example, clarification of anemia, fever of unknown origin (FUO), unexplained weight loss and elevated erythrocyte sedimentation rate (ESR). Note that when an aspirate is taken, it is known exactly what was taken out, but there is no knowledge of what was left inside!

Uni- or bilateral biopsies in patients with malignant lymphomas

With respect to bone biopsies in malignant lymphomas, the question of taking uni- or bilateral biopsies in the staging of lymphomas has not yet been decided. In our experience a large biopsy (or two smaller ones taken from the same iliac crest) is just as effective (if not more so) than bilateral biopsies. Moreover, the references dealing with this subject do not give biopsy size so that comparisons of the efficacy of the two methods are not valid. It should be stressed that our results on single biopsies include detection of the highest rates of involvement published in the literature indicating objectively that large, single biopsies are as effective as bilateral ones, and are less traumatic for the patient.

Single or double biopsies in patients with metastases

In patients with suspected skeletal metastases, particularly when imaging techniques show negative results in the bones of the pelvis, it is sometimes useful to take two biopsies from the same anesthetised site, so that a larger area is sampled. This procedure may yield one positive and one negative biopsy.

Biopsy sites

In determining the choice of site, four main considerations apply:

1. It should be easily accessible, involving a minimum of trauma and danger to the patient.

2. It should contain cortical and trabecular bone.

3. It should provide representative bone structure and turnover, and contain red hematopoietic marrow.

4. Repeat biopsies with minimal variability should be possible at this site.

The posterior (and occasionally the anterior) iliac crest is the preferred site from which bone marrow biopsies are obtained under local anesthesia (except for babies and small children from whom biopsies are sometimes taken under general anesthesia). Bone biopsies can be obtained in the operating theater under radiological guidance from almost any skeletal area, depending on the patient's condition, the indications and the diagnostic requirements. There are differences in the amounts of cortical and trabecular bone and marrow in different regions of the ilium, but these have no practical significance (Figures 1.1–1.5). Likewise, the proportions of bone, parenchyme

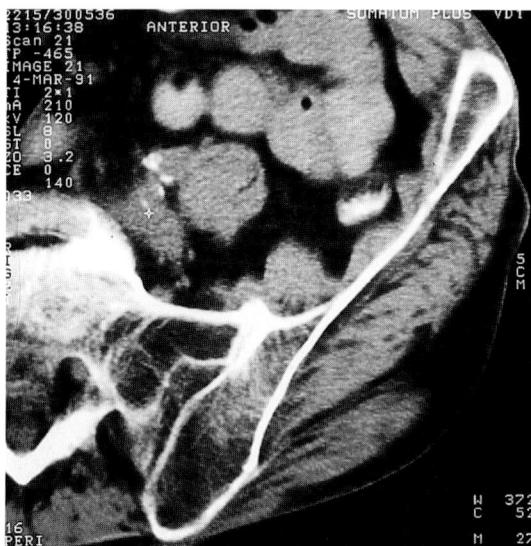

1.1 Computed tomographic scan of a pelvis at the level of the posterior superior iliac spine (processus spinosus). Note the thinner posterior than anterior cortex, upper right, and width and length of the posterior iliac intracortical space, lower left.

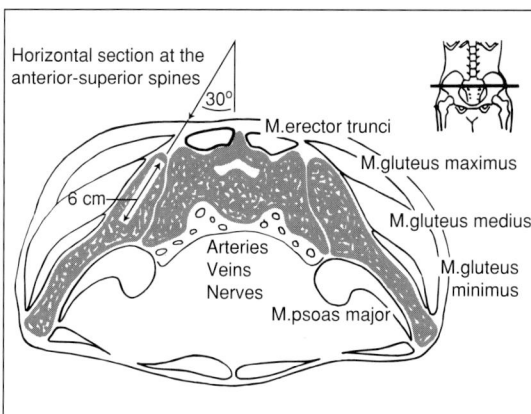

1.2 Sketch of horizontal section at the level of the anterior-superior spinous processes of the ilium (see insert). Note (a) that the posterior ilium is broader than the anterior, and (b) that long biopsies can be taken safely from the posterior ilium. In addition both external and internal surfaces of the ilium are protected by muscles.

1.3 Sketch of cortical bone as seen in bone biopsy sections. Variations are due to the site and angle at which the biopsy is taken.

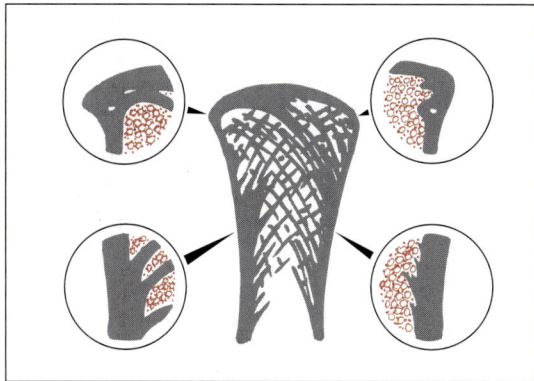

1.4 Surface of cut plastic block to illustrate variability of trabeculae as well as intertrabecular areas.

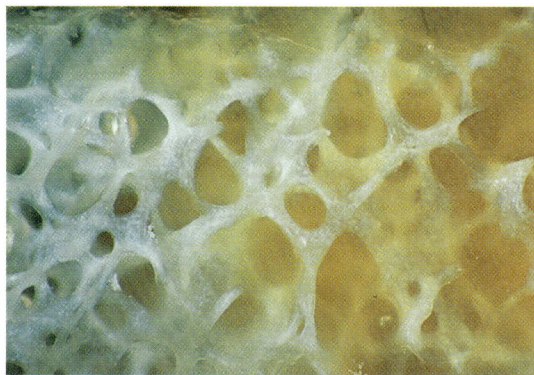

1.5 Section of plastic-embedded biopsy; Gomori's stain showing subcortical cellular, left, and deeper almost acellular areas, right, due to replacement by fat cells.

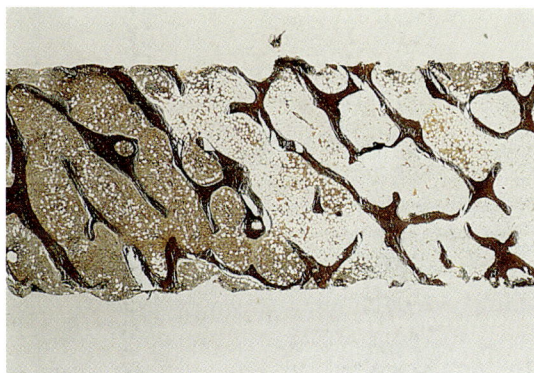

1.6 Histomorphometric data from bone marrow biopsies, taken from the iliac crest (●) and lumbar vertebra (○) correlated with age (150 autopsy cases, non-hematological and non-osseous disorders).

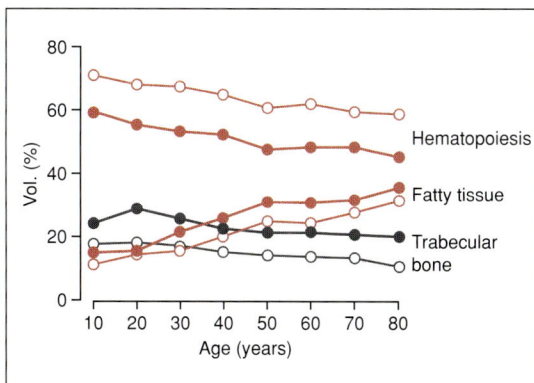

and fat vary in the different parts of the skeleton containing the red hematopoietic marrow, but the basic constituents are the same. For example, the volume percentages of trabecular bone are less, and those of the marrow cavities are greater, in sternum and vertebral bodies than in the ilium. They also have a higher parenchyme-to-fat ratio (a factor contributing to the popularity of the sternum as a site for aspiration) (Figure 1.6). Scintigraphic investigation of the ileum after bone biopsies revealed no abnormalities when the biopsies had been taken with the manual trephines.

Biopsy needles

1. The needle most commonly used (especially by hematologists) of the three main groups available is the 11 or 8 gauge 'disposable' needle which provides biopsies 2 mm in diameter, while the length varies (1–6 cm) according to the depth to which the needle is introduced in the posterior iliac crest (Figure 1.7a and b). Long biopsies can be obtained quite safely because the needle is inserted between the two cortices of the ileum, and there is no danger to the patient, even when a long biopsy core is removed. Disposable needles 4 mm × 13 or 15 cm are also available. Because of their thinner walls and wider diameter, these 'disposable' needles penetrate the bone more easily.

2. The transilial needle used for horizontal cortex-to-cortex biopsies, 8 mm diameter, taken from the anterior ileum only.

3. The electric drill used for vertical biopsies (from the anterior ileum) of about 4 mm diameter; however, this method is not used in our Institutes as biopsies obtained by the 4 mm × 13 or 15 cm manual trephines are both wide and long enough, and are suitable both for diagnostic evaluation and histomorphometric measurements if required.

The transilial biopsies are preferred by nephrologists, while the electric drill is used by some clinicians when the bone is expected to be very soft or very hard. In our Institutes the 2 or 3 mm disposable needle is used for young, especially male, patients or when hard bone is expected, and the disposable needles 3–4 mm wide by 13 or 15 cm long in all patients >50 years. Needles providing a core of 3–4 mm width are recommended when histomorphometric measurements of cortical and trabecular bone are envisaged. The longer 15 cm needles are especially recommended when the patient is obese and there is a thick layer of fat that must be traversed before the periosteum is reached. A biopsy core of 20–30 mm in length is required to ensure adequate sampling of bone and bone marrow.

Preparation of patients and taking the biopsy

1. After identification, the procedure is explained; the patient is reassured and asked to sign a printed formal consent form.

2. Knowledge of the patient's clinical condition is important so that if cardiac or pulmonary problems are present appropriate measures can be taken in advance. If there are respiratory difficulties, a biopsy may even be carried out with the patient sitting on a chair with the head resting on folded arms on a table in front.

3. A complete blood count (CBC), especially platelets, is needed; bleeding time and minimal coagulation tests should also be available.

4. Knowledge of current drug therapy (e.g. aceto-salicylic acid, (aspirin)), of allergies and sensitivities should be available, and if necessary appropriate measures should be taken, i.e. interruption of anticoagulants, administration of platelets or coagulation factors.

5. If the patient is apprehensive a tranquilising drug, e.g. 5 mg diazepam, given 30 min beforehand, may be helpful since it reduces psychological tension thereby inducing muscular relaxation, so easing the whole procedure.

6. Bone marrow biopsy must not be taken from a previously irradiated area. A suitable site on the opposite iliac crest should be selected instead.

Contraindications and potential complications

Bone biopsies are (relatively) contraindicated in patients with bleeding disorders; if neces-

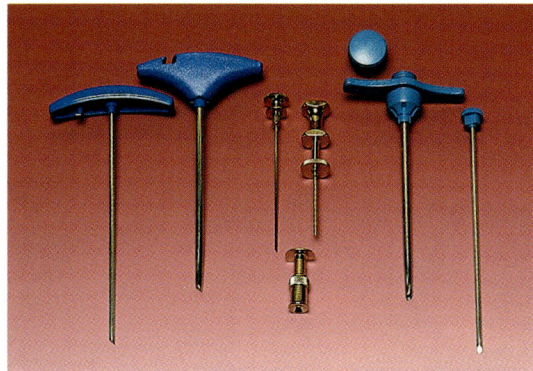

1.7a Types of manual trephines and aspirate needles; wider and longer bone biopsy needles are also available.

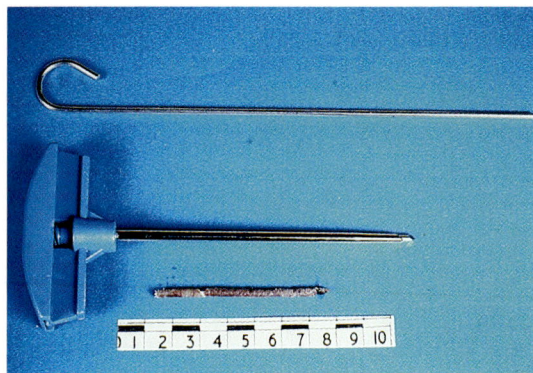

1.7b A needle frequently used, and a biopsy taken with it.

sary, the same precautionary measures must be taken as for other operations in such patients, i.e. prior administration or supplementation of the required blood products, e.g. fresh frozen plasma, platelets. Complications in our Institutes are rare, being <0.5%; they include hematoma, transient neuropathy, wound infection and osteomyelitis, drug reactions, and pain lasting more than a few days. Seeding of malignant cells along the needle track occurred once in a patient with disseminated metastases.

Position

Unless otherwise indicated, the patient is placed in the left lateral position, with legs drawn up to the chest. Alternatively, some operators prefer the patient lying on the abdomen (Figure 1.8). The posterior superior iliac spine is identified by palpation along the iliac crest and the spot marked by light pressure with a fingernail. This posterior spine is usually palpable even in fairly obese individuals. Drapes are then put in place and the area cleaned and disinfected.

Local anesthesia: infiltration

(Figure 1.9)

The injection (e.g. Lidocaine 2% without adrenalin) is started with an intradermal needle and the dermis is infiltrated so that a *peau d'orange* effect is produced. This ensures that the patient will not experience pain when a small incision is subsequently made in the skin. The needle is then exchanged for a longer one and is advanced through the layer of adipose tissue to the periosteum: an area of approximately 2 cm across is infiltrated. This procedure should be done slowly and carefully until the patient no longer feels pain when the periosteum is pricked with the needle. Careful infiltration of the periosteum goes a long way to ensure the success of the procedure. The overlying skin is massaged for increased effect and after the skin is cleaned, a small incision 4–5 mm is made in the *peau d'orange* area with a sterile scalpel.

Taking the biopsy

The biopsy is always taken before the aspirate to avoid disruption of marrow architecture and to lessen bleeding and hypocellularity in the biopsy area if taken after the aspirate.

After the area has been wiped with disinfectant, the biopsy needle is introduced and pushed through the cortex with slow, rotary movements. As the tip of the needle passes into the subcortical space a change in resistance is felt and the obdurator is immediately withdrawn (Figure 1.10). In cases where a bone disorder is suspected, the obdurator is withdrawn once the needle is firmly placed in the periosteum so that cortical bone is obtained for evaluation. The needle is advanced by slow, rotary movements till a sufficient depth is reached (Figure 1.11); the needle is then

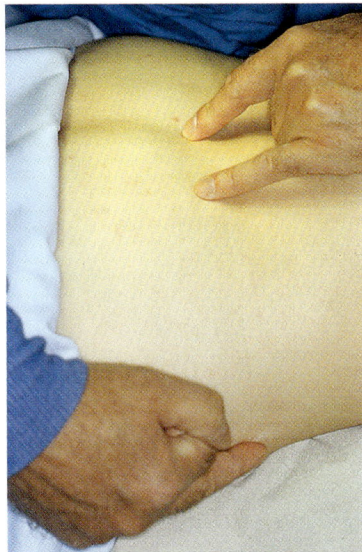

1.8 Palpation to ascertain position of iliac crest and posterior spinous process.

1.9 (left) Infiltration of biopsy site with local anesthetic.

1.10 (right) Withdrawal of obdurator after biopsy needle has penetrated the cortex.

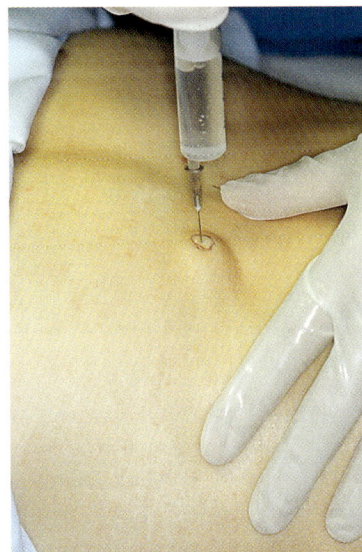

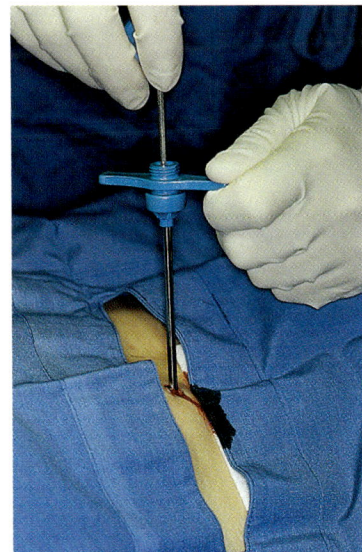

rotated 360°, withdrawn 2–3 mm, the angle is changed and the needle is advanced again for 2–3 mm, rotated completely two or three times and withdrawn gently. Pressure is exerted on the incision after application of a sterile pad.

The biopsy is removed gently by insertion of a metal probe through the front tip of the needle, so pushing the biopsy core out at the opposite end (Figures 1.12 and 1.13). Imprints are made and the core fixed as required.

Aspirate

Once the sterile pad is removed, an aspiration needle is introduced, preferably at about 1 cm from the spot where the bone marrow biopsy was taken, and marrow is aspirated into sterile test tubes with the appropriate anticoagulant or culture media. The first few drops of aspirate are collected in a separate syringe without anticoagulant and smears are made. These drops have the most marrow and are least diluted with peripheral blood (Figure 1.14). The rest of the aspirate is collected in a syringe with anticoagulant; the amount depends on the diagnostic requirements, for example, both for flow cytometry or fluorescent-activated cell sorting (FACS) (Figure 1.15) and for cytogenetics comprising conventional chromosome analysis (Figure 1.16a–d) and fluorescent *in situ* hybridisation (FISH) (Figure 1.17).

Dressing

After aspiration, the incision is again wiped clean and covered with another sterile pad and elasto-plaster. The patient is given a dated, signed sheet of instructions in case of excessive pain, bleeding or infection.

Discharge

All (ambulatory or non-hospitalised) patients stay in the daycare unit or waiting room for 0.5–1 h after completion of the procedure, and before discharge are examined for hemorrhage. In rare cases, patients stay for 1–3 h if bleeding has occurred during the procedure, aspiration or thereafter. A possible cause for such bleeding may be found in the biopsy sections which show large blood vessels or ectatic sinusoids as

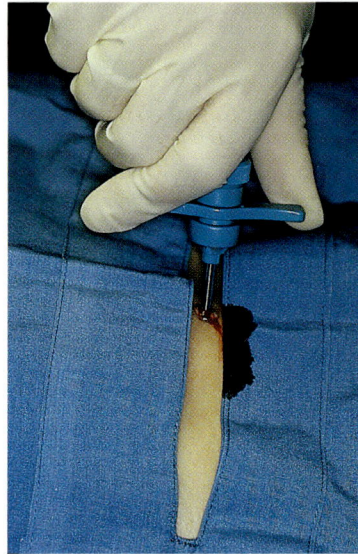

1.11 The biopsy needle is advanced by slow rotary movements till sufficient depth is reached.

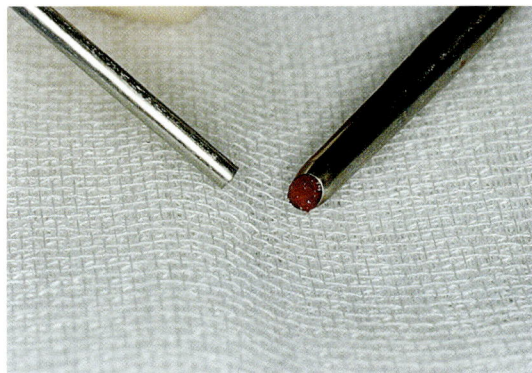

1.12 Biopsy needle (after withdrawal) with tip of biopsy showing, and probe at right.

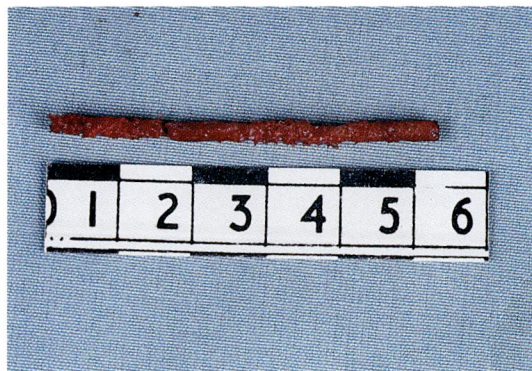

1.13 Biopsy measuring 5.5 cm in length, taken with the needle as shown in Figures 1.7–1.12.

in OMS (Figure 1.18). The patient then lies with a small sand bag on the area until the bleeding has stopped. On discharge, each patient is given a signed, dated, printed sheet of instructions for the prevention or treatment

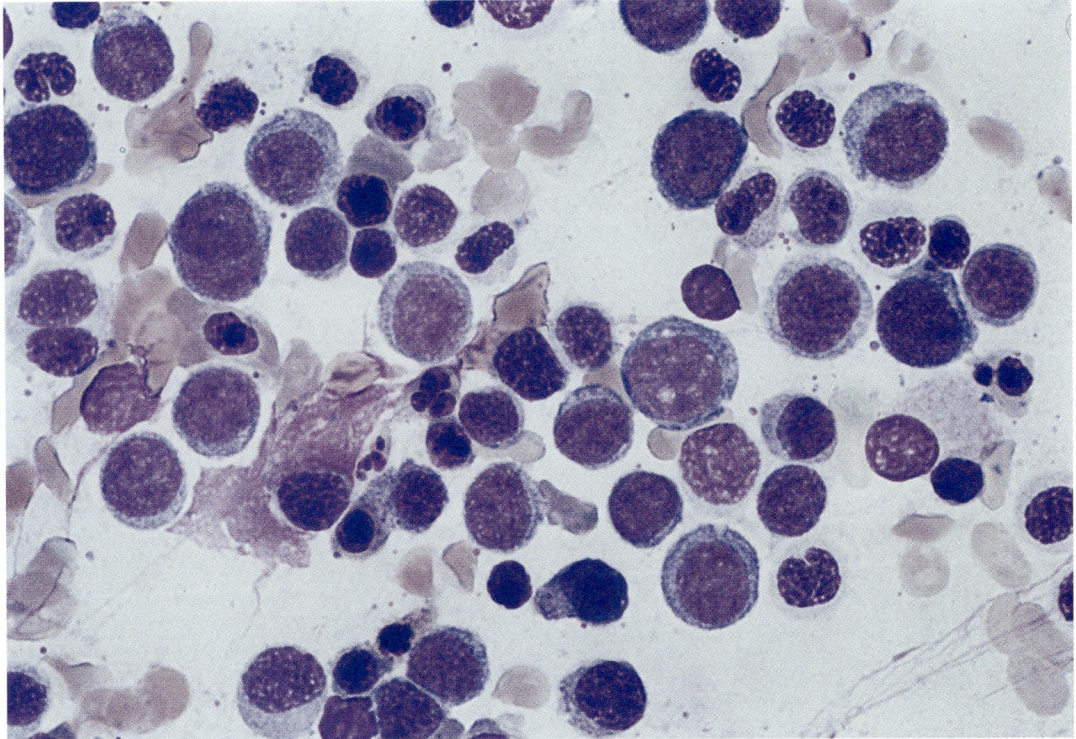

1.14 Giemsa-stained imprint of biopsy (similar to part of aspirate smear) showing bone marrow cells.

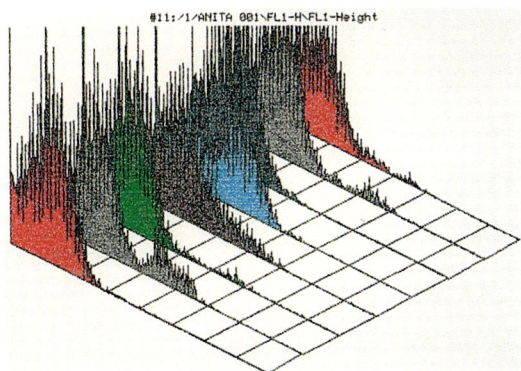

1.15 Histogram of flow cytometry of normal bone marrow, without evidence for a myelo- or lympho-proliferative disorder.

of any occurrence of bleeding, infection, swelling or exceptional pain.

Rapid processing

Biopsies that are wide enough (≥3 mm) and/or long enough (≥4 cm) may be cut and the pieces used for different purposes: fixation for both plastic and paraffin embedding, and fresh-frozen for cryostat sections. (See Appendix for precise description of methods). However, in urgent cases processing can be accomplished rapidly, with a total time of 24–26 h.

For plastic embedding

For plastic embedding the following times are used: a 4–6 h fixation, 4–6 h dehydration (two changes) infiltration 1–2 h (two changes) polymerisation 12–14 h (overnight), cut, mount and dry 0.5–1 h, stain by Giemsa or H&E (hematoxylin and eosin) and cover 0.5–1 h, total time 24–26 h (Figure 1.19).

The plastic blocks are cut in a standard histopathology microtome such as the Leica (Jung Reichert) 2055, with manual and/or automatic sectioning which is carried out with a heavy-duty tungsten-tipped knife. The sections are floated on hot water (>70°C), which straightens them; they are then picked up on glass slides from the hot water, covered with filter paper and pressure briefly applied by means of a roller to flatten and attach them to the slides.

For paraffin embedding

For paraffin embedding only about 16–24 h are required when short decalcification times are

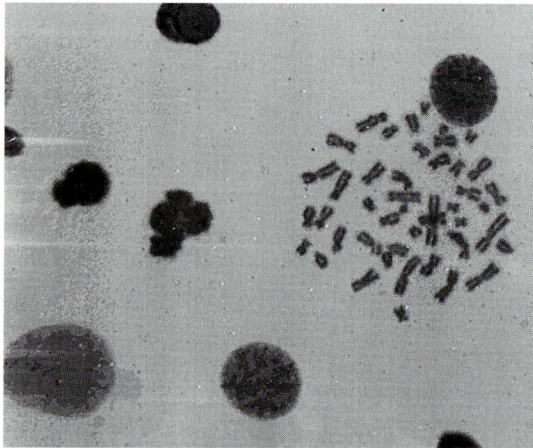

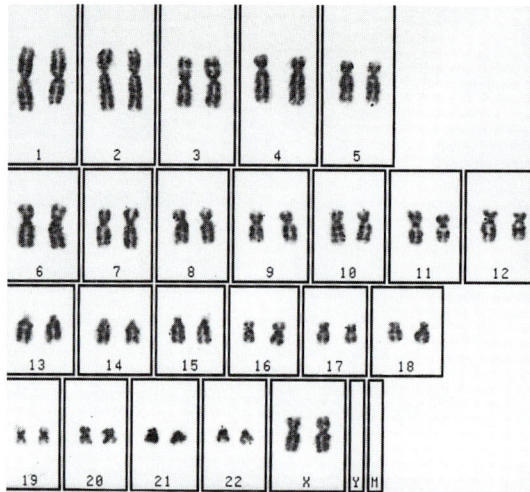

1.16a (left) Metaphase spread of good quality, suitable for conventional chromosome analysis and interphase nuclei. Both are suitable for FISH.

1.16b (right) Karyotype showing arrangement of XX chromosomes according to size and number 1–22 and 2X chromosomes: normal female karyotype.

1.16c (left) Normal male karyotype 46XY.

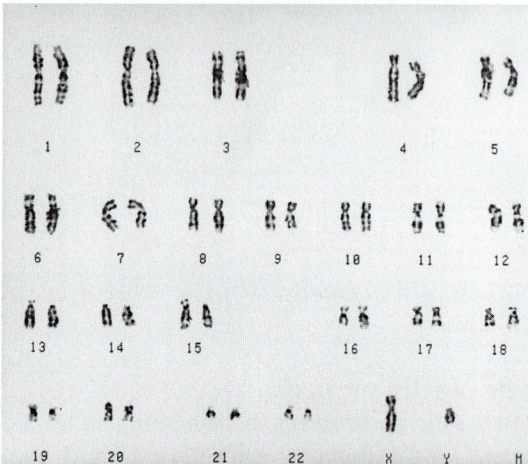

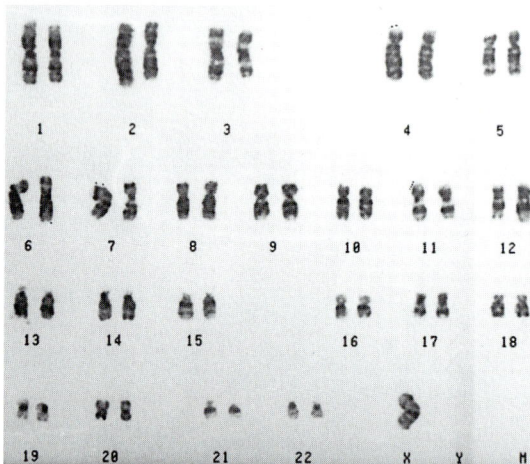

1.16d (right) Male karyotype with loss of the y chromosome, may occur in elderly people but has no known pathologic significance.

1.17 (left) Example of FISH on interphase nuclei for chromosome 8. The nuclei have two signals each.

1.18 (right) BMBS Giemsa, showing large, dilated blood vessel within biopsy, which could contribute to bleeding during and after taking the biopsy.

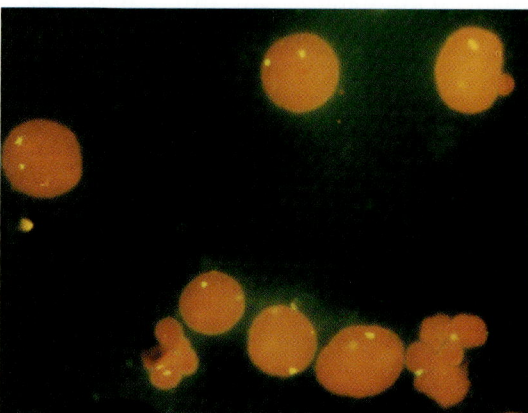

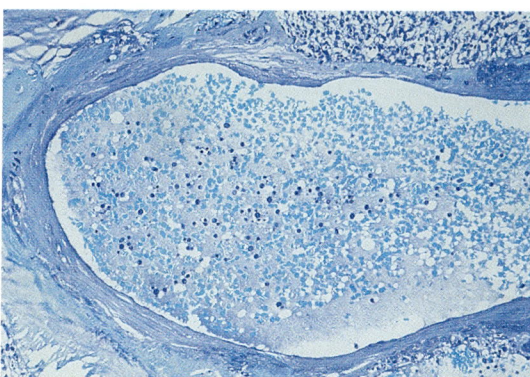

used (0.5–1 h) depending on the width of the biopsy and the amount of bone present: fixation 3–4 h, decalcification 0.5–1 h, rinse in distilled water 30 min, transfer to 70% methanol and process in an automatic tissue processor such as a Tissue-Tek (VIP300, Miles, UK), followed by cutting, mounting and staining by routine histopathologic methods. The biopsy sections, both paraffin and plastic, illustrated in this volume were processed according

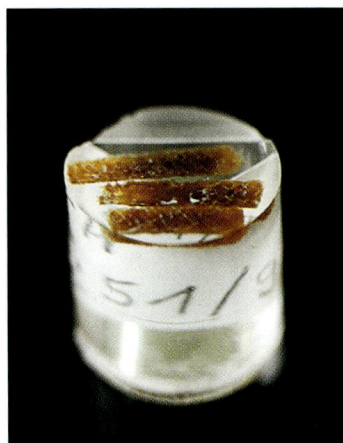

1.19 Trimmed surface of plastic block to show parallel pieces of the biopsy, embedded together.

to these rapid schedules. Immunohistology, of course, takes longer, depending on what is required, and this is decided on after microscopic evaluation of the plastic and paraffin biopsy sections stained by Giemsa and/or H&E.

Polymerase chain reaction (PCR)

This can be done on DNA from peripheral blood cells, cells of the bone marrow aspirate, and on DNA extracted from paraffin- or plastic-embedded tissue.

Check list: Biopsy of Bone and Bone Marrow

- Identity of patient.
- Is patient under any medication such as anticoagulant therapy and/or aspirin?
- Have appropriate blood tests been carried out?
- Has the patient read, understood and signed an informed consent form?
- Is there any drug sensitivity or allergy to iodine or local anesthetic?
- The patient is checked 0.5–1 h after the procedure before discharge or return to the ward.
- Has the patient received specific instructions and a printed form for avoidance of complications?
- The patient must avoid driving a car on the day of the bone marrow biopsy.
- The patient must avoid taking anticoagulants and/or aspirin for 1–2 days after the bone marrow biopsy.
- Do not wet dressing for the next 2–4 days to avoid infection.

Bibliography

Ades C.J., Ablett G.A., Collins R.J., Bunce I.H. (1989) Cell suspensions from collagenase digestion of bone marrow trephine biopsy specimens. *J. Clin. Pathol.*, **42 (4)**, 427–31.

Almeida J., Garcia-Marcos M.A., Vallejo C. *et al.* (1995) Results of a series of 104 consecutive bilateral bone marrow biopsy specimens in lymphoproliferative disorders. *Sangre (Barc)*, **40 (5)**, 365–8.

Amanao Y., Kumazaki T. (1996) Case report: serous atrophy of bone marrow and subcutaneous tissue enhancement associated with recurrent rectal carcinoma: MR appearances. *Comput Med Imaging Graph.*, **20 (3)**, 183–5.

Argiris A., Maris T., Papavasiliou G. *et al.* (1996) Radiotherapy effects on vertebral bone marrow: easily recognizable changes in T2 relaxation times. *Magn Reson Imaging*, **14 (6)**, 633–8.

Bartl R., Frisch B. (1993) *Biopsy of Bone in Internal Medicine: An Atlas and Sourcebook.* Dordrecht: Kluwer Academic.

Bartl R., Frisch B., Buchenrieder B. *et al.* (1984) Multiparameter studies on 650 bone marrow biopsy cores. Diagnostic value of combined utilisation of imprints, cryostat and plastic sections in medical practice. *Bibl. Haematologica*, **50**, 1.

Bartl R., Frisch B., Burkhardt R. (1982) *Bone Marrow Biopsies Revisited. A New Dimension*

for Haematologic Malignancies. Basel: Karger (2nd edn 1985).

Bartl R., Frisch B., Burkhardt R. (1989) Bone marrow histology. In Catovsky (ed), *Methods in Haematology. The Leukemic Cell.* Edinburgh: Churchill Livingstone.

Beckstead J.H. (1986) The bone marrow biopsy. A diagnostic strategy. *Arch Pathol Lab Med.*, **110**, 175.

Bird A.R., Jacobs P., Shuttleworth M. (1995) Bone marrow examination in clinical practice. *Hemat Rev and Comm*, **9 (2)**, 111–40.

Block M. (1976) Bone marrow examination. *Arch Pathol Lab Med.*, **100**, 454–6.

Block N. (1976) *Text Atlas of Haematology.* Philadelphia: Lea & Febiger.

Burgio V.L. (1991) Improved bone marrow biopsy technique. *Eur J Haematol,* **47,** 315–16.

Burkhardt R. (1971) Bone marrow and bone tissue. In *Colour Atlas of Clinical Histopathology.* Berlin: Springer.

Burkhardt R., Frisch B., Bartl R. (1982) Bone biopsy in haematological disorders. *J Clin Pathol.,* **35,** 257.

Colvin B.T. (1980) Practical procedures. How to biopsy the marrow. *Br J Hosptial Med,* **24,** 176–8.

Crisan D., Farkas D.H. (1993) Bone marrow biopsy imprint preparations: use for molecular diagnostics in leukemias. *Ann Clin Lab Sci,* **23 (6),** 407–22.

Duhamel G. (1974) *Histopathologie clinque de la moelle osseuse.* Paris: Masson.

Duncan H., Rao D.S., Parfitt A.M. (1980) Complications of bone biopsy. *Metab Bone Dis Rel Res.,* **2,** 475.

Ellis L.D., Jensen W.N., Westerman M.P. (1964) Needle biopsy of bone and marrow. *Arch Intern Med,* **114,** 213–21.

Estey E., Pierce S. (1996) Routine bone marrow exam during first remission of acute myeloid leukemia. *Blood,* **87 (9),** 3899–902.

Frisch B., Bartl R. (1984) *Bone Marrow Biopsies Updated.* Bibliotheca Haematologica 50. Basel: Karger.

Frisch B., Bartl R. (1990) *Atlas of Bone Marrow Pathology.* Dordrecht: Kluwer Academic.

Frisch B., Bartl R., Burkhardt R. (1982) Bone marrow biopsy in clinical medicine. An overview. *Haematologia,* **3,** 245.

Frisch B., Lewis S.M., Burkhardt R., Bartl R. (1985) *Biopsy Pathology of Bone and Bone Marrow.* London: Chapman & Hall.

Gruber H.E., Stauffer M.E., Thomson E.R., Baylink D.J. (1981) Diagnosis of bone disease by core biopsies. *Semin Hematol,* **18,** 258–78.

Grunewald K., Feichtinger H., Weyrer K. *et al.* (1990) DNA isolated from plastic embedded tissue is suitable for PCR. *Nuclear Acids Research,* **18 (20),** 6151.

Haddy T.B., Parker R.I., Magrath I.T. (1989) Bone marrow involvement in young patients with non-Hodgkin's lymphoma: the importance of multiple bone marrow samples for accurate staging. *Med Pediatr Oncol.,* **17 (5),** 418–23.

Helleberg-Rasmussen I., Sondergaard-Petersen H. (1975) Bone marrow biopsy with the Bordier trephine. *Scan J Haematol,* **14,** 123–8.

Hocking D.R. (1964) Bone marrow biopsy: a routine including marrow trephine. *Med J Aust.,* **2,** 915.

Hodgson S.F., Johnaon K.A., Muhs J.M. (1986) Outpatient percutaneous biopsy of the iliac crest: methods, morbidity, and patients acceptance. *Mayo Clin Prac.,* **61,** 28.

Hoffbrand A.V., Pettit J.E. (eds) (1995) *Essential Haematology,* 3rd edn, Oxford: Blackwell Science.

Humphries J.E. (1990) Dry tap bone marrow aspiration: clinical significance. *Am J Hematol,* **35 (4),** 247–50.

Hyun B.H., Stevenson A.J., Hanau C.A. (1994) Fundamentals of bone marrow examination. *Hematol Oncol Clin North Am.,* **8 (4),** 651–63.

Islam A. (1982) A new bone marrow biopsy needle with core securing device. *J Clin Pathol,* **35,** 359–64.

Jacobs P. (1995) Choice of needle for bone marrow trephine biopsies. *Hematol Rev and Comm,* **9 (3),** 163–8.

Jamshidi J., Swaim R.W. (1971) Bone marrow biopsy with unaltered architecture: a new biopsy device. *J Lab Clin Med.,* **77,** 335–42.

Juneja S.K., Wolf M.M., Cooper I.A. (1990) Value of bilateral bone marrow biopsy specimens in non-Hodgkin's lymphoma. *J Clin Pathol,* **44 (4),** 350–1.

Kattapuram S.V., Rosenthal D.I. (1991) Percutaneous biopsy of skeletal lesions. *Amer J Radiol.,* **157,** 935.

Krause J.R. (1981) *Bone Marrow Biopsy.* Edinburgh: Churchill Livingstone.

Lalor B., Freemont A., Carlile S. (1986) An improved transilial crest bone biopsy drill for quantitative histomorphometry. *Bone,* **7,** 273.

Landys K. (1980) A trephine for closed bone marrow biopsy. *Acta Haematol,* **64,** 216–20.

Landys K., Stenram U. (1975) Bone marrow biopsy of the posterior iliac crest with Gidlund's instrument in malignant diseases. *Scand J Haematol,* **15,** 104–8.

Luoni M., Declich P., De Paoli A. *et al.* (1995) Bone marrow biopsy for the staging of non-Hodgkin's lymphoma: bilateral or unilateral trephine biopsy? *Tumori,* **81 (6),** 410–13.

Macavei, I. and Galatar, N. (1989) Bone marrow biopsy (BMB) I. Generalities, material and method, normal structure of bone marrow, pathological conditions. *Morphol. Embryol.,* **35 (1),** 33–40.

Maung Z.T., Bown N.P., Hamilton P.J. (1993) Collagenase digestion of bone marrow trephine biopsy specimens: an important adjunct to haematological diagnosis when marrow aspiration fails. *J Clin Pathol,* **46 (6),** 576–7.

McFarland W., Dameshek W. (1958) Biopsy of bone marrow with the Vim-Silverman needle. *JAMA,* **166,** 1464–6.

Monserrat E., Villamor N., Reverter J.C. *et al.* (1996) Bone marrow assessment in B-cell chronic lymphocytic leukaemia: aspirate or biopsy? A comparative study in 258 patients. *Br J Haematol,* **93 (1),** 111–16.

Pedersen L.M., Jarner D., Winge J. (1993) Bone marrow biopsy of the iliac bone followed by severe retroperitoneal hemorrhage. *Eur J Haematol,* **51 (1),** 52.

Pedersen L.M., Nordon H., Nielsen H., Lisse I.M. (1994) Needles for bone marrow examination, *Ugeskr Laeger*, **156 (18)**, 2723–4, 2727–8.

Prasad R., Olson W.H. (1987) Bone marking for biopsy using radionuclide bone imaging. *Cancer*, **60**, 2205.

Reid M.M., Roald B. (1996) Adequacy of bone marrow trephine biopsy specimens in children. *J Clin Pathol*, **49 (3)**, 226–9.

Reid M.M. (1991) Dry tap marrow aspiration. *Am. J. Heýmatol.*, **37 (3)**, 218–19.

Rodak B.F. (1995) *Diagnostic Hematology*, Philadelphia: W.B. Saunders.

Rywlin A.M. (1976) *Histopathology of the Bone Marrow*. Boston: Little Brown.

Varma N., Dash S., Sarode R., Marwaha N. (1993) Relative efficacy of bone marrow trephine biopsy sections as compared to trephine imprints and aspiration smears in routine hematological practice. *Indian J Pathol Microbiol*, **36 (3)**, 215–26.

Westerman M.P. (1981) Bone marrow needle biopsy: an evaluation and critique. *Semin Hematol*, **18**, 293–300.

Williamson P.J., Smith A.G. (1991) Practical procedures. Bone marrow aspiration and biopsy. *Br J Hospital Med*, **46**, 328–30.

Wittels B. (1985) *Surgical Pathology of Bone Marrow – Core Biopsy Diagnosis*. Philadelphia: W.B. Saunders.

2 Evaluation of bone and bone marrow biopsies

Range of cortical and trabecular bone

Sections of biopsies illustrating the range of normal quantitative relationships between cortical and trabecular bone, hematopoietic and adipose tissue, and their topographic inter-relationships are shown in Figures 2.1 and 2.2.

Most of the cortex of the anterior part of the iliac crest is porous (Figure 2.3), about 25% void, and of varying thickness; moreover the thickness of the trabecular bone is also very variable (Figure 2.4). The same applies to the posterior part of the ilium. It is important to bear these considerations in mind, especially when histomorphometric measurements and comparative studies are made and conclusions drawn from them. However, if small and/or narrow needles have been used, there may not be any cortex present (Figure 2.5), or only shattered fragments. In many cases, a routine Giemsa and/or hematoxylin and eosin (H&E) stain will enable diagnostic evaluation. For estimation of mineralised bone, osteoid, and osseous remodeling, sections of undecalcified biopsies stained by Giemsa or toluidine blue, or other stain that shows up the mineralised bone, osteoid and cement lines should be used (Figure 2.6).

Hematopoietic and adipose tissue

The approximate relationships between hematopoietic and adipose tissues are given in Figure 2.7. However, it should be borne in mind that there are wide variations in the relative amounts of the components of the bone marrow, especially in the subcortical regions (Figures 2.8 and 2.9); so that, for example, a cellular marrow may represent an increase in hematopoiesis in a previously hypocellular region.

Immunohistology (Figures 2.10–2.14)

The purpose of immunohistology is recognition of cellular constituents – antigens – and thereby to identify and classify particular cells within a morphologically heterogeneous (or even apparently homogenous) cell population. Visualisation of the antigen–antibody complex is accomplished by attaching (conjugating) a color (fluorochrome) to the antibody, which can be seen in the microscope (Figures 2.10–2.13) or alternatively an enzyme whose reaction product may likewise be observed (Figure 2.14). In some cases, the antibodies are not entirely specific and may cross-react with more than one antigen, or there may be both false-positive as well as false-negative results, in addition to high levels of background staining and adsorption. Moreover, some cells may express antigens usually associated with a completely different type, e.g. prostate-specific antigen in pancreas and salivary glands; or lymphoid antigens in lung tumors. Because of decalcification, sections of bone marrow biopsies are particularly prone to technical dif-

2.1 (left) Bone marrow biopsy section (BMBS) plastic, Gomori, showing periosteal tissues and cortical bone, left. Note variable width of trabeculae, and subcortical hypocellular areas.

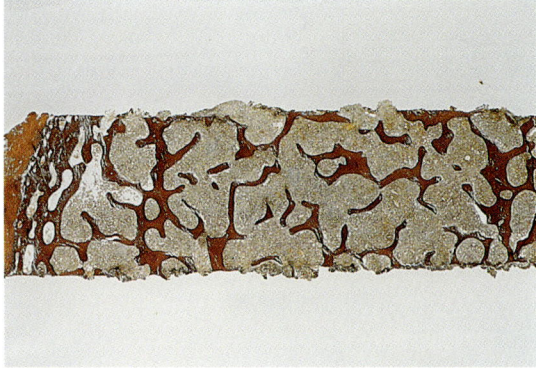

2.2 (right) BMBS paraffin, H&E; note peritrabecular fat cells.

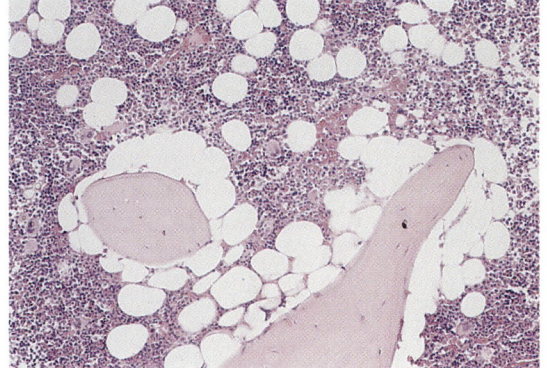

2.3 (left) BMBS plastic, Gomori, showing cortex with unusual degree of porosity.

2.4 (right) Surface of trabecular bone of iliac crest of young adult, illustrating variability in trabecular network: (a) cancellous bone consisting of fine rods anastomosing to form a meshwork, and showing narrow trabecular plates and moderate anisotropy of pattern, (b) Uneven bone architecture with variable bone volume, trabecular widths and anisotropy, and (c) dense trabecular structure consisting of plates and some rods to form a nearly isotropic network.

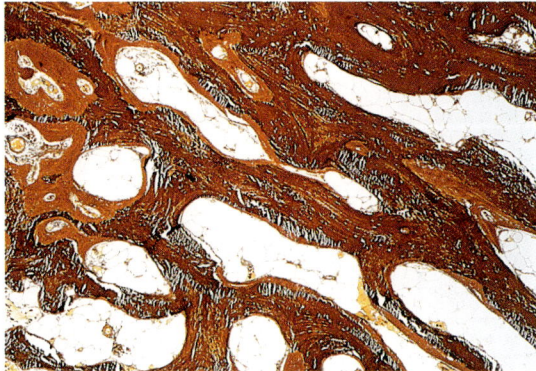

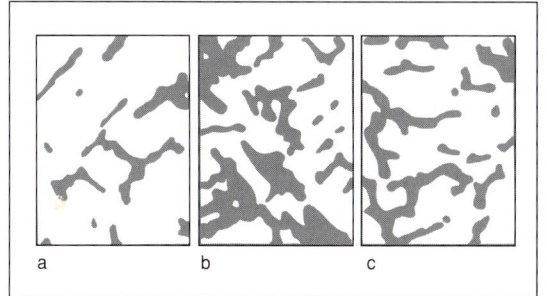

ficulties and appropriate sections of a control tissue (e.g. lymph node or tonsil for lymphoid antigens) must always be processed with the bone biopsy sections; and these controls must be checked before the bone biopsy sections are evaluated. (For methods see Chapter 32).

A relatively short list of antibodies is useful in bone and bone marrow histopathology (Table 2.1) and when the fixation, decalcification, and dehydration and embedding times are kept to the minimum and the appropriate retrieval techniques are applied (microwave, pressure-cooker, trypsin), the results are crisp with little background adsorption. Particularly useful is the distinction between T and B lymphocytes, and the demonstration of monocytes, which are often difficult to recognise in histologic sections; light chain restriction by means of antibodies to kappa and lambda is used as an indication of monoclonality in early cases of MM with minimal plasma cell infiltrations, and cytokeratin for identification

of individual metastatic cells (or other appropriate antibodies according to the particular case); Ki67 for proliferating cells.

In addition to routine stains, such as reticulin and Masson's trichrome, demonstration of blood vessels and endothelial cells with CD34, F8, and of reactive connective tissue with actin and vimentin is often useful. The relevant immunohistology especially those antibodies used in our laboratories, are given in each chapter; these are only examples – there are, of course, many others.

Histomorphometry

This refers to the quantitative evaluation of any of the components or parameters of bone and marrow. Plastic-embedded material is generally used for histomorphometry to avoid the shrinkage inherent in decalcification and subsequent paraffin embedding.

Histomorphometric measurements are

13

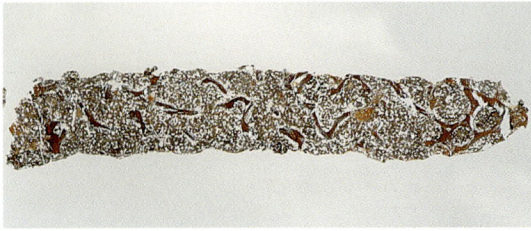

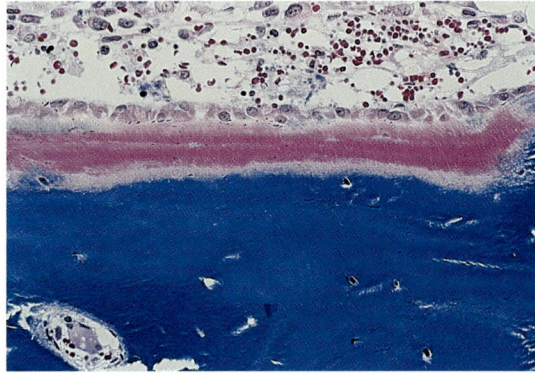

2.5 (left) BMBS plastic, Gomori, with even distribution of hematopoiesis and fat, trabecular bone but no cortex present.

2.6 (right) BMBS plastic, Ladewig's stain for bone (blue) and osteoid (red). Note layer of osteoblasts on the osteoid.

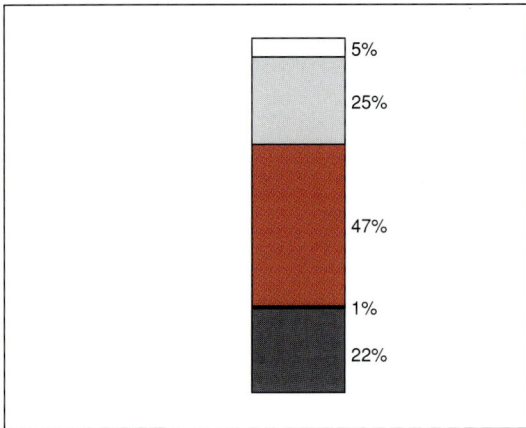

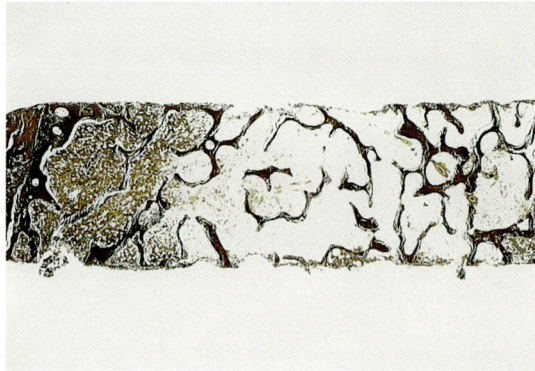

2.7 (left) Graphic representation of proportions of bone; osteoid; hematopoiesis; fat; and sinusoids.

2.8 (right) BMBS plastic, Gomori, with subcortical hematopoiesis, and fatty areas in deeper parts of the biopsy; compare with Figure 2.9.

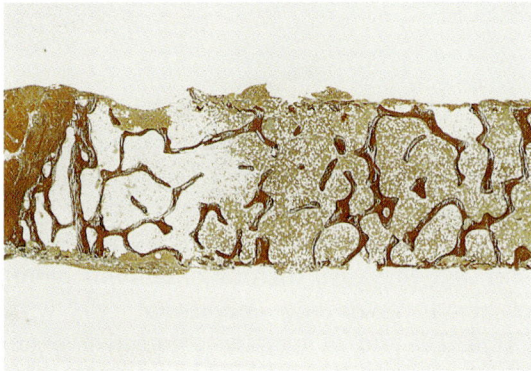

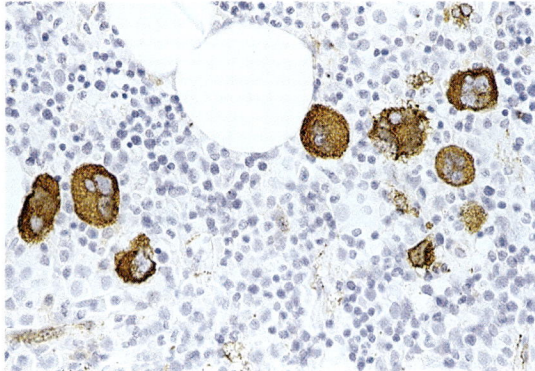

2.9 (left) BMBS plastic, Gomori, showing typical subcortical hypoplasia, frequently seen in BMBs of individuals >60 years.

2.10 (right) BMBS paraffin immunohistology(I.H.), stained by Factor VIII-related antigen. Note variably sized megakaryocytes showing cytoplasmic reaction.

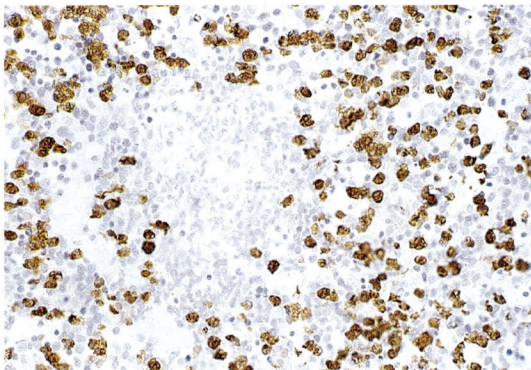

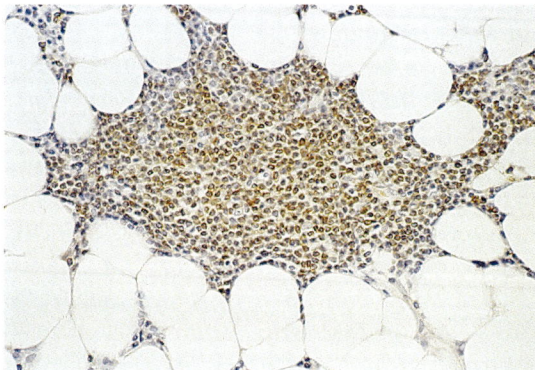

2.11 (left) BMBS paraffin immunohistology, myeloperoxidase stain in myeloid cells, but not lymphocytes in the central aggregate.

2.12 (right) BMBS paraffin immunohistology, showing nodule of lymphocytes, many stained by LCA, CD45.

2.13 (left) BMBS paraffin immunohistology, showing metastatic cancer cells stained by cytokeratin.

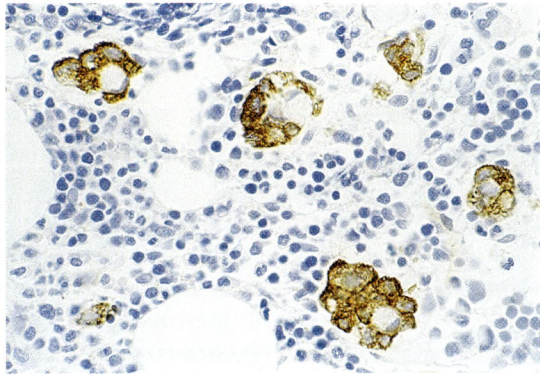

2.14 (right) BMBS plastic immunohistology, showing metastatic cancer cells, reaction with cytokeratin, visualisation of reaction product by alkaline phosphatase method.

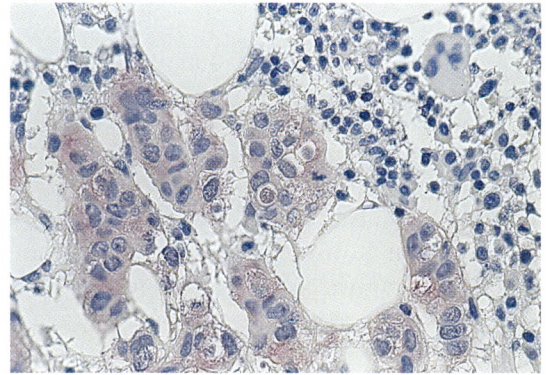

TABLE 2.1 Immunohistology: short list of antibodies

Antibody	Cell/Tissue	Source	Mono or polyclonal
Myeloperoxidase	granulocytes	Dako	P
Glycophorin	erythroid cells	Dako	M
Factor VIII Rag	megakaryocytes (MGK)	Dako	R
CD 34 (Qbend 10)	stroma, endothelium	Oxoid	M
CD 68	mononuclear phagocytes (MPs), some granulocytes	Dako	M
Lysozyme	as CD 68	Dako	P
T d T	pre B, pre T cells	Sigma	M
CD 20	B-lymphocytes	Dako	M
Ig, Kappa, Lambda	plasma cells	Dako	P
CD 45	T, B, some MPs	Dako	M
CD 79a	B cells MgK	Dako	M
CD 4	T-helper cells	Biomen	M
CD 8	T cytotoxic cells	Dako	M
BCL 2	T, some B cells	Dako	M
CD 15	Reed Sternberg R-S granulocytes	Dako	M
CD 30	R-S, B, T, MPs	Dako	M
K1 67	proliferating cells	Novocast RA	M
P 53	mutant and wild type p53	Novocast RA	M
Cytokeratin	epithelium	Becton Dickinson	M
EMA	epithelium	Dako	M
NSE	neuro endocrine tumors	Dako	P
CEA	adenocarcinoma granulocytes	Dako	
Vimentin	mesenchymal tumors, Ewing's tumor	Dako	M
Desmin	rhabdomyosarcoma	Dako	M
PSA	prostatic carcinoma	Dako	

given in Tables 2.2 and 2.3. Only sections without crushing or distortion artifacts and containing at least five but preferably more architecturally well-preserved marrow spaces should be used for qualitative and quantitative assessments. When histomorphometric measurements are planned, a surface area of 60–80 mm^2 is required for reliable and representative measurements. This may be done with or without computerised evaluation of results and calculation of their correlations and statistical significance.

There are several ways in which histomorphometry may be performed:

1. Subjective assessment by the naked eye of the structures and components of the biopsy section as observed in a number of fields in the light microscope.

2. Assessment by means of a graticule in the ocular; for example, see Figure 2.15.

3. Semi-automatic or automatic measurements with or without computerised evaluation of the results, their correlations and their statistical significance. Comparative studies have recently demonstrated the reliability of histomorphometric measurements of trabecular bone.

4. Functional studies by means of tetracycline labeling (Figure 2.16), followed by histomorphometry.

Flow cytometry (fluorescent-activated cell sorting, FACS)

A flow cytometer is an instrument used to measure physical or antigenic characteristics of single cells by means of a laser beam focused on each cell as it passes in single file in a fluid stream. Light is reflected or scattered off each cell as it passes and this light can be measured. Photomultipliers (sensitive light detectors and amplifiers) are used both for intrinsic cellular characteristics such as size, nuclei, cytoplasmic granularity, and extrinsic characteristics such as surface and nuclear antigens which must first be conjugated or attached to exogenous reagents or dyes which will emit light of a specific wavelength when the cell passes through the laser beam. A computer with the appropriate software is used to convert the light signals into histograms, as well as to calculate the relative percentage of cells stained with different dyes (Figure 2.17). Cell sorting means that subpopulations of cells may be separated from the sample stream after passing through the laser beam, and collected in tubes for further analysis or other use. The advantages of such a system are considerable: several thousand cells are rapidly analysed and accurate quantitative records are obtained as computer printouts. Technical problems may arise if the cell suspension is not properly prepared because necrotic cells or cellular fragments may cause inaccurate counts by non-specific absorption of dyes, e.g. clumps of platelets passing for megakaryocytes. Flow cytometric analysis is now considered indispensable for the diagnosis and classification of the majority of hematologic neoplasias, as morphology and cell counts of blood films and smears of aspirates are now regarded as too subjective, imprecise and unreliable to be acceptable as the only

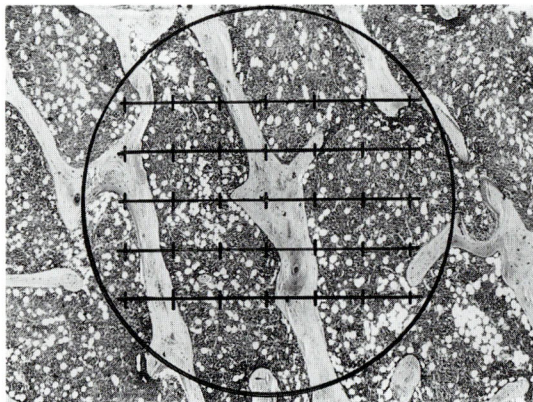

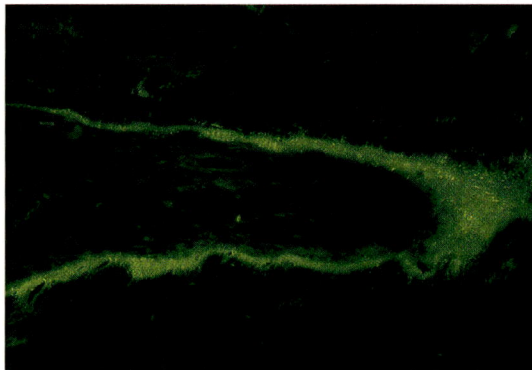

2.15 (left) Zeiss integration eyepiece (counting plate or graticule) for quantitative assessment of components of bone and bone marrow in biopsy sections.

2.16 (right) BMBS plastic, tetracycline labeling of osteoid, viewed in polarised light.

TABLE 2.2 Histomorphometric variables used in our laboratories when indicated. TV = tissue volume, BV = bone volume, MV = marrow volume, B.Ar = bone area (2D), M.Ar = marrow area (2D)

Terminology	Abbreviation	Units	Dimension
Volume			
Bone volume	BV/TV	%	3D
Lamellar bone volume	LBV/TV, LBV/BV	%	3D
Woven bone volume	WBV/TV, WBV/BV	%	3D
Osteoid volume	OV/TV, OV/BV	%	3D
Haematopoiesis volume	HV/TV, HV/MV	%	3D
Fatty tissue volume	FV/TV, FV/MV	%	3D
Sinusoid volume	SV/TV, SV/MV	%	3D
Endosteal sinusoid volume	ESV/TV, ESV/MV	%	3D
Oedema volume	EV/TV, EV/MV	%	3D
Infiltration volume	IV/TV, IV/MV	%	3D
Surface			
Bone surface	BS/BV	mm^2/mm^3	3D
Osteoid surface	OS/BV	mm^2/mm^3	3D
Osteoblast surface	Obl.S/BS	%	3D
Osteoclast surface	Ocl.S/BS	%	3D
Eroded surface	ES/BS	%	3D
Thickness			
Trabecular thickness	Tb.Th	μm	3D
Osteoid thickness	O.Th	μm	3D
Cell number			
Osteoclast number	N.Ocl/B.Ar	per mm^2	2D
Osteoblast number	N.Obl/B.Ar	per mm^2	2D
Lining cell number	N.Lin/B.Ar	per mm^2	2D
Osteocyte number	N.Ocy/B.Ar	per mm^2	2D
Megakaryocyte number	N.Meg/M.Ar	per mm^2	2D
Mast cell number	N.Mas/M/Ar	per mm^2	2D
Plasma cell number	N.Pla/M.Ar	per mm^2	2D
Vessel number			
Artery number	N.Art/M.Ar	per mm^2	2D
Arteriole number	N.Aio/M.Ar	per mm^2	2D
Capillary number	N.Cap/M.Ar	per mm^2	2D
Sinusoid number	N.Sin/M.Ar	per mm^2	2D

TABLE 2.3 Normal range of histomorphometric values at different skeletal sites (mean ± SD)

Parameters	Abbreviation	Units	Anterior iliac crest	Posterior iliac crest	Lumbar vertebra	Sternum	Calcaneus	Radius
Skeletal sites								
Bone structure								
Bone volume	BV/TV	%	22 ± 4	22 ± 4	16 ± 4	15 ± 4	20 ± 6	1.9 ± 5
Bone surface	BS/BV	mm²/mm³	2.8 ± 0.7	2.6 ± 0.8	2.3 ± 0.6	2.7 ± 0.6	3.5 ± 0.8	3.2 ± 1.8
Trabecular thickness	TB.Th	μm	175 ± 42	181 ± 40	178 ± 48	155 ± 42	157 ± 50	161 ± 44
Mineralization								
Osteoid volume	OV/BV	%	2.5 ± 2.2	2.8 ± 2.1	2.3 ± 1.8	1.6 ± 1.8	1.7 ± 1.4	1.3 ± 0.9
Osteoid surface	OS/BV	mm²/mm³	0.6 ± 0.4	0.6 ± 0.4	0.5 ± 0.3	0.4 ± 0.4	0.3 ± 0.2	0.4 ± 0.3
Osteoid thickness	O.Th	μm	4.1 ± 3.4	4.6 ± 3.3	5.4 ± 2.1	4.9 ± 3.5	4.0 ± 3.0	3.5 ± 3.6
Bone cells								
Osteoclasts	N.Ocl/B.Ar	per mm²	1.0 ± 0.9	0.9 ± 0.7	0.9 ± 0.7	1.0 ± 0.8	0.5 ± 0.4	0.4 ± 0.2
Osteoblasts	N.Obl/B.Ar	per mm²	2.5 ± 1.8	3.2 ± 1.1	2.6 ± 1.4	4.1 ± 1.6	2.2 ± 1.1	1.3 ± 0.4
Lining cells	N.Lin/B.Ar	per mm²	2.0 ± 1.3	1.9 ± 1.0	2.0 ± 1.1	1.8 ± 1.0	0.8 ± 0.6	0.9 ± 0.3
Osteocytes	N.Ocy/B.Ar	per mm²	32 ± 6	30 ± 5	24 ± 6	25 ± 6	32 ± 7	28 ± 6
Blood vessels								
Arteries	N.Art/M.Ar	per mm²	0.4 ± 0.4	0.5 ± 0.3	0.6 ± 0.4	0.5 ± 0.5	0.5 ± 0.4	0.4 ± 0.4
Arterioles	N.Aio/M.Ar	per mm²	1.3 ± 0.4	1.4 ± 0.5	1.4 ± 0.6	1.4 ± 0.9	1.4 ± 1.0	1.2 ± 0.9
Capillaries	N.Cap/M.Ar	per mm²	17 ± 5	16 ± 5	16 ± 5	16 ± 5	11 ± 3	11 ± 4
Sinusoids	N.Sin/M.Ar	per mm²	33 ± 7	35 ± 8	36 ± 9	36 ± 8	11 ± 4	11 ± 5
Endosteal sinusoid volume	ESV/TV	%	2.0 ± 1.3	2.1 ± 1.4	2.2 ± 1.4	2.3 ± 1.1	1.8 ± 0.9	1.8 ± 1.0
Stroma								
Fatty tissue volume	FV/MV	%	26 ± 8	25 ± 6	23 ± 7	28 ± 19	96 ± 4	96 ± 5
Mast cells	N.Mas/M.Ar	per mm²	2.3 ± 1.8	2.2 ± 1.9	3.7 ± 3.1	1.9 ± 2.8	0	0
Plasma cells	N.Pla/M.Ar	per mm²	30 ± 12	29 ± 10	31 ± 24	29 ± 14	0	0
Haematopoiesis								
Haematopoiesis volume	HV/MV	%	60 ± 6	62 ± 7	64 ± 7	61 ± 8	0	0
Megakaryocytes	N.Meg/M.Ar	per mm²	14 ± 4	13 ± 4	15 ± 8	16 ± 7	0	0

Terminology, abbreviations and units see Table 2.2. Histomorphometry was performed in collaboration with Dr B. Mallmann.

foundation for diagnosis and therapeutic decisions.

Cytogenetic analysis of chromosomes: karyotype

Cytogenetics is the study of genetic material at the cellular level. Mutations of the genetic material sometimes involve large parts of a chromosome, and when visible under the microscope are termed chromosome aberrations. The somatic cells involved have anomalies either on the sex or the autosomal chromosomes. The malignant cells in patients with leukemia, lymphoma or other hematologic neoplasias have acquired chromosomal abnormalities.

Cytogenetic analysis of malignant diseases

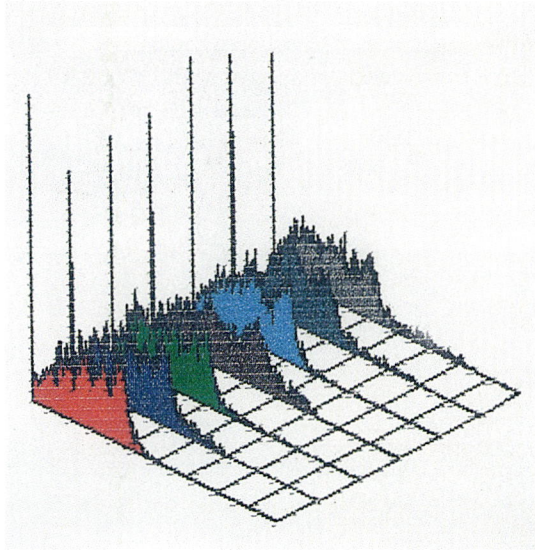

2.17 Flow cytometry of nucleated cells of marrow aspirate, case of mild cytopenia in 84-year-old man. From left to right: red control, dark blue CD20 5%, green CD3 4%, brown CD13 12%, blue CD14 1%, dark green CD34 4%, gray CD41 9%, no evidence for any lympho- or mycloproliferative disorder.

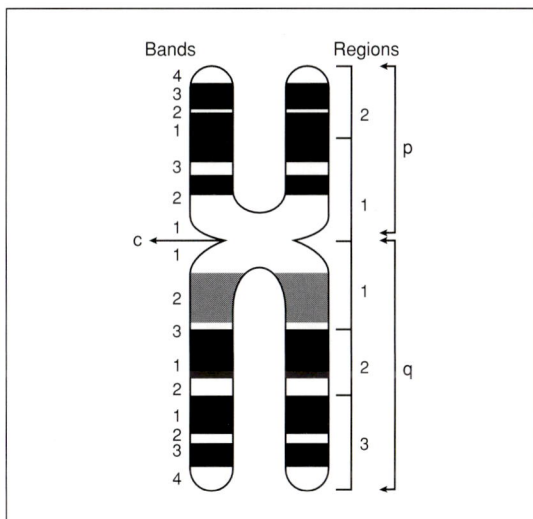

2.18 Diagram of Giemsa-banded chromosome, showing division of the chromosome into regions and bands (example of chromosome 9): c, centromere; p, short arm; q, long arm.

is made on the tumor cells themselves. In leukemia, material is usually obtained by marrow aspiration and is either processed immediately or cultured for 24–72h. When a bone marrow cannot be aspirated, cells from a marrow biopsy (bone core specimen) or a peripheral blood sample are used. Tissue samples such as lymph nodes, spleen and solid tumors can also be processed after separating cells from the samples.

Neoplastic cells often coexist with normal cells. The observation of at least two pseudo-diploid or hyperdiploid cells or three hypo-diploid cells, each showing the same abnormality, is considered evidence of an abnormal clone.

The microscopic analysis of chromosomal abnormalities is made on cells in metaphase. The basic preparatory steps are: (1) accumulation of metaphase cells (with colcemid or similar agent causing damage to spindle fibers to stop cell division; (2) swelling of the cells by a hypotonic solution; (3) fixation and washing of cells and treatment with trypsin; (4) spreading the cells on slides; and (5) staining the cells. For routine analysis, G banding (Figure 2.18) is preferred (see Appendix).

The cells in metaphase are analysed microscopically, and representative photographs are taken for karyotyping or computer-aided karyotypes are produced (Figure 2.18). A minimum of 20 cells should be fully analysed from each sample. The nomenclature used to describe cytogenetic findings follows the recommendations of the ISCN 1995 (see Appendix, Methods).

Molecular techniques, such as Southern blotting, polymerase chain reaction (PCR) or fluorescent *in situ* hybridisation (FISH) are used in the study of organisation and function of chromosomal nucleic acid sequences. FISH enables cytogenetic analysis on interphase cells as well as on metaphase cells. Cytologic smears, touch preparations, tissue sections and of course cytogenetic cultures, are all used for FISH analysis. At the present there are probes (sequences of DNA complementary to the target DNA) available for different chromosomal domains, for example centromere, as well as for whole chromosomes and unique specific sequences (Figure 2.19).

Practical uses of cytogenetics
- Evidence of clonality.
- Confirmation of diagnosis.
- Information useful in classification.
- Information relevant to staging.
- Indications of prognosis.
- Information relevant to choice of therapy.
- Evaluation post bone-marrow transplantation.

Pitfalls in histological diagnosis
(Figures 2.20–2.27)

1. Histological variation within the biopsy.
2. Subcortical hypoplasia.
3. Alternating fatty and hyperplastic areas in deeper parts of the biopsy, and concentration of one cell type in single marrow spaces.
4. Presence of misleading artifacts. It should be remembered that artifacts are easily

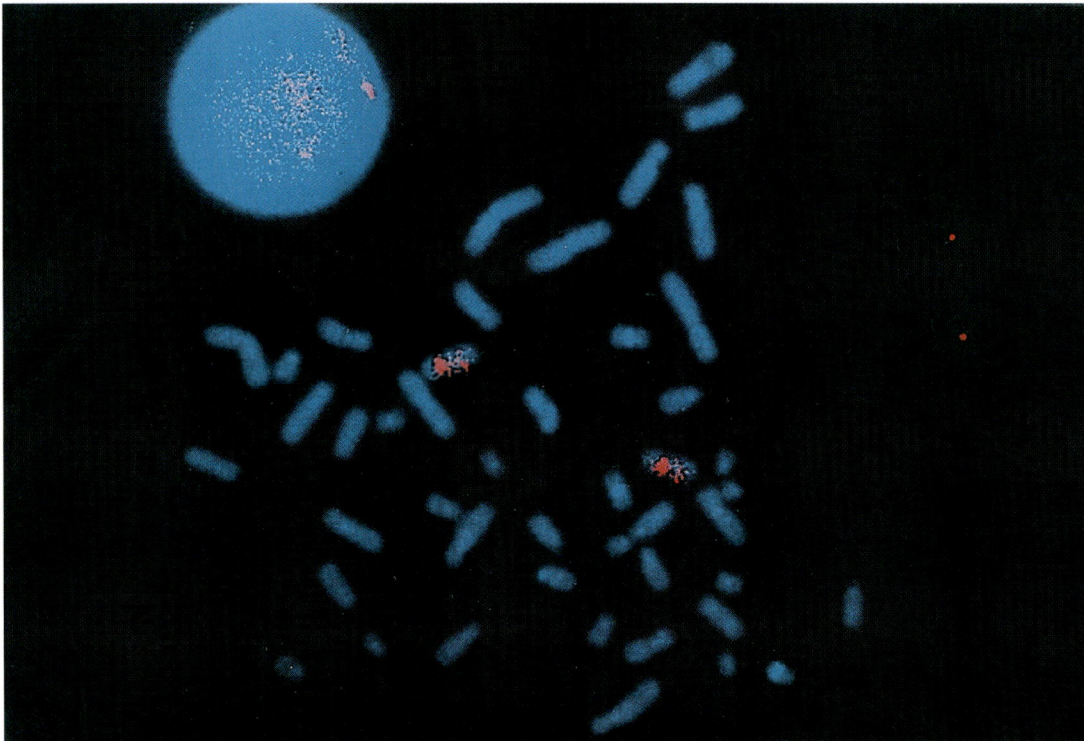

2.19 Cells of bone marrow aspirate, FISH of interphase nuclei, showing whole chromosome painting, chromosome 8 in metaphase spread.

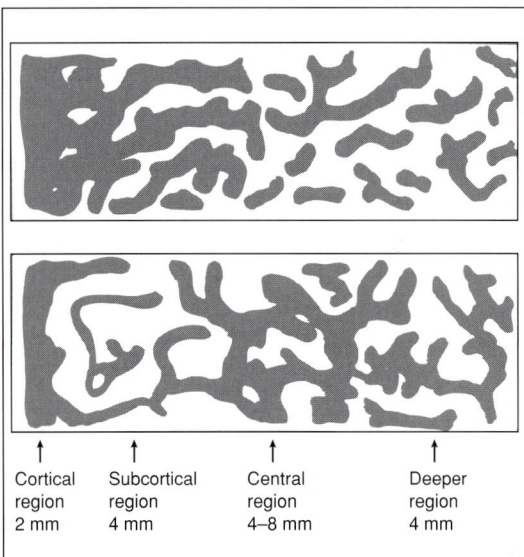

Cortical region 2 mm
Subcortical region 4 mm
Central region 4–8 mm
Deeper region 4 mm

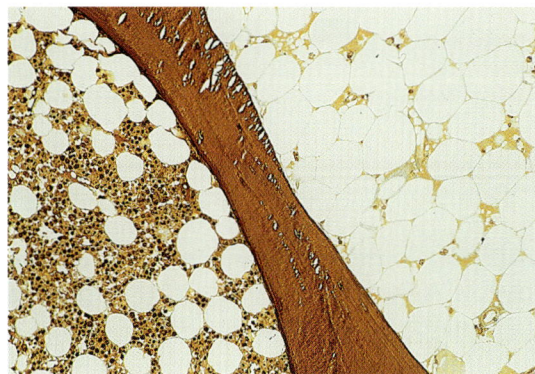

2.20 (left) Diagram of variations in trabecular bone with increasing depth from cortex. The four topographic regions and their approximate sizes are indicated on the diagram.

2.21 (right) BMBS plastic, Gomori, showing part of trabecula separating cellular from hypocellular marrow.

2.22 BMBS plastic, Giemsa, of patient with myeloproliferative disorder, showing 'compartmentalisation' of myelopoiesis, left and center, megakaryocytes, upper and lower right.

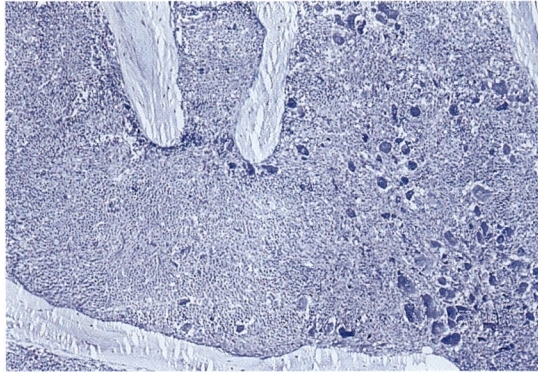

2.23 Variations encountered in the biopsy sections, due to the angle or direction of the biopsy needle: (a) vertical and between the cortical plates of the ilium; (b) vertical, but including one cortex instead of the cancellous bone between the cortices; (c) tangential, thereby penetrating the cortical bone twice.

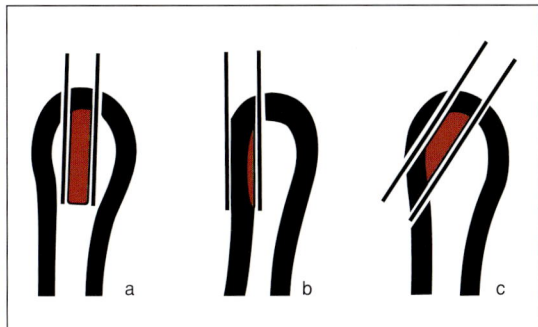

produced when taking bone biopsies; for example, pieces of epidermis, dermis, skeletal muscle, periosteum, cartilage or cortical bone may be displaced into the biopsy, and it is important to recognise them for what they are. In addition, changes in the hematopoietic cells may be due to a variety of technical errors in processing.

5. Biopsy taken from a previously biopsied site; in this case, most of the biopsy may consist of variously fibrotic granulation tissue and new bone with marked osteoblastic activity and little or no hematopoietic or adipose tissue; and/or edema.

6. Biopsy taken from a previously irradiated area, in which case the marrow may be hypocellular or even replaced almost entirely by fat cells.

Diagnostic evaluation

This is made in the first instance with respect to the histological and histopathological

2.24 (left) BMBS plastic, showing tangentially taken biopsy, much of which consists of periosteal tissues and cortical bone.

2.25 (right) BMBS plastic, biopsy taken after aspiration of bone marrow. Note hemorrhagic and hypocellular marrow.

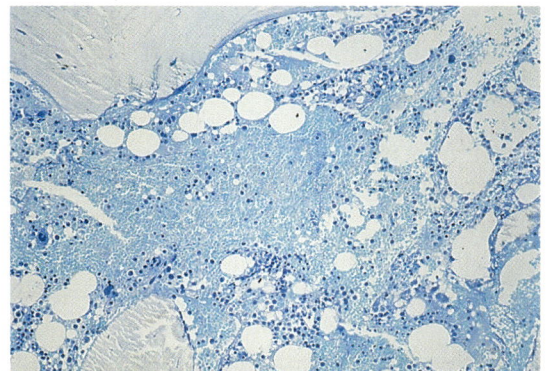

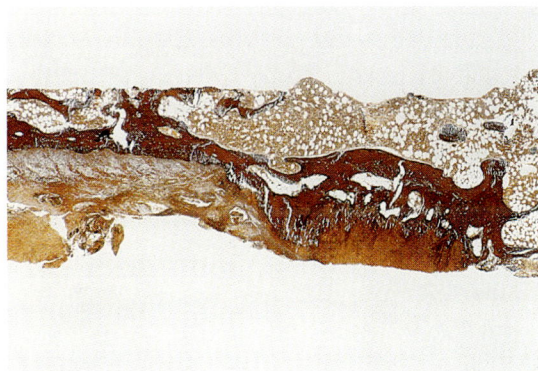

2.26 (left) BMBS plastic, Giemsa, taken from previously biopsied site, showing new bone and fibrous tissue replacing bone marrow.

2.27 (right) BMBS paraffin, H&E biopsy taken from previously irradiated area, showing marrow largely replaced by fat cells.

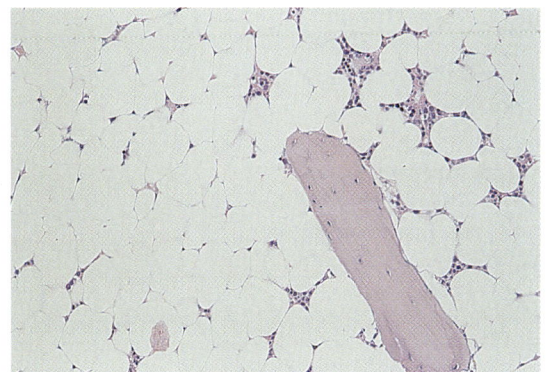

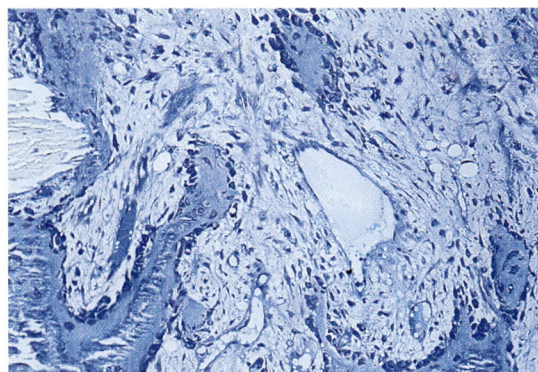

TABLE 2.4 Diagnostic evaluation of bone and bone marrow biopsy sections (BMBS)

Examination of the whole biopsy section (overview)
> Quality, artefacts
> Cortical bone and trabeculae
> Fatty tissue
> Cellularity
> Infiltration patterns?

Examination of trabecular bone
> Trabecular structure
> Osteoid
> Osteoblasts and osteocytes
> Osteoclasts
> Primitive bone?

Examination of hemopoiesis
> Eythropoiesis
> Megakaryopoiesis
> Granulopoiesis
> Topography of the cell lines
> Atypical blast forms?

Examination of bone marrow stroma
> Vasculature
> Macrophages
> Plasma cells
> Lymphocytes and lymphoid nodules
> Mast cells
> Fibers
> Iron content
> Granuloma?

Examination of malignant infiltrations
> Proliferative cell type
> Proliferative cell line(s)
> Growth pattern
> Tumor cell burden
> Stromal reactions
> Bone changes

Histopathological diagnosis
> Clinical interpretation
> Recommendations

findings and, where appropriate, immunohistological results (Table 2.4, Figure 2.28); then, taking account of the patient's clinical status and the results of other diagnostic procedures, and thirdly together with the peripheral blood picture and the smears of the bone marrow aspirate and/or the imprints of the biopsy. In addition, where necessary and available, account is also taken of enzyme and marker studies, fluorescent activated cell sorting (FACS), and cytogenetics. Occasionally chromosome analysis is useful in the confirmation of a diagnosis, as for example, the translocation t(2;5) (p23;q35) in anaplastic large cell lymphoma, but not in HD (see Chapters 27 and 28). If possible, a diagnosis (or a tentative diagnosis) is made and where appropriate, recommendations are given.

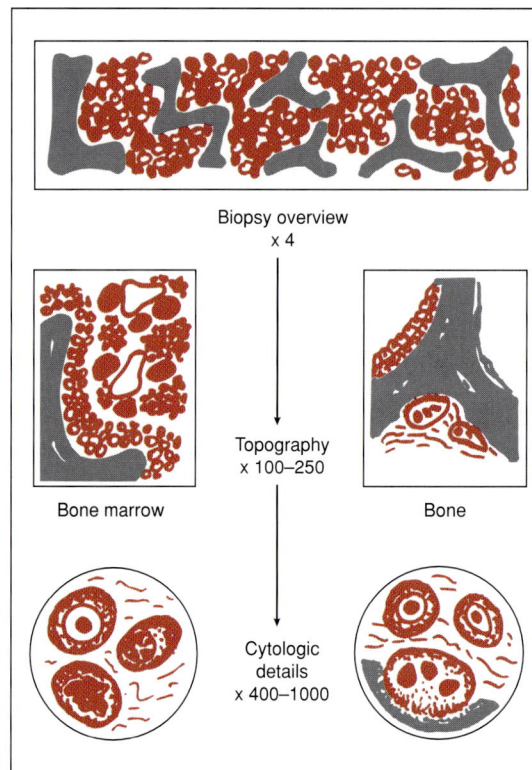

Biopsy overview x 4

Bone marrow

Topography x 100–250

Bone

Cytologic details x 400–1000

2.28 Microscopic evaluation of bone marrow biopsy: overview – cortical and trabecular bone and cellularity; topography and cytologic detail; note magnifications – these are used throughout this text.

Bibliography

Almeida J., Garcia Marcos M.A., Vallejo C. *et al.* (1995) Results of a series of 104 consecutive bilateral bone marrow biopsy specimens in lymphoproliferative disorders *Sangre (Barc)*, **40 (5)**, 365–8.

Bancroft J., Stevens A. (eds) (1990) *Theory and Practice of Histological Techniques*, 3rd edn., New York: Churchill Livingstone.

Baron R., Vignery A., Neff L. *et al.* (1991) Processing of undecalcified bone specimens for bone histomorphometry. *Bone Histomorphometry: Techniques and Interpretations.* Boca Raton: CRC Press, p. 13.

Bartl R., Frisch B., Burkhardt R. (1991) Bone marrow histology. *The Leukemia Cell*, **2**, 47–90.

Bauer K.D., Duque R.E., Shankey T.V. (1993) *Clinical Flow Cytometry*. Baltimore: Willams & Williams.

Bordier P., Matrajt H., Miravet H., Hioco D. (1964) Mesure histologique de la masse et de la resorption des travees osseuses. *Path Biol.*, **12**, 1238.

Buccheri V., Matutes E., Dyer M.J. *et al.* (1993) Lineage commitment in biphenotypic acute leukemia. *Leukemia*, **7**, 919.

Bullough P.G., Bansal M., DiCarlo E.F. (1990) The tissue diagnosis of metabolic bone disease. Role of histomorphometry. *Orthop. Clin N Amer.*, **21 (1)**, 65.

Calabrese G., Min T., Stuppia L. *et al.* (1996) Complex chromosome translocations of standard t(8;21) and t(15;17) arise from a two-step mechanism as evidenced by fluorescence in situ hybridization analysis. *Cancer Genet Cytogenet.*, **91 (1)**, 40–5.

Cantu-Rajnoldi A., Putti C., Saitta M. *et al.* (1991) Co-expression of myeloid antigens in childhood acute lymphoblastic leukaemia: relationship with the stage of differentiation and clinical signficance. *Br J Haematol.*, **79**, 40.

Chavassieux P.M., Arlot M.E., Meunier O.J. (1985) Intersample variation in bone histomorphometry: comparison between parameter values measured on two contiguous transiliac bone biopsies. *Calcif. Tissue Int.*, **37**, 345.

Chavassieux P.M., Arlot M.E., Meunier O.J. (1985) Inter-method variation in bone histomorphometry: comparison between manual and computerized methods applied to iliac bone biopsies. *Bone*, **6**, 221.

Chestnut C.H. (1988) Measurement of bone mass. *Triangle*, **27 (1/2)**, 37.

Coignet L.J., Van de Rijke F.M., Bertheas M.F. *et al.* (1996) Automated counting of in situ hybridization dots in interphase cells of leukemia samples. *Leukemia*, **10 (6)**, 1065–71.

Compston J.E., Vedi S., Stellon A.J. (1986) Inter-observer and intra-observer variation in bone histomorphometry. *Calcif Tissue Int.*, **38**, 67.

Compston J.E., Vedi S., Webb A. (1985) Relationship between toluidine blue-stained calcification fronts and tetracycline-labeled surfaces in normal iliac crest biopsies. *Calcif. Tissue*, **37**, 32.

Cotran, Kumar, Robbins (1994) *Pathologic Basis of Disease*, 5th edn. Philadelphia: W.B. Saunders.

De Wolf-Peeters C. (1991) Bone marrow trephine interpretation: diagnostic utility and potential pitfalls. *Histopathology*, **18 (6)**, 489–93.

den Ottolander G.J. (1996) The bone marrow aspirate of healthy subjects. *Br J Haematol*, **95**, 574–5.

DiCarlo E.F., Hoisington S.A., Bullough P.G. (1989) Site-dependent variation in bone volume and a relative biopsy site on the iliac crest. *Calcif. Tissue.*, **44S**, S–59 (J9).

Dunstan C.R., Evans R.A. (1980) Quantitative bone histology: a new method. *Pathology*, **12**, 255.

Elgamal A.A., Ectors N.L., Sunardhi-Widyaputra S. *et al.* (1996) Detection of prostate specific antigen in pancreas and salivary glands: a potential impact on prostate cancer overestimation. *J Urol.*, **156 (2 pt 1)**, 464–8.

Ellis H.A., Peart K.M. (1972) Quantitative observations on mineralised and non-mineralised bone in the iliac crest. *J Clin Pathol.*, **25**, 277.

Eriksen E.F., Steiniche T., Mosekilde L., Melsen F. (1989) Histomorphometric analysis of bone in metabolic bone disease. *Endocrinol. Metab Clin N Amer.*, **18 (4)**, 919.

Faugere M.C., Malluche H.H. (1983) Comparison of different bone biopsy techniques for qualitative and quantitative diagnosis of metabolic bone diseases. *J Bone Jt Surg.*, **65**, 1314.

Frisch B., Bartl R. (1990) *Atlas of Bone Marrow Pathology*. Dordrecht: Kluwer Academic.

Frisch B., Lewis S.M., Burkhardt R., Bartl R. (1985) *Biopsy Pathology of Bone and Bone Marrow*. London: Chapman & Hall.

Frost H.M. (1989) Some effects of basic multicellular unit–based remodelling on photon absorptiometry of trabecular bone. *Bone Miner.*, **7**, 47.

Garner A., Ball J. (1966) Quantitative observations on mineralised and unmineralised bone in chronic renal azotaemia and intestinal malabsorption syndrome. *J Pathol Bacteriol.*, **91**, 545.

Giroux J.M., Courpron P., Meunier P. (1975) *Histomorphometrie de l'osteopenie physiologique senile*. Lyon: Monographie de Laboratoire de Researches sur l'Histodynamique Osseuse.

Givan A.L. (ed) (1992) *Flow Cytometry: First principles*. Chichester: Wiley-Liss.

Hodgson S.V., Maher E.R. (1993) A practical guide to human cancer genetics.

Hoffman R., Benz E.J. Jr., Shattil S.J. *et al.* (1995) *Hematology: Basic Principles and Practice*, 2nd edn. Edinburgh: Churchill Livingstone.

Hyun B.H., Stevenson A.J., Hanau C.A. (1994) Fundamentals of bone marrow examination. *Hematol Oncol Clin North Am*, **8 (4)**, 651–63.

Ioachim H.L., Pambuccian S.E., Hekimgil M. *et al.* (1996) Lymphoid monoclonal antibodies reactive with lung tumors. *Am J Surg Pathol.*, **20 (1)**, 64–71.

Keren D.F., Hanson C.A., Hurtubise P.E. (eds) (1994) *Flow Cytometry and Clinical Diagnosis*, ASCP Press.

Kerndrup G., Pallesen G., Melsen F., Mosekilde L. (1980) Histomorphometrical determination of bone marrow cellularity in iliac crest biopsies. *Scand J Haematol.*, **24**, 110.

Kita K., Nakase K., Miwa H. *et al.* (1992) Phenotypic characteristics of acute myelocytic leukemia associated with the t(8;21) (q22;q22) chromosomal abnormality; frequent expression of immature B-cell antigen CD19 together with stem cell antigen CD34. *Blood*, **80**, 470.

Kotylo P. (1995) Flow cytometric analysis in diagnostic hematology. In *Diagnost Haematol*. Rodak: Saunders, pp. 425–35.

Malluche H.H., Faugere M.C. (1986) *Atlas of Mineralized Bone Histology*. Basel: Karger.

Malluche H.H., Faugere M.C. (1991) Bone biopsies: histology and histomorphometry of bone. Avioli and Krane, *Metabolic Bone Disease*. Philadelphia: W.B. Saunders, p. 283.

Malluche H.H., Meyer W., Sherman D., Massry S.G. (1972) Quantitative bone histology in 84 normal American subjects. Micromorphometric analysis and evaluation of variance in iliac bone. *Calcif. Tissue Int.*, **34**, 449.

McCluggage W.G., Clarke R., Bharucha H. (1995) Non-neoplastic glandular structures in bone marrow: a technical artefact. *J Clin Pathol.*, **48 (12)**, 1141–2.

Melsen F., Melsen B., Mosekilde L. (1978) An evaluation of the quantitative parameters applied to bone histology. *Acta Pathol Microbiol.*, **86**, 63.

Melsen F., Melsen B., Mosekilde L., Bergman S. (1978) Histomorphometric analysis of normal bone from the iliac crest. *Acta Pathol Microbiol Scand.*, **86**, 70.

Merz W.A., Schenk R.K. (1970) Quantitative structural analysis of human cancellous bone. *Acta Anat.*, **75**, 54.

Moore R.J., Durbridge T.C., Woods A.E., Vernon-Roberts B. (1989) Variation in histomorphometric estimates across different site of the iliac crest. *J Clin Pathol.*, **42**, 814.

Nacheva E., Holloway T., Brown K. *et al.* (1994) Philadelphia-negative chronic myeloid leukaemia: detection by FISH of BCR-ABL fusion gene localized either to chromosome 9 or chromosome 22. *Br J Haematol.*, **87 (2)**, 409–12.

Naish S.J. (ed) (1989) *Handbook of Immunochemical Staining Methods*. Carpinteria: Ca. Dako Corp.

Parfitt A.M. (1983) The physiological and clinical significance of bone histomorphometric data. In Recker (ed), *Bone Histomorphometry, Techniques and Interpretation*. Boca Raton: CRC Press, pp. 143–223.

Parfitt A.M. (1988) Bone histomorphometry: standardization of nomenclature, symbols and units. Summary of proposed system. *Bone Miner.*, **4**, 1.

Perez Losada A., Sole F., Woessner S. *et al.* (1996) Cytogenetic study of 121 patients suffering from various hematologic neoplasms using the in situ hybridization technique. *Sangre (Barc)*, **41 (3)**, 201–9.

Rao S. Practical approach to bone biopsy. Becker: *Bone Histomorphometry: Techniques and Interpretation*. Boca Raton: CRC Press, p. 3.

Reading C.L., Estey E.H., Huh Y.O. *et al.* (1993) Expression of unusual immunophenotype combinations in acute myelogenous leukemia. *Blood*, **81**, 3083.

Recker R.R. (1983) *Bone Histomorphometry: Techniques and Interpretation*. Boca Raton: CRC Press.

Rothe G., Schmitz G. for Working Group on Flow Cytometry and Image Analysis.

Consensus protocol for the flow cytometric immunophenotyping of hematopoietic malignancies. *Leukemia*, **10**, 877.

Rozman C., Woesnner S., Feliu E. *et al.* (1993) *Cell Ultrastructure for Hematologists*. Doyma.

Savill J. (1997) Role of molecular cell biology in understanding disease. *BMJ*, **314**, 203–8.

Schwonzen M., Pohl C., Steinmetz T. *et al.* (1993) Immunophenotyping of low-grade B-cell lymphoma in blood and bone marrow: poor correlation between immunophenotyping and cytological/histological classification. *Br J Haematol.*, **83**, 232.

Shi S.R., Cote R.J., Taylor C.R. (1997) Antigen retrieval immunohistochemistry: past, present, and future. *J Histochem Cytochem.*, **45 (3)**, 327–43.

True L.D. (ed) (1990) *Atlas of Diagnostic Immunohistopathology*. New York: Gower Medical.

Tuzuner N., Cox C., Rowe J.M., Bennett J.M. (1994) Bone marrow cellularity in myeloid stem cell disorders: impact of age correction. *Leuk Res*, **18 (8)**, 559–64.

Vedi S., Compston J.E., Webb A., Tighe J.R. (1982) Histomorphometric analysis of bone biopsies from the iliac crest of normal British subjects. *Bone*, **4**, 231.

Whitehouse W.J. (1977) Cancellous bone in the anterior part of the iliac crest. *Calcif. Tissue Res.*, **23**, 67.

Whyte M.P., Bergfeld M.A., Murphy W.A. *et al.* (1982) Postmenopausal osteoporosis: a heterogeneous disorder as assessed by histomorphometric analysis of iliac crest bone from untreated patients. *Am J Med.*, **72**, 193–202.

Willman C.L. (1992) Flow cytometric analysis of hematologic specimens. In D.M. Knowles (ed), *Neoplastic Hematopathology*. Baltimore: Williams and Wilkins, p. 169.

Yates J.R.W. (1996) Medical genetics. *BMJ*, **312**, 2021–5.

Yunis J.J. (1976) High resolution of human chromosomes. *Science*, **191**, 1268–70.

3 Normal bone

The skeleton

Owing to the calcification of its extracellular compartment, bone is converted into an extremely hard structure enabling optimal implementation of its three major functions: (1) it constitutes the means for direct locomotion and movement, while providing support and protection for softer, vulnerable tissues; (2) it participates in the homeostasis of minerals, and (3) it houses the bone marrow which provides the formed elements of the blood. The ilium (along with other flat, long or short irregular bones) consists of an outer frame – the cortex, and an interior network of bone – ossicles: the trabecular, spongy or cancellous bone. Undecalcified biopsies embedded in plastic are the most suitable for bone and its cells and for histomorphometry.

Osteogenesis

Bone may be detected by 8 weeks in the human fetus. Histogenesis of bone proceeds by the initial formation of primary woven bone which is later replaced by secondary lamellar bone. Bone formation occurs by one of two pathways: intramembranous or enchondrial ossification. Increases in length occur at the epiphyseal growth plate (Figures 3.1 and 3.2) within which five zones are distinguished: (1) resting cells; (2) cell proliferation; (3) cell maturation; (4) cell hypertrophy and (5) provisional calcification.

The shape and size of bone, i.e. the skeleton, is determined by bone modeling which stops at adulthood. Remodeling occurs throughout life and is essential for maintenance of normal bone structure (Figures 3.3–3.6) (see page 32).

Bone structure

Cortical bone (cortex)

The cortex (Figures 3.7 and 3.8) is seen in BMB as a layer of compact bone of variable thickness to which the periosteum is attached on the outside and which is lined by a single layer of cells, the endosteum, on the inside. About 80% of the total bone volume is cortical compact bone and about 20% is cancellous bone. Over 90% of compact bone consists of matrix and <10% is soft tissue.

Bone matrix consists mainly of fibers of collagen type I and the amorphous ground substance between them contains proteins and proteoglycans specific for bone, e.g. osteocalcin, thrombospodin, and bone sialoprotein I and II. Bone morphogenic proteins (BMPs) are also present in bone matrix. About 65% of normal bone is mineral, mainly hydroxyapatite; the rest is amorphous calcium phosphate.

Osteons

These are the functional units of cortical and compact bone. They are cylindrical structures (which may be branching) composed of concentric layers (or lamellae) of bone disposed around a central (Haversian) canal within which are capillaries and venules (Figure 3.9). Osteons are found in compact bone, and as they are oriented along the long axis of the bones, they provide mechanical strength along the stress lines. Osteons are lined by endosteal cells, or osteoblasts on layers of osteoid, and may have osteoclasts in erosion cavities. Osteons are the units responsible for the maintenance and remodeling of cortical bone.

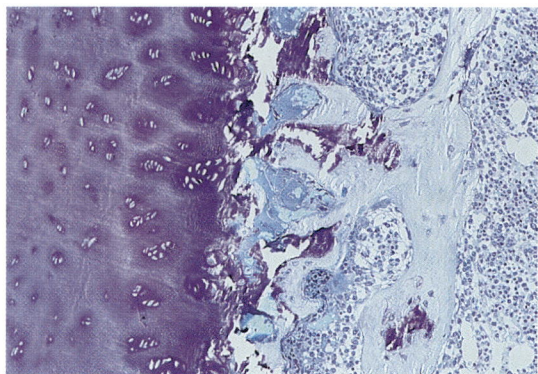

3.1 (left) BMBS plastic, Giemsa, showing growth plate; cartilage, left, bone with residual islands of cartilage, lower center.

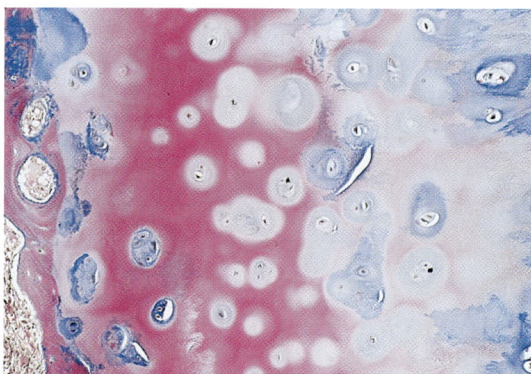

3.2 (right) BMBS paraffin, Masson's stain, showing cartilageous growth plate.

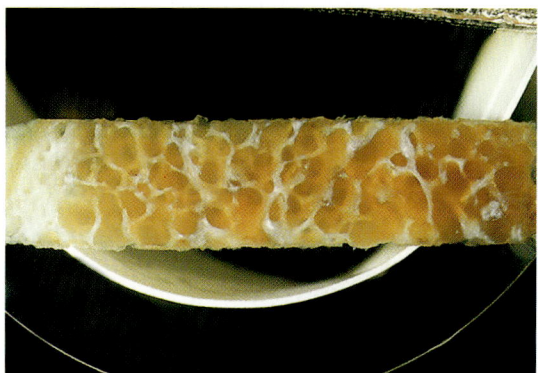

3.3 (left) Cut surface of plastic block showing trabecular network and intertrabecular spaces.

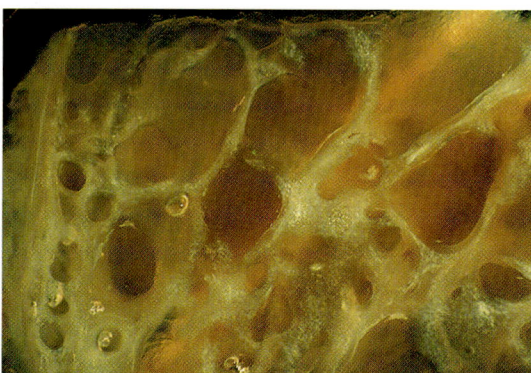

3.4 (right) As for Figure 3.3; higher magnification showing variable thickness of trabecular network.

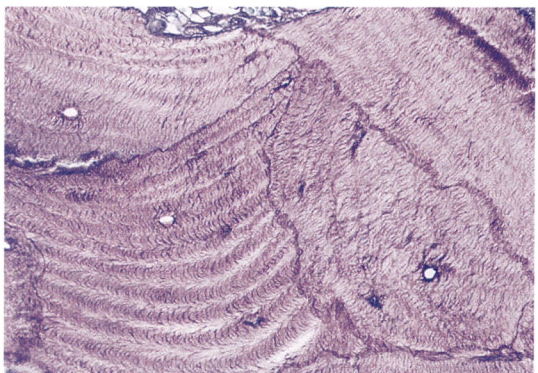

3.5 (left) BMBS plastic, H&E showing lamellar bone structure, lower left, and scalloped edge of area of previous remodeling, right of center.

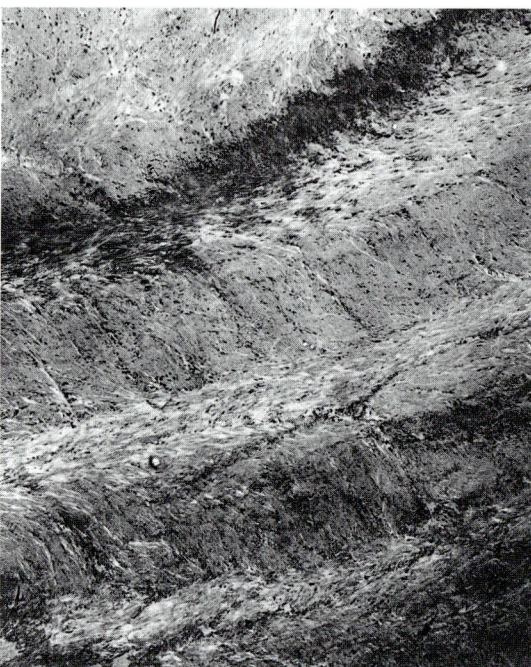

3.6 (right) BMB EM section to show lamellar bone structure.

Trabecular bone (cancellous bone, trabeculae, ossicles)

This refers to the honeycomb of bones that partitions the space enclosed by the cortical bone and which is lined by the endosteum continuous with that of the cortices (Figures 3.10 and 3.11). Most trabeculae (or ossicles) are <0.2 mm thick and do not contain blood vessels. Trabeculae consist of segments formed by parallel layers – lamellae (Figure 3.12). As with compact bone, cement lines hold the lamellae together. The few trabeculae thicker than 0.2 mm may contain a central osteon-like structure lined by endosteal cells (Figure 3.13) with circular rings of lamellae surrounding a blood vessel. About 10% of the trabecular surface is covered by osteoid, of which about half shows the mineralisation or calcification front (Figure 3.14), which is the interphase between calcified bone and osteoid, at which mineralisation starts; in some sections this may be seen as a thin line between the calcified bone and the osteoid.

A nucleation site, possibly provided by osteonectin or proteoglycans, may initiate deposition of calcium. Alternatively, alkaline phosphatase together with matrix vesicles may be the chief initiators and mediators of calcification of osteoid.

3.7 BMBS plastic, Gomori, showing porous cortex with blood vessels.

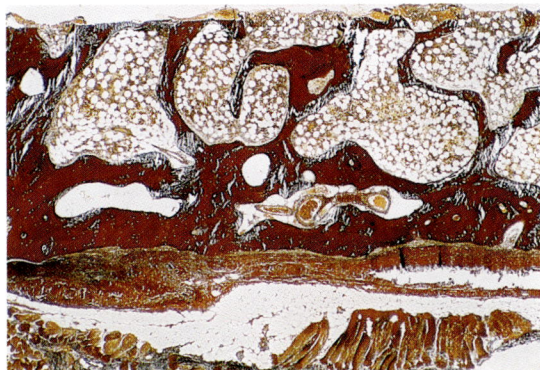

3.8 (left) BMB plastic, Gomori, cortex showing circular lamellae of Haversian systems.

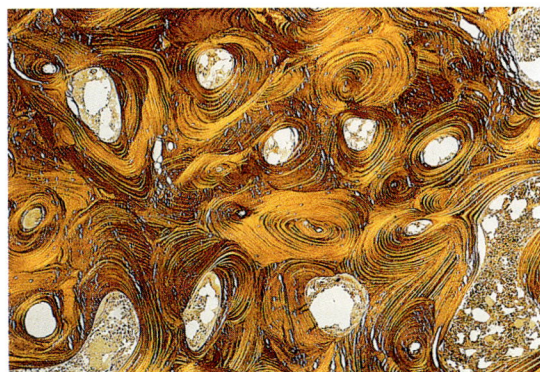

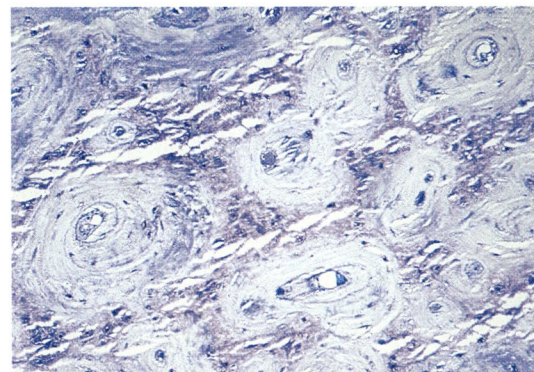

3.9 (right) BMBS paraffin showing Haversian systems, central canals within which are capillaries and venules.

3.10 and 11 Plastic Gomori and paraffin H&E, showing network of cancellous (trabecular) bone, of variable thickness which does not contain blood vessels, and which is better preserved in subcortical than in the deeper parts of the biopsies.

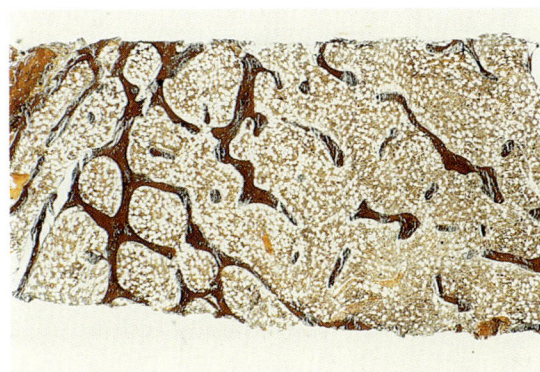

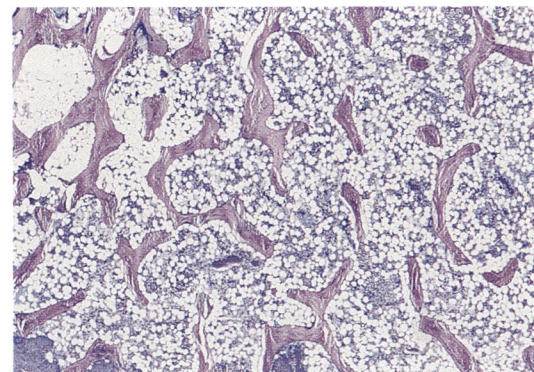

Osseous remodeling

Osseous remodeling, as indicated by the presence of osteoclasts in the scalloped niches (Howship's lacunae) and by a row of cuboidal osteoblasts on a layer of osteoid (unmineralised bone) on the trabecular surface, is often present in the subcortical regions even when the deeper cancellous bone is almost devoid of it. There is a delicate balance between bone formation and resorption of bone in which highly complex regulatory mechanisms are involved.

Osteoblasts

These are the cells that produce bone matrix (Figure 3.15). They arise, or develop, out of progenitor cells in the stroma 'mesenchyme' of the bone marrow, and also from the endosteal cells lining the surfaces of the cancellous bone (Figures 3.16 and 3.17). Indeed, they are looked on as a resting form of osteoblasts. When activated they become cuboidal, and fibers and blood vessels in the vicinity appear more prominent. Occasionally (with the light microscope) there appears to be direct continuity as well as contiguity between the endosteal cells and the endothelial cells of the paratrabecular sinusoids. Recently, a lineage pathway derived from stromal stem cells with the capacity to differentiate into reticular cells, fibroblasts, adipocytes and osteogenic cells has been proposed. In this context it is worth noting that both the endosteal and endothelial cells in their proximity have PAS-positive

droplets in their cytoplasm while they are absent from the endothelial cells of the sinusoids further away. Endosteal cells also stain positively with the antibody to actin. In areas of increased osseous remodeling, especially obvious in tangential cuts, the osteoblasts may form several layers. Osteoblasts lay down the bone matrix, osteoid, which later becomes

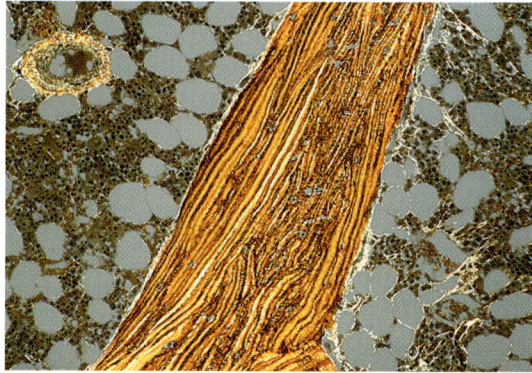

3.12 BMBS plastic, Gomori stain viewed in polarised light; note reticular fibers around blood vessels, sinus, and near the trabecula which consists of parallel layers – lamellae.

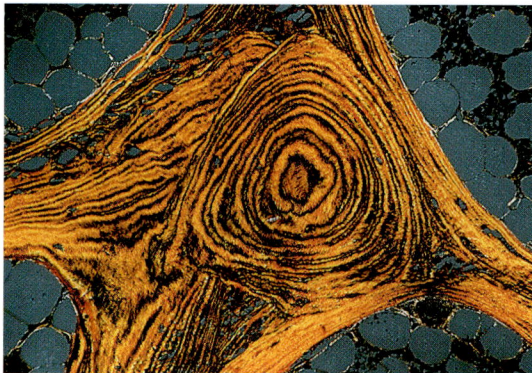

3.13 BMBS plastic, Gomori stain viewed in polarised light, showing lamellar bone and a Haversian system in a trabecular intersection.

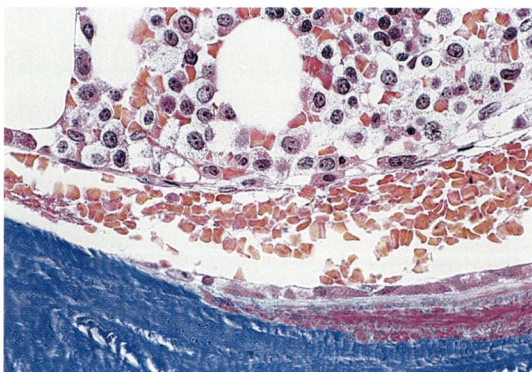

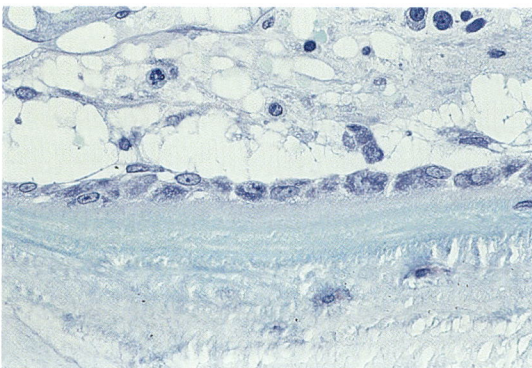

3.14 (left) BMBS plastic, Ladewig, bone in blue, osteoid red, lower right, with layer of osteoblasts and paratrabecular sinus; erythrocytes – yellow.

3.15 (right) BMBS plastic, Giemsa, layers of osteoid (green) on paler bone; note osteoblasts and osteocytes.

3.16 (left) BMBS EM showing endosteal lining cell on collagen fibers, calcification bottom and right.

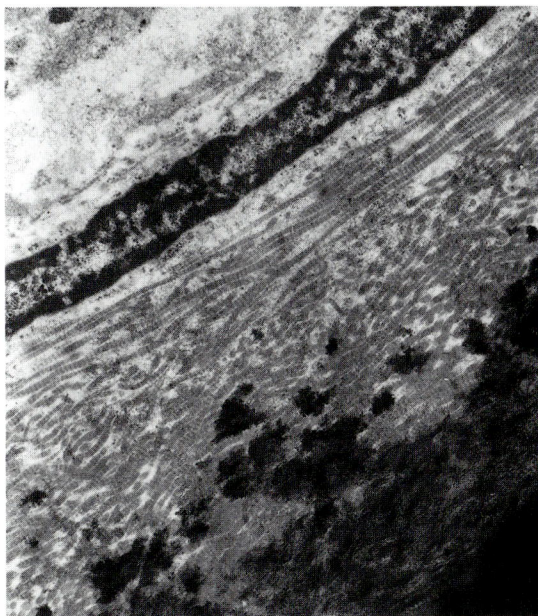

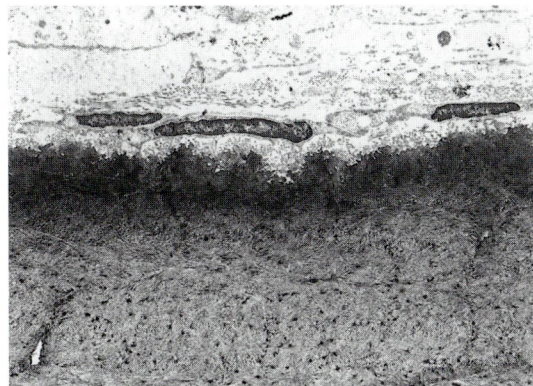

3.17 (right) BMBS EM showing three endosteal lining cells on bone.

3.18 BMBS plastic H&E, lamellar bone, cement lines, osteocytes and canaliculi.

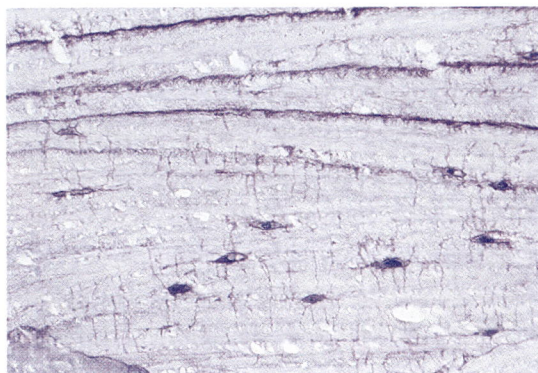

mineralised to form lamellar bone. Osteoblasts also produce osteocalcin and alkaline phosphatase which enter the blood stream and are used as specific bone markers in many metabolic bone disorders. Osteoblasts are target cells and possess receptors for parathyroid hormone and $1,25(OH)_2$ vitamin D. Other hormones, factors and mediators acting on bone cells include estrogens, glucocorticoids, growth factors, insulin, prostaglandins, cobalamin and cytokines released by reabsorbing osteoclasts. Osteoblasts also possess an autocrine pathway for self-stimulation resulting in increased production of collagen, osteonectin, alkaline phosphatase and osteocalcin. In addition, they also secrete collagenase and participate in the regulation of osteoclast activity.

Osteocytes

Following deposition of osteoid and its mineralisation, the osteoblasts in that layer are enclosed and embedded in their own matrix and thus become osteocytes (Figures 3.18–3.20) with lacunae whose processes connect by means of the canaliculi with those of other osteocytes and with the osteoblasts on the surface of the bone (Figure 3.21). Thus, an osseous circulatory system is formed (Figures 3.22 and 3.23); this guarantees the sustenance of the osteocytes, exchange and transfer between bone and the intercellular (interstitial) fluid and the bloodstream. Moreover, it is thought that this is one mechanism by which the osteocytes participate in the homeostasis of minerals, and respond to stimuli, e.g. to initiate osteocytic osteolysis (resorption of lacunar walls), though this is not accepted by some investigators.

Osteoclasts

These are the cells that resorb bone (Figure 3.24). They range from 20 to >100 mm in

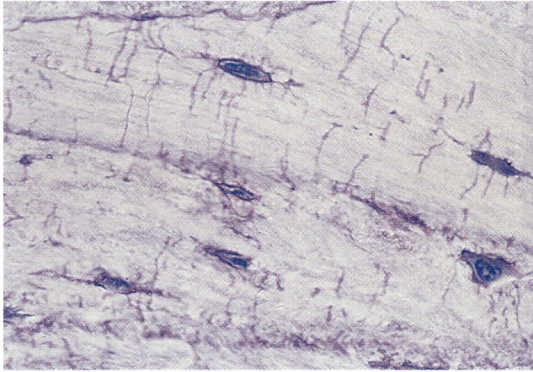

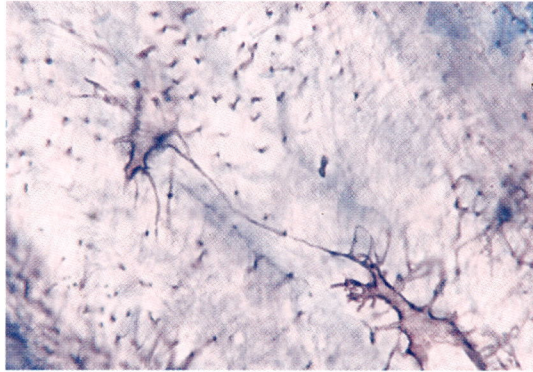

3.19 and 20 BMBS as for Figures 3.18, 3.19 higher magnification showing osteocytes and 3.20 showing connecting osteocytic canaliculi.

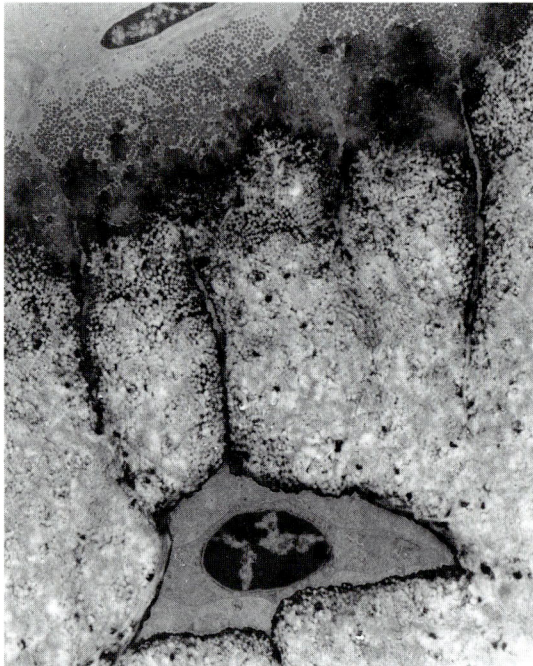

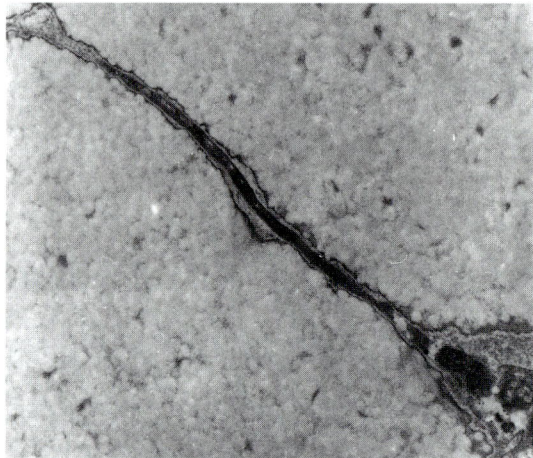

3.21 (left) BMBS EM showing osteocyte in bone with canaliculus extending to the surface (top).

3.22 (right) BMBS EM osteocyte process in canaliculus; these processes are often connected to osteocyte nuclei. Longitudinal cut.

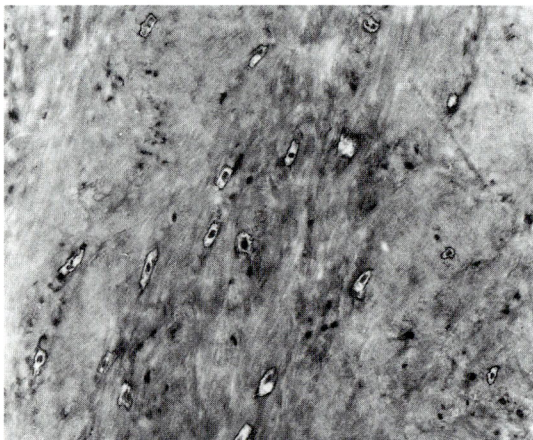

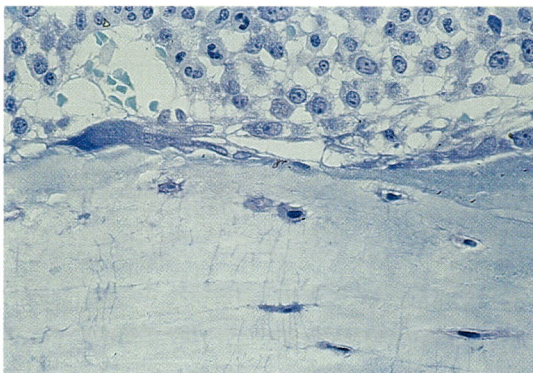

3.23 (left) As for Figure 3.22 EM showing osteocytic canaliculi and processes cut in cross-section.

3.24 (right) BMBS plastic, Giemsa, showing focus of remodeling, osteoclast, left, and osteoblasts, right. Note rather flat and elongated osteoclast.

diameter and may have one or 2–100 nuclei (Figure 3.25). Osteoclasts are formed by cell fusion, and they are found on the trabecular bone surface, in association with the endothelia of blood vessels, and in the erosion cavities (Howship's lacunae) on both cortical and cancellous bone where resorption occurs (Figure 3.26). This area of contiguity between osteoclast and bone is the 'attachment zone' mediated by integrin-type receptors. It is here

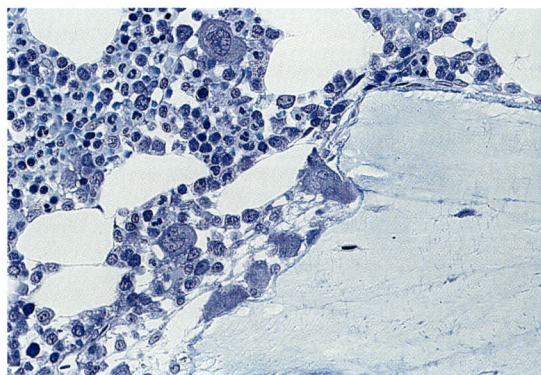

3.25 BMBS plastic, Giemsa, focus of osteoclastic remodeling; group of osteoclasts in erosion cavity.

that resorption takes place and the resorption bays (Howship's lacunae) are formed: proteinases remove the organic matrix and hydrogen ions dissolve the hydroxyapatite crystals. In addition, osteoclasts also release noncollagenous proteins from bone, such as a variety of growth factors, including transforming growth factor β (TGF-β). Osteoclasts also possess receptors for mediators of their function, such as integrins and vitronectin.

Osteoclasts may be observed interposed between adjacent endothelial and endosteal cells as well as between bone and endothelium on the trabecular and subcortical bone surfaces, especially on the resorbing surfaces.

In some disease states and after certain physiological stimuli there appears to be an association between the number of nuclei and activity. It is now believed, however, that the relatively flat and uninucleated osteoclasts resorb bone. Osteoclastic resorption is accompanied by increase in blood vessels and blood flow (a classic example is Paget's disease). Recent experimental studies appear to have

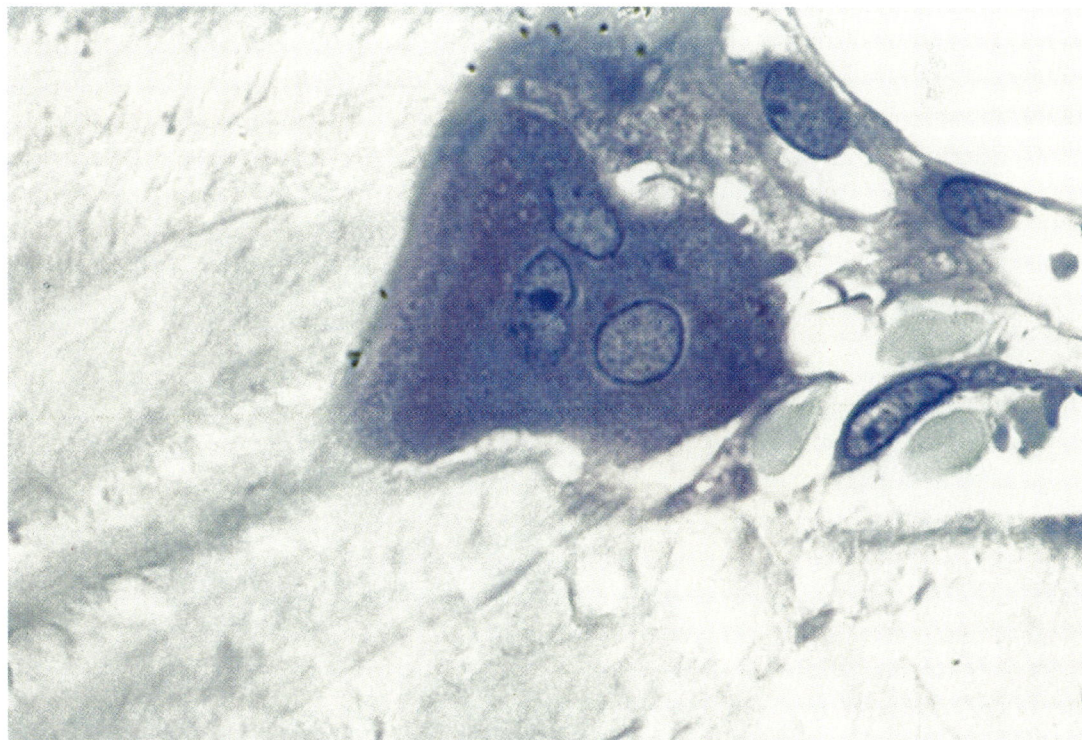

3.26 BMBS plastic, Giemsa, ruffled membrane of osteoclast on bone, left.

elucidated the origin of osteoclasts – they are now thought to develop from a precursor of the monocytic series, i.e. they belong to the hematopoietic cell lines. However, from a morphological point of view, cells with the cytological characteristics of osteoclasts may be seen in areas of stimulated mesenchyme, as well as in close proximity to blood vessels and their endothelium. In these situations there appears to be a close association between the developing mesenchymal cells, the endothelial cells of the blood vessels, the endosteal cells, the osteoblasts and the osteoclasts. It should be noted that mitotic figures in cells that are identified unequivocally as osteoclasts are extremely rare and it is assumed that these multinucleated cells arise by means of coalescence; endomitosis may also contribute to osteoclast multinuclearity. Whether osteoclasts derive exclusively from the monocytic series, or also from local precursors or progenitors in the stimulated mesenchyme, is not fully clarified. However, as noted earlier, physiological processes in the bone marrow are extremely rapid, may leave little or no trace and therefore extreme caution should be exercised in the interpretation of, and drawing conclusions from, one-time snapshot observations made on bone marrow morphology.

The concept of bone remodeling

Remodeling involves a balanced sequence of resorption and formation (Figures 3.27–3.29). Overall, 5–10% of the existing bone is replaced annually, though the turnover of trabecular bone is probably nearer 20%. Remodeling is not uniform and varies greatly throughout the skeleton. The concept of bone remodeling was first formulated by Frost in 1964: the following stages are distinguished – A, osteoclast activation; R, resorption; Rev, reversal and deposition of cement line; F, osteoblast activation and formation of osteoid; and Rest, resting phase after mineralisation of osteoid. A complete trabecular remodeling cycle takes about 200 days, and there are about 35 million basic multicellular units (BMVs) operative at any given time in the skeleton.

Regulation of bone remodeling

There are highly complex mechanisms and pathways of regulation involved in bone remodeling, as indicated in Tables 3.1 and 3.2. However, a detailed account of the current ideas on different factors, mediators, modulators, inhibitors and targets as well as their complex interactions are beyond the scope of this text; comprehensive reviews are available.

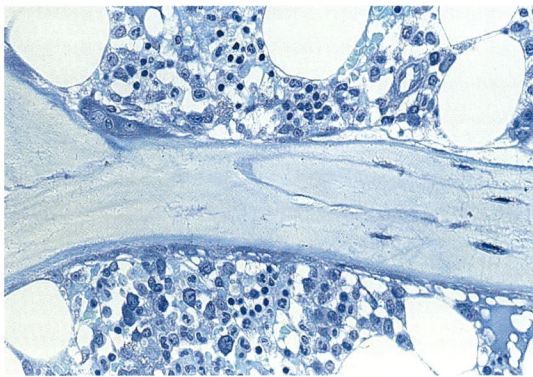

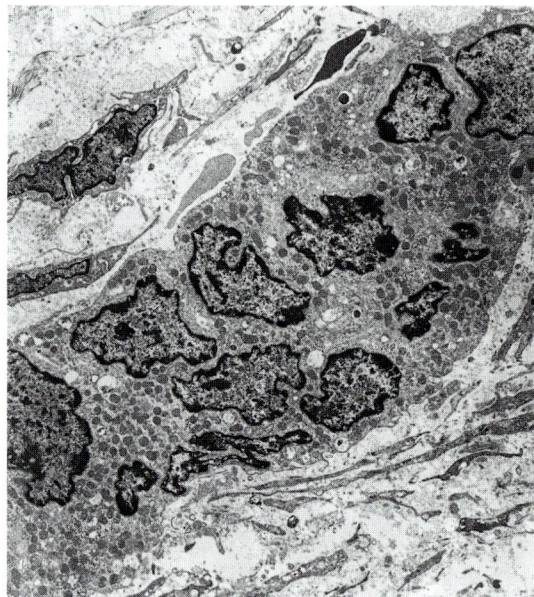

3.27 (left) As for Figure 3.26; trabecula showing resorption on the upper surface and formation on the lower.

3.28 (right) BMBS EM showing multinucleated osteoclast. Note also numerous cytoplasmic organelles.

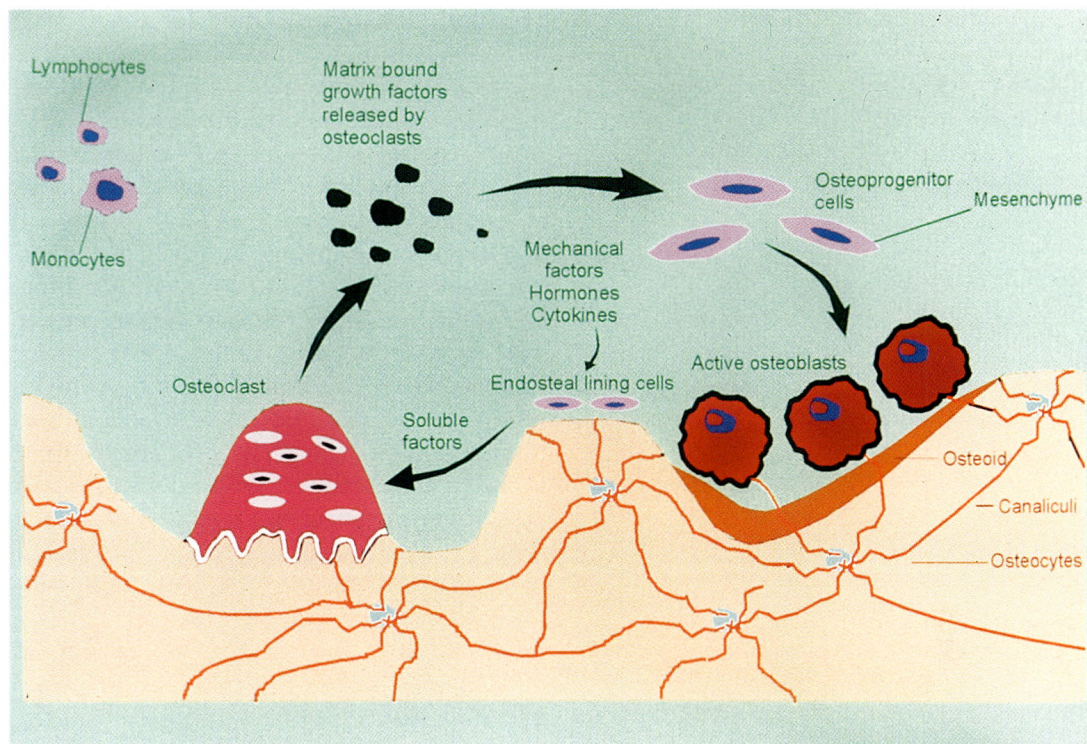

3.29 Sketch of precursor cells and bone cells, and their presumptive pathways of development.

TABLE 3.1 Factors in bone metabolism

Hormones	Growth factors	Cytokines
Parathyroid hormone	Fibroblast growth factors (FGF)	M-CSF
Calcitonin	Platelet-derived growth factors (PDGF)	GM-CSF
Vitamin D	Transforming growth factors (TGF)	IL-1
Glucocorticoids	Insulin-like growth factors (IGF)	IL-6
Estrogens	Binding proteins (BP)	TNF-α
Androgens	Beta-2-microglobulin (β_2-M)	Interferon
Thyroxine	Osteoinductive factors (OIFs)	
Insulin	Parathyroid hormone-related protein (PTH-rP)	
Growth hormone	Epidermal growth factor (EGF)	
	Oxygen-derived free radicals (ODFR)	
	Plasminogen tissue activator (PTA)	
	Bone morphogenic proteins (BMP)	
	Macrophage-derived growth factor (MDGF)	
	Inhibitors of collagenase and metallo-proteinases	

TABLE 3.2 Bone matrix: osteoblast factors

Collagen Type I

Fibronectin, osteopontin, thrombospondin (CAMs)
Osteonectin, sialoprotein (Ca-binding proteins)
Osteocalcin (mineralisation)
Alkaline phosphatase (osteoid)
Collagenase (matrix breakdown)
IGF-1, TGF-β, PDGF (growth factors)
Interleukins 1, 6 and others (cytokines)

IGF-1, insulin-like growth factor-1; TGF-β, transforming growth factor-beta; PDGF, platelet-derived growth factor; CAMs, cell adhesion molecules.

In brief, systemic circulating substances such as parathyroid hormones, calcitonin and metabolites of vitamin D are among the most important of the numerous factors participating in the intricate mechanisms controlling calcium metabolism and the integrity of bone.

In addition, a variety of locally produced growth factors, cytokines, and cellular connections between bone cells themselves and other connective tissue cells in their vicinity participate in the regulation of bone remodeling. Moreover, there is a close association between bone and marrow and the interactions and interdependence of these two organs must be taken into account. For example, diseases of the marrow affect the bone – hair on end skull in thalassemia, osteolyses in multiple myeloma and disorders of bone affect the marrow – anemia in osteopetrosis and in Paget's disease. Furthermore, stromal abnormalities may affect both bone and marrow – hematopoietic hypoplasia and osteopenia in angiopathies; and finally, bone and marrow may be altered by pathological changes in other organs – anemia and osteodystrophy in renal disease.

Bibliography

Aaron J.E., Makins N.B., Sagreiya K. (1987) The microanatomy of trabecular bone loss in normal ageing men and women. *Clin Orthop.*, **215**, 260.

Anderson H.C. (1989) Biology of disease: mechanism of mineral formation. *Lab Invest.*, **60**, 320.

Arey L.B. (1965) *Developmental Anatomy: A Textbook and Laboratory Manual of Embryology.* Philadelphia: W.B. Saunders.

Arnaud C.D. (1988) Mineral and bone homeostasis. Wyngaarden and Smith (eds), *Cecil Textbook of Medicine.* Philadelphia: W.B. Saunders, p. 1469.

Arnett T.R., Dempster T.W. (1990) Protons and osteoclasts. *J Bone Miner Res.*, **5**, 1099.

Arnold J.S. (1970) Focal excess endosteal resorption in ageing and senile osteoporosis.

in U.S. Brazel (ed), *Osteoporosis.* New York: Grune & Stratton, p. 80.

Athanasou N.A., Quinn J., Horton M.A., Mcgee I.D. (1990) New sites of cellular vitronectin receptor immunoreactivity detected with osteoclast reacting mononuclear antibodies 13C2 and 23C6. *Bone Miner.*, **8 (1)**, 7.

Atkinson P.J. (1965) Changes in resorption spaces in femoral cortical bone with age. *J Pathol Bacteriol.*, **89**, 173.

Atkinson P.J. (1967) Variation in the trabecular structure of vertebrae with age. *Calcif Tissue Res.*, **1**, 24.

Avioli L.V., Hruska K., Civitelli R. (1990) Activation of the (Ca2+) I message system by parathyroid-hormone-related protein in osteoblastic cells. *Adv. Second Mess. Phosphoprotein Res.*, **24**, 529.

Avioli L.V., Krane S.M. (1990) *Metabolic Bone Disease.* Philadelphia: W.B. Saunders.

Baron R. (1989) Molecular mechanisms of bone resorption by the osteoclast. *Anat Rec.*, **224**, 317.

Bartl R., Frisch B. (1993) *Biopsy of Bone in Internal Medicine: An Atlas and Sourcebook.* Dordrecht: Kluwer Academic.

Birkenhaeger-Frenkel D.H., Coupron P., Clermont E. (1986) Trabecular thickness, intertrabecular distance and age related bone loss. *Bone*, **6**, 402.

Bouvier M. (1989) The biology and composition of bone. In Cowin (ed), *Bone Mechanics.* Boca Raton: CRC Press, p. 1.

Brown D.C., Gatter K.C. (1993) The bone marrow trephine biopsy: a review of normal histology. *Histopathology*, **22 (5)**, 411–22.

Canalis E., McCarthy T., Centrella M. (1988) Growth factors and regulation of bone remodeling. *J Clin Invest.*, **81**, 277.

Canalis E., McCarthy T.L., Centrella M. (1991) Growth factors and cytokines in bone cell metabolism. *Ann Rev Med.*, **42**, 17.

Canalis E., McCarthy T.L., Centrella M. (1993) Factors that regulate bone formation. In G.R. Mundy and T.J. Martin (eds), *Physiology and Pharmacology of Bone. Handbook of Experimental Pharmacology*, **107**, 249–66.

Carter D.H., Sloan P., Aaron J.E. (1991), Immunolocalization of collagen types I and III, tenascin, and fibronectin in intramembranous bone. *J. Histochem. Cytochem.*, **39 (5)**, 599–606.

Centrella M., McCarthy T., Canalis E. (1991) Current concepts review: transforming growth factor-beta and remodeling of bone. *J Bone Jt. Surg.*, **73A**, 1418.

Centrella M., McCarthy T.L., Canalis E. (1992) Growth factors and cytokines. In Hall (ed), *Bone Metabolism and Mineralization.* Boca Raton: CRC Press. p. 47–72.

Chambers T.J., Hall T.J. (1991) Cellular and molecular mechanisms in the regulation and function of osteoclasts. *Vitam. Horm.*, **46**, 41.

Chatterji S., Wall J.C., Jeffrey J.W. (1981) Age-related changes in the orientation and particle size of the mineral phase in human femoral cortical bone. *Calcif Tissue Int.*, **33**, 567.

Chow J., Tobias J.H., Colston K.W., Chambers T.J. (1992) Estrogen maintains trabecular bone volume in rats not only by suppression of bone resorption but also by stimulation of bone formation. *J Clin Invest.*, **89**, 74.

Coe F.L., Favus M.J. (eds) (1992) *Disorders of Bone and Mineral Metabolism.* New York: Raven Press.

Colvard D.S., Eriksen E.F., Keeting P.E. *et al.* (1989) Identification of androgen receptors in normal human osteoblast-like cells. *Proc., Natl. Acad. Sci.,***86**, 854.

Dempster D.W. (1992) Bone remodeling. In Coe and Favus (eds), *Disorders of Bone and Mineral Metabolism.* New York: Raven Press, pp. 355–80.

Editorial (1990) Fibroblast growth factors: time to take note. *Lancet*, **336**, 777.

Editorial (1992) New bone? *Lancet*, **339**, 463.

Editorial (1992) Pyridinium crosslinks as markers of bone resorption. *Lancet*, **340**, 278.

Evans D.B., Thavarajah M., Kanis S.A. (1990) Involvement of prostaglandin E2 in the inhibition of osteocalcin synthesis by human osteoblast-like cells in response to cytokines and systemic hormones. *Biochem Biophys Res Commun.*, **167**, 194.

Eventov I., Frisch B., Cohen Z., Hammel I. (1991) Osteopenia, hematopoiesis, and bone remodeling in iliac crest and femoral biopsies: a prospective study of 102 cases of femoral neck fractures. *Bone*, **12**, 1.

Favus M.J. (ed) (1993) *Primer on the Metabolic Bone Diseases and Disorders of Mineral Metabolism*, 2nd edn. New York: Raven Press.

Frisch B., Bartl R. (1990) *Atlas of Bone Marrow Pathology.* Dordrecht: Kluwer Academic.

Frost H.M. (1969) Tetracycline based histological analysis of bone remodeling. *Calcif. Tissue Res.*, **3**, 211–37.

Frost H.M. (1973) *Bone Remodeling and its Relationship to Metabolic Bone Diseases.* Springfield: Thomas.

Frost H.M. (1989) Tetracyclin-based histological analysis of bone remodeling. *Calcified Tissue Res.*, **3**, 211.

Garn S.M. (1972) Calcium requirements for bone building and skeletal maintenance. *Amer J Clin Nutr.*, **23**, 1149.

Gowen M. (1994) Cytokines and cellular interactions in the control of bone remodeling. In Heersche and Kanis (eds), *Bone and Mineral Research.* Amsterdam: Elsevier, pp. 77–114.

Gronthos S., Graves S.E., Ohto S., Simmons P.J. (1994) The STRO-1+ fraction of adult human bone marrow contains the osteogenic precursors. *Blood*, **84 (12)**, 3164–73.

Gruber H.E. (1991) Bone and the immune system. *Proc. Soc. Exp. Biol. Med.*, **197**, 219.

Hall, T.J., Schaeublin, M., Chambers, T.J. (1993) The majority of osteoclasts require mRNA and protein synthesis for bone resorption in vitro. *Biochem. Biophys. Res. Comm.*, **195 (3)**, 1245–53.

Hanaoka H., Yabe H., Bun H. (1989) The origin of the osteoclast. *Clin Orthop.*, **239**, 286.

Holick M.F., Krane S.M., Potts J.T. (1991) Calcium, phosphorus, and bone metabolism: calcium-regulating hormones. In Wilson (ed), *Harrison's Principles of Internal Medicine.* New York: Mcgraw-Hill, p. 1888.

Hufter W.E. (1988) Morphology and biochemistry of bone remodelling: possible control by vitamin D., parathyroid hormone, and other substances. *Lab Invest.*, **59 (4)**, 418.

Ishizaka H., Horikoshi H., Inoue T. *et al.* (1995) Bone marrow cellularlity: quantification by chemical-shift misregistration in magnetic resonance imaging and comparison with histomorphometric techniques. *Australas Radiol.*, **39 (4)**, 411–4.

Jandinsli J.J. (1988) Osteoclast activation factor is now interleukin-1 beta: historical perspective and biological implications. *J Oral Pathol.*, **17**, 145.

Junth G., Berghauser K.H., Termine J.D., Schulz A. (1987) Osteonectin – a differentiation marker of bone cells. *Cell Tissue Res.*, **248**, 409.

Kassem M., Mosekilde l., Eriksen E.F. (1994) Growth hormone stimulates proliferation of normal human bone marrow stromal osteoblast precursor cells in vitro. *Growth Regul.*, **4 (3)**, 131–5.

Katz E.P., Li S.T. (1973) Structure and function of bone collagen fibrils. *J Mol Biol.*, **80**, 1.

Kelly P.J., Eisman J.A., Sambrook P.N. (1990) Interaction of genetic and environmental influences on peak bone density. *Osteoporosis Int.*, **1**, 56.

Kelly P.J., Montgomery R.J. (1990) Circulation in bone. In McCollister Evarts (ed), *Surgery of the Musculoskeletal System*, 2nd edn. New York: Churchill Livingstone, p. 71.

Khokher M.A., Dandona P. (1989) Diphosphonates inhibit human osteoblast secretion and proliferation. *Metabolism*, **38**, 184.

Kiebzak G.M. (1991) Age-related bone changes. *Exp Gerontol.*, **26**, 171.

Kragstrup J., Melsen F., Mosekilde L. (1983) Thickness of lamellae in normal human iliac trabecular bone. *Metab Bone Dis Rel Res.*, **4**, 291.

Lomri A., Marie P.J., (1990) Changes in cytoskeletal proteins in response to parathyroid hormone and 1,25-dihydroxy vitamin D in human osteoblastic cells. *Bone Miner.*, **10 (1)**, 1.

Long M.W., Robinson J.A., Ashcraft E.A., Mann K.G. (1995) Regulation of human bone marrow-derived osteoprogenitor cells by osteogenic growth factors. *J Clin Invest.*, **95 (2)**, 881–7.

Majumdar S., Newitt D., Jergas M. *et al.* (1995) Evaluation of technical factors affecting the quantification of trabecular bone structure using magnetic resonance imaging. *Bone*, **17 (4)**, 417–30.

Malluche H.H., Faugere M.C. (1991) Bone biopsies: histology and histomorphometry of bone. In Avioli and Krane (eds), *Metabolic Bone Disease*. Philadelphia: W.B. Saunders p. 283.

Manolagas S.C., Jilka R.L. (1995) Bone marrow, cytokines, and bone remodeling. *N Engl J Med.*, **332**, 305–11.

Marcus R. (1987) Normal and abnormal bone remodeling in man. *Ann Rev Med.*, **38**, 129.

Martin T.J., Ng K.W., Suda T. (1989) Bone cell physiology. *Endocrinol Metab Clin N Amer.*, **18 (4)**, 833.

Matkovic V. (1991) Calcium metabolism and calcium requirements during skeletal modeling and consolidation. *Am J Clin Nutr.*, **54**, 245–60.

Mazess R.B. (1982) On aging bone loss. *Clin Orthop Rel Res.*, **165**, 239.

McCalden R.W., Mcgeough J.A., Barker M.B., Court-Brown C.M. (1991) Mechanical changes in aging cortical bone: the role of changes in porosity, mineralisation and microstructure. *J Bone Jt Surg.*, **73-B**, 103.

Meier D.E., Orwoll E.S., Jones J.M. (1983) Marked disparity between trabecular and cortical bone loss with age in healthy men. *Ann Intern Med.*, **101**, 605.

Mosekilde L. (1990) Consequences of the remodeling process for vertebral trabecular bone structure: a scanning electron microscopic study (uncoupling of unloaded structures) *Bone Miner.*, **10**, 13.

Mosekilde L., Mosekilde L. (1990) Sex differences in age-related changes in vertebral body size, density and biomechanical competence in normal individuals. *Bone*, **11**, 67–73.

Mundy G.R. (1995) Bone remodeling and its disorders. London: Martin Dunitz.

Mundy G.R., Bonewald L.F. (1990) Role of TGFβ in bone remodeling. *Ann N Y Acad Sci.*, **593**, 91.

Mundy G.R., Martin T.J. (eds) (1993) *Physiology and Pharmacology of Bone. Handbook of Experimental Pharmacology*, **107**. Berlin: Springer.

Noda M. (ed) (1993) *Cellular and Molecular Biology of Bone*. San Diego: Academic Press.

Owen M. (1985) Lineage of osteogenic cells and their relationship to the stromal system. In Peck (ed), *Bone and Mineral Research*, vol. 3. Amsterdam: Elsevier, p. 1.

Parfitt A.M. (1988) Bone histomorphometry: standardization of nomenclature, symbols and units. Summary of proposed system. *Bone Miner.*, **4**, 1.

Parfitt A.M., Matthews C.H.E., Villanueva A.R. *et al.* (1983) Relationships between surface, volume and thickness of iliac trabecular bone in ageing and in osteoporosis. Implications for the microanatomic and cellular mechanisms of bone loss. *J Clin Invest.*, **72 (1)**, 396.

Pellegrini W., Facchetti F., Marocolo D. *et al.* (1995) Assessment of cell proliferation in normal and pathological bone marrow biopsies: a study using double sequential immunophenotyping on paraffin sections. *Histopathology*, **27 (5)**, 397–405.

Pierce A.N., Lindskog S., Hammerstrom L. (1991) Osteoclasts: structure and function. *Electronmicrosc Rev.*, **4**, 1.

Podenphant J., Gotfredsen A., Nilas L. *et al.* (1986) Iliac crest biopsy: representativity for the amount of mineralized bone. *Bone*, **7**, 427.

Power M.J., Fottrell P.F. (1991) Osteocalcin: diagnostic methods and clinical applications. *Crit Rev Clin Lab Sci.*, **28**, 287.

Recker R.R., Davies M., Hinders M. *et al.* (1992) Bone gain in young adults. *J Am Med Assoc.*, **268**, 2403–8.

Recker R.R., Kimmel D.B., Parfitt A.M. *et al.* (1988) Static and tetracycline based bone histomorphometric data from 34 normal postmenopausal females. *J Bone Miner Res.*, **3**, 133–44.

Rees R.C. (1992) Cytokines as biological response modifiers. *J Clin Pathol.*, **45**, 93.

Rodan G.A. (1991) Autocrine/paracrine regulation of osteoblast growth and differentiation. *Lab Invest.*, **64 (5)**, 593.

Roodman G.D. (1991) Osteoclast differentiation. *Crit Rev Oral Biol Med.*, **2**, 389.

Schreiber, W.E., Gorecki, T., Bernstein, V. (1991) A unique bone-like variant of alkaline phosphatase. *Am. J. Clin. Pathol.*, **95 (5)**, 749–53.

Thompson D.D. (1980) Age changes in bone mineralisation, cortical thickness, and Haversian canal area. *Calcif Tissue Int.,* **31**, 5.

Trueta J. (1963) The role of vessels in osteogenesis. *J Bone Joint Surg.,* **45 B**, 402.

Vernejoul S., Kuntz D., Miravet L. *et al.* (1981) Bone histomorphometric reproducibility in normal patients. *Calcif Tissue Int.,* **33**, 369.

Wallach S., Carstens J.B., Avioli L.V. (1990) Calcitonin, osteoclasts and bone turnover. *Calcif. Tissue Int.,* **47**, 388.

Weinstein R.S., Hutson M.S. (1987) Decreased trabecular width and increased trabecular spacing contribute to bone loss with aging. *Bone,* **8**, 137.

Wlodarsky K.H. (1990) Properties and origin of osteoblasts. *Clin Orthop.,* **252**, 276.

Zheng M.H., Nicholson G.C., Warton A., Papadimitriou J.M. (1991) What's new in osteoclast ontogeny. *Path Res Pract.,* **187**, 117.

4 Normal bone marrow

Definition and biology

This term is generally used to refer to the tissue occupying the cavities between the trabecular bone. Normal marrow is either red, containing the hematopoietic elements, or yellow, composed mainly of adipose tissue (fat cells). In the adult, red marrow is found in the cavities of the skull, sternum, scapulae, vertebrae, ribs, pelvic bones and the proximal ends of the long bones, such as femora and humeri. The red hematopoietic marrow is the organ that produces the mature blood cells, which have a finite life span and must be constantly replenished. The weight of the bone marrow is 1600–3700 g, approximately the same as that of the liver. The red marrow weighs about 1000 g. Why hematopoiesis in the adult is normally confined to these bones is not clear; for example, expansion into the shafts of the long bones may occur if required. Stem cells circulate in the peripheral blood and 'home' to the bone marrow. Therefore, the hematopoietic marrow itself is not a static organ and, in the confines of its bony cage, it can expand or contract as required by means of an increase or decrease in the proportion of adipose tissue present, as well as by changes in the microcirculation. Under special circumstances other bones and organs – liver, spleen, lymph nodes – also support hematopoiesis.

A continuous supply of precursor cells is provided by the pluripotent stem cell compartment capable of self-renewal and also having the ability to differentiate into the progenitor cells committed to erythro-, granulo-, mono- and megakaryopoiesis. The bone marrow is also a site for lymphopoiesis and maturation of plasma cells; however, stem and progenitor cells are not recognisable as such by the usual morphological techniques and are therefore not visualised on smears of aspirates and sections of biopsies. The dynamics of hematopoiesis, as well as the multiplicity of interacting regulatory factors involved in the normal (as well as abnormal) production of blood cells, is beyond the scope of this text, which deals with the clinical interpretation of bone marrow biopsy histology and histopathology.

Age-related changes

With advancing age there is a reduction in the trabecular bone volume and the numbers of associated endosteal cells, osteocytes and paratrabecular sinusoids (Table 4.1). Hematopoietic tissue is also decreased, accompanied by an increase in fat cells, particularly in the subcortical regions. However, there is great individual variability in these age- (and sex-) related changes. They are not consistently observed, and they may be influenced by numerous other factors. In addition, other cells normally present in the bone marrow, such as lymphocytes, plasma cells and mast cells, may show increases in the bone marrows of older people. Stromal changes are also found: increase in fibers and changes in walls of blood vessels especially sclerosis.

Marrow cellularity

This refers to both hematopoietic and fat cells and it indicates the relative amounts of these two components. Normocellular (Figure 4.1)

TABLE 4.1 Histomorphometric parameters measured in posterior iliac crest biopsies according to age groups

Parameters	Abbreviation	Units	Age groups (years)							
			–9	10–19	20–29	30–39	40–49	50–59	60–69	70–
Bone structure										
Bone volume	BV/TV	%	20 ± 4	25 ± 5	24 ± 5	22 ± 4	21 ± 5	20 ± 5	17 ± 3	13 ± 1
Bone surface	BS/BV	mm²/mm³	2.9 ± 0.4	2.8 ± 0.6	3.1 ± 0.3	2.9 ± 0.6	3.0 ± 0.6	3.0 ± 0.9	2.6 ± 0.7	2.1 ± 0.5
Trabecular thickness	TB.Th	μm	172 ± 30	222 ± 53	195 ± 44	173 ± 52	179 ± 49	177 ± 39	173 ± 33	171 ± 44
Mineralisation										
Osteoid volume	OV/BV	%	7.7 ± 2.4	5.2 ± 4.8	3.4 ± 3.4	2.0 ± 2.4	1.0 ± 1.1	1.9 ± 1.5	2.3 ± 2.3	1.7 ± 2.0
Osteoid surface	OS/BV	mm²/mm³	0.8 ± 0.4	0.9 ± 3.7	0.9 ± 0.5	0.5 ± 0.4	0.3 ± 0.2	0.5 ± 0.5	0.4 ± 0.4	0.5 ± 0.4
Osteoid thickness	O.Th	μm	11 ± 4	6 ± 4	4 ± 3	4 ± 9	4 ± 2	4 ± 5	5 ± 3	3 ± 3
Bone cells										
Osteoclasts	N.Ocl/B.Ar	per mm²	3.1 ± 1.3	1.2 ± 1.0	0.7 ± 0.4	1.0 ± 0.8	0.8 ± 0.5	1.0± 0.9	2.1 ± 0.9	1.3 ± 0.9
Osteoblasts	N.Obl/B.Ar	per mm²	3.6 ± 2.9	4.0 ± 2.6	1.7 ± 0.9	1.5 ± 1.3	0.7 ± 0.6	1.7 ± 2.0	1.6 ± 2.1	1.1 ± 1.2
Lining cells	N.Lin/B.Ar	per mm²	5.4 ± 2.8	2.0 ± 1.2	1.9 ± 1.3	1.8 ± 0.9	1.0 ± 0.8	0.9 ± 0.7	1.4 ± 1.0	1.8 ± 1.3
Osteocytes	N.Ocy/B.Ar	per mm²	24 ± 5	18 ± 5	17 ± 6	20 ± 8	18 ± 8	16 ± 6	18 ± 6	13 ± 3
Blood vessels										
Arteries	N.Art/M.Ar	per mm²	0.3 ± 0.4	0.5 ± 0.6	0.4 ± 0.4	0.4 ± 0.4	0.4 ± 0.4	0.4 ± 0.4	0.5 ± 0.6	0.3 ± 0.4
Arterioles	N.Aio/M.Ar	per mm²	1.3 ± 1.2	1.7 ± 0.9	1.3 ± 0.7	1.3 ± 0.7	1.0 ± 1.0	0.8 ± 0.7	1.2 ± 0.8	1.4 ± 1.2
Capillaries	N.Cap/M.Ar	per mm²	13 ± 4	17 ± 6	18 ± 6	18 ± 6	18 ± 4	20 ± 7	18 ± 8	19 ± 5
Sinusoids	N.Sin/M.Ar	per mm²	37 ± 5	31 ± 8	30 ± 7	34 ± 10	31 ± 7	33 ± 9	39 ± 5	36 ± 7
Endosteal sinusoids	ESV/TV	%	2.5 ± 0.9	2.7 ± 1.0	2.5 ± 1.5	3.0 ± 3.3	1.7 ± 1.7	1.8 ± 0.7	1.7 ± 0.7	1.5 ± 0.5
Stroma										
Fatty tissue	FV/MV	%	12 ± 7	17 ± 5	19 ± 9	26 ± 9	28 ± 11	30 ± 10	31 ± 9	44 ± 14
Mast cells	N.Mas/M.Ar	per mm²	0.4 ± 0.7	0.7 ± 0.8	2.1 ± 1.9	2.2 ± 1.9	2.2 ± 2.4	2.2 ± 1.4	2.6 ± 2.1	3.9± 3.8
Plasma cells	N.Pla/M.Ar	per mm²	19 ± 6	32 ± 11	30 ± 9	31 ± 9	29 ± 9	33 ± 9	34 ± 8	30 ± 9
Hematopoiesis										
Haematopoiesis	HV/MV	%	78 ± 13	72 ± 11	70 ± 12	62 ± 11	61 ± 14	59 ± 13	58 ± 11	45 ± 14
Megakaryocytes	N.Meg/M.Ar	per mm²	20 ± 8	16 ± 4	15 ± 6	14 ± 6	15 ± 4	14 ± 5	13 ± 5	10 ± 6

For terminology, abbreviations and units, see Table 2.2. Histomorphometry was performed in collaboration with Dr B. Mallmann. *Post-mortem* biopsies from 100 normal subjects, 10 or more cases in each age group.

implies marrow with approximately the proportions given in Table 4.1. Hypocellular (Figure 4.2) indicates a reduction in hematopoiesis and a corresponding increase in fat cells. A concomitant reduction in hematopoietic tissue and trabecular bone is frequently observed: hypoplasia plus osteopenia. Hypoplasia in the subcortical marrow spaces frequently may be found in older individuals. Moreover, variable marrow cellularity, hypocellular intertrabecular spaces alternating with hyper- or normocellular ones may be found in normal as well as pathological marrow conditions. Hypercellular (Figure 4.3) is used when the fat is decreased and replaced by other elements.

Topography and bone marrow architecture

The hematopoietic tissue is distributed in the marrow spaces in the extravascular

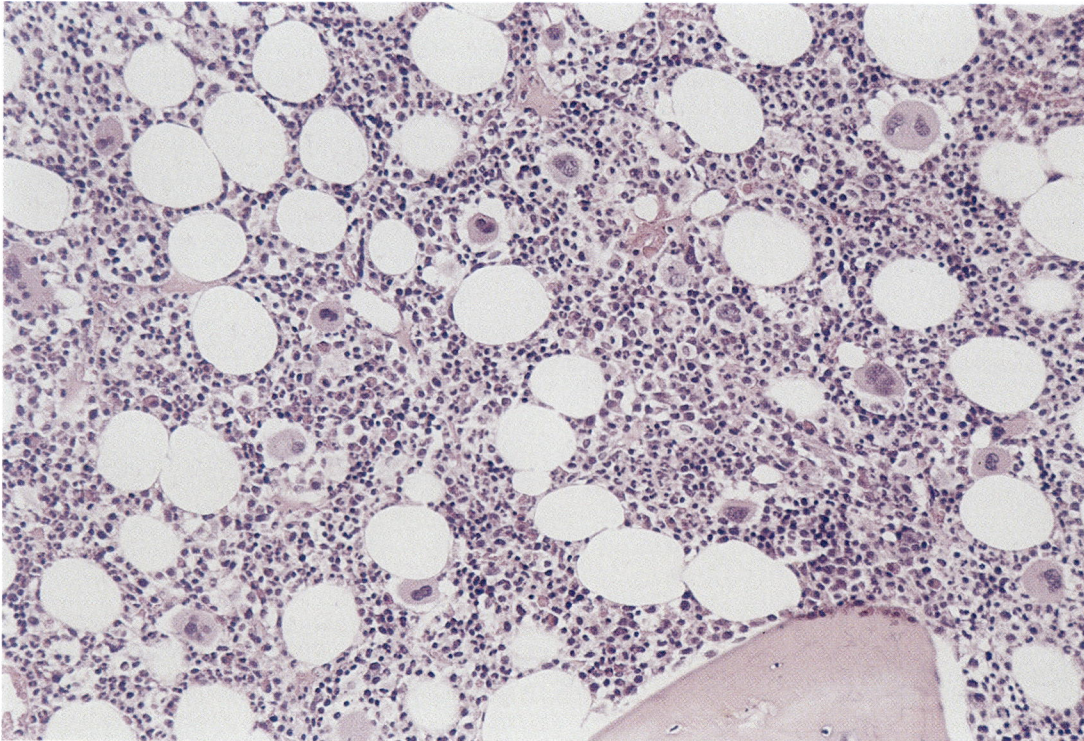

4.1 BMBS paraffin, H&E, showing hematopoiesis, normocellular bone marrow.

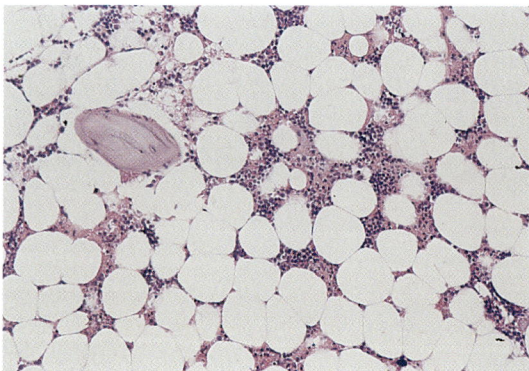

4.2 (left) BMBS paraffin, H&E, showing hypocellular bone marrow, fat cells increased.

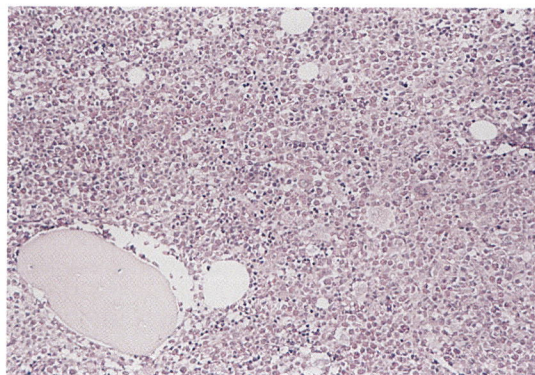

4.3 (right) BMBS paraffin, H&E, showing hypercellular bone marrow, few residual fat cells.

compartment, erythropoietic islands and megakaryocytes are associated with the marrow sinusoids in the central regions of the marrow cavities, early myeloid precursors lie close to the endosteal surfaces and to the arterioles, while the more mature forms of the granulocytic series are also found in the central intertrabecular areas (Figure 4.4). There are, however, normally considerable variations in the quantitative and qualitative distribution of the components of the bone marrow; alterations are especially prone to occur in hyper- and hypoplastic conditions, and when osseous changes are present. Moreover, these spatial differences represent potential pitfalls, as mentioned earlier, especially the subcortical hypoplasia which occurs frequently in older individuals. Selective hypoplasia in the iliac crest has also been observed in certain conditions such as autoimmune states, and it may be seen after radiotherapy to that region.

Cellular constituents of marrow

Hematopoiesis

This is the term applied to the process of production of the formed elements of the blood; it takes place in the extravascular compartments of the marrow within the intertrabecular cavities; there are cords, islands or clusters of precursor cells between the sinusoids through whose walls the erythrocytes, leucocytes and platelets enter the lumina of the blood vessels. The normal values in the peripheral blood are maintained by the hematopoietic tissues in the bone marrow. Stem cells, the earliest cells capable of hematopoiesis, possess the capacity for self-renewal and the potential for multilineage differentiation. The stem cell compartment gives rise to the pluripotent cells for both myeloid and lymphoid cell lines, which in turn produce progenitor cells of progressively restricted potential. In addition to erythrocytes, granulocytes, lymphocytes, megakaryocytes and platelets, the stem cells give rise to mast cells, macrophages and osteoclasts, but not to the bone marrow fibroblasts and osteoblasts whose origin is in the mesenchyme.

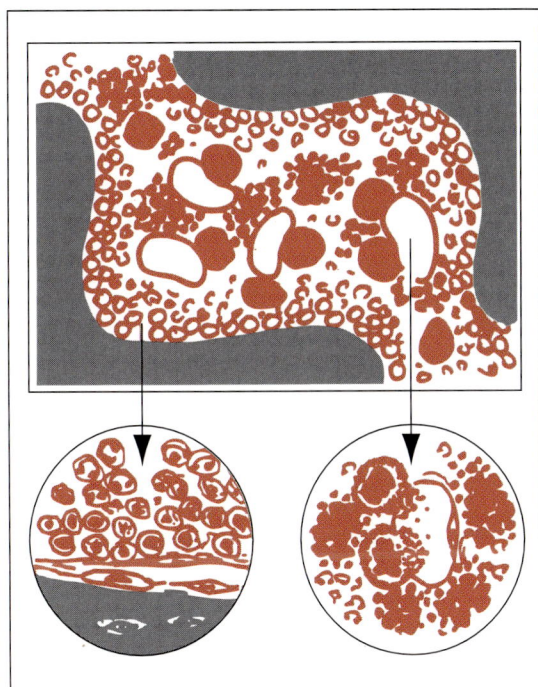

Erythropoiesis – red blood cells
(immunohistory [I.H.] glycophorin, hemoglobin)

The nucleated precursors of the red cells are found in small and large clusters of cells exhibiting the range of maturational sequences from the earliest recognisable erythroblast to normoblast (Figures 4.5–4.7). A macrophage (reticular cell) with long cytoplasmic processes, and containing hemosiderin and possibly some cellular or nuclear debris is usually located in the middle or the vicinity of a medium to large cluster of six or more erythroid cells at different maturational stages. The macrophage appears to play a supporting role in normal red cell production. However, the classical appearance of an erythropoietic island with a central macrophage (the erythron) is rarely seen in the light microscope in biopsy sections, possibly due to the plane of sectioning. Morphologically normal erythroid

4.4 Normal architecture of the bone marrow, with granulopoietic precursors at endosteal surface (left circle), erythrons and megakaryocytes around the central sinusoids (right circle).

4.5 (left) BMBS plastic, Giemsa, sinus with erythroblasts and megakaryocyte, upper right, and myeloid precursors, lower right.

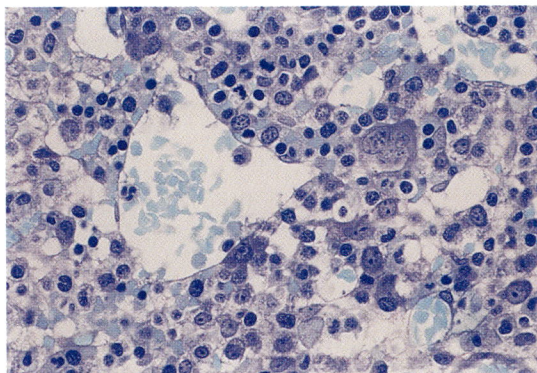

4.6 (right) BMBS paraffin, H&E, cellular bone marrow erythroid islands, myelocytes and granulocytes clearly distinguishable.

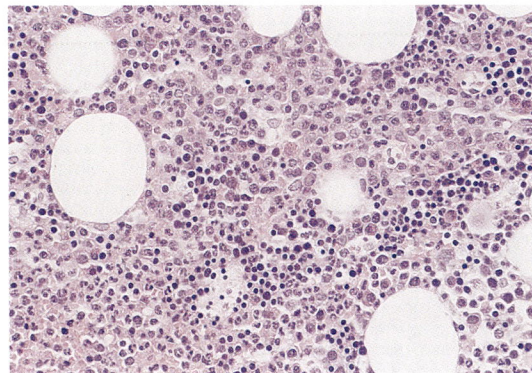

maturation (normoblastic) is observed in the clusters and usually there is a mixed population from early to late normoblasts ready to extrude their nuclei. It takes approximately 5 days from erythroblasts to reticulocytes, though this process may be accelerated in acute conditions. The myeloid : erythroid ratio is 1.5 : 1 to 3 : 1 in bone marrow biopsies (BMB). A decreased ratio found in normo- or hypocellular marrow indicates erythroid hyperplasia in the absence of decreases in the other elements. When one considers the astronomical numbers of erythrocytes produced per unit time (millions per mm^3 per s) it is astonishing that extruded nuclei and macrophages containing them are so rarely observed in normal BMB. This strongly indicates that the engulfment and/or lysis of normoblast nuclei must be remarkably efficient and fast. In contrast, cellular debris reminiscent of granulocytic nuclei may be found within macrophage cytoplasm much more frequently.

Myelopoiesis – granulocytes (I.H. myeloperoxidase, CD11, CD13, CD15, CD33, and CD34, QBEND10 for progenitors)

The granulocytic series consists of neutrophils, eosinophils and basophils. Myeloblast, promyelocyte, myelocyte, metamyelocyte, band and segmented forms are all identifiable in sections of the bone marrow (Figures 4.8–4.10). An increase in the myeloid : erythroid (M : E) ratio in a normocellular or hypocellular marrow, in the absence of a decrease in erythroid precursors, indicates granulocytic hyperplasia. There may be normal proportions of cells in the maturational stages, or a 'shift to the left', i.e. a preponderance of immature forms, or a 'shift to the right' with a greater number of mature polymorphonuclear leukocytes present. The paratrabecular and periarteriolar regions constitute the granulocytic generation zones, but precursors are also scattered throughout the rest of the marrow.

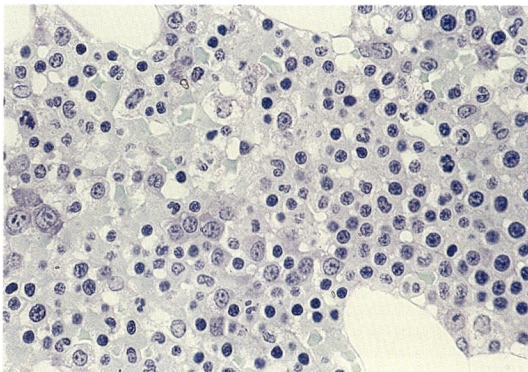

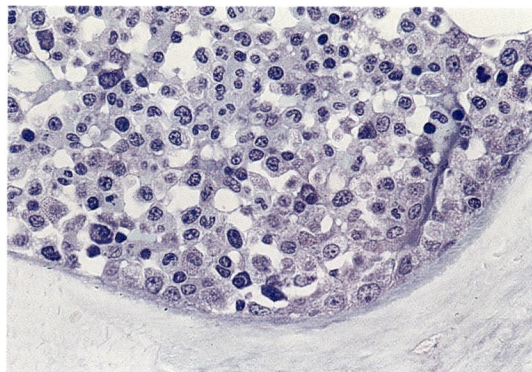

4.7 (left) BMBS plastic, Giemsa, showing cellular bone marrow with large erythroid islands, right, in patient with hepatic cirrhosis.

4.8 (right) BMBS plastic, Giemsa, myeloid precursors at trabecular surface, bottom right.

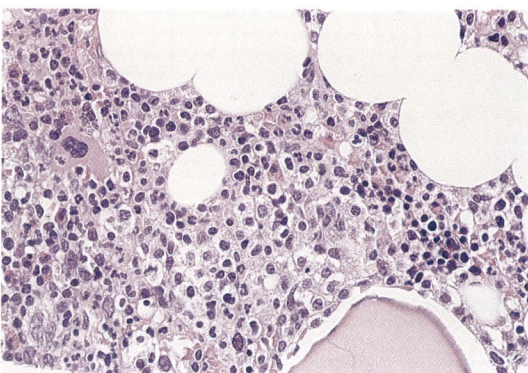

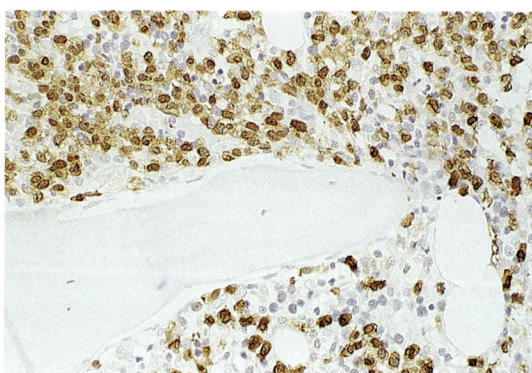

4.9 (left) BMBS paraffin, H&E, myeloid precursors left, and erythroid island right of trabecula.

4.10 (right) BMBS paraffin, I.H., myeloperoxidase highlighting myeloid precursors.

Neutrophilic (punctuate, brownish) granules and eosinophilic (slightly larger and yellowish-red) granules are readily distinguished, even in early myelocyte development. Basophils (having partially water-soluble granules) are recognised infrequently though mature basophils are occasionally seen. They have fewer, larger and dark red granules and must be distinguished from mast cells. Under normal circumstances granulopoiesis is very effective, so that practically all the cells produced reach the circulation. Mature granulocytes migrate through the endothelium into the sinusoids. The normal neutrophil : erythroid ratio in bone marrow sections is about 1.5 ± 0.07.

Mast cells – basophils (I.H. IgE)
(Figure 4.11)
These are best recognised in plastic embedded biopsies and are thought to arise from the same granulocyte precursors that produce the basophilic leukocyte. Mast cells lie adjacent to the endothelial cells of sinusoids, at the endosteal surface of the trabecular bone, in the periosteum, in the walls of small arteries, scattered in the bone marrow and frequently at the edges of and in lymphoid aggregates or nodules. Mast cells are characterised by oval-to-round nuclei and cytoplasm densely packed with bright red granules in Giemsa-stained sections of undecalcified BMBs. Mast cells may be round, oval or spindle shaped with abundant cytoplasm, or thin and elongated resembling fibroblasts, in which case they are best identified in sections stained by

toluidine blue and under high magnification as only a few granules may be present. Small accumulations of mast cells and histiocytes, sometimes in association with endothelial cells (previously designated fibrohistiocytic lesions) may also be found in the bone marrow; their significance is unknown. They may be increased in infections or occur as reactions to drugs.

Megakaryocytes and thrombopoiesis
(I.H. platelet peroxidase, Factor VIII-related antigen, CD41, CD61, CD79a, PAS stain)
These are the largest cells normally present in the bone marrow (Figures 4.12–4.14). Their size ranges from 12 to 150 μm; they show considerable variation in shape as well as size and in nuclear configuration. The smaller ones may be difficult to identify at first, so that occasionally (particularly in hematopoietic neoplasias) enzymic or marker techniques are required. Three stages are recognised in megakaryocytes at maturation:

1. The megakaryoblast, 15–20 μm, with an oval- or kidney-shaped nucleus and basophilic cytoplasm. These measurements are approximate and related to the method of preparation, i.e. whether smears or sections, paraffin or plastic embedding.

2. The promegakaryocyte, 20–80 μm, cytoplasm less basophilic, but with a zone of developing granules, especially perinuclear.

3. Mature megakaryocytes, with eosinophilic cytoplasm, and with variable granularity. The nucleus is coarsely cerebriform, multi-

4.11 (left) BMBS plastic, Giemsa, mast cells at trabecular surface; disorganisation of marrow architecture in bone biopsy of patient with MDS.

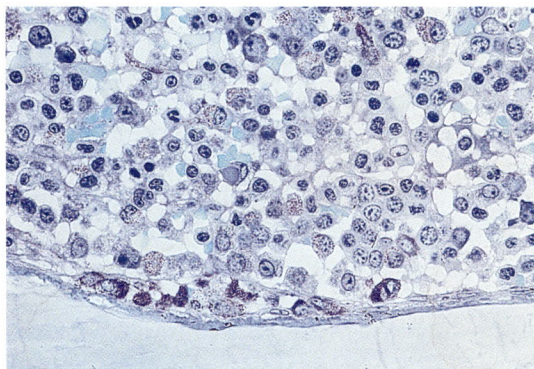

4.12 (right) BMBS plastic, Giemsa, megakaryocytes adjacent to sinusoids.

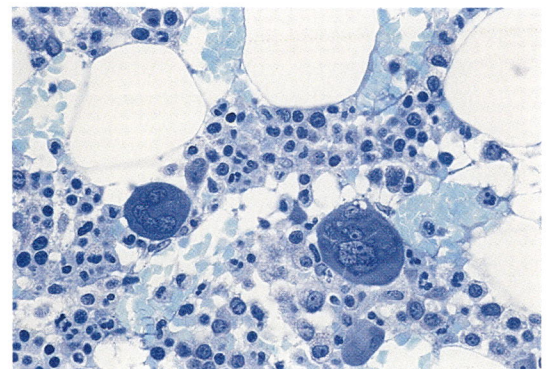

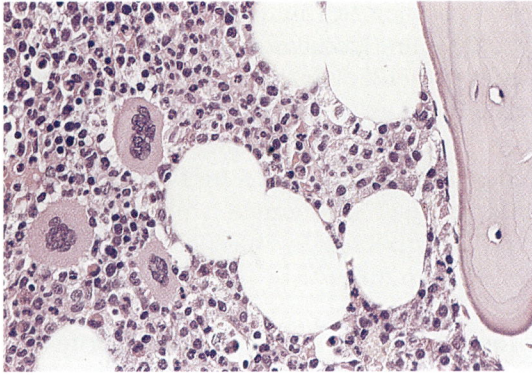

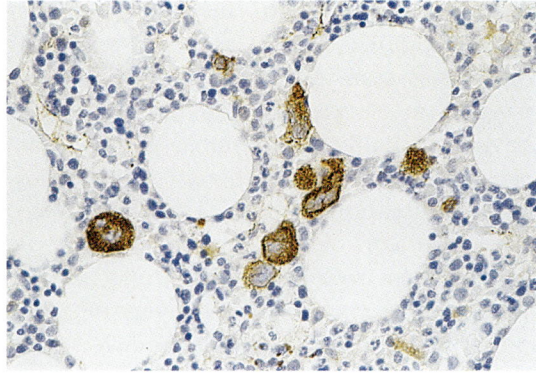

4.13 (left) BMBS paraffin, H&E, megakaryocytes and erythroid precursors (left) but sinusoids not clearly visible.

4.14 (right) BMBS paraffin, I.H., with Factor VIII-related antigen, demonstrating variably sized megakaryocytes.

lobed, but not necessarily so. DNA synthesis proceeds as polyploidy goes through 8, 16, 32 or 64 n, while lobulation may continue after that, though there is no definite correlation between ploidy and lobulation of the nucleus and the extent of cytoplasmic differentiation. However, there is some link, as 95% of plateletsshedding megakaryocytes are 16–32 n. Differentiation of the cytoplasm commences after DNA synthesis has ceased (in most cases) and three cytoplasmic zones are distinguished in the mature megakaryocyte: perinuclear, intermediate and marginal. The first contains the synthetic apparatus, the second the developing demarcation membranes and the third, which is found only in non-platelet-releasing megakaryocytes, contains filaments. In cases of extreme demand or pathologic conditions, large megakaryocyte fragments are released into the circulating blood – megaplatelets or megathrombocytes. Emperipolesis – the presence of other cells within megakaryocyte cytoplasm – may be found in megakaryocytes of any size, though it is more frequently observed in the larger ones, and also when there are more megakaryocytes in the section, i.e. in hyperplasia of megakaryocytes. The cells within may be granulocytes, lymphocytes, erythroblasts and erythrocytes and they are not apparently phagocytosed.

Examples of megakaryocytes of various sizes and nuclear configurations are shown in Figures 4.12–4.14. Megakaryocytes typically appear to abut on or project into the sinusoids, and the platelets are shed directly into their lumina. Whole megakaryocytes or portions of their cytoplasm may also enter the sinuses and fragment in the vascular system. Megakaryocytes frequently appear to be connected with or interposed between endothelial cells. In the light microscope and even more so in the electron microscope, megakaryocytes have a variably granular cytoplasm, with clear and dense areas; occasional denuded megakaryocyte nuclei are also found in normal bone marrows. Groups or clusters of megakaryocytes are usually found only in unusual situations (see Chapters 22 and 23). In normal bone marrow megakaryocytes are dispersed singly in the intertrabecular spaces, near or partly in, the sinusoids. Interleukins known to act on megakaryocytes include 1, 3, 4, 6 and 11, as well as thrombopoietin.

Monocytes, macrophages and iron-containing reticular cells M-PIRE (mononuclear phagocyte immunoregulatory effector system)
(I.H. CD14, CD68, lysozyme and others)

Monocytes (though produced in the bone marrow) are not often encountered, even in optimal histological sections. Perhaps the problem is one of recognition as they are easily confused with granulocytic precursors, though they are larger, but like the latter they have oval- to kidney-shaped vesicular nuclei; and they have abundant eosinophilic cytoplasm with no or variable granulation. They are recognised in greater quantities in immune histology than in conventionally stained sections.

Macrophages (histiocytes, reticular cells)

Macrophages (histiocytes, reticular cells) are discussed separately from monocytes because there is still some uncertainty about their derivation in the bone marrow. Macrophages appear to be a heterogeneous population and there are several views as to their origin, which may be from the fixed reticular cells or their derivatives, from the granulocyte–monocyte precursors, or from mature monocytes. Macrophages may be very large, with nuclei which resemble those of histiocytes, and their abundant cytoplasm may contain granules, vacuoles, lipid, cellular and nuclear debris. Typical bone marrow macrophages (reticular cells) containing hemosiderin and/or cellular debris are shown in Figure 4.15. These cells form part of the reticuloendothelial system (RES) or the mononuclear phagocyte system, which is responsible for the breakdown of senescent red cells and the storage of iron. Iron stains on bone marrow sections demonstrate overload, depletion and normal storage. Iron stores in bone marrow sections may be graded: none; small particles in a few reticulin cells; more numerous particles in more cells; and large particles as well as deposition on osteoid seams. Up to 50% of erythroid precursors may contain iron, though unevenly distributed and not in the form of 'ring' sideroblasts. There is generally a good correlation between serum ferritin levels, iron absorption and marrow stores, except in cases of sideroblastic anemia, hemosiderosis, some cases of neoplasia, infec-

tions and hepatic diseases. There are about 16 iron-containing macrophages per mm^2 of bone marrow. Lipo-macrophages and foam cells, sea blue histiocytes and pseudo-Gaucher cells, as well as Gaucher cells as seen in the storage diseases, are also thought to develop out of reticular or adventitial cells (or even endothelial cells). Tissue histiocytes are derived partly by recruitment of monocytes and partly by mitotic division of local histiocytes. This term is used for cells that take up vital dyes and are capable of phagocytosis. Tissue histiocytes have oval- or kidney-shaped vesicular nuclei, with variable amounts of cytoplasm and inclusions. Histiocytes in different situations may have different properties.

Some subgroups of histiocytes are recognised. Littoral cells are the sinus histiocytes that line the venous sinuses of the bone marrow (and other organs); they are spindle shaped with cytoplasmic processes. Epithelioid histiocytes have nuclei similar to those of histiocytes, and abundant eosinophilic and granular cytoplasm. Giant cells are thought to be derived from the histiocyte–monocyte series by endomitosis and/or by fusion or coalescence.

Lymphocytes and lymphopoiesis

(I.H. B cells, CD19, CD20, CD74, CD75, CD79a; T cells, CD2, CD3, CD5. LCA-leucocyte common antigen, both B and T cells, progenitors CD10, TdT)

Some measure of lymphopoietic function (as in the embryo) is most probably retained by the adult bone marrow. Whether or not lymphoid cells belong to the normal marrow population, they may constitute up to 15–20% of the nucleated cell population of the bone marrow. On immunohistology, most are T cells (Figure 4.16), reflecting the proportions in the peripheral blood: T cells 65–75%, B cells 10–15%, NK cells 10–20%. They are dispersed among the hematopoietic and fat cells, or aggregated as lymphoid nodules whose incidence increases with age (Figures 4.17–4.22). Such nodules are found in 1 to >40% of bone marrow biopsies with the higher incidence in the older age groups. The nodules or aggregates, especially when small, are more readily

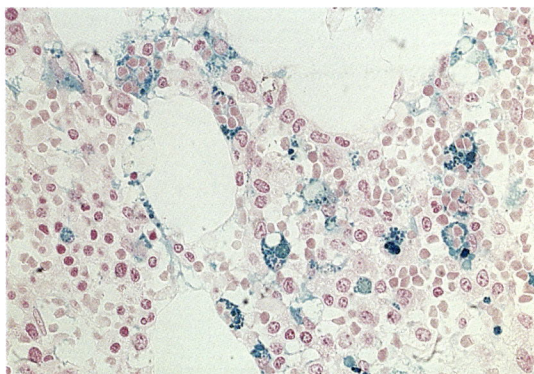

4.15 BMBS plastic, stain for iron, macrophages and some endothelial and endosteal cells show blue-stained cytoplasm and cytoplasmic inclusions; note erythrocytes in macrophage cytoplasm – hemaphagocytosis.

observed in sections stained for reticulin fibers, as they contain more fibers than their surroundings. Capillaries, reticular cells, a few plasma cells and mast cells may also be associated with these lymphoid nodules. On immunohistology the aggregates or nodules consist of a heterogeneous population of T and B cells, though mainly T cells.

Four configurations of lymphoid aggregates have been described: (1) nodules with germinal centres (Figures 4.23 and 4.24); (2) sharply

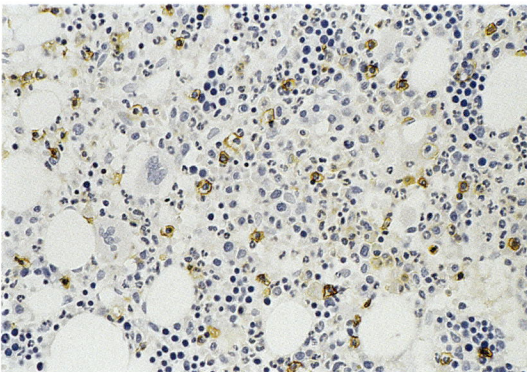

4.16 BMBS paraffin, I.H., for T cells which show an interstitial distribution.

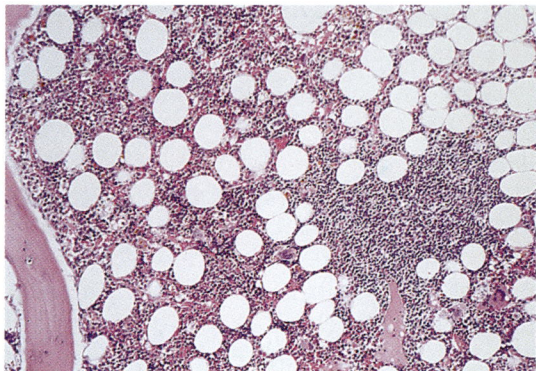

4.17 (left) BMBS paraffin, H&E, partly perivascular lymphocytic aggregate, at low magnification.

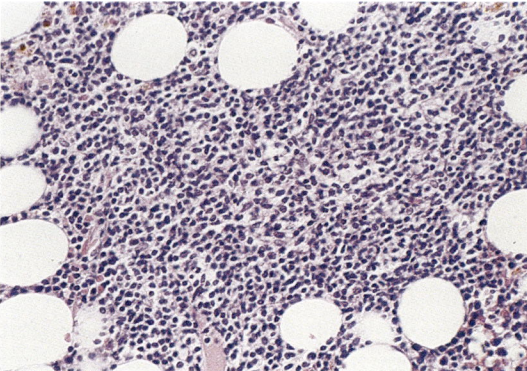

4.18 (right) As for Figure 4.17, higher magnification lymphocytic aggregate, showing fairly homogeneous cell population.

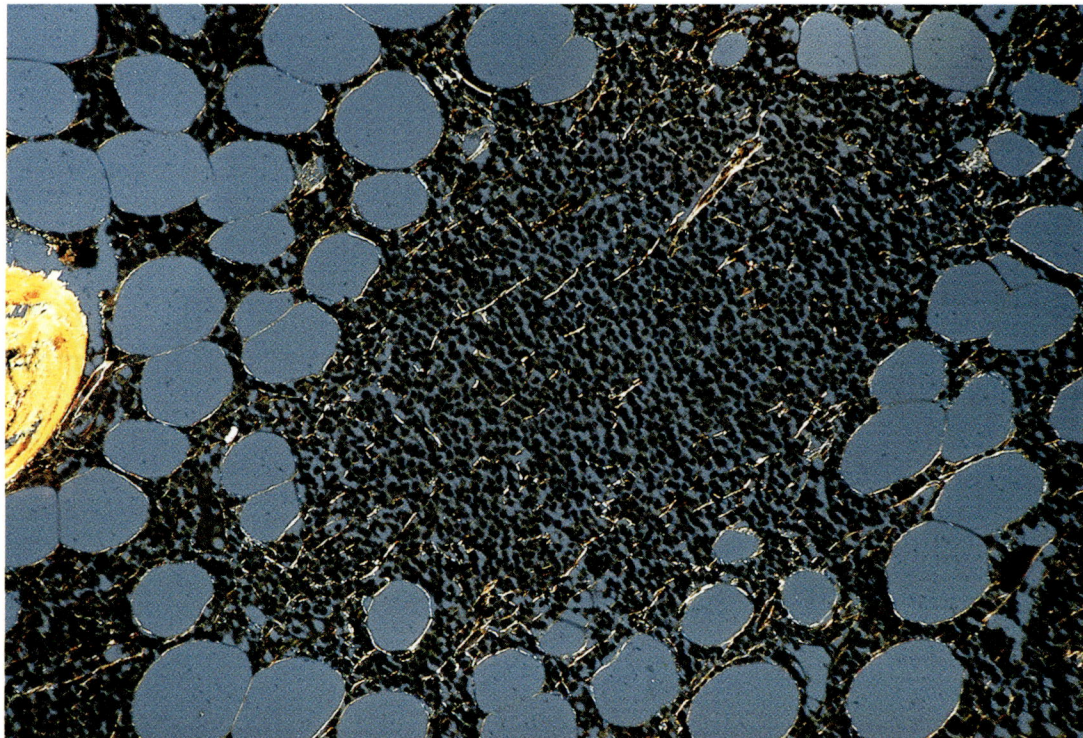

4.19 BMBS plastic, Gomori, polarised light showing reticular fibers in lymphocytic nodule.

4.20 (left) BMBS paraffin, I.H., myeloperoxidase positive cells around lymphoid nodule.

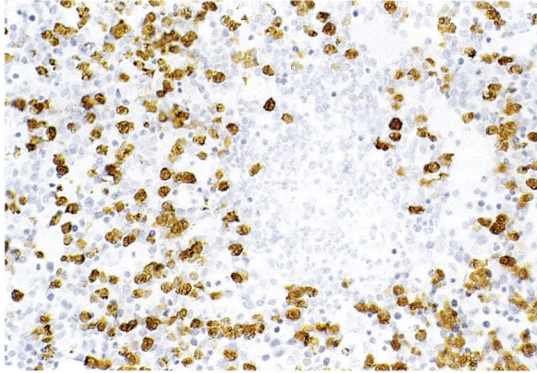

4.21 (right) BMBS paraffin, I.H., for T cells, many lymphocytes in the nodule are positive.

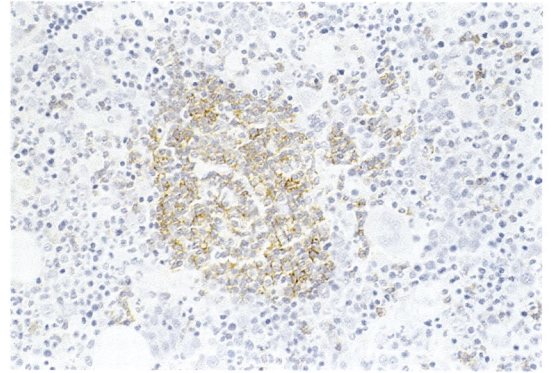

4.22 (left) BMBS paraffin, I.H., for B cells, which shows fewer positive cells in the nodule than with the T cell antigen.

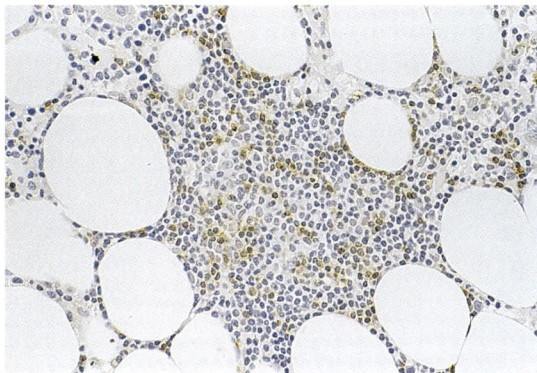

4.23 (right) BMBS plastic, Giemsa, lymphoid nodule with a central area of larger lymphocytes surrounded by smaller ones.

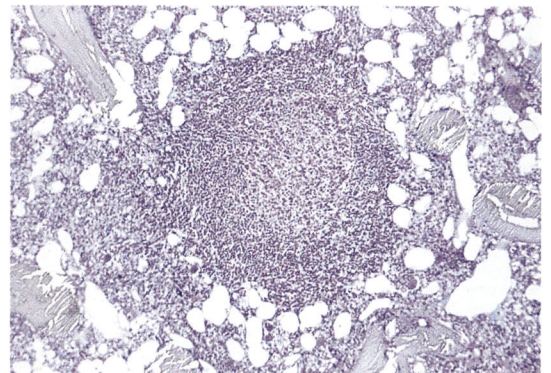

4.24 BMBS plastic, Giemsa, lymphoid nodule, with a cuff of small lymphocytes around a germinal center.

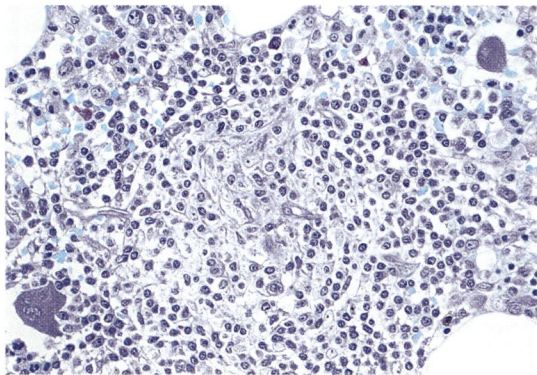

demarcated nodules; (3) nodules with irregular borders; and (4) small aggregates of lymphoid cells (Chapter 25). When multiple nodules are found in a section, immunohistology may be required to rule out or to confirm involvement by a neoplastic lymphoproliferative disorder. Immunohistology is required for identification of B and T cells in the bone marrow (Figures 4.21 and 4.22). There are relatively few B cells in normal bone marrows; the number of T cells is higher and may increase considerably in reactive conditions. In benign conditions, lymphoid cell aggregates are found mainly in the intertrabecular and perivascular regions. Paratrabecular aggregates are more characteristic of a neoplastic infiltration. Regulation of the migration, localisation and function of lymphocytes is also partly controlled by cellular adhesion molecules (CAM), broadly divided into three groups: immunoglobulins, integrins and selectins. Adhesion molecules also play a part in the homing, attachment and differentiation of hematopoietic stem and precursor cells, as well as in pathologic processes; for example, in multiple myeloma (Chapter 29), as well as in the lymphomas (Chapter 26) and metastatic invasion of the bone marrow (Chapter 14).

Plasma cells (I.H. kappa, lambda CD 79a and CD138 in flow cytometry)

These belong to the normal cell population of the bone marrow and represent the final developmental stage, i.e. the effector cells of the B cell lineage. They constitute about 1% of the nucleated cells of aspirates of normal adult marrow with a range of 0.5–4.0%. Plasma cells are equally distributed throughout the red marrow with no significant differences between various skeletal sites, i.e. iliac crests, sternum and vertebrae; while they are almost absent from the yellow marrow. Possibly, they are produced and mature in the bone marrow, as well as at other sites in the body. Table 4.1 gives the numbers of plasma cells in sections, according to age groups. These data imply that there are >100 million plasma cells in the red marrow, producing >90% of the serum immunoglobulins.

When B lymphocytes differentiate to plasma cells, large amounts of rough endoplasmic reticulum (RER) are synthesised, assembled and occupy the cytoplasm, often dilated by accumulation of immunoglobulins. Other variably sized inclusions may also be enclosed by the RER; these likewise consist of immunoglobulins, while Russell-bodies probably consist of light chains. As indicated by the labeling index with tritiated thymidine, plasma cells and their immediate precursors have a very low proliferative activity.

There are normally two types of bone marrow plasma cells:

The reticular plasma cells ('Marschalko')

This is the predominant plasma cell (80%) in normal marrow and reactive plasmacytosis from whatever cause. In aspirate smears these plasma cells are usually oval, 8–25 mm in diameter, with abundant basophilic cytoplasm, a paranuclear 'hof' and, in sections more than smears, a 'spoke-wheel' nuclear pattern; nucleoli are rare. Electron microscopy shows the typical RER, Golgi apparatus, vacuoles and lysosomes. Plasma cells exhibit acid phosphatase, β glucuronidase and non-specific esterase activity. Plasma cells are normally found in close apposition to capillaries (Figure 4.25) and small blood vessels as well as singly and in clusters of two or three within the bone marrow. Demonstration of light chain restriction, i.e. reactivity with either kappa or lambda antibodies (Figure 4.26) is a useful indicator of possible monoclonality.

The 'lymphoplasmacytoid' plasma cells

These derive directly from IgM-bearing B1 lymphocytes and produce low-affinity IgM. They are smaller, have a less eccentric nucleus, a narrower rim of cytoplasm and a poorly defined Golgi zone; they often appear in viral infections and may be found in peripheral blood as well as dispersed in the bone marrow.

Bone marrow stroma: cells, fibers and extracellular matrix (I.H. actin, vimentin, reticulin stains, Mason's trichrome stain)

Stromal cells

The stroma provides the supporting framework for hematopoiesis which takes place in the

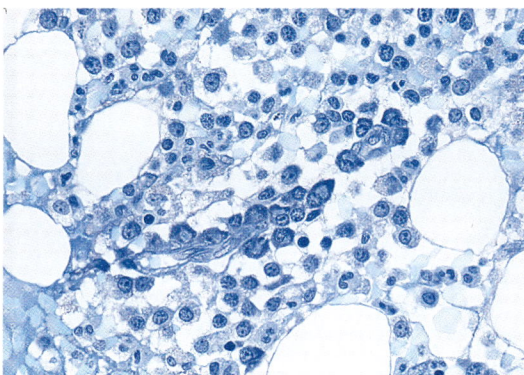

4.25 BMBS plastic, Giemsa, showing mainly myeloid precursors and perivascular plasma cells; arteriole cut lengthways, center left, and cross-section, right.

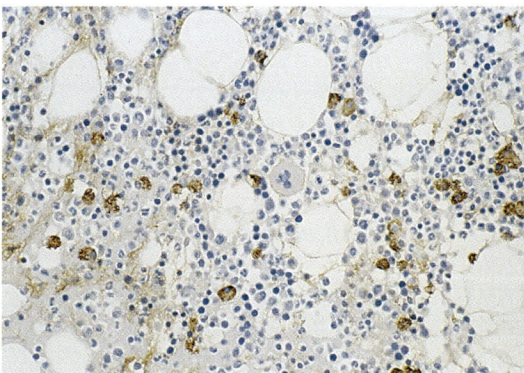

4.26 BMBS, I.H., plasma cells positive for kappa light chains.

extravascular compartment and is supported by the reticular cells, fat cells, fibroblasts and their fibrils and by the extensive network of blood vessels, including the sinusoids, and their accompanying nerves. Together, these components constitute the bone marrow hematopoietic microenvironment. Adhesion molecules are responsible for stem cell adhesion to stromal cells. Fat cells occupy about one-third of the marrow volume in the iliac crest biopsy. They serve a supporting, filling and metabolic function as shown, for example, by their ability to participate in steroid aromatisation. There are close associations between the mesenchymal elements – the endothelium, the advential cells, fibroblasts and osteoblasts, and the endosteal lining cells as well as reticular cells and macrophages. Fibroblasts, elongated cells with elongated nuclei, may be indistinguishable from the so-called reticular cells. Fibroblasts produce the reticular fibers of which the normal bone marrow has few,

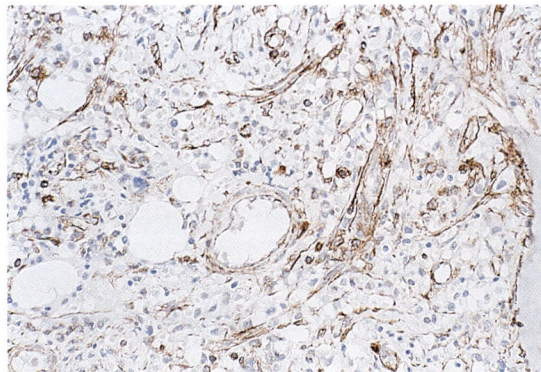

4.27 BMBS paraffin, I.H., connective tissue positive for vimentin.

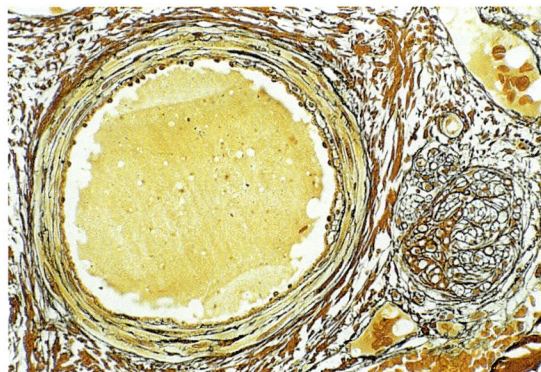

4.28 BMBS plastic, Gomori, showing large blood vessels accompanied by nerve, lower right.

mainly in association with blood vessels and endosteum.

Extracellular matrix
This consists of a variety of components – mainly proteins – produced by the stromal cells. These proteins include cell adhesion molecules (CAMs), collagen, fibronectin, vitronectin, proteoglycans as well as growth, and other factors involved in the highly complex regulatory mechanisms controlling the production of the formed elements of the blood.

Fibers
The normal bone marrow contains only thin reticular fibers (near bone and blood vessels), best visualised by the Gomori stain for reticulin or similar stains and by polarised light. Fibrosis in the marrow may involve reticulin fibers only, or also collagen (i.e. bundles of reticulin). An increase in fibers (Figure 4.27), i.e. myelofibrosis may occur in numerous conditions, which are described in the appropriate sections of this book (Chapter 23). All these components of the bone marrow stroma constitute the microenvironment which provides the niches for the stem cells and the inductive influences which direct them to one or other line of differentiation, support their maturation and facilitate their egress from the extravascular compartment into the systemic circulation.

Nerves
These are rarely found; occasionally may be seen next to blood vessels in the periosteum (Figure 4.28).

Blood vessels (I.H. CD34, Factor VIII, actin and vimentin)
The medullary arteries (Figures 4.29 and 4.30) enter via the cortical bone and branch within the marrow and the trabeculae, accompanied by nerve fibers (Figure 4.28). The smaller branches divide into arterioles (Figures 4.31 and 4.32), and then into capillaries which frequently have a cuff of plasma cells around them, and lead into the sinusoids (Figures 4.33–4.36). These form a system of channels of variable width and length whose walls consist

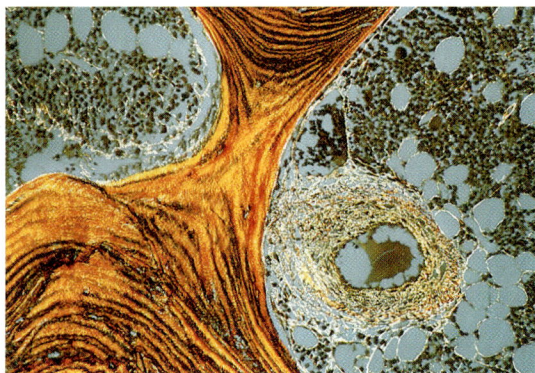

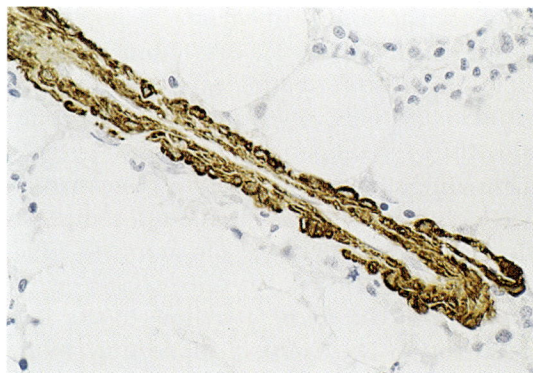

4.29 (left) BMBS plastic, Gomori, seen in polarised light, showing reticular fibers around sinus, upper left, and blood vessels, right.

4.30 (right) BMBS paraffin, I.H., vimentin, small artery strongly positive.

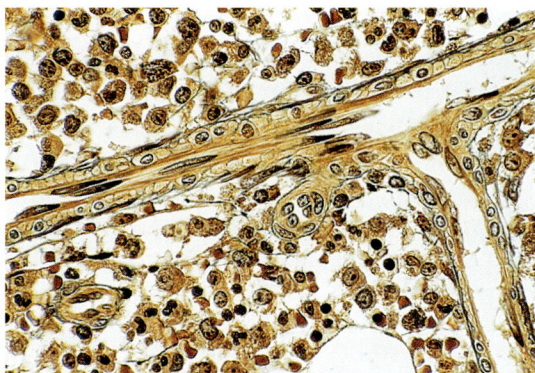

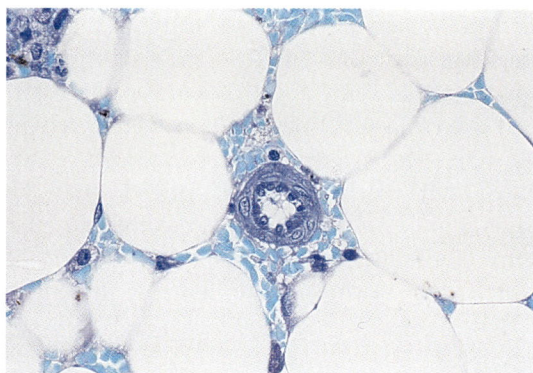

4.31 (left) BMBS plastic, Gomori, branching arteriole.

4.32 (right) BMBS plastic, Giemsa, small arteriole with adjacent sinusoid in hypocellular marrow.

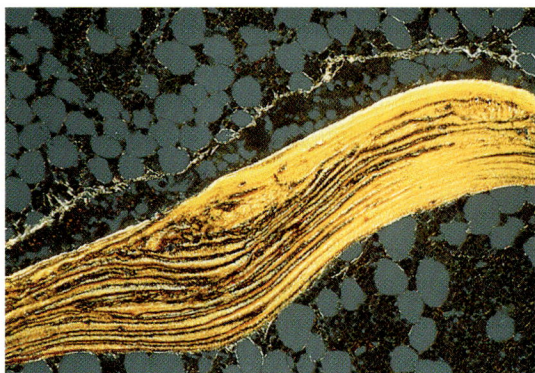

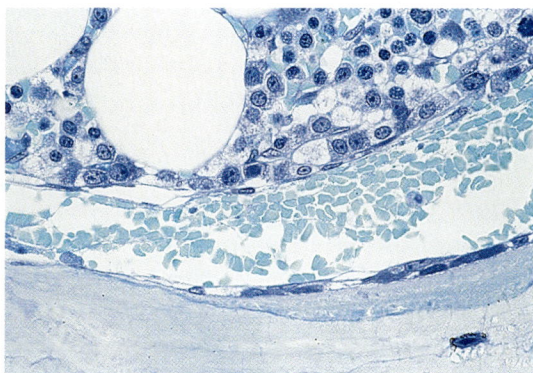

4.33 (left) BMBS plastic, Gomori, polarised light, reticular fibers on paratrabecular sinusoid wall.

4.34 (right) BMBS plastic, Giemsa, large paratrabecular sinus; note osteoblastic remodeling, right.

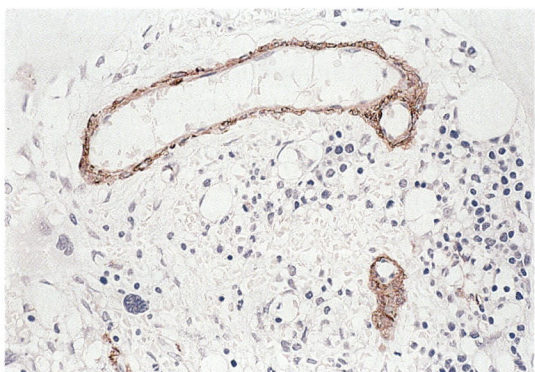

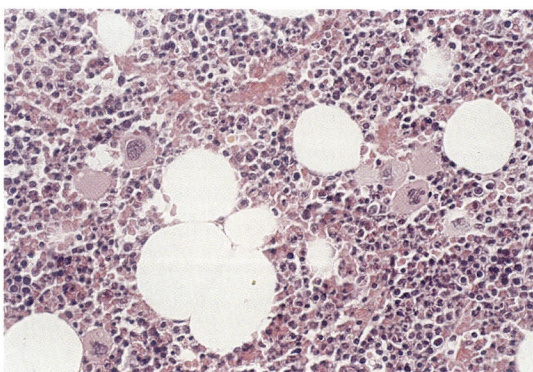

4.35 (left) BMBS paraffin, I.H., blood vessels highlighted by Factor VIII-related antigen.

4.36 (right) BMBS paraffin, H&E, sinusoids, upper center, visible because of the erythrocytes (yellow) in the lumen.

of a single layer of endothelial cells, an incomplete outer covering of adventitia and, when large, a loose network of reticulin fibers. The sinusoids in turn drain into the periosteal veins. The endothelial cells of post-capillary or post-sinusoidal venules may be plump, with vesicular nuclei and distinct nucleoli. This layer forms the interface between the intra- and extravascular compartments, which must be traversed by the blood cells for entry into the circulation. Thus a BMB provides a cut

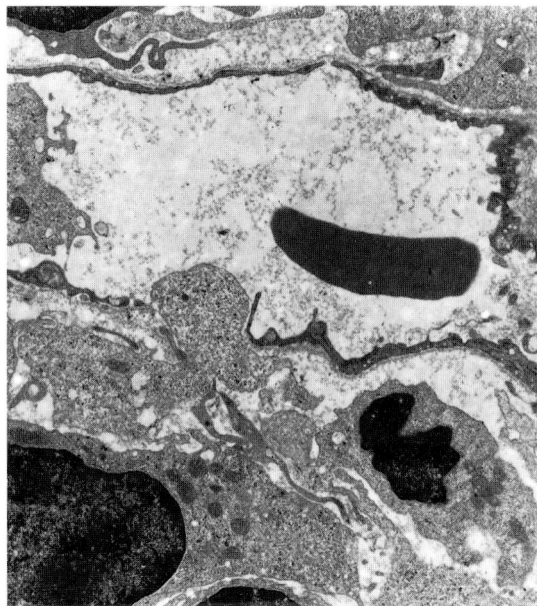

4.37 BMBS, EM, passage of part of megakaryocyte cytoplasm through endothelium into lumen of sinusoid.

through the vascular system and may therefore supply additional information in diseases which affect it, such as arteriosclerosis, arteritis and amyloidosis. Physiologically, portions of the sinusoidal channels are collapsed at any one time and the expansion and contraction of the vascular system within the rigid bony cage enclosing the marrow, contribute (together with quantitative changes in fat cells) to the extreme fluctuations in the production of blood cells of which the marrow is capable. When the need arises, an increase of up to 10-fold its usual capacity is possible. It should be remembered that the parenchyme of the bone marrow is at all times composed of a rapidly evolving, highly mobile population so that a section of a biopsy is comparable with a still of a motion picture. This helps to account for the great variety seen in biopsy sections, which are nevertheless within the 'normal' range. Moreover, many processes in the bone marrow are highly efficient and fast and leave few traces, as witness the disposal of normoblast nuclei and the transendothelial passage of reticulocytes and granulocytes, which is so rarely observed, in contrast with megakaryocytes (Figures 4.37–4.39).

Hematopoietic microenvironment

The components of the normal bone marrow as described above are in reality closely packed

4.38 (left) BMBS, EM, megakaryocyte adjacent to sinusoid.

4.39 (right) BMBS, EM, example of so-called 'naked' megakaryocyte nucleus in bone marrow. Note narrow rim of cytoplasm surrounding the nucleus.

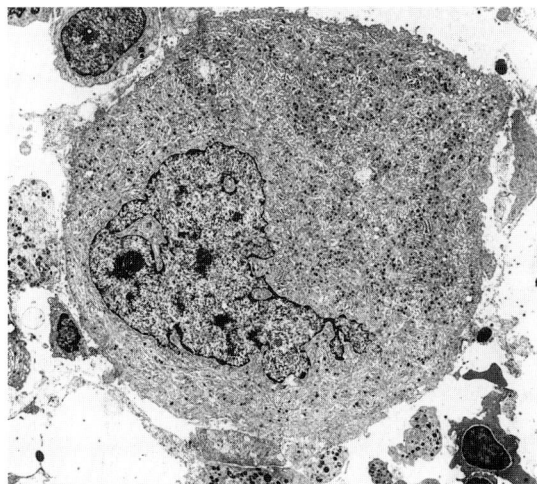

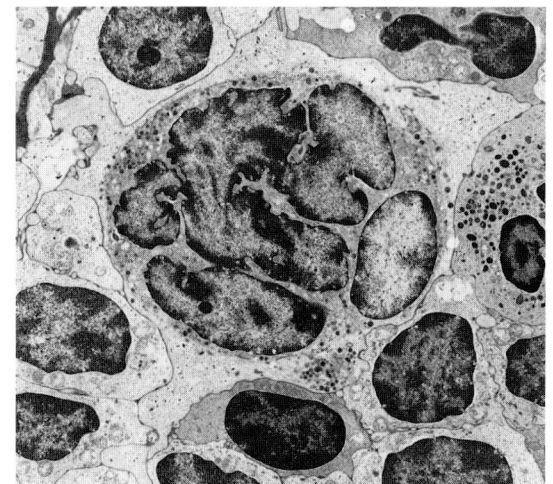

51

together in a hard bony cage. The stromal elements form an extensive, closely woven network in which the hematopoietic precursors are embedded, attached in various ways and to different components by adhesive proteins such as integrins, and by other cells, such as the central macrophages in the erythroid islands. The integrins are transmembrane glycoproteins that mediate cell–cell and cell–matrix interactions. Through the extracellular matrix and fluid these differentiating hematopoietic cells receive their nutrients, vitamins, hormones, regulatory factors, cytokines, modulators and any other cell–cell substance that in any way influences their activity. Indeed, the correct processing of signals from the extracellular matrix (ECM) contributes to the regulation of the cell cycle, cellular differentiation and apoptosis. All cells of a particular organism have the same genetic information, but there are striking differences in morphology and function of different types, e.g. a leucocyte and a liver cell. Remove a cell from its normal microenvironment and it loses many of its distinguishing characteristics. Thus, the ECM is an essential factor in normal cell survival and activity and in tissue integrity. Interruption of the signals traveling the two directional information highway between a cell and its microenvironment may contribute to malignant transformation. Moreover, interactions involving adhesion molecules, vascular endothelium and the malignant cells play an important part in dissemination of leukemic cells, in intra- and extravasation of tumor cells and in the establishment of metastases. An enormous amount of experimental and other work has already been done on the hematopoietic microenvironment and its contribution to the normal, balanced production of the formed elements of the peripheral blood.

However, most of it is not yet directly applicable to the interpretation of bone and bone marrow biopsy sections, though this may well happen in the not too distant future, especially with the ever-increasing possibilities of immunohistology due to the rapid development of new antibodies.

Diagnostic evaluation

A systematic survey is made, beginning with a scan of the whole biopsy section at low power (see Chapter 2, Figure 2.28) and ending with examination at high power, under oil if necessary, of individual cells and structures (see Chapter 2, Table 2.4). It is important to consider the bone and marrow together as a single system, because alterations in the one are almost invariably accompanied by changes in the other.

Pitfalls in histologic diagnosis

The most important pitfalls in histological diagnosis are: (1) histological variation within the biopsy: (a) subcortical hypoplasia, and (b) alternating fatty and hyperplastic areas in deeper parts of the biopsy and accumulation of one cell type in single intertrabecular areas; (2) non-representative tangentially taken biopsies; and (3) presence of misleading artefacts – displaced pieces of epidermis, skeletal muscles, periosteal tissues, cartilage or bone, or blood and clots within the biopsy. Moreover, changes in hematopoietic cells due to technical factors should also be recognised, for example swelling or shrinkage due to inadequate fixation, insufficient dehydration, incomplete penetration of paraffin or plastic embedding medium, and inadequate staining, either too weak or too strong.

Bibliography

Abrahamsen J.F., Lund-Johansen F., Laerum O.D. et al. (1995) Flow cytometric assessment of peripheral blood contamination and proliferative activity of human bone marrow cell populations. *Cytometry*, **19 (1)**, 77–85.

Algino K.M., Thomason R.W., King D.E. et al. (1996) CD20 (pan-B cell antigen) expression on bone marrow-derived T cells. *Am J Clin Pathol*, **106 (1)**, 78–81.

Almeida Porada G., Ascensao J.L. (1996) Isolation, characterization, and biologic features of bone marrow endothelial cells. *J Lab Clin Med.*, **128 (4)**, 399–407.

Arkin S., Naprstek B., Guarini L. *et al.* (1991) Expression of intercellular adhesion molecule-1 (CD54) on hematopoietic progenitors. *Blood*, **77 (5)**, 948–53.

Beresford J.N. (1989) Osteogenic stem cells and the stromal system of bone and marrow. *Clin. Orthop.*, **240**, 270–80.

Boque C., Pujol-Moix N., Linde M.A. *et al.* (1989) Use of monoclonal anti-actin as a megakaryocyte marker in paraffin wax embedded bone marrow biopsy specimens. *J Clin Pathol*, **42 (9)**, 982–4.

Bradstock K., Bianci A., Makrynikola V. *et al.* (1996) Long-term survival and proliferation of precursor-B acute lymphoblastic leukemia cells on human bone marrow stroma. *Leukemia*, **10 (5)**, 813–20.

Burgio V.L., Pignoloni P., Baroni C.D. (1991) Immunohistology of bone marrow: a modified method of glycolmethacrylate embedding. *Histopathology*, **18 (1)**, 37–43.

Carter D.H., Sloan P., Aaron J.E. (1991) Immunolocalization of collagen types I and III, tenascin, and fibronectin in intramembranous bone. *J. Histochem. Cytochem.*, **39 (5)**, 599–606.

Cheong S.K., Lim Y.C. (1990) Frozen bone marrow trephine biopsy – a technical evaluation. *Malays. J. Pathol.*, **12 (1)**, 51–6.

Clark B.R., Keating A. (1995) Biology of bone marrow stroma. *Ann N Y Acad Sci.*, **770**, 70–8.

Clark P., Normansell D.E. (1990) Phenotype analysis of lymphocyte subsets in normal human bone marrow. *Am J Clin Pathol.*, **94 (5)**, 632–6.

deBruyn P.P.H., Breen P.C., Thomas T.B. (1970) The microcirculation of the bone marrow. *Anat Rec.*, **168**, 55.

Delikat S.E., Galvani D.W., Zuzel M. (1995) The metabolic effects of interleukin 1 beta on human bone marrow adipocytes. *Cytokine*, **7 (4)**, 338–43.

Dolcetti R., Giardini R., Doglioni C. *et al.* (1997) α4β7 integrin expression is associated with the leukemic evolution of human and murine T-cell lymphoblastic lymphomas. *Am J Pathol.*, **150 (5)**, 1595.

Elfenbein G.J., Janssen W.E., Perkins J.B. (1995) Relative contributions of marrow microenvironment, growth factors, and stem cells to hematopoiesis in vivo in man. Review of results from autologous stem cell transplant trials and laboratory studies at the Moffitt Cancer Center. *Ann N Y Acad Sci.*, **770**, 315–38.

Farhi D.C. (1989) Germinal centers in the bone marrow. *Hematol Pathol*, **3 (3)**, 133–6.

Gulati G.L., Ashton J.K., Hyuan B.H. (1988) Structure and function of the bone marrow and hematopoiesis. *Hematol Oncol Clin N Amer.*, **2 (4)**, 495.

Hirsch K., Zaontz M., Marchildon M. *et al.* (1993) Immunophenotyping of pediatric bone marrow. Preliminary report of normal reference ranges. *Ann N Y Acad Sci.*, **677**, 410–2.

Hoffkes H.G., Schmidtke G., Schmucker U. *et al.* (1995) Immunophenotyping of B lymphocytes by multiparametric flow cytometry in bone marrow aspirates of healthy adults. *Ann Hematol*, **71 (3)**, 123–8.

Horny H.P., Engst U., Walz R.S., Kaiserling E. (1989) In situ immunophenotyping of lymphocytes in human bone marrow: an immunohistochemical study. *Br J Haematol*, **73 (4)**, 576–7.

Horny H.P., Wehrmann M., Griesser H. *et al.* (1993) Investigation of bone marrow lymphocyte subsets in normal, reactive, and neoplastic states using paraffin-embedded biopsy specimens. *Am J Clin Pathol*, **99 (2)**, 142–9.

Invernizzi R., Cazzola M., De Fazio P. *et al.* (1990) Immunocytochemical detection of ferritin in human bone marrow and peripheral blood cells using monoclonal antibodies specific for the H and L subinit. *Br. J. Hematol.*, **76 (3)**, 427–32.

Lichtman M.A. (1981) The ultrastructure of the hematopoietic environment of the marrow: a review. *Exp Hematol.*, **9 (4)**, 391.

Lips P., VanGinkel F.C., Netelenbos J.C. (1985) Bone marrow and bone remodelling. *Bone*, **6**, 343.

Lisovsky M., Braun S.E., Ge Y. *et al.* (1996) FltS ligand production by human bone marrow stromal cells. *Leukemia*, **10 (6)**, 1012–18.

Macavei I., Galatar N. (1989) Bone marrow biopsy (BMB). I. Generalities, material and method, normal structure of bone marrow, pathological conditions. *Morphol Embryol*, **35 (1)**, 33–40.

Marie J.P., Brophy N.A., Ehsan M.N. *et al.* (1992) Expression of multidrug resistance gene mdr1 mRNA in a subset of normal bone marrow cells. *Br J Haematol.*, **81 (2)**, 145–52.

Merville P., Dechanet J., Desmouliere A. *et al.* (1996) Bcl-2+ tonsillar plasma cells are rescued from apoptosis by bone marrow fibroblasts. *J Exp Med.*, **183 (1)**, 227–36.

Naeim F., Moatamed F., Sahimi M. (1996) Morphogenesis of the bone marrow: fractal structures and diffusion-limited growth. *Blood*, **87 (12)**, 5027–31.

Nagao T. (1987) Characteristics of bone marrow fibroblasts and their significance in hematopoiesis. *Tokai J. Exp. Clin. Med.*, **12 (1)**, 1–6.

Navone R., Angeli G., Ramponi A., Viberti L. (1987) Bone marrow in the elderly: normal and pathological patterns frequently encountered. Study of biopsy and autopsy case records. *Pathologica*, **79 (1063)**, 571–9.

O'Donnell L.R., Alder S.L., Balis U.J. *et al.* (1995) Immunohistochemical reference ranges for B lymphocytes in bone marrow biopsy paraffin sections. *Am J Clin Pathol*, **104 (5)**, 517–23.

Papayannopoulou T., Craddock C. (1997) Homing and trafficking of hemopoietic progenitor cells. *Acta Haematol*, **97 (1–2)**, 97–104.

Peled A., Kalai M., Toledo J., Zipori D. (1991) Stroma-cell dependent hematopoiesis, *Semin., Hematol.*, **28 (2)**, 132–7.

Pellegrini W., Facchetti F., Marocolo D. *et al.* (1995) Assessment of cell proliferation in normal and pathological bone marrow biopsies: a study using double sequential immunophenotyping on paraffin sections.

Pich A., Gastaldi M., Tragni G., Naývone R. (1991) Lymphocyte subsets in bone marrow lymphoid nodules and malignant lymphoma nodular involvement. *Eur. J. Basic. Appl. Histochem.*, **35 (1)**, 81–9.

Pujuget P., Bissel M. (1997) Dynamic Reciprocity. *Helix*, **6 (2)**, 16–25.

Rao S.G., Chitnis V.S., Deora A. *et al.* (1996) An ICAM-1 like cell adhesion molecule is responsible for CD34 positive haemopoietic stem cell adhesion to bone-marrow stroma. *Cell Biol Int*, **20 (4)**, 255–9.

Rozman C., Reverter J.C., Feliu E. *et al.* (1990) Variations of fat tissue fraction in abnormal human bone marrow depend on both size and number of adipocytes: a stereologic study. *Blood*, **76 (5)**, 892–5.

Salisbury J.R., Deverell M.H., Cookson M.J. (1996) Three-dimensional reconstruction of benign lymphoid aggregates in bone marrow trephines. *J Pathol*, **178 (4)**, 447–50.

Santucci M.A., Lemoli R.M., Tura S. (1997) Peripheral blood mobilization of hematopoietic stem cells: cytokine-mediated regulation of adhesive interactions within the hematopoietic microenvironment. *Acta Haematol*, **97 (1–2)**, 90–6.

Schmitt-Graff A., Skalli O., Gabbiani G. (1989) Alpha-smooth muscle actin is expressed in a subset of bone marrow stromal cells in normal and pathological conditions. *Virchows Arch. B. Cell. Pathol.*, **57 (5)**, 291–302.

Schweitzer K.M., Vicart P., Delouis C. *et al.* (1997) Characterization of a newly established human bone marrow endothelial cell line: distinct adhesive properties for hematopoietic progenitors compared with human umbilical vein endothelial cells. *Lab Invest.*, **76 (1)**, 25–36.

Simmons P.J., Masinovsky B., Longenecker B.M. *et al.* (1992) Vascular cell adhesion molecule-1 expressed by bone marrow stromal cells mediates the binding of hematopoietic progenitor cells. *Blood*, **80 (2)**, 388–95.

Singh T., Kochar R., Gaiha M. (1989) Estimation of marrow iron stores, biopsy vs. aspirate. *J Assoc Physicians India*, **37 (11)**, 705–6.

Sletvold O., Smaaland R., Laerum O.D. (1991) Cytometry and time-dependent variations in peripheral blood and bone marrow cells: a literature review and relevance to the chronotherapy of cancer. *Chronobiol Int.*, **8 (4)**, 235–50.

Tavassoli M., Friedenstein A. (1983) Haematopoietic stromal microenvironment. *Amer J Hematol.*, **15**, 195.

Terstappen L.W., Johnsen S., Segers-Nolten I.M.J. *et al.* (1990) Identification and characterization of plasma cells in normal human bone marrow by high resolution flow cytometry. *Blood*, **76**, 1739.

Terstappen L.W., Loken M.R. (1990) Myeloid cell differentiation in normal bone marrow and acute myeloid leukemia assessed by multi-dimensional flow cytometry. *Anal. Cell Pathol.*, **2 (4)**, 229–40.

van Furth R. (1989) Origin and turnover of monocytes and macrophages. *Curr. Top. Pathol.*, **79**, 125–50.

Wulfhekel U., Dullman J. (1990) The diagnostic value of bone marrow iron. *Folia Hematol. (Leipz)*, **117 (3)**, 419–34.

Zamboni L., Pease D.C. (1961) The vascular bed of red bone marrow. *Ultrastruct. Res.*, **5**, 65.

5 Major aspects of bone biopsy pathology

Types of osteopathies

Bone undergoes dynamic changes throughout life: acquisition of shape by modeling, increase in size during growth, adaptation to physical stress, repair of damage and maintenance of structural integrity. Abnormalities of bone cells and/or regulatory factors may result in impaired bone turnover with unbalanced bone production or destruction. Hence osteopathies are characterised by four main manifestations: (1) abnormalities of bone mass; (2) undermineralisation; (3) abnormal bone architecture; and (4) abnormal bone remodeling (Figure 5.1).

Abnormalities of bone mass

Osteopenia
Osteopenia (or osteoporosis) signifies a reduced trabecular bone volume, mostly due to attenuation (rarefaction) with the consequent enlargement of the marrow cavities. It may be focal or widespread (Figures 5.2 and 5.3).

Osteosclerosis
Osteosclerosis is a thickening and alteration of the structure of the cancellous bone resulting in a decrease in size of the intertrabecular cavities (or marrow spaces). This also may be generalised or focal. Osteosclerosis may also involve the cortical bone, so that the transition between cortex and trabeculae is blurred and they appear as a continuous structure (Figure 5.4).

Undermineralisation

This is an excess of osteoid, of which there are two types: (1) hyperosteoidosis in which there is defective mineralisation of the increased osteoid (osteomalacia) (Figure 5.5); and (2) hyperosteoidosis with normal calcification.

Abnormal bone architecture

This includes such abnormalities as woven bone, mosaic structures, changes in trabecular shape or in the cancellous network, particularly discontinuities which weaken it since bone strength depends on the architectural arrangements of the trabecular network (Figure 5.6). Two main types of changes are recognised: (1) attenuated trabeculae but with preservation of the trabecular connections and network; and (2) thick or thin trabeculae but with disruption of the trabecular network and formation of large marrow spaces, and isolated osseous trabecular profiles or 'button' phenomenon.

Abnormal bone remodeling

When osseous remodeling is balanced the amount formed is equal to that resorbed. When 'decoupling' occurs, this balance is lost and the ratio between resorption and formation of bone is altered, resulting in osteopenia or osteosclerosis, or mixtures of the two (Figure 5.6).

The bone turnover rate may be estimated by the density of active osteoclasts and osteoblasts and the extent of resorption and formation surfaces; for example, high and low turnover values indicate active and inactive forms of osteoporosis that require different therapeutic approaches such as calcitonin and/or bisphosphomates in the former, and vitamin D and/or fluoride in the latter. Classic examples of abnormal unbalanced bone remodeling are seen in Paget's disease of bone, renal osteodystrophy, primary hyperparathyroidism and metastatic bone disease (Figures 5.7–5.10).

Aging and bone structure

Predisposing factors

Bone loss throughout life is regarded as a universal feature of aging called 'physiological osteopenia'. The skeleton weighs approximately 100 g at birth, and increases rapidly till approximately 18 years of age, but at this time the weight is lower in females than in males. 'Peak' (maximal) bone mass is acquired by the end of the second decade. It is influenced by many factors: genes, sex, race, weight, lifestyle (alcohol, physical activity, smoking, type of nutrition), drugs and diseases.

Bone loss (Figure 5.11)

This may begin during the third decade and though possibly genetically determined may be influenced by other factors also: these

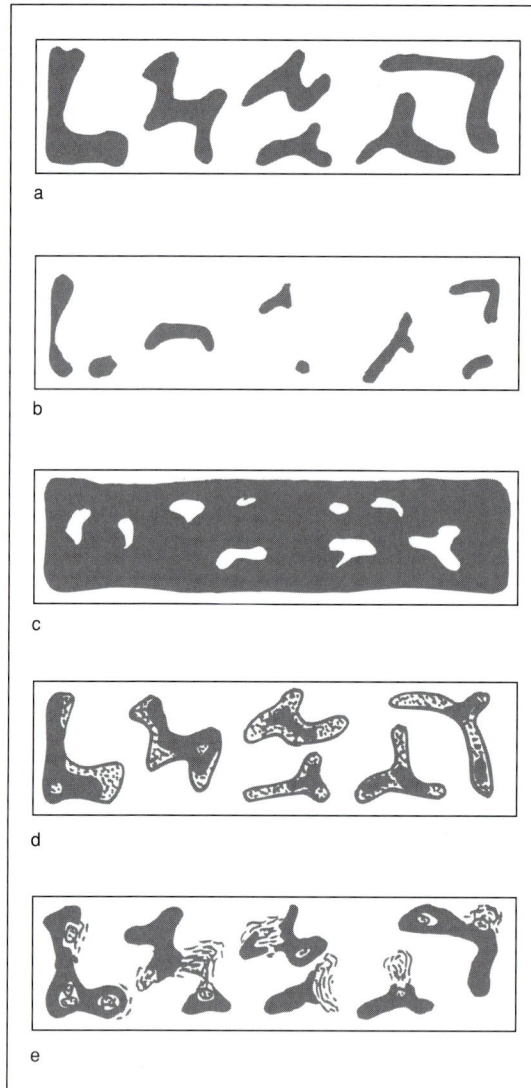

5.1 Sketch of four major aspects of bone biopsy pathology. Normal bone structure (a) is given for comparison: osteoporosis (b), osteosclerosis (c), osteomalacia (d) and disordered osseous remodeling as in hyperparathyroidism (e).

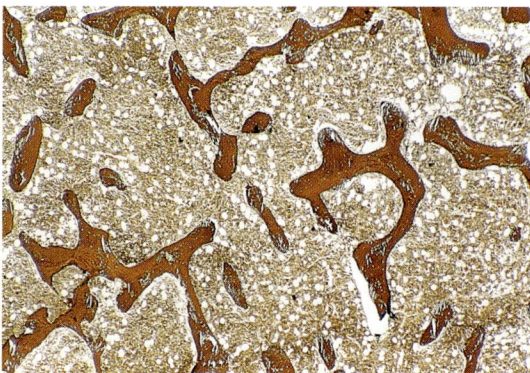

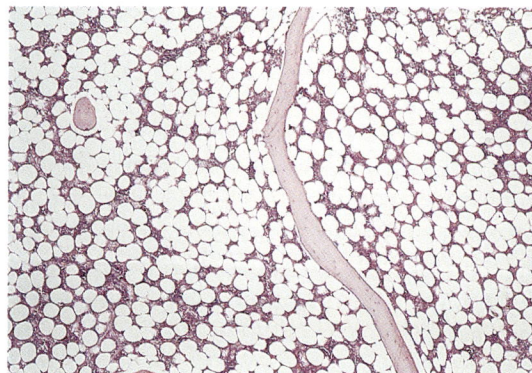

5.2 (left) BMBS plastic, Gomori, showing normal trabecular network and bone marrow, with incipient patchy osteoporosis.

5.3 (right) BMBS paraffin, H&E, osteoporotic trabecular bone and hypocellular bone marrow. Note 'button' phenomenon, upper left.

5.4 (left) BMBS paraffin, H&E, osteosclerotic bone with greatly reduced marrow spaces, containing fibrotic marrow with little hematopoiesis.

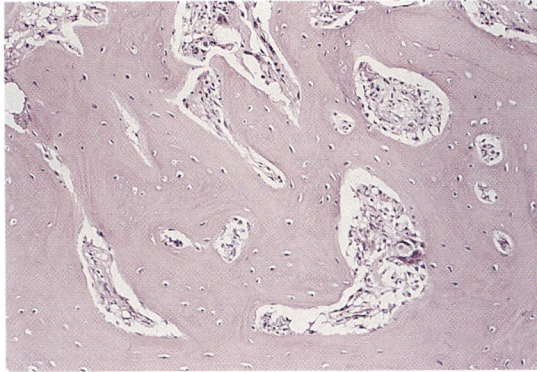

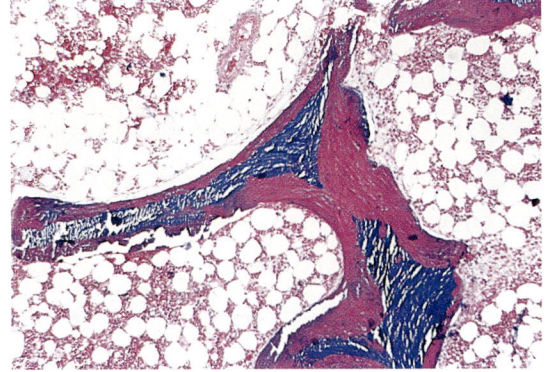

5.5 (right) BMBS plastic, Ladewig, osteoid red, bone blue, and hypocellular bone marrow. Extent and width of osteoid seams indicate osteomalacia.

5.6 (left) BMBS plastic, Gomori, showing patchy disorganisation of trabecular architecture: thin and thick trabeculae.

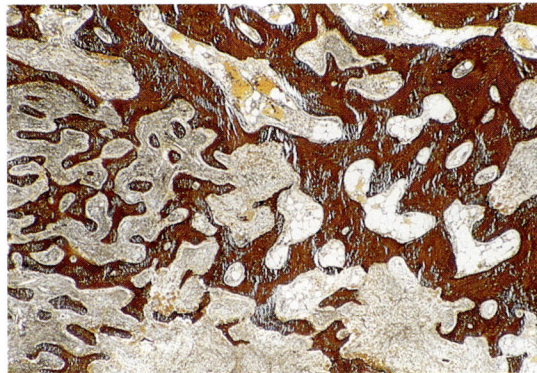

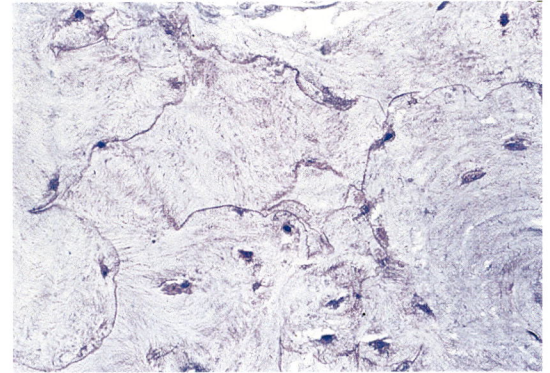

5.7 (right) BMBS plastic H&E, cortical bone showing mosaic pattern typical of Paget's disease of bone.

5.8 (left) BMBS plastic, Giemsa, trabecular bone showing osteoblasts and osteoid seam, as well as osteoclastic erosion, left and lower right. Renal osteodystrophy.

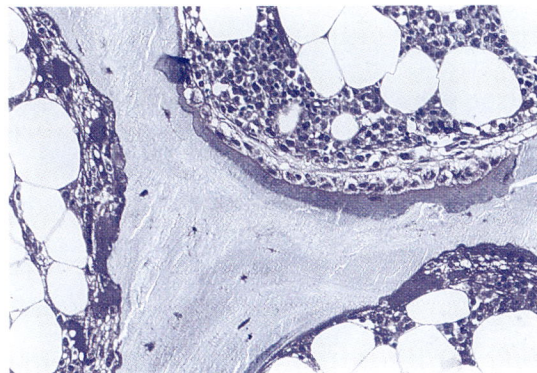

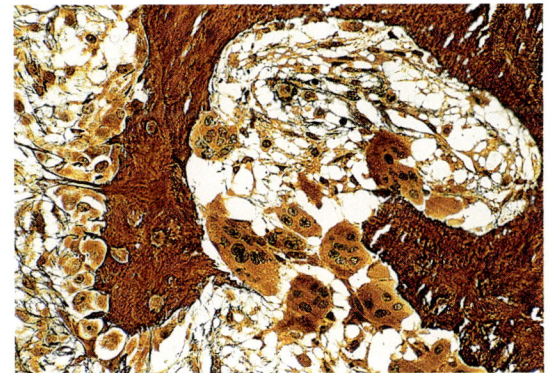

5.9 (right) BMBS plastic, Gomori, cluster of osteoclasts near and on bone, center; osteoblasts, left. Primary hyperparathyroidism.

include changes in absorption and excretion of calcium and in concentrations of its systemic regulating hormones and local growth factors, decrease in calcitonin levels, decrease in osteoblastic function, changes in quality or alterations in immune surveillance of remodeling and changes in bone marrow cellularity and composition. Though men and women reach peak bone mass at between 20 and 30 years, women have lower values than men and the difference increases with age. In summary, bone mass depends on the amount of bone produced, its peak value and its subsequent rate of loss (Figure 5.12). But in addition to the aspects mentioned above, qualitative bone defects also play a part: (1) age-related changes

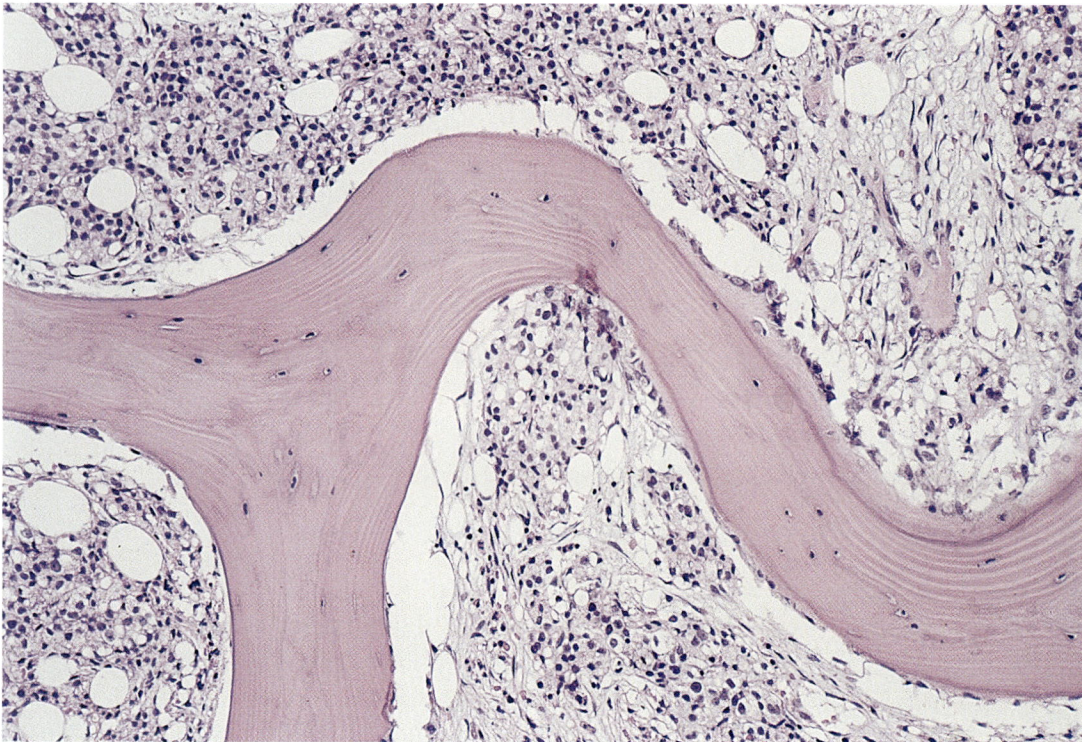

5.10 BMBS paraffin, H&E, showing osteoblastic remodeling, right. Note cement line and layer of new bone. Case of metastatic involvement of bone marrow.

in collagen arrangement and linking; (2) defective and/or unbalanced remodeling and repair of bone; (3) increase in bone fragility due to decrease in thickness, number and connectivity of trabeculae; (4) the osteoid produced is not mineralised ('poromalacia'); and (5) overall decrease in bone formation resulting from 'uncoupling' of the remodeling.

Bone loss at different skeletal sites

There are marked differences of bone loss at different skeletal sites (Figure 5.13) and between cortical and trabecular bone, so that measurements of serum and urinary indicators of resorption and formation can provide only generalised information, and a particular skeletal site requires individual investigation, by whatever of the appropriate means available. It follows from the above that three points in particular must be borne in mind:

1. Changes in bone are site-specific and cannot be extrapolated from one area to another.

2. Cortical bone behaves differently from trabecular bone.

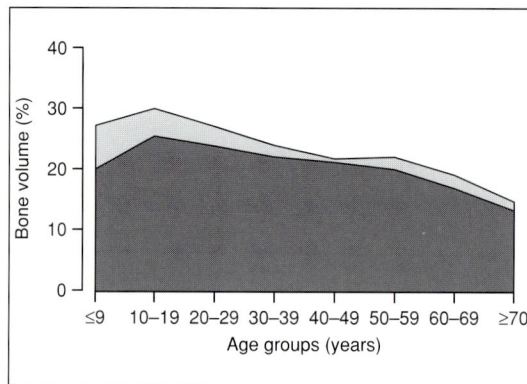

5.11 Peak bone mass and progressive decrease in trabecular bone volume with increasing age in posterior iliac crest biopsies. Note peak in osteoid volume in childhood; another smaller peak occurs in the older age groups.

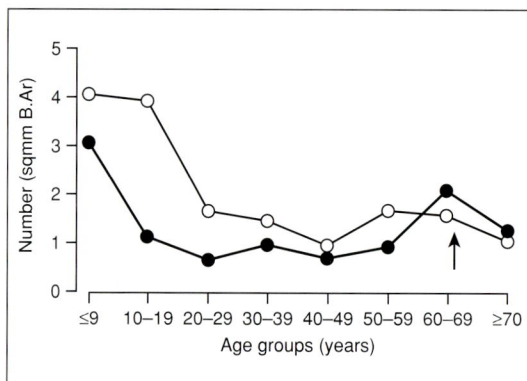

5.12 Number of osteoblasts (○) and osteoclasts (●) according to age groups in posterior iliac crest biopsies.

understood, including changes in endocrine, intestinal and renal functions at the systemic level and alterations in bone matrix, mineralisation, architecture and blood supply at the local level.

Osteodystrophies

These occur in congenital disorders of connective tissue, of cartilage and of bone, in vitamin D-resistant rickets, in gastrointestinal disorders and hepatic disorders, in chronic metabolic acidosis, as a consequence of drug therapy (for example administration of anti-convulsants in epilepsy, corticosteroids in asthma and rheumatic disorders). Classic examples of osteodystrophy are primary hyperparathyroidism and renal osteodystrophy. All the above are dealt with in the following chapters.

5.13 Trabecular bone volume according to age groups and different skeletal sites. At iliac crest (●), sternum (△), radius (○), lumbar vertebra (□) and calcaneus (▫).

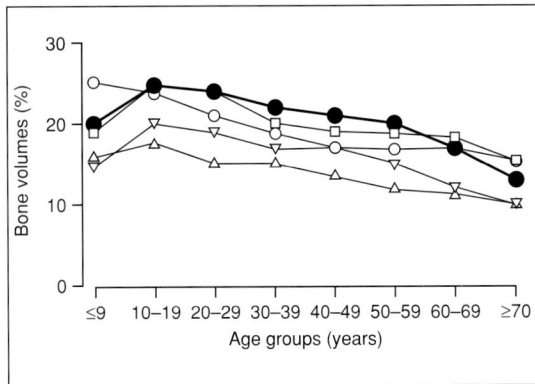

3. Changes in the axial skeleton do not necessarily relate closely to those in the appendicular skeleton.

Moreover, bone loss in the elderly has a multifactorial etiology, as yet only partly

Bibliography

Altman R.D., Gray R.G. (1988) Bone disease. In Katz (ed), *Diagnosis and Management of Rheumatic Diseases*, 2nd edn. Philadelphia: Lippincott.

Alvioli L., Krane S.M. (1990) *Metabolic Bone Disease*. Philadelphia: W.B. Saunders.

Bartl R., Frisch B. (1993) *Biopsy of Bone in Internal Medicine: An Atlas and Sourcebook*. Dordrecht: Kluwer Acaemic.

Boyce B.F. (1988) Uses and limitations of bone biopsy in management of metabolic bone disease. In Martin (ed), *Metabolic Bone Disease*, vol. 31. London: Baillière Tindall.

Bullough P.G., Bansal M., DiCarlo E.F. (1990) The tissue diagnosis of metabolic bone disease. *Orthop. Clin N Amer.*, **21** (1), 65.

Burr D.B., Martin R.B. (1989) Errors in bone metabolism toward a unified theory of metabolic bone disease. *Amer J Anat.*, **186** (2), 186.

Canalis E., McCarthy T.L., Centrella M. (1993) Factors that regulate bone formation. In G.R. Mundy and T.J. Martin (eds), *Physiology and*

Pharmacology of Bone. Handbook of Experimental Pharmacology, **107**, 249–66.

Chestnut C.H. (1988) Measurement of bone mass. *Triangle*, **27** (1/2), 37.

Coe F.L., Favus M.J. (eds) (1992) *Disorders of Bone and Mineral Metabolism*. New York: Raven Press.

Cormier C. (1991) Metabolic bone disease associated with systemic disorders. *Curr Opin Rheumatol.*, **3**, 463.

Favus M.J. (ed.) (1993) *Primer on the Metabolic Bone Diseases and Disorders of Mineral Metabolism*, 2nd edn. New York: Raven Press.

Fleisch H. (1995) *Bisphosphonates in Bone Disease – From the Laboratory to the Patient*. New York: Parthenon.

Frisch B., Bartl R. (1990) *Atlas of Bone Marrow Pathology*. Dordrecht: Kluwer Academic.

Frisch B., Lewis S.M., Burkhardt R., Bartl R. (1985) *Biopsy Pathology of Bone and Bone Marrow*. London: Chapman & Hall.

Frost H.M. (1973) *Bone Remodeling and its Relationship to Metabolic Bone Diseases*. Springfield: Thomas.

Gowen M. (1994) Cytokines and cellular interactions in the control of bone remodelling. In J.N.M Heersche and J.A. Kanis (eds), *Bone and Mineral Research*, 77–114.

Jensen G.F., Meinecke B., Boesen J., Tansbol I. (1985) Does 1,25(OH)$_2$D$_3$ accelerate spinal bone loss? A controlled therapeutic trial on 70-year-old women. *Clin Orthop.*, **192**, 215–21.

Kanis J.A., Meunier P.J. (1984) Should we use fluoride to treat osteoporosis? *Quart J Med.*, **53**, 145–64.

Malluche H.H., Faugere M.C. (1986) *Atlas of Mineralized Bone Histology*. Basel: Karger.

Milgram J.W. (1990) *Radiologic and Histologic Pathology of Nontumorous Diseases of Bones and Joints*. South Lane Northbrook: Northbrook.

Mundy G.R. (1995) *Bone Remodeling and its Disorders*. London: Martin Dunitz.

Navone R., Angeli G., Ramponi A., Viberti L. (1987) Bone marrow in the elderly: normal and pathological patterns frequently encountered. Study of biopsy and autopsy case records. *Pathologica*, **79 (1063)**, 571–9.

Noda M. (ed.) (1993) *Cellular and Molecular Biology of Bone*. San Diego: Academic Press.

Raisz L.G. (1981) What marrow does to bone. *N Engl J Med.*, **304**, 1485.

Revell P.A. (1986) *Pathology of Bone*. Berlin: Springer.

Rosenberg A.E. (1991) The pathology of metabolic bone disease. *Radiol Clin N Amer.*, **29 (1)**, 19.

Tam C.S. (1989) The pathogenesis of metabolic bone disease – an overview. In Tam, Heersche and Murray (eds), *Metabolic Bone Disease: Cellular and Tissue Mechanisms*, vol. 19. Boca Raton: CRC Press.

Verloog H., DeRoo M., Mortelmans L., Dequeker J. (1991) Common features of bone in osteomalacia, secondary hyperparathyroidism and renal osteodystrophy. *Clin Nucl Med.*, **16**, 372.

6 Osteoporosis

General aspects: primary osteoporosis

Osteoporosis is the commonest metabolic disorder of bone and, when established, one of the most difficult to treat. It is defined as a condition in which bone mass (both trabecular and cortical) and strength are decreased to levels below those required for mechanical support, and thus it leads to an increased incidence of fractures either spontaneous, or due to minimal trauma. Clinically, a diagnosis of osteoporosis is usually made when fractures and/or deformities have already occurred. Patients with osteoporotic fractures have 30–50% less bone mass than normal young adults. Osteoporosis is called 'primary' or age-related when no other disease causing bone loss is found. Osteoporosis is also a consequence of, or associated with, many other conditions (Table 6.1). Some parts of the skeleton are more liable to osteopenia than others; for example, the vertebrae and the femoral neck. This is because osteoporosis affects the more metabolically active trabecular bone in these skeletal sites. In iliac crest biopsies a value of <16% trabecular bone is defined as osteopenia and four different histological patterns have been found in iliac crest biopsies (Figure 6.1): (1) an irregular rarefaction of trabeculae with marked differences in various regions of the biopsy (39%); (2) overall trabecular attenuation (29%); (3) reduction in trabecular number resulting in broad ossicles and wide marrow spaces (11%); and (4) presence of small islands of bone (button phenomenon) (21%) (Figures 6.2 and 6.3).

High and low turnover

Heterogeneity in bone turnover is also seen, and is divided into two main groups: (1) low turnover (inactive), and (2) high turnover (active) (Figures 6.4–6.7). The second group may also have significantly higher values for osteoid volume and surface, i.e. osteoporosis plus osteomalacia (poromalacia) (Figures 6.8–6.10). The relationship between hematopoiesis, adipose tissue, bone remodeling and osteopenia has received relatively little attention. Increase in fat cells was seen in 60% of biopsies of osteoporotic patients; there were four topographic patterns: diffuse (48%); patchy (31%); peritrabecular (4%); and complete (7%) (Figures 6.11–6.15). Concomitantly, there was a decrease in the amount of hematopoiesis and of sinusoids, thickening of the walls of small vessels and a relative increase in plasma and mast cells, lymphocytes and lymphoid nodules. If rarefied trabeculae with resorption lacunae are present, osteoclastic activity may be observed, especially if serial sections are cut. But osteoblasts and osteoid seams are few and far between unless an element of 'poromalacia' is also present.

Primary osteoporosis

Type I and Type II

Type I osteoporosis occurs mainly in women (85%) approximately 10 years after the menopause, and is also called the vertebral crush fracture syndrome. However, bone loss may start well before the menopause, may be intermittent and is subject to modification by many factors – diet, exercise, hormones – so that both the manifestations and the response to therapy are varied.

Type II osteoporosis (senile or involutional) occurs mainly in older patients with fractures of the proximal femur. Reduction in cortical and trabecular bone is involved, resulting in cortical thinning, porosity and loss of trabecular microarchitecture. Usually very few

TABLE 6.1 Main causes of osteopenia

Primary
Postmenopausal (type I)
Senile (type II)
Juvenile
Idiopathic

Congenital
Osteogenesis imperfecta
Marfan syndrome
Ehlers–Danlos syndrome
Homocystinuria

Endocrine
Hyperparathyroidism
Hyperthyroidism
Cushing syndrome
Hypogonadism
Hyperprolactinaemia

Nutritional
Malnutrition
Scurvy
Anorexia nervosa

Gastrointestinal
Gastrectomy
Primary biliary cirrhosis
Liver transplantation
Pancreatic disease

Immobilisation
Bed rest
Paraplegia
Space flight

Hematopoietic
Hemolytic anaemias
Aplastic anaemia
Myelodysplastic syndrome
Chronic myeloproliferative
    disorders
Acute leukemias
Chronic
lymphoproliferative
    disorders
Multiple myeloma
Systemic masotcytosis

Metabolic
Diabetes mellitus
Gaucher disease

Metastatic
Diffuse bone metastasis

Drugs/toxins
Corticosteroids
Heparin
Anticonvulsants
Excess of thyroid hormone
    replacement
Methotrexate
Excess of alcohol

Miscellaneous
Rheumatic and
    autoimmune disorders
Renal disease

osteoblasts or osteoclasts are found, and there is little or no osteoid.

Functionally one defect is thought to be a disturbance of the balance between resorption and formation, in favor of the former, but in primary osteoporosis the cause is most likely to be multifactorial. Exercise may have a beneficial effect even in established osteoporosis.

Though osteoporosis is considered a condition mainly affecting women, it does also occur in men. According to recent studies the risk of hip fracture by age and bone density is similar in men and women. However, in men it occurs 5 years later than in women, which could be explained by different bone density distributions at these ages, as well as differences in levels of hormones. In the course of a lifetime, men lose about 30% of cortical bone and about 30% of trabecular bone. Androgens stimulate bone formation – osteoblasts have receptors for androgens. As in the case of estro-

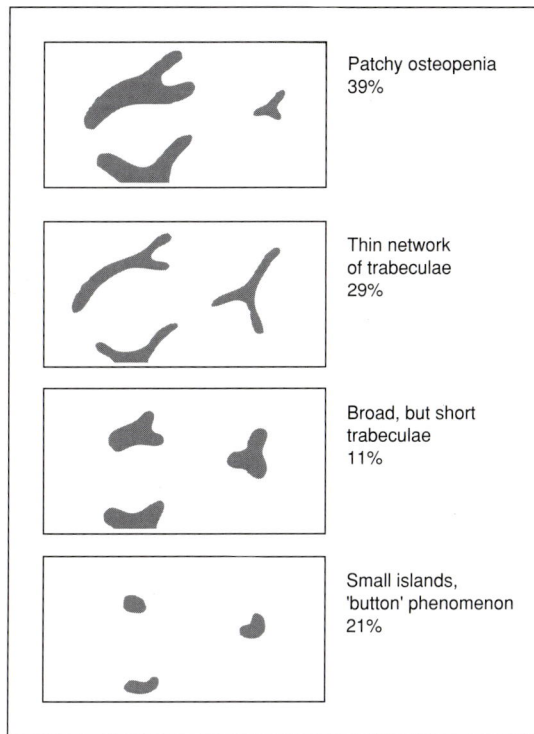

6.1 The four histological patterns of osteopenia.

Patchy osteopenia
39%

Thin network
of trabeculae
29%

Broad, but short
trabeculae
11%

Small islands,
'button' phenomenon
21%

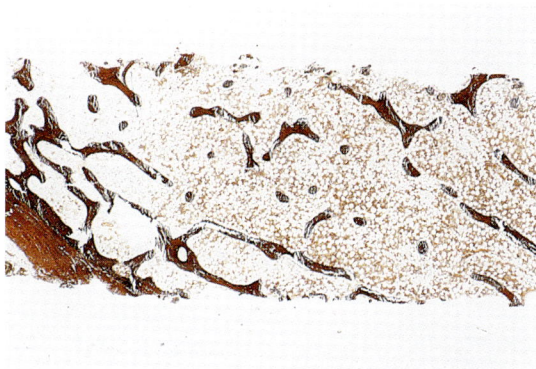

6.2 BMBS plastic, Gomori, showing great reduction in trabecular bone, discontinuous network, 'button phenomenon' and hypocellular bone marrow with increase in fat cells especially in the subcortical area.

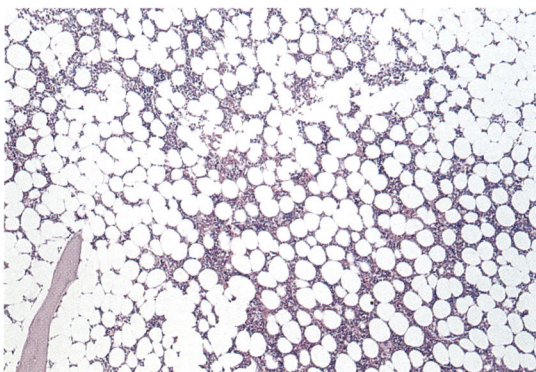

6.3 BMBS paraffin, H&E, great reduction in trabecular bone, only a single thin trabecula, lower left, remaining in a large part of the biopsy section. Hypocellular marrow.

gens, bone resorption may be inhibited by androgens by way of alterations of IL-1 and IL-6.

Causes of osteoporosis in men, other than age, include glucocorticoid therapy, gastric resection and ethanol abuse.

Idiopathic osteoporosis

This may occur in relatively young men and women, is localised to the spine and no cause is found. There is no histologic evidence of increased resorption but possibly activity of osteoblasts is impaired.

Juvenile osteoporosis

This is rare, occurs at puberty and involves the axial skeleton. It is self-limited and with time bone mass is restored. It must be distinguished from osteogenesis imperfecta (see p. 68).

Endocrine osteoporosis

Metabolic bone disease occurs frequently in patients with endocrine disorders. Moreover, some endocrine disturbances may exist in patients with age-related osteoporosis and aggravate the bone loss, as may be seen, for example, in hyperthyroidism and hypercorticosteroidism. In the former osteoclasts are stimulated directly, resulting in greater resorption than formation, thus accelerating the already-present tendency to bone loss.

Hyperthyroidism and osteoporosis

Thyroid hormone activates osteoclasts so that mineral content of bone is decreased, and resorption is greater than formation, though mineralisation is normal. The picture observed is one of rarefaction of the trabecular bone with mildly increased osseous remodeling. Hyperthyroidism should be considered in cases with accelerated age-related osteoporosis. Changes in bone density in women receiving long-term thyroxine therapy are minimal and are not a contraindication to therapy.

63

Corticosteroids and osteoporosis

Corticosteroids have two main actions on bone cells: they stimulate resorption and inhibit osteoid synthesis. Osteoporosis has been observed in >80% of patients with Cushing's disease. Excess of glucocorticoid may lead to aseptic bone necrosis. Iliac crest biopsies of patients on long-term steroid therapy confirm the decrease in trabecular and cortical bone (Figure 6.14), the low turnover,

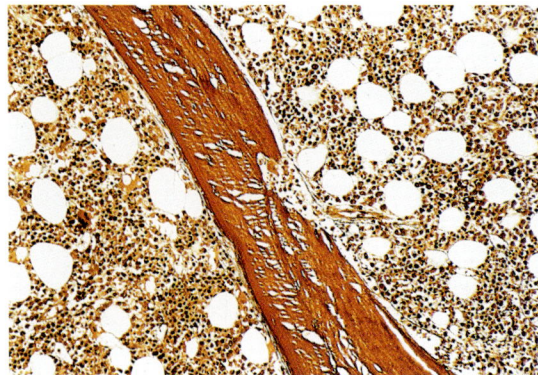

6.4–6.7 BMBS plastic, illustrating steps in transection of a trabecula by osteoclastic activity.

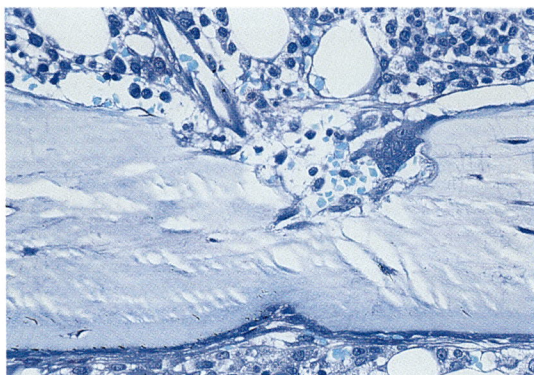

6.4 Initial erosion cavity near blood vessel.

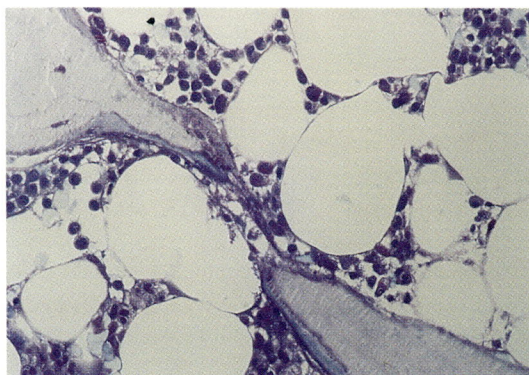

6.5 (left) Deeper cavity with several osteoclasts. Note paratrabecular sinus and arteriole, left of center, and mast cells; osteoblasts on opposite side of trabecula.

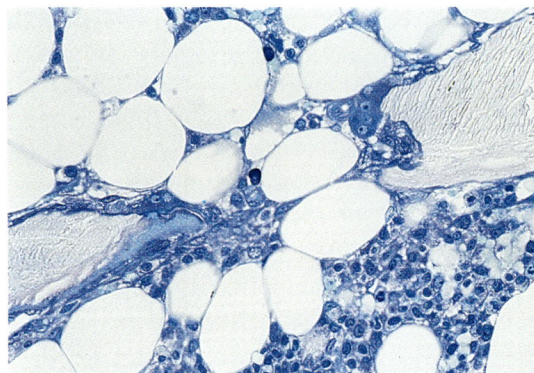

6.6 (right) Transection almost complete, only a connective tissue strand connects the two ends of the trabecula.

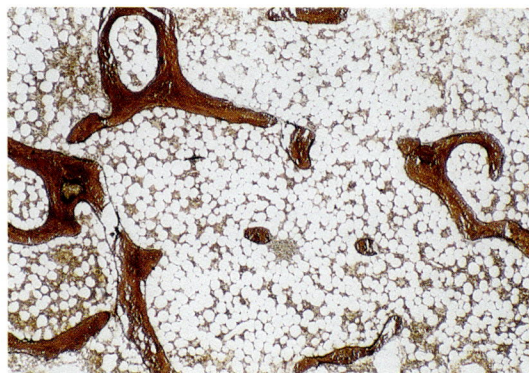

6.7 (left) Transection complete with bone eroded by osteoclasts.

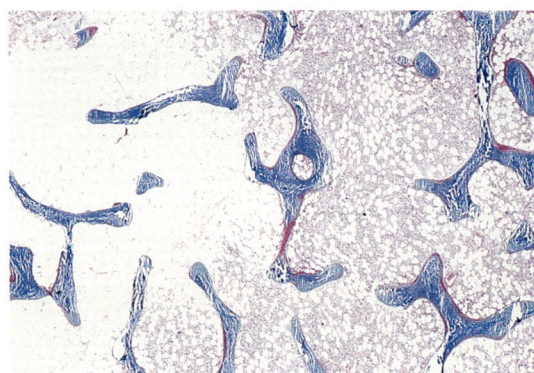

6.8 (right) BMBS plastic, Gomori, showing result of trabecular transection: discontinuous network and 'button phenomena'. Overall decrease in hematopoiesis and in bone, and increase in fat cells.

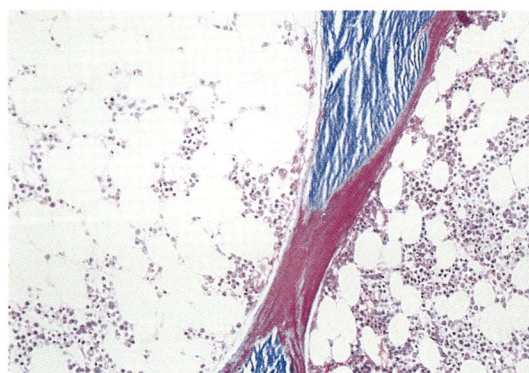

6.9 and 6.10 BMBS plastic Ladewig, low and high magnifications.

6.9 (left) Osteopenia and osteomalacia-poromalacia, bone blue, osteoid red.

6.10 (right) Note demineralisation across width of the trabecula.

6.11 (left) BMBS plastic, Gomori, peritrabecular fat in cellular marrow, thought to be a contributory cause in incipient osteopenia.

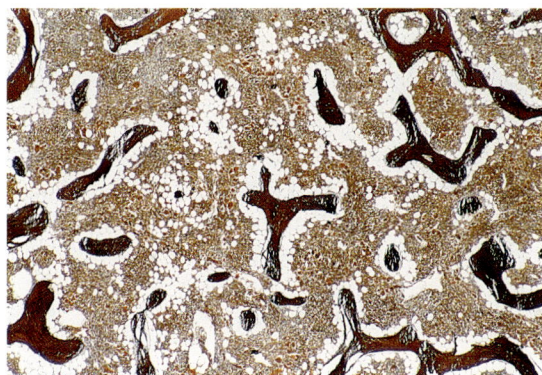

6.12 (right) BMBS plastic, Giemsa, attenuated trabecula with osteoid at thinnest part.

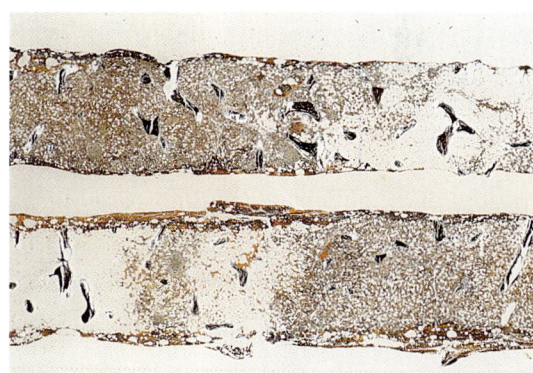

6.13 (left) Patterns of distribution and extent of fatty tissue in iliac crest biopsies of patients with osteoporosis.

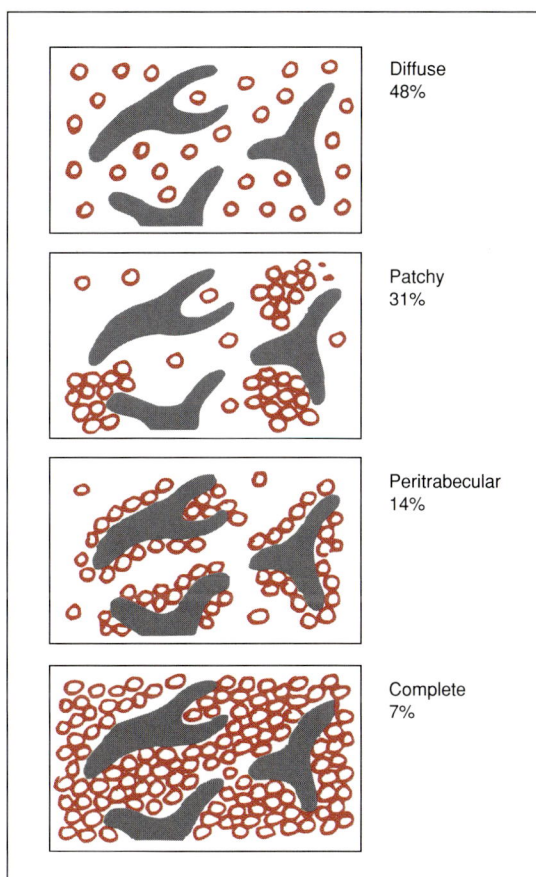

Diffuse 48%

Patchy 31%

Peritrabecular 14%

Complete 7%

6.14 (right top) BMBS plastic, Giemsa, low magnification showing only a single, long, thin trabecula, with more fat cells on one side than on the other.

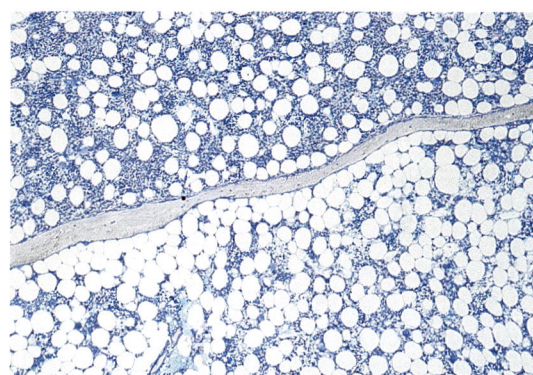

6.15 (right bottom) BMBS plastic, Gomori, showing marked osteopenia and large areas of hypocellularity.

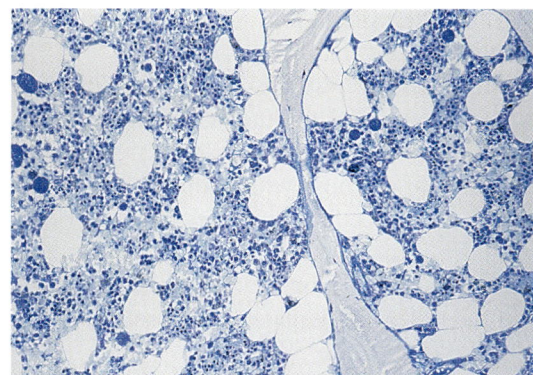

increase in marrow fatty tissue and inflammatory vascular changes. However, in some patients bone loss may be due to the primary disease and its complications (e.g. rheumatoid arthritis, asthma and immobilisation) as well as the therapeutic administration of steroids. Additional causes of endocrine osteoporosis are listed in Table 6.1.

Nutritional osteoporosis

This may be due to four main causes:

1. Inadequate dietary intake (e.g. anorexia nervosa, gastrectomy) (Figure 6.16).
2. Impaired absorption.
3. Increased loss of nutrients.

4. Hepatobiliary and pancreatic disorders involving intestinal malabsorption.

All four may result in inadequate calcium uptake. Additional risk factors for osteoporosis are excessive dietary protein, caffeine, alcohol, nicotine, and drugs which may cause a decrease in trabecular thickness. Bone disease related to nutritional factors may therefore be a combination of osteoporosis, osteomalacia and secondary hyperparathyroidism.

Hepatic osteoporosis

In hepatic osteoporosis, decreased bone formation is due to inhibition of osteoblastic activity possibly because of the liver disease itself, and/or the toxic effects of alcohol, iron, aluminum fluoride or copper. Osteoclastic activity is increased. The net result is trabecular plate thinning. Pathogenesis of osteoporosis after liver transplantation is multifactional and includes immobilisation and steroid therapy.

Immobilisation osteoporosis

Since maintenance of bone mass depends on skeletal stress and weight-bearing, reduction in physical activity as in bed-rest is accompanied by bone loss, about 4% of bone mass per month, due to osteoclastic resorption. With resumption of normal activity, bone mass is restored. Children are particularly susceptible to this type of loss (Figure 6.17). Astronauts may suffer a severe generalised bone loss because of weightlessness during space flight.

Diabetic osteoporosis

This type of osteoporosis may affect children as well as adults. Mechanisms of bone loss in diabetes include decreased formation due to insulin deficiency, increased excretion of calcium due to glycosuria, decreased physical activity and increased bone resorption. Diabetic microangiopathy in the bone marrow may also contribute (Figure 6.18). The resulting reduction in bone mass is associated with an increased risk of fracture. If and when the kidneys are affected, hyperparathyroid bone disease may occur.

Rheumatic osteoporosis

Both localised and generalised osteoporosis may occur in rheumatic disorders; many factors may contribute – non-specific such as decreased activity and steroid therapy and possibly more specific such as production of osteoclast activating factors by T lymphocytes.

Transient osteoporosis

This is a rare condition in which osteoporosis develops in periarticular bone areas. It may be regional, affecting mainly the hip joint, or migratory with sequential involvement of multiple joints. Neural, mechanical and circulatory mechanisms have been implicated.

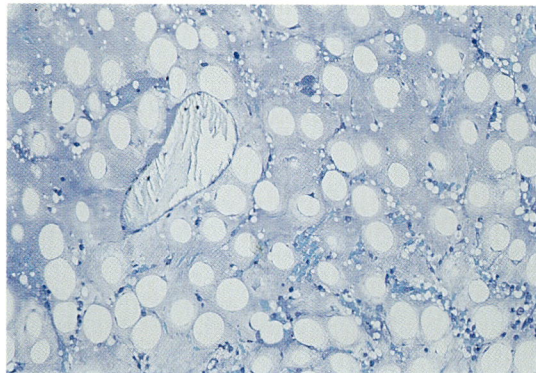

6.16 BMBS plastic, Giemsa, showing osteopenia with serous (or gelatinous) atrophy, as in anorexia nervosa or malnutrition from any other cause.

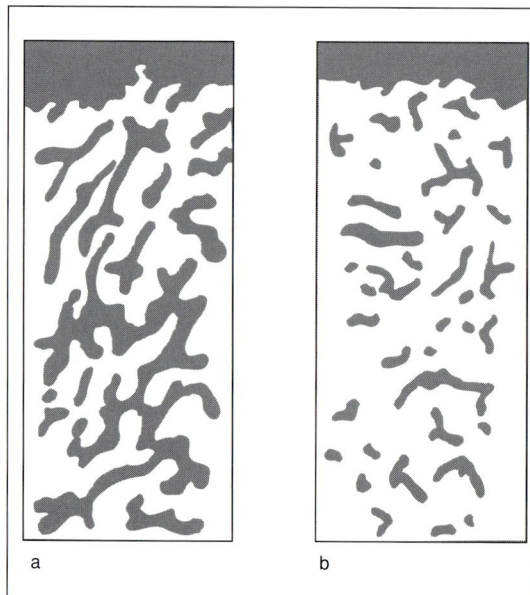

6.17 Iliac crest biopsy of child before (a) and after (b) 17 weeks of immobilisation. There is a marked reduction in trabecular volume.

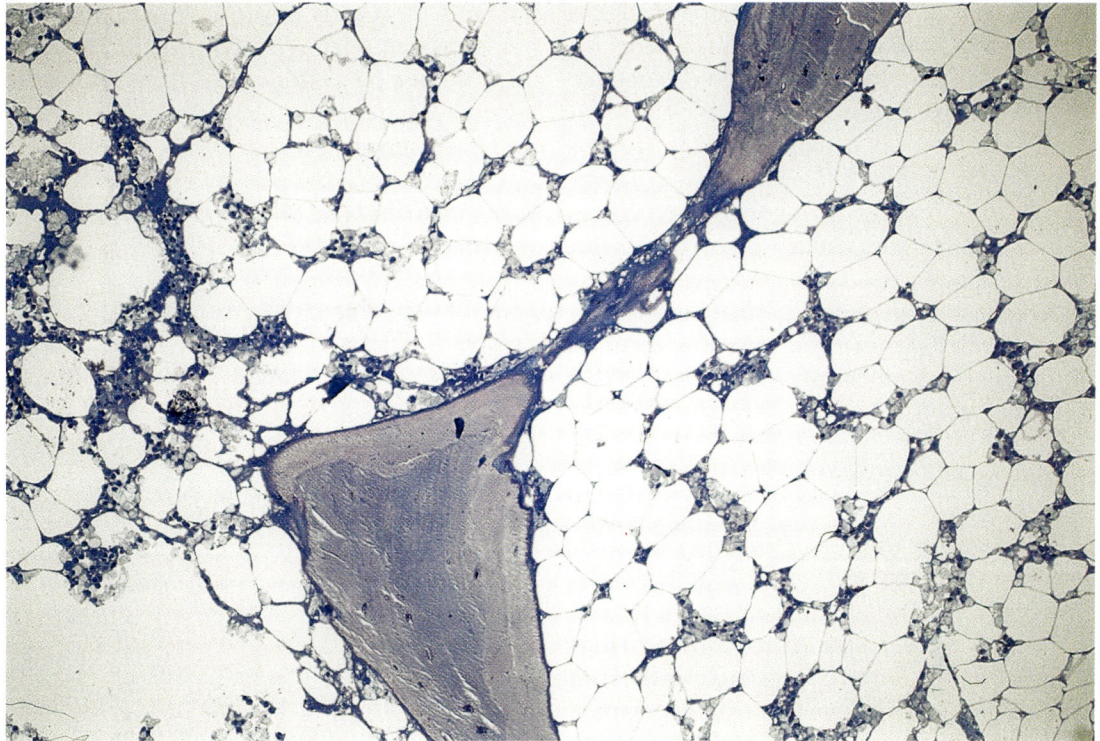

6.18 Diabetes BMBS paraffin, Giemsa. Osteopenia with trabecular erosion and hypocellularity, histologic type A osteoporosis.

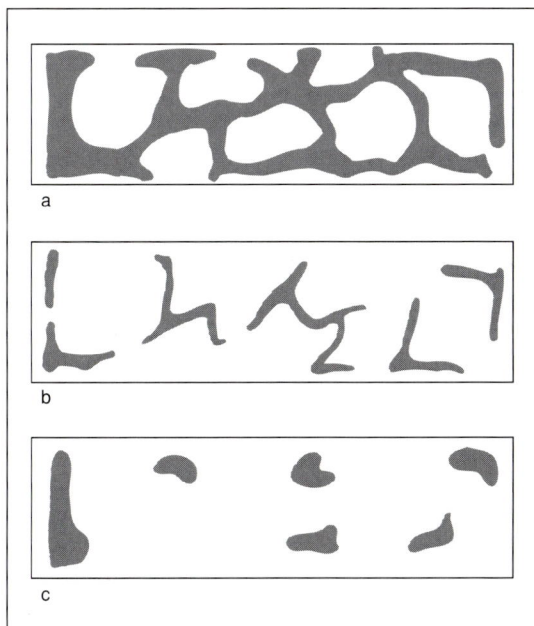

6.19 Comparison of normal cortical and trabecular bone (a) in iliac crest biopsies with osteoporosis, histological types A (b) and B (c).

Hematopoietic osteoporosis

Bone and marrow are closely inter-related organs and therefore diseases of the one affect the other (Table 6.1). Myelogenous osteopathy is used for osteolysis and osteosclerosis occurring in diseases of the marrow, and osteogenous myelopathy for the suppression of hematopoiesis in diseases of the bones.

Three histologic aspects of osteopenia depend on the underlying condition of the marrow:

1. Low turnover or high turnover osteopenia. Low turnover osteopenia is found in hypo and aplastic bone marrow conditions, as well as hyperplastic ones accompanied by absence of endosteal sinusoids, osteoclasts and osteoblasts. High turnover occurs in hematologic malignancies with diffuse spread (acute leukemias, diffuse myelomatosis) and is due to production of osteoclast activating factors (OAFs) by leukemia, myeloma or lymphoma cells.

2. Thin or coarse trabecular osteopenia. In the former the trabeculae are attenuated but the connections and network preserved. In the latter the trabeculae are fewer, thicker, and separate larger marrow spaces, and the trabecular network is not preserved (Figures 6.19 and 6.20).

3. Generalised and focal osteopenia. The mode of spread of marrow infiltrations affects

the pattern of the osseous lesions: diffuse processes in bones with trabecular networks and red marrow cause generalised osteopenia; while focal, paratrabecular or patchy infiltrations induce focal osteopenia or osteolytic lesions (as in granulomatous disorders, Hodgkin's disease, nodular lymphomas, etc.). These hematopoietic osteopenias will be dealt with in the appropriate sections.

Osteoporosis may also occur in iron overload. Deposition of iron can be seen in endothelial and endosteal cells, on osteoid and around osteocytic lacunae.

Osteogenesis Imperfecta (O.I.)

This refers to a group of disorders caused by defective synthesis of collagen Type I, causing changes in its structure and function. It is an autosomal, usually dominant, disorder. However, there are numerous collagen genes, at least 20, scattered over 10 chromosomes, including chromosomes 7 and 17, which contain the two genes that code for the two components of collagen Type I. Glycosaminoglycans and other matrix proteins may be involved. O.I. is also called 'Brittle Bone Disease': there is inadequate bone formation and a reduced calcification rate. Clinical manifestations are highly variable and range from stillbirth to late adult onset of fractures, which is why the condition is mentioned here, as patients may be misdiagnosed as having primary osteoporosis. In the mild form there is normal stature and only a slightly higher rate of fractures. Though four main types of osteogenesis imperfecta are recognised, many patients are difficult to classify. Basically, there is 'too little bone' with thin cortices and thin trabeculae. Iliac crest biopsies of young patients show abnormalities in the transitional region from cartilage to bone (Figure 6.21), and in the trabeculae: islands of cartilage surrounded by rims of woven bone 'popcorn calcification', thereby reducing mechanical strength and support. Osteoblasts, osteoid-covered surfaces and osteocytes are increased (Figure 6.22). Osteogenesis imperfecta is characterised not only by the propensity of bones to break, but also by an inability to repair the fractures adequately, suggesting a failure of the modeling–remodeling system. In the juvenile form it must be distinguished from idiopathic juvenile osteoporosis. Rehabilitation is especially important.

Rare connective tissue disorders with osteoporosis

Other rare connective tissue disorders that involve skeletal abnormalities include: Ehlers–Danlos syndrome, Marfan syndrome, Homo-

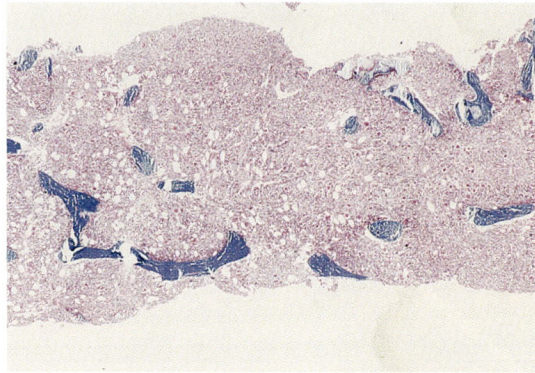

6.20 BMBS Ladewig, bone blue, osteoid red, case of hypercellular MDS, showing histologic type B osteoporosis.

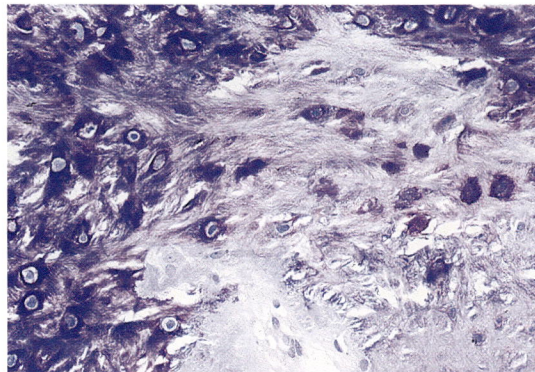

6.21 BMBS plastic, Giemsa, of a young patient with osteogenesis imperfecta, showing disorganisation and irregularity of transitional zones of cartilage and bone.

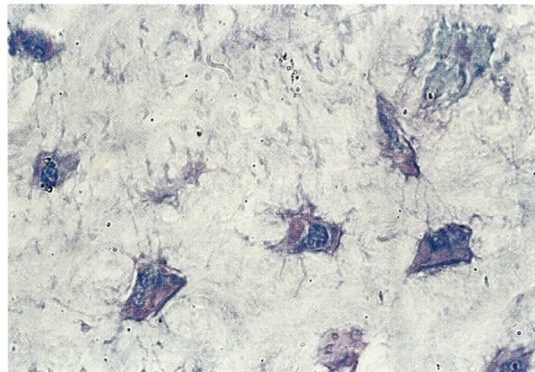

6.22 As for Figure 6.21 area of cortex showing relatively high density of osteocytes, but no parallel lamellae of bone.

cystinuria and Menckes syndrome. All may have an osteoporotic component, though the major defect may cause multiple abnormalities affecting other systems. For example, in the Marfan syndrome there are musculoskeletal, cardiovascular and ocular (lens dislocation and myopia) disorders. It is caused by anomalies of a gene on chromosome 15 which encodes Fibrillin I, a major constituent of extracellular matrix and of microfibrils of elastic.

Check list: Osteoporosis

- Is bone marrow biopsy adequate in width and length?
- Cortex: thin or porous?
- Subcortical remodeling: present, osteoblasts, osteoclasts, balanced?
- Trabecular bone and microarchitecture: overall volume decreased?
- Network, attenuated network, no network, patchy osteopenia?
- Widely separated ossicles, thick or thin, button phenomenon, whole or part of biopsy affected?
- Remodeling: activity of osteoblasts, osteoclasts, flat endosteal lining cells, high or low turnover?
- Hematopoiesis: increased, normal, decreased?
- Peritrabecular layers of fat?
- Blood vessels: sclerosis of walls?
- Osteoid: none, present, normal, increased?
- Infiltrations of the bone marrow: present?
- Immunohistology (I.H.) LCA, CD68, acid phosphatase and TRAP for osteoclasts, alkaline phosphatase for osteoblasts.
- Stromal alterations: atrophy, amyloidosis, fibrosis? I.H.: vimentin, actin; and reticulin stain.
- Grade of osteopenia: low, intermediate, high?
- *Example.* Bone biopsy 3 × 40 mm
  - Cortex present: thin and porous.
  - Trabecular microarchitecture disrupted.
  - Presence of button phenomenon.

- Mineralisation: no defect.
- Osteopenia, massive (9 vol% bone), very few osteoblasts or osteoclasts. Flat endosteal lining cells.
- Low turnover type.
- Hypocellular bone marrow – all cell lines equally reduced, fat increased.
- Normal stroma, no sclerosis of vessel walls.
- Malignant infiltration not detected. Conclusion: Bone biopsy showing high grade osteopenia (osteoporosis) low turnover type, and hypocellular bone marrow.

Clinical correlations

- Older age groups; females 60, males 70; osteopenia on imaging techniques.
- Frequent back pain, propensity to fractures, e.g. vertebral, with minimal stress.
- Diagnosed by bone mineral density (BMD) or bone mineral content (BMC)
- Severe osteoporosis (i.e. plus fracture) diagnosed by BMD measurement plus X-rays.
- Hip fractures before or as a result of a fall.
- In early osteoporosis – hydroxyproline and pyridinoline crosslinks in urine may indicate an active phase.
- Alkaline phosphatase and osteocalcin may also be elevated in blood if bone formation is increased, e.g. during and after therapy.
- Exclusion (and treatment) of other disorders likely to cause or exacerbate osteoporosis.
- Exclusion of an osteomalacia component – levels of vitamin D, exposure to sunlight, diet?
- Prevention of further bone loss, e.g. by therapy with osteoclast inhibiting agents such as bisphosphonates.
- The saying 'prevention is better than cure' applies, *par excellence*, to osteoporosis since it can now be prevented, but once established cannot be cured.

Bibliography

Anon (1993) Consensus development conference: diagnosis, prophylaxis and treatment of osteoporosis. *Am J Med.*, **94**, 646–50.

Arlot M.E., Delmas P.D., Chappard D., Meunier P.J. (1990) Trabecular and endocortical bone remodelling in postmenopausal osteoporosis: comparison with normal postmenopausal women. *Osteoporosis Int.*, **1(1)**, 41.

Avioli L.V. (1991) Heterogenity of osteoporotic syndromes and the response to calcitonin therapy. *Calcif Tissue Int.*, **49**, S16.

Avioli L.V., Lindsay R. (1990) The female osteoporotic syndrome(s). In Avioli and Krane (eds), *Metabolic Bone Disease.* Philadelphia: W.B. Saunders, p. 397.

Bachrach L.K., Katman D.K., Litt I.F. *et al.* (1991) Recovery from osteopenia in adolescent girls with anorexa nervosa. *J Clin Endocrinol Metab.*, **72**, 602.

Baron R., Gertner J.M., Lang R., Vignery A. (1983) Increased bone turnover with decreased bone formation by osteoblasts in children with osteogenesis imperfecta. *Pediatr Res.*, **17**, 204.

Bisballe S., Eriksen E.F., Melsen F. (1991) Osteopenia and osteomalacia after gastrectomy: interrelations between biochemical markers of bone remodelling, vitamin D metabolites and bone histomorphometry. *Gut*, **32**, 1303.

Bonadio J., Byers P.H. (1985) Subtle structural alterations in the chains of type I procollagen produce osteogenesis imperfecta type II. *Nature*, **316**, 363.

Bouillon R. (1991) Diabetic bone disease. *Calcif Tissue Int.*, **49**, 155.

Buchanan J.R., Myers C., Lloyd T. (1988) Early vertebral trabecular bone loss in normal premenopausal women. *J Bone Miner Res.*, **3**, 583.

Byers P.H., Wallis G.A., Willing M.C. (1991) Osteogenesis imperfecta: translation of mutation to phenotype. *J Med Genet.*, **28**, 433.

Chappard D., Plantard B., Petitjean M. *et al.* (1991) Alcoholic cirrhosis and osteoporosis in men: a light and scanning electron microscopic study. *J Stud Alcohol.*, **52**, 269.

Chatterji S., Wall J.C., Jeffrey J.W. (1972) Changes in the degree of orientation of bone materials with age in the human femur. *Experimentia*, **28**, 156.

Chesnut C.H. (1991) Theoretical overview: bone development, peak bone mass, bone loss, and fracture risk. *Amer J Med.*, **91 (5B)**, 2S.

Chesnut C.H. (1992) Osteoporosis and its treatment. *New Engl J Med.*, **326**, 406.

Christiansen C. (ed) (1993) *Proceedings of the Consensus Development Conference on Osteoporosis*, Hong Kong. *Am J Med.*, **95 (5A)**, 1S–78S.

Christiansen C., Riis B. (1990) *The Silent Epidemic. Post-Menopausal Osteoporosis.* Vedbaeck.

Cole W.G. (1988) Osteogenesis imperfecta. *Clin Endocrinol Metab.*, **2 (1)**, 243.

Compston J.E., Vedi S., Croucher P.I. (1991) Low prevalence of osteomalacia in elderly patients with hip fracture. *Age Ageing*, **20**, 132.

Consensus Development Conference (1993) Diagnosis, prophylaxis and treatment of osteoporosis. *Am J Med.*, **94**, 646–50.

Cuthbert J., Pak C.Y.C., Zerwekh J.E. *et al.* (1984) Bone disease in primary biliary cirrhosis: increased bone resorption and turnover in the absence of osteoporosis or osteomalacia. *Hepatology*, **4 (1)**, 1.

De Laet C.E.D.H., van Hout B.A., Burger H. *et al.* (1997) Bone density and risk of hip fracture in men and women: cross sectional analysis. *BMJ*, **315**, 221–5.

DeLuca H.F. (1990) Osteoporosis and the metabolites of vitamin D. *Metabolism*, **4 (1)**, 3–9.

Dequeker J., Remans J., Franssen R., Waes J. (1971) Ageing patterns of trabecular and cortical bone and their relationship. *Calcil Tissue Res.*, **7**, 23.

Diamond T., Stiel D., Luncer M. *et al.* (1990) Osteoporosis and skeletal fractures in chronic liver disease. *Gut*, **31**, 82.

Diebold J., Batge B., Stein H. *et al.* (1991) Osteoporosis in longstanding acromegaly: characteristic changes of vertebral architecture and bone matrix composition. *Virch Archiv B.*, **4**, 209.

Dunhill M.S., Anderson J.A., Whitehead R. (1966) Quantitative histological studies on age changes in bone. *J Pathol Bacteriol.*, **94**, 275.

Eastell R., Riggs B.L., (1987) Calcium homeostasis and osteoporosis. *Endocrinol Metab Clin N Amer.*, **16 (4)**, 829.

Epstein S., Bryce G., Hinman J.W. (1986) The influence of age on bone mineral regulating hormones. *Bone*, **7**, 421.

Eriksen E.F., Mosekilde L. (1990) Estrogens and bone. In Heersche and Kanis (eds), *Bone and Mineral Research*, vol. 7. Amsterdam: Elsevier, pp. 273–312.

Eriksen E.F., Mosekilde L., Melsen F. (1985) Effects of sodium fluoride, calcium phosphate and vitamin D_2 on bone balance and remodelling in osteoporotics. *Bone*, **6**, 381–90.

Eventov I., Frisch B., Cohen Z., Hammel I. (1991) Osteopenia, hematopoiesis, and bone remodelling in iliac crest and femoral biopsies: a prospective study of 102 cases of femoral neck fractures. *Bone*, **12**, 1.

Ferris B.D., Klenerman L., Dodds R.A. (1987) Altered organisation of noncollagenous bone matrix in osteoporosis. *Bone*, **8**, 288.

Finkelstein J.S., Neer R.M., Biller B.M.K. *et al.* (1992) Osteopenia in men with a history of delayed puberty. *N Engl J Med.*, **326**, 600.

Foldes J., Parfitt A.M., Shih M.S. *et al.* (1991) Structural and geometric changes in iliac bone: relationship to normal aging and osteoporosis. *J Bone Miner Res.*, **6**, 759.

Francis R.M. (1990) *Osteoporosis: Pathogenesis and Management.* Dordrecht: Kluwer Academic.

Francis R.M., Peacock M., Aaron J.E. *et al.* (1986) Osteoporosis in hypogonadal men: role of decreased plasma 1,25-dihydroxyvitamin D, calcium malabsorption and low bone formation. *Bone,* **7**, 261–8.

Frisch B., Bartl R. (1990) *Atlas of Bone Marrow Pathology.* Dordrecht: Kluwer Academic.

Frisch B., Eventov I. (1986) Hematopoiesis in osteoporosis–preliminary report comparing biopsies of the femoral neck and iliac crest. *Isr J Med Sci.*, **22**, 380.

Gallagher J.C., Goldgar D., Moy A. (1987) Total bone calcium in normal women: effect of age and menopause status. *J Bone Miner Res.*, **2**, 491.

Gertner J.M., Root L. (1990) Osteogenesis imperfecta. *Orthop Clin N Amer.*, **21 (1)**, 151.

Goldman A., Davidson D., Pavlov H., Bullough P.G. (1980) 'Popcorn calcifications': a prognostic sign in osteogenesis imperfecta. *Radiology,* **136**, 351.

Hahn T.J., Halstead L.R., Strates B. *et al.* (1980) Comparison of subacute effects of oxacort and prednisone on mineral metabolism in man. *Calcif Tissue Int.*, **31**, 109–15.

Hansen M., Overgaard K., Riis B., Christiansen C. (1991) Role of peak bone mass and bone loss in postmenopausal osteoporosis: 12 year study. *BMJ,* **303**, 961–4.

Heany R.P., Recker R.R., Saville P.D. (1978) Menopausal changes in bone remodeling. *J Lab Clin Med.*, **92**, 964.

Hedlund L.R., Gallagher J.C. (1989) The effect of age and menopause on bone mineral density of the proximal femur. *J Bone Miner Res.*, **4**, 639.

Hodgson S.F. (1990) Corticoid-induced osteoporosis. *Endocrinal Metab Clin N. Amer.*, **19 (1)**, 95.

Hoffman G.S., Filie J.D., Schumacher H.R. *et al.* (1991) Intractable vasculitis, resorptive osteolysis and immunity to type I collagen in type VIII Ehlers–Danlos Syndrome. *Arthritis Rheum.*, **34**, 1466.

Jackson J.A., Kleerekoper M. (1990) Osteoporosis in men: diagnosis, pathophysiology, and prevention. *Medicine (Baltimore),* **69**, 137–52.

Khairi M.R.A., Johnston C.C. (1978) What we know – and don't know – about bone loss in the elderly. *Geriatrics,* **67**.

Kiezbak G.M. (1991) Age-related bone changes. *Exp Gerontol.*, **26**, 171.

Kim G.S., Kim C.H., Park J.Y. *et al.* (1996) Effects of vitamin B12 on cell proliferation and cellular alkaline phosphatase activity in human bone marrow stromal osteoprogenitor cells and UMR106 osteoblastic cells. *Metabolism,* **45 (12)**, 1443–6.

Kirsch E., Krieg T., Nerlich A. *et al.* (1987) Compositional analysis of collagen from patients with diverse forms of osteogenesis imperfecta. *Calcif., Tissue Int.*, **41**, 11.

Kleerekoper M., Peterson E.L., Nelson D.A. *et al* (1990) A randomized trial of sodium fluoride as a treatment for postmenopausal osteoporosis. *Osteoporosis Int.*, **1**, 155–61.

Lepore L., Pennesi M., Barbi E., Pozzi R. (1991) Treatment and prevention of osteoporosis in juvenile chronic arthritis with disodium clodronate. *Clin Exp Rheumatol.*, **9 (6)**, 33–5.

Lindsay R. (1990) Fluoride and bone-quantity versus quality. *N Engl J Med.*, **322 (12)**, 845.

Lindsay R. (1991) Estrogens, bone mass, and osteoporotic fracture. *Amer J Med.*, **91 (5B)**, 105.

Lindsay R., Cosman F. (1992) Primary osteoporosis. In Coe and Favus (eds), *Disorders of Bone and Mineral Metabolism.* New York: Raven Press, pp. 831–88

Lips P., Netelenbos J.C., Jongen M.J.M. *et al.* (1982) Histomorphometric profile and vitamin D status in patients with femoral neck fracture. *Metab Bon Dis Rel Res.*, **4**, 85–93.

LoCascio V., Bonucci E., Imbimbo B. *et al.* (1984) Bone loss after glucocorticoid therapy. *Calcif Tissue Int.*, **36**, 435–8.

Lukert B.P., Johnson B.E., Robinson R.G. (1992) Estrogen and progesterone replacement therapy reduces glucocorticoid-induced bone loss. *J Bone Miner Res.*, **7**, 1063–9.

Mack R.M., Ross P.K. (1990) A current perception of HRT risks and benefits. In DeLuca and Mazess (eds), *Osteoporosis: Physiological Basis, Assessment and Treatment.* Amsterdam: Elsevier, pp. 161–78.

Manolagas S.C., Bellido T., Jilka R.L. (1995) Sex steroids, cytokines and the bone marrow: new concepts on the pathogenesis of osteoporosis. *Ciba Found Symp.*, **191**, 187–96.

Marcus R. (1992) Secondary forms of osteoporosis. In Coe and Favus (eds), *Disorders of Bone and Mineral Metabolism.* New York: Raven Press, pp. 889–904.

Marcus R., Kosec J., Pfefferbaum A. (1983) Age-related loss of trabecular bone in premenopausal women: a biopsy study. *Calcif Tissue Int.*, **35**, 406.

Marcus R., Madvig P., Young G. (1984) Age-related changes in parathyroid hormone and parathyroid hormone action in normal humans. *J Clin Endocrinol Metab.*, **58**, 223.

Marini J.C., Gerber N.L. (1997) Osteogenesis imperfecta. Rehabilitation and prospects for gene therapy. *JAMA (United States),* **277 (9)**, 746–50.

Martin R.B., Pickett J.C., Zinaich S. (1980) Studies of skeletal remodeling in aging man. *Clin. Orthop. Rel Res.*, **149**, 268.

Mazess R.B. (1982) On aging bone loss. *Clin Orthop Rel Res.*, **165**, 239.

McDonald J.A., Dunstan C.R., Dilworth P. *et al.* (1991) Bone loss after liver transplantation. *Hepatology,* **14**, 59.

Melton L.J. (1990) Fluoride in the prevention of osteoporosis and fractures. *J Bone Miner Res.*, **5 (1)**, S163–7.

Melton L.J. (1991) Differing patterns of osteoporosis across the world. In C.H. III Chesnut (ed), *New Dimensions in Osteoporosis in the 1990s*. Hong Hong: Excerpta Medica, pp. 13–18.

Melton L.J. (1993) Hip fractures: a worldwide problem today and tomorrow. *Bone*, **14**, 1–8.

Melton L.J., Atkinson E.J., O'Fallon W.M. *et al.* (1991) Long-term fracture risk prediction with bone mineral measurements made at various skeletal sites. *J Bone Min Res.*, **6 (1)**, S136.

Meunier P., Courpron P., Edouard C. (1976) Physiological senile involution and patho-logical rarefaction of bone. *Clin Endocrinol Metab.*, **2**, 239.

Mosekilde L., Eriksen E.F., Charles P. (1990) Effects of thyroid hormones on bone and mineral metabolism. *Endocrinol Metab Clin N Amer.*, **19 (1)**, 35.

Mörike M., Windsheimer E., Brenner R. *et al.* (1993) Effects of transforming growth factor beta on cells derived from bone and callus of patients with osteogenesis imperfecta. *J. Orthoped. Res.*, **11 (4)**, 564–72.

Neaton J.D., Wentworth D. For the Multiple Risk Factor Intervention Trial Research Group (1992) Serum cholesterol. Blood pressure, cigarette smoking and death from coronary artery disease. Overall findings and differences by age for 316099 white men. *Arch Intern Med.*, **152**, 56–64.

Newton-John H.F., Morgan D.B. (1970) The loss of bone with age, osteoporosis, and fractures. *Clin Orthop.*, **71**, 229–52.

Nilas L., Christiansen C. (1987) Bone mass and its relationship to age and the menopause. *J Clin Endocrinol Metab.*, **65**, 697.

Nilsson B.E., Westlin N.E. (1973) Changes in bone mass in alcoholics. *Clin Orthop Rel Res.*, **90**, 229.

Nordin B.E.C., Heaney R.P. (1990) Calcium supplementation of the diet: justified by the present evidence. *BMJ*, **300**, 1056–9.

Parfitt A.M., Mathews C., Rao D. *et al.* (1981) Impaired osteoblast function in metabolic bone disease. In DeLuca, Frost, Jee, Johnston and Parfitt (eds), *Osteoporosis: Recent Advances in Pathogenesis and Treatment*. Baltimore: University Park Press, pp. 321–30.

Pocock N.A., Eisman J.A., Hopper J.L. (1987) Genetic determinants of bone mass in adults. A twin study. *J Clin Invest.*, **80**, 706.

Raisz L.G. (1988) Local and systemic factors in the pathogenesis of osteoporosis. *N Engl J Med.*, **318**, 818.

Raisz L.G., Shourki K.C. (1993). Pathogenesis of osteoporosis. In Mundy and Martin (eds), *Physiology and Pharmacology of Bone. Hand-book of Experimental Pharmacology*, **107**, 299–331.

Ralston S.H. (1997) Science, medicine and the future: Osteoporosis. *Br. Med. J.*, **315**, 469–72.

Recker R.R., Kimmel D.B., Parfitt A.M. *et al.* (1988) Static and tetracycline based bone histomorphometric data from 34 normal postmenopausal females. *J Bone Miner Res.*, 3, 133–44.

Reginster J.Y., Sarlet N., Deroisy R. *et al.* (1992) Minimal levels of serum estradiol prevent postmenopausal bone loss. *Calcil. Tissue Int.*, **51**, 340–3.

Remagen W. (1989) *Osteoporosis*. Basle: Sandoz.

Riggs B.L., Melton L.J.III (1986) Involution osteoporosis. *N Engl J Med.*, **314**, 1676–86.

Riggs B.L., Melton L.J.III (1992) The prevention and treatment of osteoporosis. *N Engl J Med.*, **327**, 620–7.

Riggs B.L., Wahner H.W., Melton L.J. (1986) Rates of bone loss in the appendicular and axial skeletons of women. *J Clin Invest.*, **77**, 1487.

Rigotti N.A., Nussbaum S.R., Herzog D.B., Neer R.M. (1984) Osteoporosis in women with anorexia nervosa. *N Engl J Med.*, **311**, 1601.

Rowe D.W., Shapiro J.R. (1990) Osteogenesis imperfecta. In Avioli and Krane (eds), *Metabolic Bone Disease*. Philadelphia: W.B. Saunders, p. 659.

Sanguinetti C., Greco F., Depalma L. *et al.* (1990) Morphological changes in growth-plate cartilage in osteogenesis imperfecta. *J Bone Jt Surg.*, **72B**, 475.

Smith E.L., Gilligan C. (1990) Calcium and exercise in prevention of bone loss in age. *Clin Nutr.*, **9**, 17.

Ste Marie L.G., Charhon S.A., Edouard C. *et al.* (1984) Iliac bone histomorphometry in adults and children with osteogenesis imperfecta. *J Clin Pathol.*, **37**, 1081.

Stevenson J.C. (1988) Pathophysiology of osteoporosis. *Triangle*, **27 (1/2)**, 47.

Stevenson J.C., Lees B., Devenport M. *et al.* (1989) Determinants of bone density in normal women: risk factors for future osteoporosis? *Br Med J.*, **298**, 924.

Suominen H., Heikkinen E., Vainio P., Laitinen T. (1984) Mineral density of calcaneus in men at different ages: a population study with special reference to life-style factors. *Age Ageing*, **13**, 273.

Termine J.D. (1990) Cellular activity, matrix proteins and aging bone., *Exp Gerontol.*, **25**, 217.

Tsipouras P., DelMastro R., Sarfarazi M. (1992) Genetic linkage of the marfan syndrome, ectopia lentis, and congenital contractual arachnodactyll to the fibrillin genes on chromosomes 15 and 5. *N Engl J Med.*, **326**, 905.

Vanberkum F.N.R., Beukers R., Birkenhager J.C. *et al.* (1990) Bone mass in women with primary biliary cirrhosis: the relation with histological stage and use of glucocorticoids. *Gastroenterology*, **99**, 1134.

Vigorita V.J., Suda M.K., Lane J.M. (1983) Osteoporosis with idiopathic nodular lymphoid hyperplasia of the marrow. *Arch Pathol Lab Med.*, **107**, 276.

Wasnich R., Davis J., Ross P., Vogel J. (1990) Effect of thiazide on rates of bone mineral loss: a longitudinal study. *BMJ,* **301**, 1303–5.

WHO Study Group (1994) *Assessment of Fracture Risk and its Application to Screening for Postmenopausal Osteoporosis*. Geneva: WHO Technical Report Series, 843.

Whyte M.P. (1990) Heritable metabolic and dysplastic bone disease. *Endocrinol Metab Clin N Amer.*, **19**, 133.

Whyte M.P., Bergfeld M.A., Murphy W.A. *et al.* (1982) Postmenopausal osteoporosis: a heterogeneous disorder as assessed by histomorphometric analysis of iliac crest bone from untreated patients. *Am J Med.*, **72**, 193–202.

Wilson A.J., Murphy W.A., Hardy D.C., Totty W.G. (1988) Transient osteoporosis: transient bone marrow edema? *Radiology,* **167**, 757.

7 Osteosclerosis

General aspects

Osteosclerosis (hyperostosis) may be localised, multifocal or generalised, usually involving both cortical and cancellous bone and is caused by increased bone formation, reduced bone resorption or both, and may be either inherited or acquired as a result of metabolic, inflammatory toxic or neoplastic disorders (Table 7.1) Osteosclerosis, therefore, may occur with disturbances in bone growth, in bone modeling (i.e. shaping of the bones) and in remodeling, i.e. turnover of bone.

Osteopetrosis (marble bone disease)

There are two main forms of inherited osteopetrosis:

1. An autosomal-recessive variant, affecting juveniles and frequently lethal because of hematopoietic failure.

2. An autosomal dominant late onset, milder form.

Osteopetrosis is characterised by an increase in bone mass, both cortical and trabecular (Figures 7.1–7.4), so that the distinction between them is blurred as the marrow spaces are diminished, or completely obliterated, causing osseous fragility and propensity to fractures, hematopoietic failure and neurologic complications.

The condition is due to defective osteoclasts that do not resorb bone, possibly due to defects in local signals, chemotactic factors, adhesion molecules, or other mechanisms intrinsic to osteoclasts. The exact pathogenesis is unknown, though various possibilities have been suggested:

1. Morphologic or biochemical abnormalities of the osteoclasts.

2. Abnormalities of the hematopoietic system, thus producing defective osteoclasts.

3. Abnormalities of the bone marrow stromal system.

4. Abnormalities of humoral factors; hormones, cytokines, chemotactic and other signals involved in bone resorption. A viral etiology has also been suggested. In juvenile cases, early transplantation with compatible bone marrow may induce production of normally functioning osteoclasts and thereby restore the equilibrium between formation and resorption, thus remodeling the marrow cavities and restoring hematopoiesis.

Fluorosis

Fluoride is incorporated into bone matrix and stimulates osteoblastic activity (Figures 7.5–7.7). Fluoride is lost very slowly from the skeleton – about 50% over 20 years. Bones throughout the skeleton are affected, especially the vertebrae and pelvis. Fluoride-induced effects include increased remodeling, trabecular bone and osteoid, so that a combination of osteosclerosis and osteomalacia may result, but the lamellar orientation is disordered so that the overall picture has some similarity to Paget's disease of bone. A definitive diagnosis is made by the clinical history and chemical analysis of a small piece of the biopsy.

Drugs, chemicals, vitamins and osteosclerosis

Other substances may also cause an increase in bone density: bisphosphonates, lead, bismuth, phosphorus and mercury, and retinoids. In children hypervitaminosis A and D may cause osteosclerosis.

TABLE 7.1 Main causes of osteosclerosis

Congenital disorders and dysplasias
Osteopetroses
Carbonic anhydrase II deficiency
Pycnodysostosis
Progressive diaphyseal dysplasia*
Hyperphosphatasia

Chemicals and toxins
Fluorosis
Hypervitaminosis A, D
Heavy-metal poisoning
Biphosphonate intoxication

Endocrine disorders
Primary hyperparathyroidism
Secondary hyperparathyroidism
Acromegaly
Hypothyroidism
Healing osteomalacia
Previous fractures

Inflammatory disorders
'Sclerosing myelitis'
Sarcoidosis*
Radiation*
Osteomyelitis* (followed by osteosclerosis)

Hematopoietic disorders
Sickle cell disease
Osteomyelosclerosis
Malignant lymphomas*
Multiple myeloma (sclerotic variant)*
Systemic mastocytosis*

Osteoblastic metastases
Prostate carcinoma*
Breast carcinoma*

Paget's disease (sclerotic phase)

* May occur as widespread or as patchy osteosclerotic lesions.

7.1 and 7.2 BMBS plastic, Gomori, low and high magnification, showing osteosclerosis.
7.1 (left) No clear separation of cortex and trabeculae.
7.2 (right) Greatly reduced intratrabecular spaces, containing loose connective tissue without hematopoiesis.

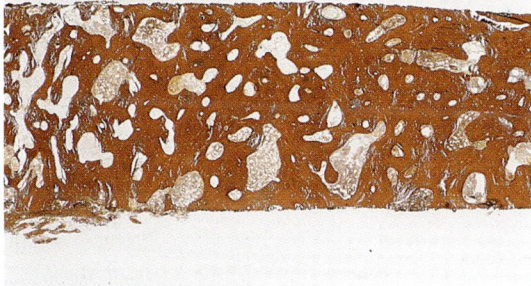

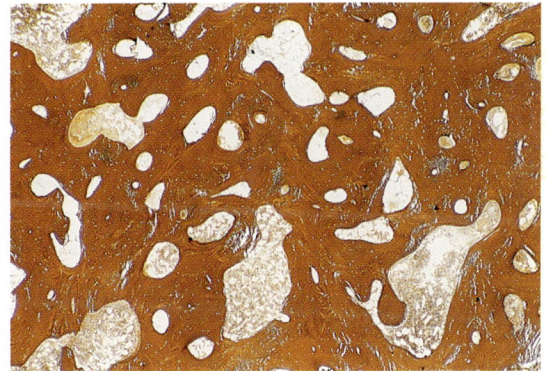

7.3 and 7.4 BMBS plastic, Haversian systems in osteosclerotic bone.
7.3 (left) Low magnification showing tetracycline labeling of Haversian system and osteocytic lacunae.
7.4 (right) Giemsa at higher magnification, Haversian system with narrow lumen containing blood vessels.

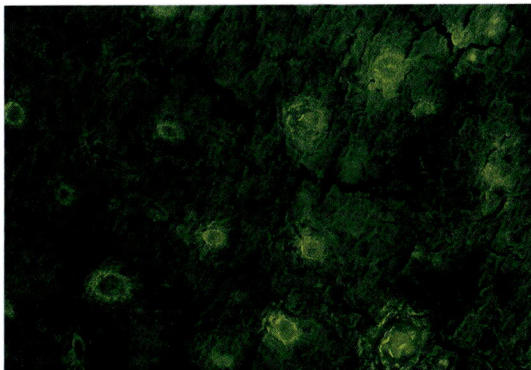

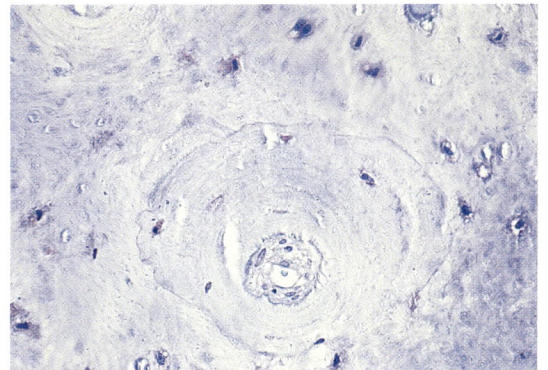

Dysplasias and osteosclerosis

Other rare conditions may cause osteosclerosis, but the ilium is affected only in very severe cases, e.g. Camurati–Engelman disease, progressive diaphyseal dysplasia, a developmental disorder, transmitted as an autosomal dominant trait. New bone formation involves both periosteal and endosteal surfaces of the diaphyses of long bones, but bones of the axial skeleton are only rarely affected. Age of onset, rate of progression and severity of disease are variable. There are characteristic radiologic and bone scan findings.

Hematologic disorders causing osteosclerosis are dealt with in the appropriate chapters.

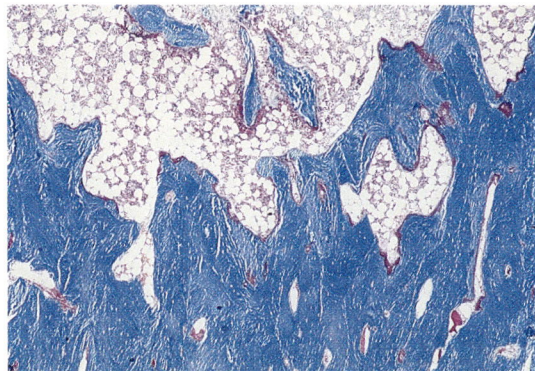

7.5 (left) BMBS plastic, Ladewig, low power view of osteosclerosis due to fluorosis; much of the bone is unmineralised (osteoid red).

7.6 (top right) BMBS plastic, Ladewig, osteosclerosis due to fluorosis. Mainly cortical bone, with little osteoid and subcortical hematopoiesis.

7.7 (bottom right) BMBS plastic, Gomori, showing sclerotic bone with extreme reduction in marrow spaces.

Clinical correlations

- Patient's age and history, manifest in infancy?
- Increase in skeletal mass: both cortical and trabecular, typical radiologic findings.
- Increased fragility and fracture rate; poor development in infants.
- Increased frequency of osteomyelitis, hepatosplenomegaly.
- Neurologic disorders due to pressure on nerves: compression of optic, oculomotor and facial nerves.
- Cytopenias due to encroachment of bone on marrow cavities and consequent hematopoietic failure.
- Complications due to cytopenias: infections and bleeding.
- In pharmacological osteosclerosis: history of drug intake; identification of causative substance, e.g. fluoride, bisphosphonates.
- Predisposing conditions in osteosclerosis, e.g. osteoblastic metastases; long-term strenuous physical activity.
- Dietary influences.

Check list: Osteosclerosis

- Adequate, non-tangential biopsy.
- Increase in cortical and trabecular bone mass (vol%)
- Apparent extension of cortex into trabecular region.
- Diminution and/or obliteration of marrow spaces.
- Drastic decrease in hematopoiesis, no infiltrations present.
- Little osteoclastic activity, the few osteoclasts present appear morphologically normal.
- On I.H. (immunohistology) osteoclasts are positive with acid phosphatase and with TRAP (tartrate resistant acid phosphatase).
- Mineralisation is normal.

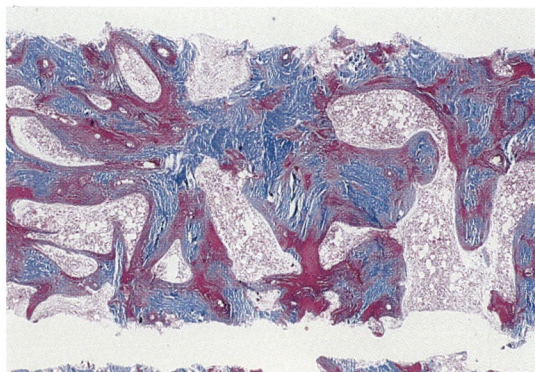

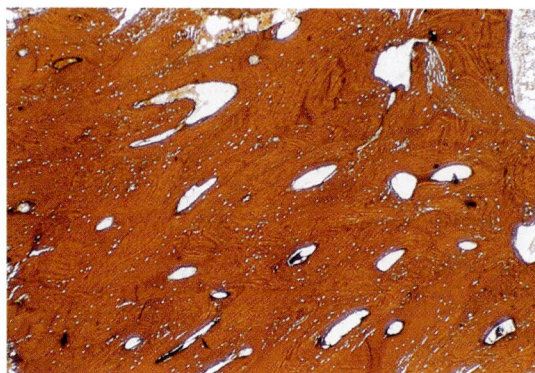

Bibliography

Beighton P., Horan F., Hammersma H. (1977) A review of the osteoscleroses. *Postgrad Med J.*, **53**, 507.

Bollersley J., Nielsen H.K., Storm T., Mosekilde L. (1988) Serum vitamin D metabolites and nuclear uptake of (3H)-1,25 dihydroxyvitamin D 3 in monocytes from patients with autosomal dominant osteopetrosis: a study of two radiological types. *Calcif Tissue Int.*, **43** (2), 67.

Bowley N.B. (1984) Osteosclerosis. Nordin: *Metabolic Bone and Stone Disease.* Edinburgh: Churchill Livingstone.

Coccia P.F., Krivit W., Cervenka J. *et al.* (1980) Successful bone marrow transplantation for infantile malignant osteopetrosis. *N Engl J Med.*, **302**, 701.

Evans R.A., Hughes W.G., Dunstan C.R. *et al.* (1983) Adult osteopetrosis. *Metab Bone Dis Rel Res.*, **5**, 111.

Glorieux F.H., Pettifor J.M., Marie P.J. *et al.* (1981) Induction of bone resorption by parathyroid hormone in congenital malignant osteopetrosis. *Metab Bone Dis Rel Res.*, **3**, 143.

Gruber H.E., Baylink D.J., (1991) The effects of fluoride on bone. *Clin Orthop.*, **267**, 264.

Khoker M.A., Dandona P. (1990) Fluoride stimulates (3D) thymidine incorporation and alkaline phosphatase production by human osteoblasts. *Metabolism*, **39 (11)**, 1118.

Labat M.L., Milhaud G. (1986) Osteopetrosis and the immune deficiency syndrome. In Peck (ed.), *Bone and Mineral Research*, vol. 4. Amsterdam: Elsevier, pp. 131.

Marks S.C. (1987) Osteopetrosis – multiple pathways for the interception of osteoclast function. *Appl Pathol.*, **5**, 172.

Marks S.C., McGuire J.L. (1989) Primary bone cell dysfunction II-osteopetrosis. In Tam, Heersche and Murray (eds), *Metabolic Bone Disease: Cellular and Tissue Mechanism.* Boca Raton: CRC Press, pp. 49.

Meunier P.J., Femenias M., Duboeuf F. *et al.* (1989) Increased vertebral bone density in heavy drinkers of mineral water rich in fluoride. *Lancet*, **45 (1)**, 152.

Milgram J.W., Jasty M. (1982) Osteopetrosis: a morphological study of twenty-one cases. *J Bone Joint Surg.*, **64 A**, 912.

Milhaud G., Labat M.L., Litwin I. *et al.* (1981) Osteopetro-rickets: a new congenital bone disorder. *Metab Bone Dis Rel Res.*, **3**, 91.

Mills B.G., Yake H., Singer F.R. (1988) Osteoclasts in human osteopetrosis contain viral nucleocapsid-like nuclear inclusions. *J Bone Miner Res.*, **3 (1)**, 101.

Reeves J., Arnaud S., Gordon S. *et al.* (1981) The pathogenesis of infantile malignant osteopetrosis: bone mineral metabolism, and complications in five infants. *Metab Bone Dis Rel Res.*, **3**, 135.

Silvestrini G., Ferraccioli G.F., Quaini F. *et al.* (1987) Adult osteoporosis: study of two brothers. *Appl Pathol.*, **5 (3)**, 184–9.

Whyte M.P. (1990) Heritable metabolic and dysplastic bone disease. *Endocrinol Metab Clin N Amer.*, **19 (1)**, 133.

Zerwekh J.E., Morris A.C., Padalino P.K. *et al.* (1990) Fluoride rapidly and transiently raises intracellular calcium in human osteoblasts. *J Bone Mineral Res.*, **5 (1)**, 131.

8 Osteomalacia

General aspects

Osteomalacia is the skeletal manifestation of defective bone formation and mineralisation, such that osteoid takes up 10% of the total bone volume and >25% of the trabecular surface is covered by osteoid. In children it is called 'Rickets'. The 'softness' of this defective bone results in progressive deformity and pain under normal stresses.

Severe osteomalacia results in increased width of osteoid seams and in patchy periosteocytic and intratrabecular areas of demineralisation; there is augmented bone remodeling together with anomalies of tetracycline labeling as revealed by bone biopsies. Biochemically a combination of low calcium (Table 8.1) and phosphate concentrations together with high levels of osseous alkaline phosphatase confirm the diagnosis. Nutritional, gastrointestinal and renal factors should be checked; the main causes of osteomalacia are given in Table 8.2. Since X-rays cannot distinguish osteoid tissue, a bone biopsy is mandatory if osteomalacia is suspected on biochemical or clinical grounds.

Process of mineralisation

To understand osteomalacia, it is necessary to consider the process of mineralisation (Figure 8.1). Approximately 90% of bone matrix is composed of collagen, while the remaining 10% consists primarily of organic non-collagenous proteins, proteoglycans and others, of which several, such as osteonectin, appear to control the orientation and growth of mineral crystals in osteoid. Following maturation for 8–20 days after synthesis, deposition of mineral starts at the osteoid–mineralised bone interface – the mineralisation front and most (80%) of the mineral is laid down within 3–4 days and the rest is deposited distally during the next 3–4 months until 95% saturation is reached. The mineralisation front is also the site of tetracycline binding. Double tetracycline labeling is used to investigate and quantitate dynamic bone formation. It involves oral administration of two short courses of tetracycline, which is deposited along the calcification front as two distinct lines which can be seen in the biopsy sections under fluorescent microscopy. A typical labeling schedule is: 300 mg tetracycline twice daily for 2 days, 10-day interval, with no tetracycline, then 300 mg tetracycline twice daily for 4 days. A bone biopsy is then taken 4–8 days later.

Diagnosis of osteomalacia

A diagnosis of osteomalacia is made when:

1. >25% of the trabecular surface is covered by osteoid (Figures 8.2 and 8.3).
2. Osteoid seams are increased in width >15 mm (Figures 8.4 and 8.5).
3. Periosteocytic zones of demineralisation are present (Figure 8.6).

In some cases, osteomalacia may be associated with osteosclerosis and with secondary hyperparathyroidism (Figures 8.7 and 8.8), especially in younger age groups. Moreover, subclinical osteomalacia may be more frequent in the elderly than previously suspected, particularly in house-bound patients with poor nutrition, and can be diagnosed only by bone biopsy. Osteomalacia may also be seen in the osteosclerotic phase of a myeloproliferative disorder (Figure 8.9; see also Chapter 23).

Axial osteomalacia
Axial osteomalacia is a rare disorder involving only the axial skeleton and affecting adult men.

TABLE 8.1 Causes of hypocalcemia

Hypoparathyroid

Renal
Acute renal failure
Chronic renal failure
Nephrotic syndrome

Gastrointestinal
Vitamin D deficiency
Malnutrition
Malabsorption
Acute pancreatitis
Hepatic disease

Metabolic
Alkalosis
Magnesium deficiency
Phosphate administration

Neoplastic
Osteoblastic metastases

Infectious
Measles

Drugs
Calcitonin
Bisphosphonates
Chelating agents
Aminoglycosides
Anticonvulsant drugs
Antineoplastic drugs

Postsurgical
Acute tissue necrosis
Massive blood transfusions
Toxic shock syndrome

Pregnancy

TABLE 8.2 Main causes of osteomalacia and rickets

Congenital
Hypophosphataemic rickets
Hypophosphatasia
Vitamin D-dependent rickets, types I and II
Primary renal tubular defects
Axial osteomalacia

Nutritional
Low dietary intake
Lack of exposure to the sun
Parenteral alimentation

Gastrointestinal
Postgastrectomy
Malabsorption syndrome
Hepatobiliary diseases
Chronic pancreatic insufficiency

Renal
Chronic renal failure
Dialysis bone disease
Renal tubular acidosis
Nephrotic syndrome

Tumor-associated
Mesenchymal tumors
Metastatic carcinomas
Acute leukemias
Malignant lymphomas
Multiple myeloma

Drugs/toxins
Fluoride
Bisphosphonates
Anticonvulsants
Barbiturates
Cholestyramine
Aluminum
Lead

Oncogenic (tumor-induced) osteomalacia

Oncogenic (tumor-induced) osteomalacia may accompany benign (mesenchymal) as well as malignant (prostatic, breast and other) tumors. Excision of the tumor, or effective treatment of the metastases, is followed by disappearance of the osteomalacia. In some cases, the osteomalacia may precede the detection of the tumor or the metastases.

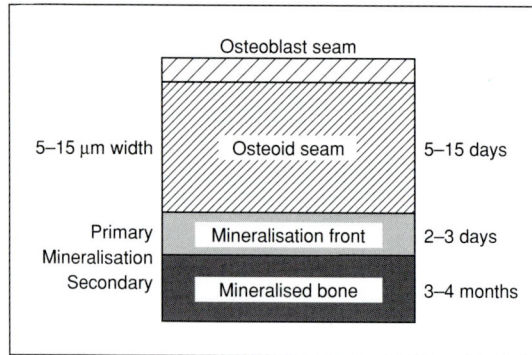

8.1 Steps in mineralisation showing the zones and the duration of the various steps in the process.

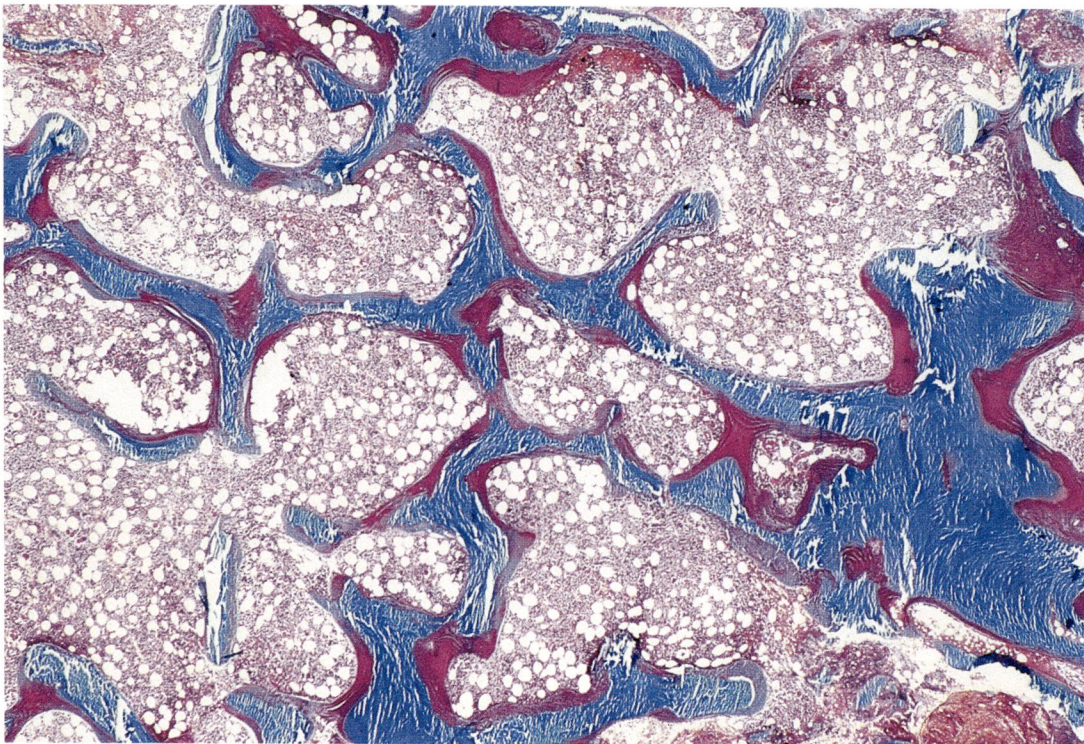

8.2 BMBS plastic, Ladewig, bone blue, osteoid red; trabecular volume not increased, but extensive osteoid seams present, overall structure preserved.

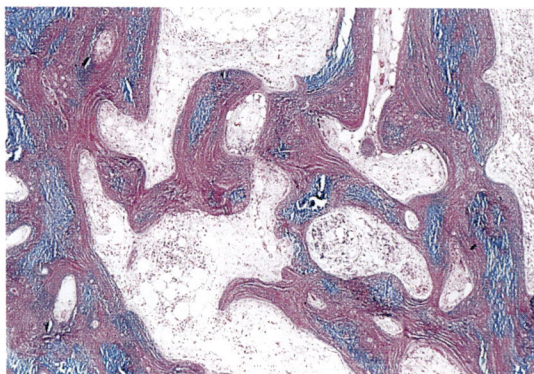

8.3 (left) BMBS plastic, Ladewig, trabecular volume increased, structure of network not preserved and more osteoid than bone present.
8.4 (right) BMBS plastic Giemsa, showing line of osteoblasts on osteoid (dark green) separated from the bone (pale green) by irregular cement lines.

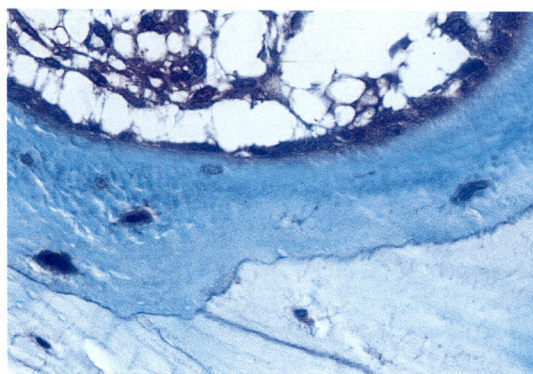

8.5 (left) BMBS plastic, Ladewig, showing demineralisation of large area of trabecular lamellae, red, bone blue.

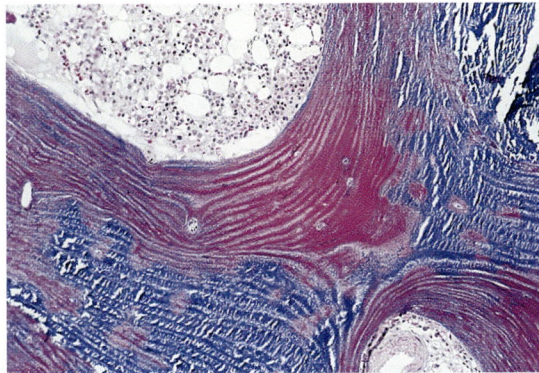

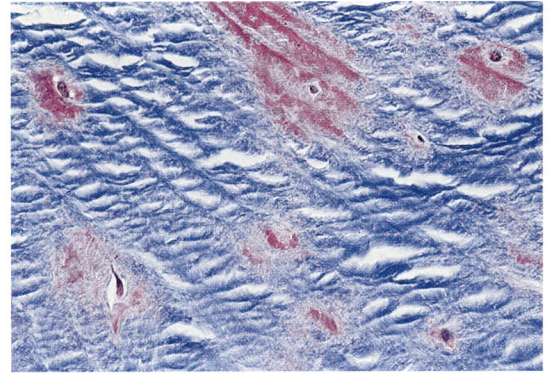

8.6 (right) BMBS plastic, Ladewig, showing periosteocytic osteoid, red.

8.7 (left) BMBS plastic, Giemsa, showing osteoid on trabecular surface and in tunnel underneath. Note osteoclast (left) surrounding osteoid seam.

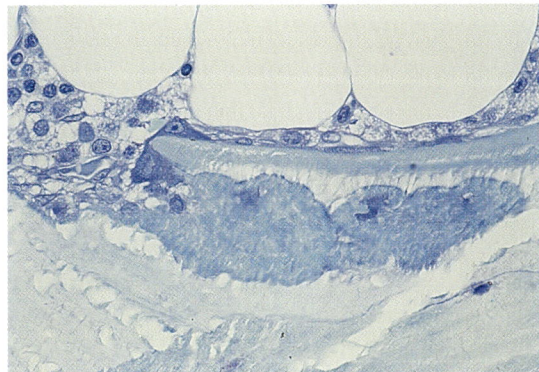

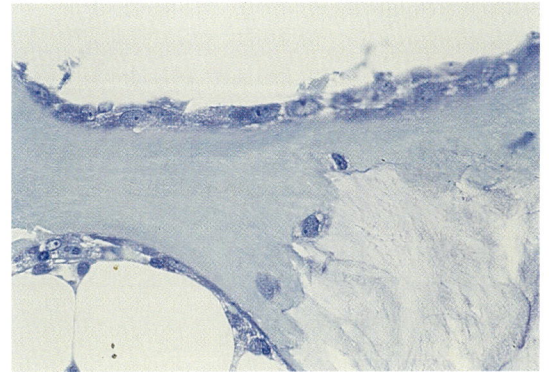

8.8 (right) BMBS plastic Giemsa, osteoid (left) spanning width of trabecula, lined by osteoblasts. Bone on right.

8.9 BMBS plastic, Ladewig, showing osteomalacia component in OMS, osteoid red.

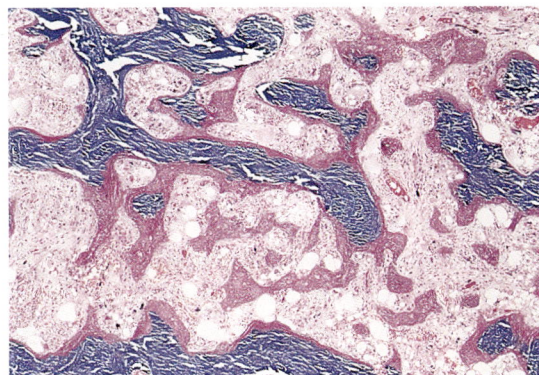

Drug-induced osteomalacia

Drug-induced osteomalacia is not rare and may be symptomless or lead to clinically apparent bone disease. Anticonvulsant and other toxic substances, acidosis and aluminum have been implicated. Treatment is usually effective, providing that the underlying cause can be treated, removed or reversed.

X-linked hypophosphatemia (XLH)

This is the most common form of inherited vitamin D-resistant rickets, and iliac crest biopsy shows an elevated bone volume: osteoid and mineralised bone are both increased.

Hypophosphatasia

This is also a heritable form of rickets due to the non-specific tissue alkaline phosphatase isoenzyme. The clinical manifestations vary from lethal to asymptomatic, occurring in four age groups: (1) perinatal (lethal), (2) infantile, (3) childhood and (4) adult.

Serum levels of calcium phosphate and $1,25\ (OH)_2D_3$ are not reduced, and therefore administration of these substances should be avoided. Prognosis improves with age after infancy.

Check list: Osteomalacia

- Undecalcified, plastic embedded biopsy.
- Adequate non-tangential biopsy.
- Appropriate stain to distinguish osteoid from calcified bone: toluidine blue, Ladewig, Goldner, Masson's trichrome.
- Cortex and trabecular bone present?
- Increased extent and width of osteoid seams?
- Periosteocytic and intratrabecular areas of demineralisation?
- Extension of osteoid through the width of a trabecula, from one side to the other?
- In several areas, alteration of trabecular microarchitecture, and large areas of the trabecular network consist of osteoid?
- Increased bone remodeling, resorption lacunae?
- State of hematopoiesis?

Clinical correlations

- Extremes of age: children and older people.
- Clinical symptoms related to bone and muscle pain, deformity and fractures.
- Weakness of muscles; and hypotonia in children.
- Characteristic biochemistry and radiology, hypocalcemia, Looser's zones in shafts of long bones.
- When secondary hyperparathyroidism occurs, subperiosteal resorption; osteoclastic activity.
- Predisposing condition(s) present; exposure to drugs and/or toxins.
- Inadequate diet and/or sunlight.
- If causative agent identified and removed, treatment of osteomalacia is effective.

Bibliography

Balsan S., Garabedian M. (1991) Rickets, osteomalacia and osteopetrosis. *Curr Opin Rheumat.*, **3**, 496.

Brunet J.A. (1986) Drug-induced osteomalacia. In Uhthoff and Stahl (eds), *Current Concepts of Bone Fragility*. Berlin: Springer, pp 271.

Brunette M.G. (1985) The X-linked hypophosphatemic vitamin D resistant rickets: old and new concepts. *Int J Pediatr Nephrol.*, **6**, 55.

Canalis E., Mccarthy T.L., Centrella M. (1993) Factors that regulate bone formation. In Munday and Martin (eds), *Physiology and Pharmacology of Bone. Handbook of Experimental Pharmacology*, **107**. Berlin: Springer, pp 249–66.

Cheng C.L., Ma J., Wu P.C. (1989) Osteomalacia secondary to osteosarcoma. *J Bone Joint Surg.*, **71A**, 288.

Condon J.R., Nassim J.R. (1971) Axial osteomalacia. *Postgrad Med J.*, **47**, 817.

Eisman J.A. (1988) Osteomalacia. *Clin Endocrinol Metab.*, **2** (1), 125.

Frymoyer J.W., Hodgkin W. (1977) Adult-onset vitamin D-resistant hypophosphatemic osteomalacia. *J Bone Jt Surg.*, **59A**, 101.

Garrick R., Ireland A.W., Posen S. (1971) Bone abnormalities after gastric surgery. *Ann Intern Med.*, **75**, 221.

Gruber H.E., Baylink D.J. (1991) The effects of fluoride on bone. *Clin Orthop.*, **267**, 264–77.

Hanna J.D., Niimi K., Chan J.C. (1991) X-linked hypophosphatemia. Genetic and clinical correlates. *Amer J Dis Child.*, **145**, 865.

Harrison N.A., Bateman J.M., Ledingham J.G., Smith R. (1991) Renal failure in adult onset hypophosphatemic osteomalacia with Fanconi syndrome: a family study and review of the literature. *Clin Nephrol.*, **35**, 148.

Hewison M. (1992) Vitamin D and the immune system. *J Endocrinol.*, **132**, 173.

Hughes M.R., Macloy P.J., O'Malley B.W. *et al.* (1991) Genetic defects of the 1,25-dihydroxyvitamin D3 receptor. *J Receptor Res.*, **11**, 699.

Itoi E., Sakurai M., Honma T. *et al.* (1991) Adult-onset vitamin D-resistant osteomalacia. *J Bone Jt Surg.*, **73A**, 932.

Kleerekoper M., Peterson E.L., Nelson D.A. *et al.* (1990) A randomized trial of sodium fluoride as a treatment for postmenopausal osteoporosis. *Osteoporosis Int.*, **1**, 155–61.

Mankin H.J. (1990) Rickets, osteomalacia, and renal osteodystrophy: an update. *Orthop Clin N Amer.*, **21** (1), 81.

McGuire M.H., Merenda J.T., Etzkorn J.R. (1989) Oncogenic osteomalacia. *Clin Orthop.*, **244**, 305.

Melton L.J. (1990) Fluoride in the prevention of osteoporosis and fractures. *J Bone Miner Res.*, **5 (1)**, S163–7.

Murray T.M. (1989) PTH-like substances. Tam, Heersche and Murray: *Metabolic Bone Disease: Cellular and Tissue Mechanisms*, vol. 125. Boca Raton: CRC Press.

Parfitt A.M. (1990) Osteomalacia and related disorders. In Avioli and Krane (eds), *Metabolic Bone Disease*, vol. 71. Edinburgh: Churchill Livingstone.

Pitt M.J. (1991) Rickets and osteomalacia are still around. *Radiol Clin N Amer.*, **29 (1)**, 97.

Reid I.R., Murphy W.A., Hardy D.C. *et al.* (1991) X-linked hypophosphatemia: skeletal mass in adults assessed by histomorphometry, computed tomography, and absorptiometry. *Amer J Med.*, **90**, 63.

Ronin D.I., Wu Y.C., Sahgal V., MacLean I.C. (1991) Intractable muscle pain syndrome, osteomalacia, and axonopathy in long-term use of phenotoin. *Arch Phys Med Rehabil.*, **72**, 755.

Siris E.S., Clemens T.L., Dempster D.W. *et al.* (1987) Tumor-induced osteomalacia. *Amer J Med.*, **82**, 307.

Sitrin M., Meredith S., Rosenberg I.H. (1978) Vitamin D deficiency and bone disease in gastrointestinal disorders. *Arch Intern Med.*, **138**, 886.

Taylor H.G., Hothersall T.E. (1991) Hypo-phosphatemic rickets and pyrophosphate arthropathy. *Clin Rheumatol.*, **10**, 155.

Tovey F.I., Karamanolis D.G., Godfrey J. (1987) Screening for early post-gastrectomy osteomalacia. *Practitioner*, **231**, 817.

Verge C.F., Lam A., Simpson J.M. *et al.* (1991) Effects of therapy in X-linked hypophosphatemic rickets. *N Engl J Med.*, **325**, 1843-B.

Weidner H. (1991) Review and update: oncogenic osteomalacia-rickets. *Ultrastruct Pathol.*, **15**, 317.

9 Primary hyperparathyroidism (PHPT)

Hypercalcemia and PHPT

PHPT is a disorder that usually comes to light when hypercalcemia is found, because hyperparathyroidism (HPT) and malignancy (leukemias, lymphomas and metastases) are the two most common causes for the increased calcium. More rarely, vitamin D intoxication, thyrotoxicosis, sarcoidosis and tuberculosis may also give rise to hypercalcemia (Table 9.1).

Groups of PHPT

HPT is characterised by overproduction of parathyroid hormones and may be classified into five groups (Table 9.2): the elevated parathyroid hormone levels act on bone and kidney and indirectly on the intestine and thereby cause the hypercalcemia. Alterations in vitamin D metabolism also participate in determining the clinical presentation of HPT. Though some pathways have been investigated, the precise mechanisms by which parathyroid hormone (PTH) stimulates bone remodeling are not yet known. PTH increases production of local growth factors such as TGF-β, PGE and IL-6. 1,25-(OH)$_2$ D$_3$ enhances effectiveness of PTH and is itself more rapidly catabolised, so that its level is decreased in overt HPT. Other substances such as corticosteroids, estrogens and thyroid hormones may influence the osseous manifestations of HPT. A direct effect of parathyroid hormone on osteoclasts has not yet been demonstrated – possibly it exerts its effect via osteoblast stimulation.

Primary HPT occurs mainly in young adults (20–40 years) and its expression is extremely varied. About 20% of patients have kidney stones and high levels of 1,25-(OH) vitamin D$_3$ levels, while <10% of patients have severe bone disease resulting in the 'osteitis fibrosa cystica' with relatively low levels of 1,25-(OH) vitamin D, but higher levels of serum calcium and PTH, with lower urinary calcium values than patients with kidney stones (Table 9.3). However, due to early detection because of more widespread biochemical screening, 60% of patients may be asymptomatic. Most cases (85%) of PHPT are due to one or more adenomas; the rest are caused by diffuse hyperplasia or parathyroid carcinoma. Secondary HPT develops in response to chronic stimulation – as in renal failure or intestinal malabsorption. If prolonged this may lead to tertiary HPT because of hyperplasia of the parathyroid glands, and this condition may be indistinguishable from PHPT. Recent radiologic analysis showed osteopenia in 62%, vertebral compression in 53% and subperiosteal resorption in only 21% of patients.

Histology of PHPT

Increased bone turnover (osseous remodeling) is the most consistent feature found in iliac crest biopsies (Figures 9.1–9.7, Table 9.4). There is a lack of orderly arrangement and balance between formation and resorption. Both osteoclastic and osteoblastic activities are closely associated with the blood vessels, especially the sinusoids and their endothelial lining cells. There is paratrabecular fibrosis in the affected areas, extending inwards into the marrow spaces, when severe the fibrosis may replace hematopoiesis in large areas of the biopsy. Osteoclastic remodeling usually outpaces osteoblastic bone production so that the trabeculae become excavated with cystic formations as well as exhibiting areas of

9.1–12 Aspects of osseous remodeling and bone marrow in PHPT.

9.1 BMBS plastic, Gomori, low-power view illustrating patchy, uneven distribution of affected trabecular network.

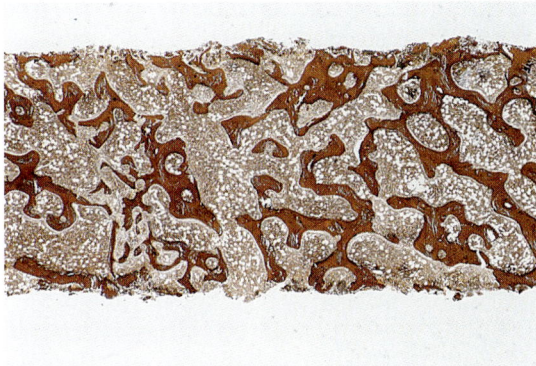

TABLE 9.1 Causes of hypercalcemia

Common
Malignant disease
Primary hyperparathyroidism

Uncommon
Thyrotoxicosis
Vitamin D intoxication
Sarcoidosis
Tertiary hyperparathyroidism
Hemodialysis
Immobilisation (not in the elderly)
Addison's disease
Phaeochromocytoma
Milk alkali syndrome
Thiazide diuretics
Lithium therapy
Parenteral nutrition
Vitamin A intoxication
Hypereosinophilic syndrome
Berylliosis
Tuberculosis

9.2 BMBS plastic, Giemsa, incipient excavating osteoclastosis, surface erosion.

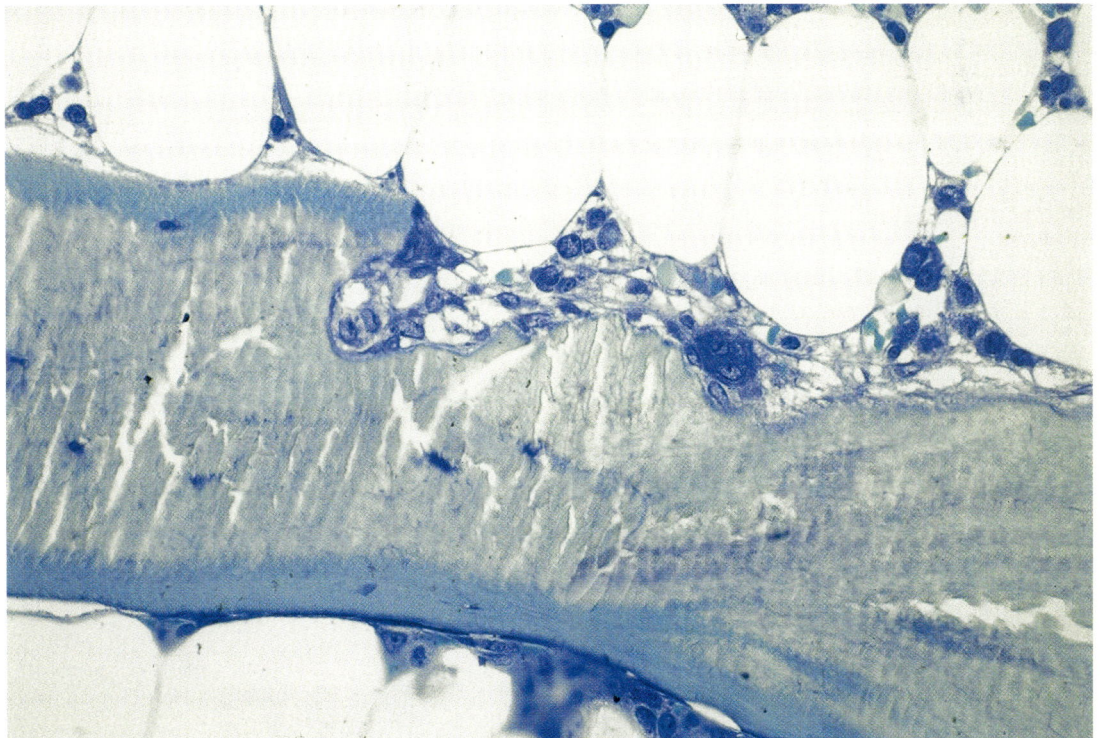

TABLE 9.2 Types of hyperparathyroid syndrome

Primary hyperparathyroidism
Parathyroid adenoma(s)
Parathyroid hyperplasia
Parathyroid carcinoma

Secondary hyperparathyroidism
Chronic renal failure
Gastrointestinal diseases
Pseudohypoparathyroidism

Tertiary hyperparathyroidism

Ectopic hyperparathyroidism

PTH-like substances (oncogenic)
'Pseudohyperparathyroidism'
Oncogenic osteomalacia

TABLE 9.3 Clinical and histological data in patients with PHPT disease: bone versus stone disease

Variant of PHPT	Stone disease	Bone disease
Number of patients	43	36
Trabecular bone (vol%, BV/TV	26	21
Osteoid (vol%)	2	11
Fibrosis (vol%)	0	31
Hematopoiesis (vol%)	45	21
Osteoclasts (no./mm^2)	1	11
Osteoblasts (no./mm^2)	3	19
Age of patients (years), median	44	55
Size of adenoma(s) (mm^2)	90	143
Renal calculi	+++	0
Osteolyses (X-ray)	0	+++
Serum ALP, increased	normal	+++

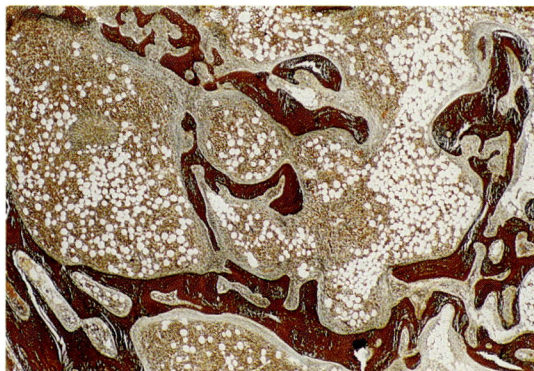

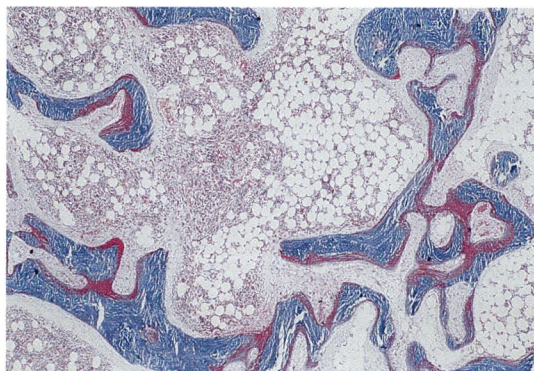

9.3 (left) BMBS plastic, Gomori, destruction of trabecular network, marked, extensive paratrabecular fibrosis, but some remaining hematopoiesis and fat cells.

9.4 (right) BMBS plastic, Ladewig, osteoid red, bone blue. Section similar to Figure 9.3, but showing extent of component of unmineralised bone.

TABLE 9.4 Histomorphometry of iliac crest biopsies in PHPT

Parameters*	Units	PHPT mean (maximum)	Normal mean
Lamellar bone	LBV/TV, %	19 (62)	22
Woven bone	WBV/TV, %	5 (32)	–
Osteoid	OSV/TV, %	3 (24)	1
Howship's lacunae	HOV/TV, %	5 (29)	–
Osteoclasts	No./mm^2 bone area	16.3 (143)	1.0
Osteoblasts	No./mm^2 bone area	9.5 (4)	2.5
Hematopoiesis	HAV/TV, %	32 (61)	45
Fatty tissue	FAV/TV, %	22 (55)	28
Fibrous tissue	FIV/TV, %	6 (71)	–
Sinusoids	SIV/TV, %	4 (15)	3
Edema	EDV/TV, %	4 (21)	1

* Derived from 139 cases.

9.5 (left) BMBS plastic, Gomori, part of a trabecula with hematopoiesis on one side and paratrabecular fibrosis on the other, and excavating osteoclastosis, upper right, typical of PHPT.

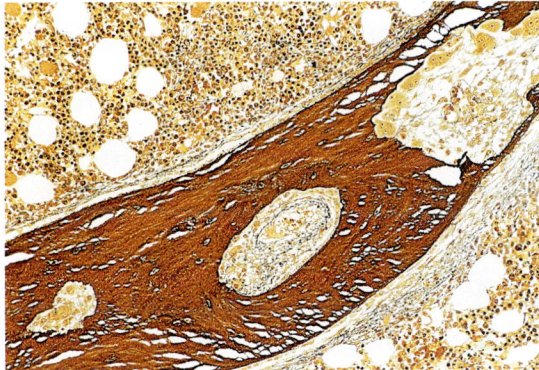

9.6 (right) BMBS plastic, Giemsa, tunneling osteoclastosis, large cavity filled by loose connective tissue containing developing osteoclasts. Note osteoclasts on inside of bone, upper left, center and lower right.

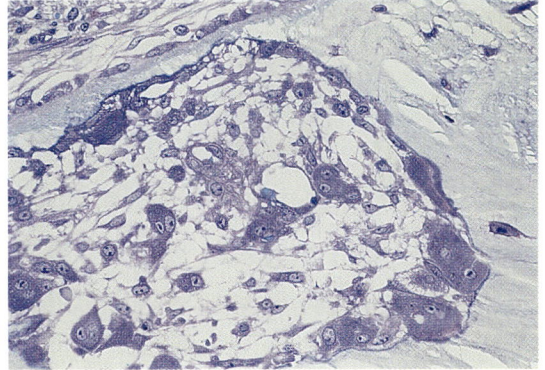

9.7 (left) BMBS plastic, Gomori, more advanced stage of osteoclastic erosion with fragmentation of trabecula, right.

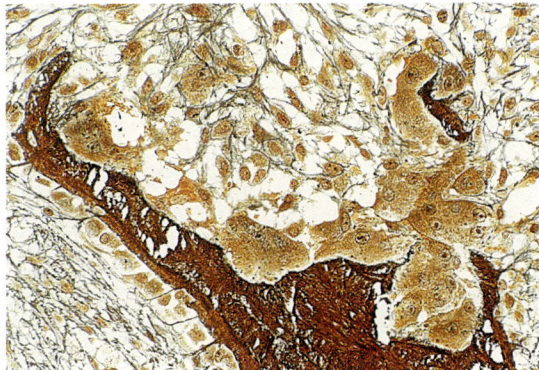

9.8 (right) BMBS plastic, Gomori. The trabecular junction has been reabsorbed and replaced by fibrosis. Note cellular bone marrow.

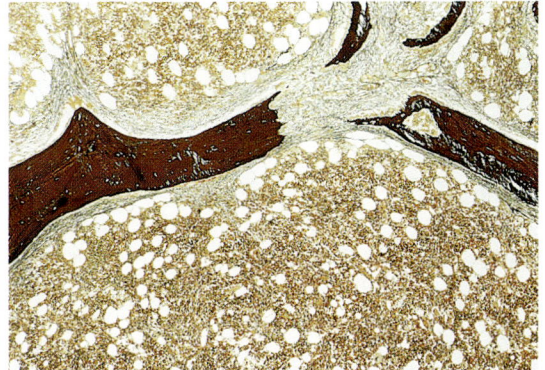

rarefaction and of wide osteoid seams (Figures 9.8–9.12) The cortical bone is likewise affected, and a variety of alterations has been observed (Figure 9.13). However, it should be borne in mind that the skeleton is not equally or evenly affected, so that iliac crest biopsies may show a spectrum of histologic manifestations from normal histologic parameters to the full-blown picture of osteitis fibrosa cystica with massive osteoclastic resorption, trabecular replacement by poorly mineralised woven bone and fibrosis of the bone marrow. There are small and large foci of resorption containing highly vascularised connective tissue, and areas of hemorrhage with hemosiderin-laden macrophages, as well as multinucleated giant cells brown tumors (Figures 9.14–9.16). Some degree of hyperparathyroidism may also contribute to

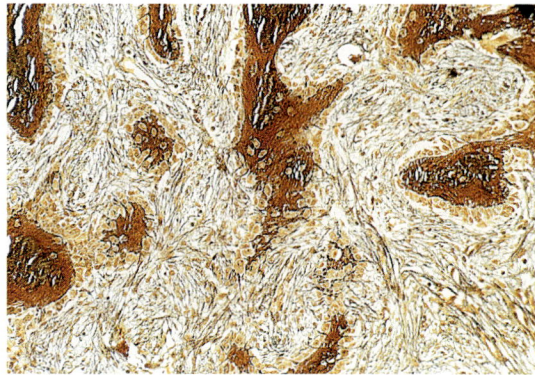

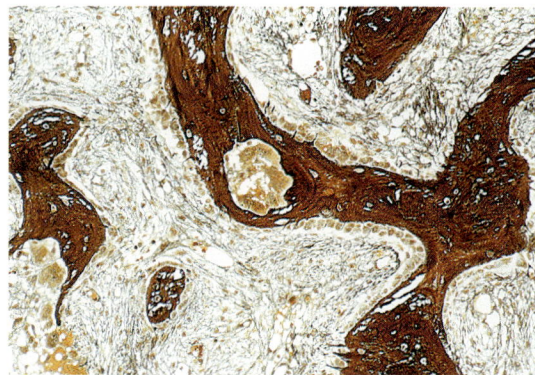

9.9 (left) BMBS plastic, Gomori, low-power view, extensive replacement of normal trabecular network and hematopoiesis, massive osseous remodeling and fibrosis of bone marrow.

9.10 (right) BMBS plastic, Gomori, high-power view, showing both osteoclastic and osteoblastic activity, and fibrous connective tissue but no hematopoiesis.

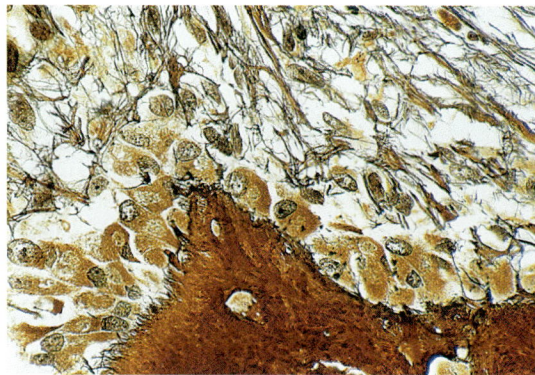

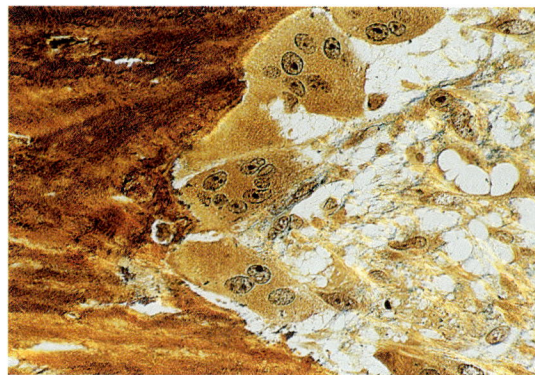

9.11 (left) BMBS plastic, Gomori, subcortical area, endosteal bone surface with pronounced osteoclastic activity.

9.12 (right) As for Figure 9.11, high-power view showing osteoclasts on the endosteal surface.

9.13 (left) Cortical bone in iliac crest biopsy in PHPT.

9.14 (right) BMBS plastic, Gomori, development of 'brown tumor' – accumulations of macrophages loaded with iron and hemosiderin.

Normal 41%		Spongiosa-like 17%	
Thin 8%		Dissecting osteoclasia 11%	
Broad 18%		Interrupted 5%	

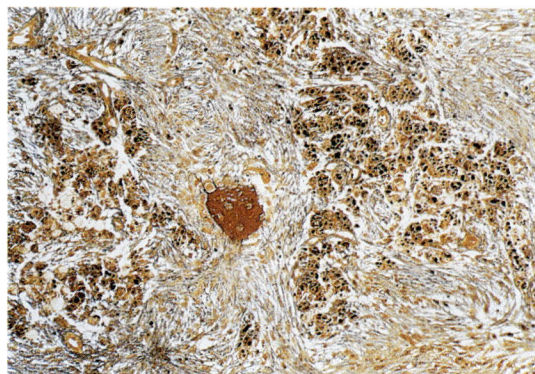

9.15 (left) BMBS plastic, Giemsa 'brown tumor' macrophages, left; note residual trabecula with osteoclastic remodeling, right; marrow replaced by connective tissue.

9.16 (right) BMBS plastic, Gomori, low-power view showing typical picture of full-blown PHPT including the features illustrated above.

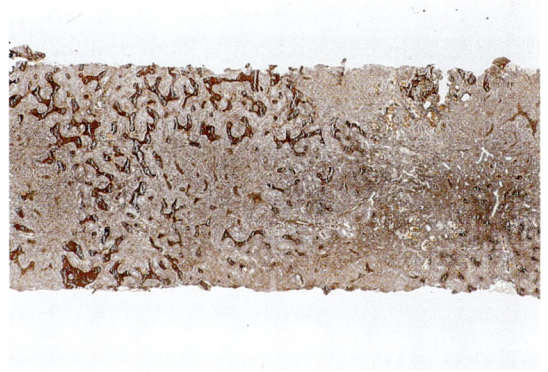

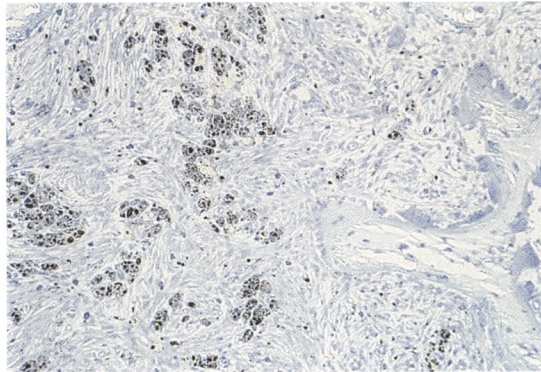

9.17 BMBS plastic, Gomori, showing calcified wall of blood vessel.

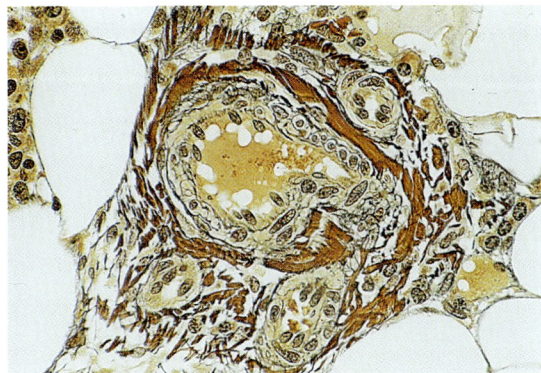

the osteopenia and 'osteoporotic' fractures of older people. Calcification of the walls of blood vessels also occurs (Figure 9.17).

Primary HPT may also occur in infants, and in cases of suspected or biochemically and radiologically supported HPT, a bone biopsy will reveal the exact type of osteodystrophy involved.

Nephrolithiasis and PHPT

In PHPT, two types of bone changes have been reported: striking lesions in patients without renal calculi, and minimal effects in those with kidney stones.

Differential diagnosis

Giant cell tumor of bone (also called osteoclastoma) must be considered in the differential diagnosis of histological findings in the bone biopsy interpreted as 'brown tumor' due

to hyperparathyroidism. The clinical picture and biochemical spectrum must always be taken into account. The great majority of giant cell tumors occur in the long bones, but rare instances of their occurrences in other locations, including the pelvis, have been reported. In addition, metastasis of giant cell tumors may be found in that region (see Chapter 12).

Hypoparathyroidism

Patients with low levels of parathyroid hormones showed no changes in iliac crest biopsies. However, in pseudo hypoparathyroidism (due to PTH resistance) there may be signs of secondary HPT, established previously.

Check list: Primary Hyperparathyroidism

- Adequate bone biopsy with cortical bone and trabecular network: cortex and trabeculae altered or not, cortical thinning, splits in cortex, subperiosteal remodeling?
- Increased bone turnover?
- Excavating and dissecting osteoclastosis?
- Surface erosion cavities?
- Numerous osteoclasts, most morphologically normal? Positive with acid phosphatase and tartrate resistant acid phosphate TRAP on immunohistology.

Continued

- Irregular cement lines, but not mosaic pattern?
- Para- and intertrabecular fibrosis, may replace bone marrow? Reticulin stain.
- Replacement of trabecular network by connective tissue?
- Aggregates of hemosiderin-laden macrophages, 'brown tumor'? Stain for iron. On immunohistology, CD68-positive cells increased.
- Mild-to-massive histologic alterations may occur; hematopoiesis present but reduced.
- Note: excavating or dissecting osteoclastosis in the cortex or the trabeculae is typical for PHPT, one or two such foci are enough to raise the possibility of increased secretion of parathyroid hormone.

Clinical correlations

- Fortuitous discovery due to biochemical screening.
- Occurs frequently in young adults 20–40 years.
- Very varied symptomatology; presenting feature may be nephrolithiasis.
- Subperiosteal resorption on radiology.
- Biochemical profile: hypercalcemia and high levels of 1,250H vitamin D, in some cases.
- Osteopenia and/or osteosclerosis on radiology; vertebral compression in many cases.
- Possibly PTH has a preferential effect on cortical bone: reduction in width and splits on radiology.
- Fractures in severe cases.
- Hematopoietic impairment in severe cases.
- PHPT may be cause of hip fracture in older people.

Bibliography

Benhamow C.L., Chappard D., Ganvain J.B. et al. (1991) Hyperparathyroidism in proximal femur fractures: biological and histomorphometric study in 21 patients over 75 years old. *Clin Rheumatol.*, **10**, 144.

Bianco P., Bonucci E. (1991) Endosteal surfaces in hyperparathyroidism: an enzyme cytochemical study on low-temperature processed, glycol methacrylate embedded bone biopsies. *Virch Arch A.*, **419**, 425.

Breslau N.A., Pak C.Y.C. (1992) Asymptomatic primary hyperparathyroidism. In Coe and Flavus (eds), *Disorders of Bone and Minerals Metabolism*. New York: Raven Press, pp. 523–38.

Byers P.D., Smith R. (1971) Quantitative histology of bone in hyperparathyroidism: its relation to clinical feature, x-ray, and biochemistry. *Quart J Med.*, **160**, 471.

Charon S.A., Edouard C.M., Arlot M.E., Meunier P.J. (1982) Effects of parathyroid hormone on remodeling of iliac trabecular bone packets in patients with primary hyperparathyroidism. *Clin Orthop Rel Res.*, **162**, 255.

Christiansen P., Steinicke T., Mosekilde L. et al. (1990) Primary hyperparathyroidism: changes in trabecular bone remodeling following surgical treatment – evaluated by histomorphometric methods. *Bone*, **11 (2)**, 75.

Delling G. (1987) Bone morphology in primary hyperparathyroidism. A qualitative and quantitative study of 391 cases. *Appl. Pathol.*, **5**, 147,

Editorials (1988) Acquired vitamin D deficiency and hyperparathyroidism. *Lancet*, **i**, 451.

Editorials (1991) Primary hyperparathyroidism and 1,25 dihydroxyvitamin D. *Lancet*, **337**, 768.

Eriksen E.F., Mosekilde L., Melsen F. (1986) Trabecular bone remodeling and balance in primary hyperparathyroidism. *Bone*, **7**, 213.

Genant H.K., Baron J.M., Straus F.H. et al. (1975) Osteosclerosis in primary hyperparathyroidism. *Amer J Med.*, **59**, 104.

George D.C., Incavo S.J., Devlin J.T., Kristiansen T.K. (1990) Histology of bone after parathyroid adenectomy. *J Bone Joint Surg.*, **72-A**, 1558.

Habener J.F., Potts J.T. (1990) Fundamental considerations in the physiology, biology, and biochemistry of parathyroid hormone. In Avioli and Krane (eds), *Metabolic Bone Disease*. Philadelphia: W.B. Saunders, pp. 69.

Hayes C.W., Conway W.F. (1991) Hyper-parathyroidism. *Radiol Clin N Amer.*, **29 (1)**, 85.

Lips P., Wiersinga A., van Ginkel F.C. *et al.* (1988) The effect of vitamin D supplementation on vitamin D status and parathyroid function in elderly subjects. *J Clin Endocrinol Metab.*, **67**, 644–50.

Mergenthaler H.G., Fink M., Sauer H. *et al.* (1989) Multiple brown tumours in a patient with nutritional secondary hyper-parathyroidism. *Klin Wschr.*, **67**, 42.

Morris C.A., Mitnick M.E., Weir E.C. *et al.* (1990) The parathyroid-related protein stimulates human osteoblast-like cells to secrete a 9,000 dalton bone-resorbing protein. *Endocrinology*, **126 (3)**, 1783.

Mosekilde L., Nelsen F. (1978) A tetracycline-based histomorphometric evaluation of bone resorption and bone turnover in hyperthyroidism and hyperparathyroidism. *Acta Med Scand.*, **204**, 97.

Mundy G.R. (1990) Primary hyperparathyroidism. Other causes of hypercalcemia. In Munday (ed), *Calcium Homeostasis: Hypercalcemia and Hypocalcemia.* London: Martin Dunitz, vol. 2, pp. 137–95.

Peacock M. (1993) Hyperparathyroid and hypoparathyroid bone disease. In Munday and Martin (eds), *Physiology and Pharmacology of Bone. Handbook of Experimental Pharmacology*, vol. 107. Berlin: Spinger, pp. 443–83.

Stewart A.F., Broadus A.E. (1990) Clinical review 16: parathyroid mormone-related proteins: coming of age in the 1990s. *J Clin Endocrinol Metab.*, **71**, 1410–14.

Wang J.C., Steiner W., Aung M.K., Tobin M.S. (1978) Primary hyperparathyroidism and chronic lymphatic leukaemia. *Cancer*, **42**, 1964.

Wendelaar Bonga S.E., Pang P.K.T. (1991) Control of calcium regulating hormones in the vertebrates: parathyroid hormone, calcitonin, prolactin and stanniocalcin. *Int Rev Cytol.*, **128**, 139–213.

10 Renal bone disease

General aspects and pathogenesis of renal bone disease

Abnormalities of cortical and trabecular bone and remodeling occur to a greater or lesser extent in patients with impairment of the function of the kidney. Such patients are, of course, subject to the same circumstances that affect the skeleton in other individuals; sex, age, activity, endocrine status, immobilisation, diseases such as diabetes, toxic substances such as ethanol, drugs and other aspects of life-style. In addition, the skeleton in renal disease is also influenced by the type of disease, degree of uremia and of secondary hyperparathyroidism (HPT), changes in vitamin D metabolism, type of therapy (dialysis and/or drugs), and osseous accumulation of toxic products (aluminum, fluoride, iron). Thus, renal osteodystrophy is caused by derangements in metabolic and homeostatic control of minerals (Tables 10.1–10.3). It represents a progressive form of bone disease that presents histologically as a mixture of osteosclerosis, osteoporosis, osteomalacia and osteitis fibrosis cystica; reduction in hematopoiesis and edema of the marrow contribute to the anemia of chronic renal failure. In areas of very active HPT there may be no residual hematopoietic tissue, its place having been taken by stimulated connective tissue and blood vessels, particularly arterioles. However, such mesenchymal activation is not exclusive to primary and secondary HPT, as it may occur in Paget's disease of bone and in osteomyelitis. In many instances there is a prominent population of infiltrating cells such as lymphocytes, plasma cells, macrophages and mast cells, especially in association with the angiogenesis and the osteogenesis which characterise the activated mesenchyme.

Main components of renal bone disease

The differences in activity of these factors and their interactions account for the considerable heterogeneity of renal osteodystrophy. There are three main components: (1) changes in bone remodeling, (2) changes in mineralisation, and (3) changes in bone mass, i.e. osteoporosis and osteosclerosis. Every degree of osteomalacia and of HPT may be seen, while osteoporosis and osteosclerosis may coexist in the same patient. When chronic renal failure occurs in children, growth retardation may become a major problem. There appears to be an increased risk of femoral neck fractures in patients with renal insufficiency receiving fluorides.

There are two broad categories of renal bone disease: high turnover (e.g. secondary HPT) and low turnover bone disease (e.g. osteomalacia and osteopenia), which can be divided into groups, though overlapping and transformations occur. The five groups may be briefly described below.

Hyperparathyroid uremic bone disease (Figures 10.1 and 10.2)

In uremic patients the hypocalcemia caused by phosphate retention, altered vitamin D metabolism, partial skeletal resistance to PTH, and impaired degradation of PTH metabolites,

TABLE 10.1 Pathophysiology of the bone lesions

Chronic renal failure:
- Phosphate retention → hyperphosphatemia
  ↵
- Hypocalcemia → secondary hyperparathyroidism
  ↓
- Decreased conversion of 25-(OH)-D3 → 1,25-(OH)$_2$-D3 (due to damaged kidneys)
  ↑
- High phosphorus → inhibits renal hydroxylase
- Low levels of 1,25-(OH)$_2$-D3
  ↓
- Reduced intestinal absorption of calcium

TABLE 10.2 Pathophysiology of the bone lesions

Chronic renal failure:
- Low levels of 1,25-(OH)$_2$-D
  ↵
- Bone unresponsive to parathyroid hormone
  ↵
- Parathyroids stimulated to increase secretion
  ↵
- Increased osteoclastic activity
- Parathyroid glands more sensitive to ↓ serum-ionised calcium levels
- Breakdown and excretion of PTH ↓
- Low 1,25-(OH)$_2$-D3 and low serum calcium
  ↵
- Osteomalacia

10.1 and 10.2
Hyperparathyroid uremic bone disease.

10.1 BMBS plastic, Gomori, showing greatly increased osseous remodeling, excavating osteoclastosis, paratrabecular fibrosis and some encroachment on the intertrabecular marrow spaces.

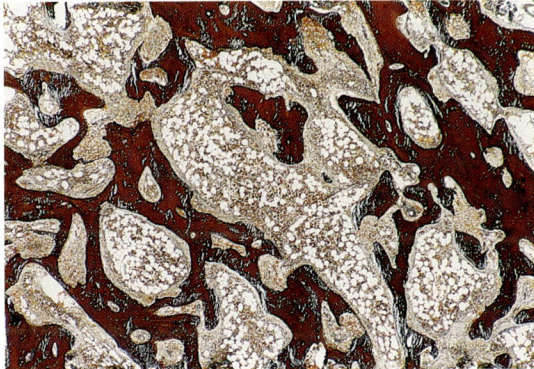

TABLE 10.3 Renal osteodystrophy

Contributing factors
- Hyperphosphatemia
- Metabolic acidosis
- Iron accumulation in bone
- Aluminium deposition in bone on calcification front → osteomalacia

10.2 BMBS plastic, Gomori, high power view of more advanced stage, showing lysis of trabecula and marked fibrosis.

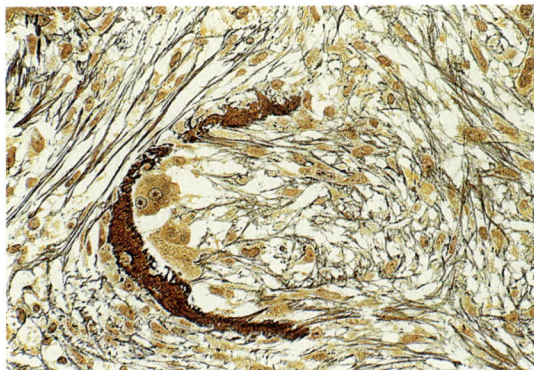

enhances PTH secretion. Eventually, complete resistance of bone to PTH may develop. Histologically there is increased osteoclastic bone resorption with dissecting, excavating and transecting osteoclasia, while increased osteoblastic activity accounts for increased formation of osteoid, not lamellar but 'woven'. Together, these changes undermine the strength of bone, and when extensive cause mechanical difficulties. Peritrabecular and medullary fibrosis encroach on hematopoiesis

93

and contribute to cytopenias in these patients. Subperiosteal resorption and dissecting osteoclasia lead to cortical thinning and porosity. Bone biopsy sections show minimal aluminum staining.

Osteomalacic uremic bone disease

(Figures 10.3–10.5)

This is characterised by hyperosteoidosis. Studies with tetracycline labeling demonstrate an impaired mineralisation and prolonged mineralisation lag time. Deposits of aluminum (occasionally iron) found at the mineralisation front apparently prevent mineralisation and inhibit hydroxyapatite crystal formation. This type of osteodystrophy most frequently causes bone pain and pathological fractures. A low turnover type of osteomalacia also occurs, with few active osteoblasts and low serum alkaline phosphatase.

Mixed uremic bone disease

(Figures 10.6–10.8)

There are characteristics of both HPT and osteomalacia, to varying degrees: increased osteoid, increased remodeling and patchy marrow fibrosis, abnormalities in tetracycline

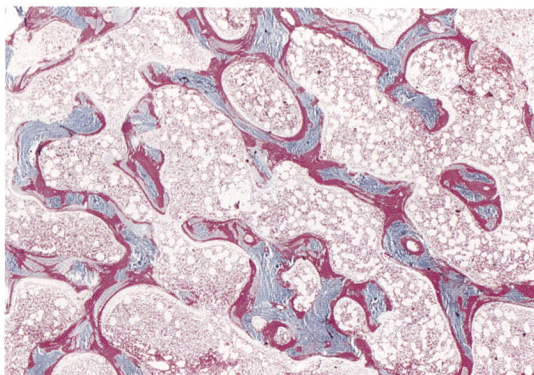

10.3–10.5 Osteomalacic uremic bone disease.

10.3 BMBS plastic, Ladewig, low power view to show degree of osteoid (red) in the trabecular network.

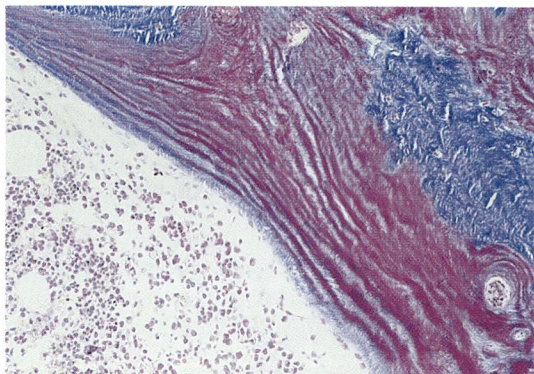

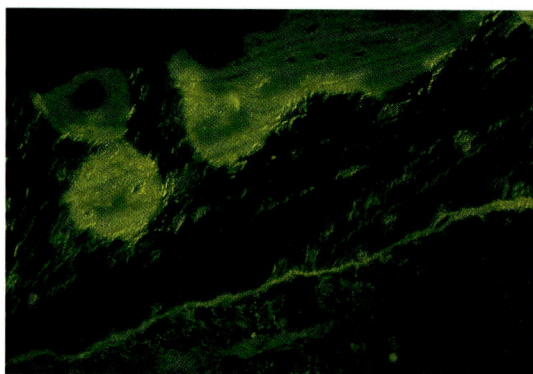

10.4 (left) BMBS plastic, Ladewig, endosteal surface of cortical bone showing osteoid (red).

10.5 (right) BMBS plastic, tetracycline labeling illustrating mineralisation defect.

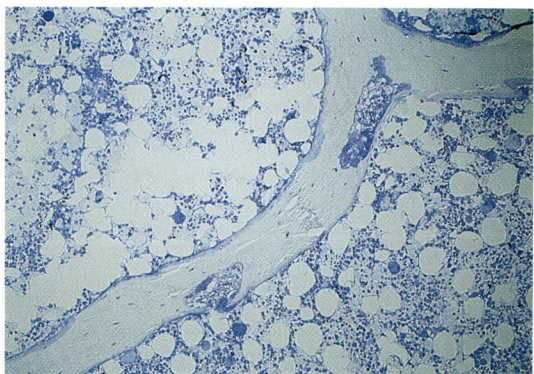

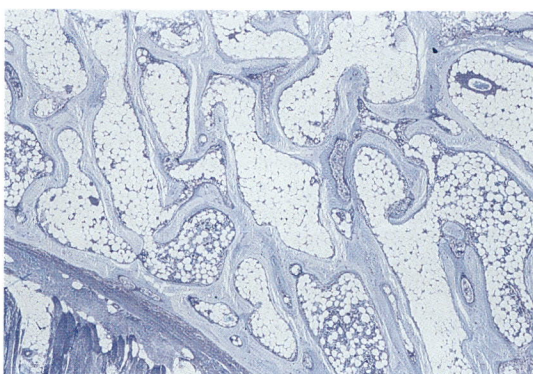

10.6–10.8 Mixed uremic bone disease.
10.6 (left) BMBS plastic, Giemsa, showing foci of osteoclastosis as in HPT.

10.7 (right) BMBS plastic, Giemsa, trabecular bone volume increased, extensive osteoid seams.

10.8 (left) BMBS plastic, Ladewig, showing attenuated trabecula, little osteoid but foci of osteoclastic remodeling.

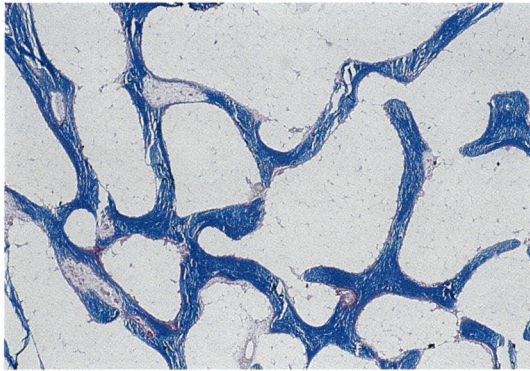

10.9 (right) BMBS paraffin, H&E showing osteopenic trabecular bone with little remodeling and hypocellular bone marrow.

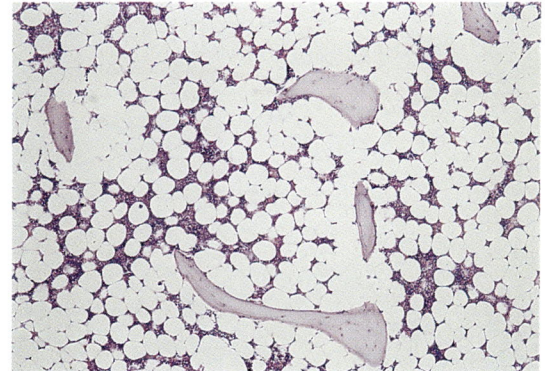

10.10 BMBS plastic, Giemsa, high magnification to show trabecula with only little bone cell activity, and fatty bone marrow.

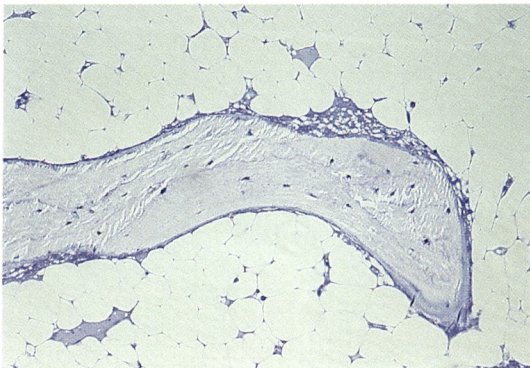

10.11–10.14 BMBS plastic, Giemsa, of a patient with congenital polycystic kidney disease who developed evidence of impairment of renal function at 70 years of age.

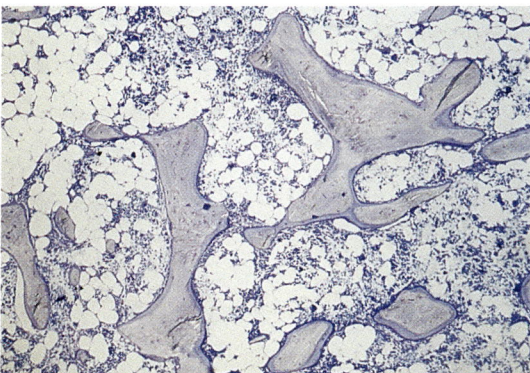

10.11 Low-power view showing trabecular bone with extensive osteoid seams.

labeling and significant aluminum and possibly iron deposition.

Low turnover uremic bone disease.
(Figure 10.9)
Remodeling, osteoid and bone mass are low; aluminum deposition is variable. Tetracycline

uptake demonstrates impaired bone formation rate.

Mild uremic bone disease (Figure 10.10)
This is found when the abnormalities of mineral metabolism in patients with renal failure have been treated. Bone biopsy reveals only a slight increase in remodeling, no mineralisation defect and a normal bone mass.

Congenital renal disorders

One example is polycystic kidney (Figures 10.11–10.14). In autosomal-dominant polycystic kidney disease (ADPKD) the gene has been located to chromosome 16p(13.3). This condition may be quiescent for long periods and only leads to problems late in adult life, when some degree of renal functional impairment occurs and consequent renal osteodystrophy. Erythropoietin production is usually not affected until later in life if and when the renal parenchyme is reduced and erythropoietin production is decreased.

Oxalosis (synonym: primary hyperoxaluria)

This rare metabolic disorder is characterised by increased urinary excretion of oxalic acid. Hyperoxalemia and hyperoxaluria cause recurrent kidney stones and progressive renal failure. Bone biopsy reveals the generalised

95

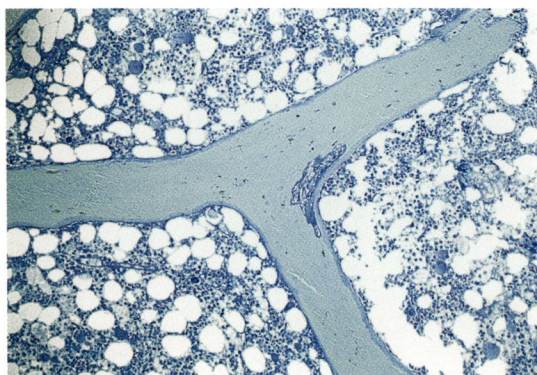

10.12 (left) Trabecular bone with focus of excavating osteoclastosis.

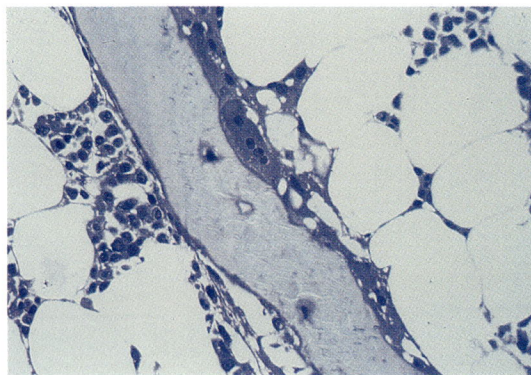

10.13 (right) Trabecular bone with surface erosion.

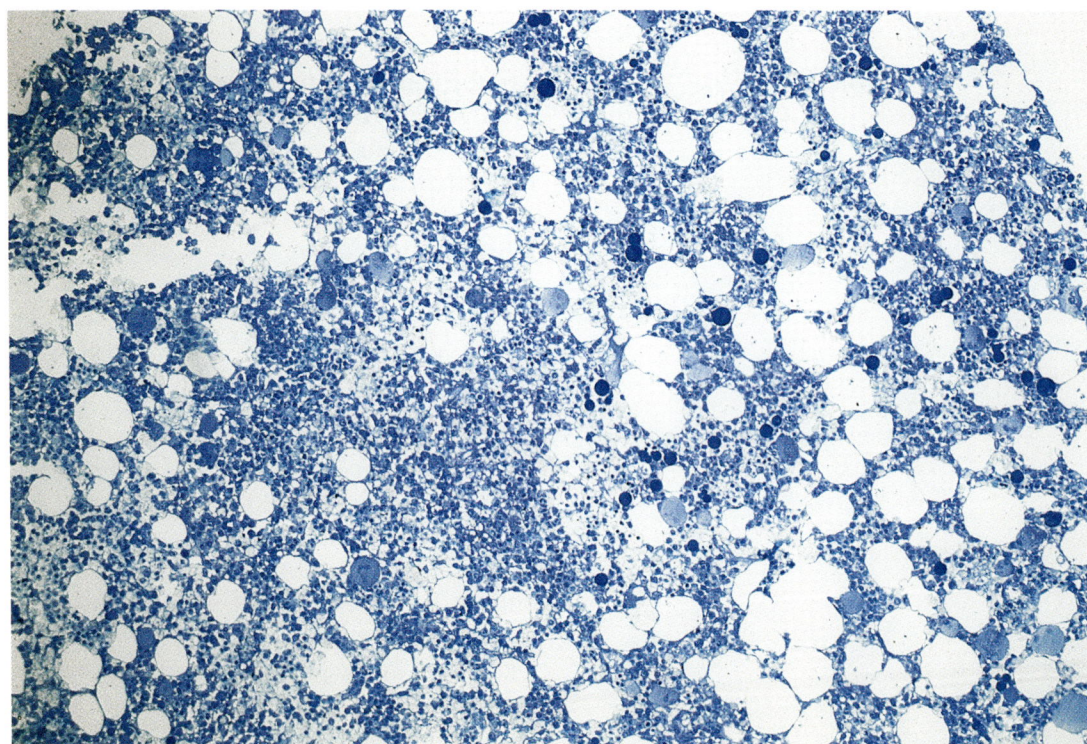

10.14 Another part of the same biopsy showing normocellular bone marrow with hematopoietic precursors and plasmacytosis. Large plasma cells with Russell bodies (dark blue).

depositions of calcium oxalate crystals in the periosteum and in the marrow cavities (Figure 10.15). Cystic rarefaction with marginal sclerosis may be present in the trabecular bone. Osseous changes due to secondary hyperparathyroidism may also be evident in cases of renal insufficiency.

Dialysis bone disease

The incidence of low turnover bone disease increases with duration of dialysis, and aluminum deposition is now implicated as the main cause for refractory osteomalacia (Figure 10.16). The additional osseous manifestations

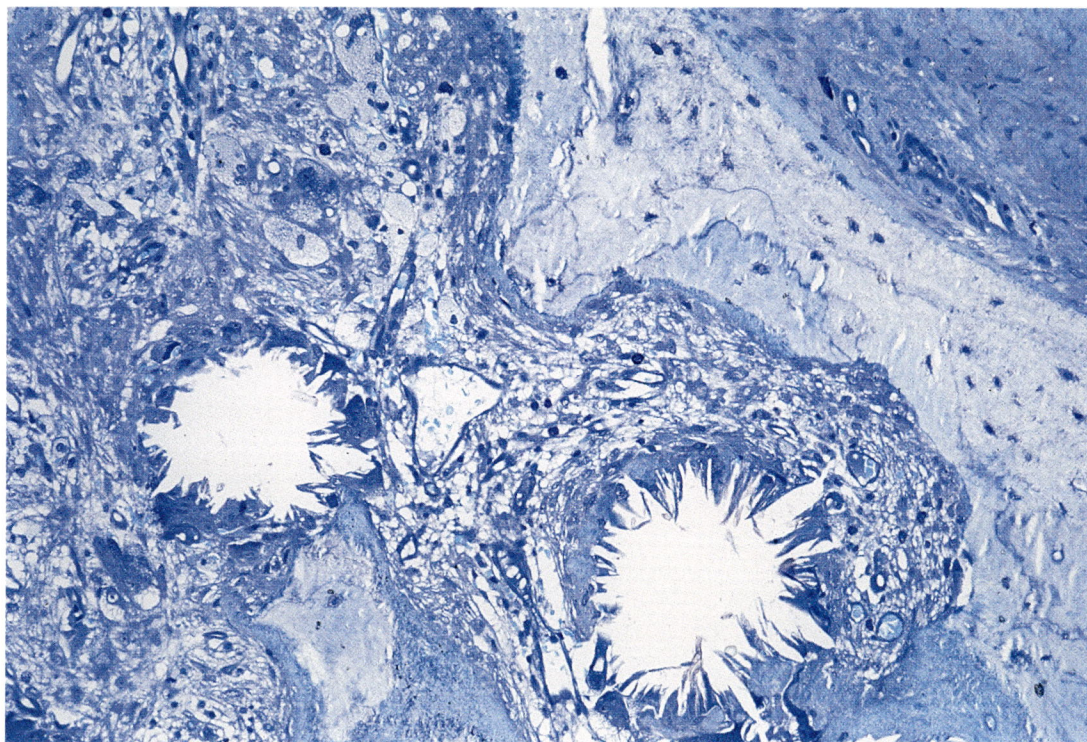

10.15 BMBS plastic, Giemsa, showing variably sized rosettes of calcium oxalate needles in a patient with hereditary oxalosis and renal disease.

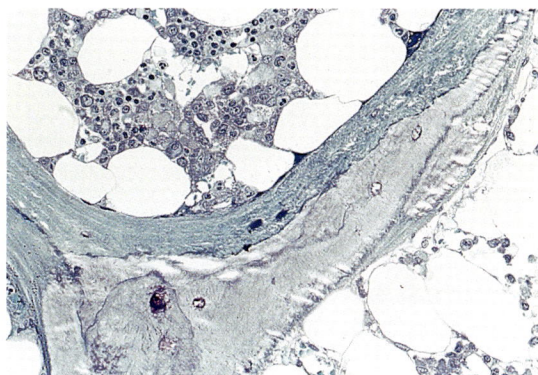

10.16 BMBS plastic, Giemsa, of a young patient on dialysis showing osteoid seam without osteoblasts.

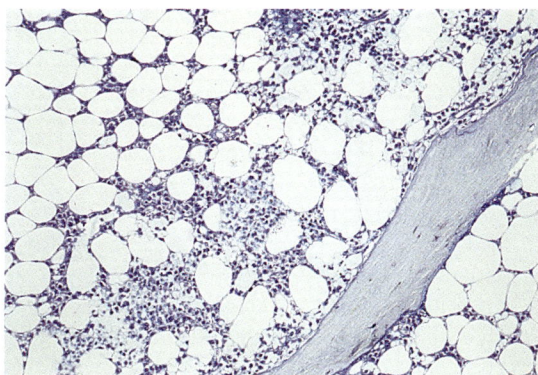

10.17 Bone biopsy 3 months after renal transplantation. BMBS plastic, Giemsa, showing trabecula with indication of previous osteoclastic remodeling, upper right, and somewhat hypocellular bone marrow containing hematopoietic precursors.

of patients on long-term dialysis, including continuous ambulatory peritoneal dialysis (CAPD) have been ascribed to vascular and interstitial deposits of amyloid composed of β_2 microglobulin. These changes include pathological fractures, periarthritis, pain in joints and carpal tunnel syndrome.

Bone disease after renal transplantation

With restoration of renal function, there is improvement in pre-existing bone disease, though effects of HPT may persist (Figure 10.17). Aluminum is rapidly excreted the associated bone disease also resolves after successful renal transplantation (see also Chapter 31). In contrast, the immunosuppressive therapy required in these patients results in progressive bone loss, i.e. osteoporosis, if not counteracted by, for example, therapy with bisphosphonates. Patients who had undergone parathyroidectomy before renal transplantation had a slower rate of bone loss.

97

Check list: Renal Bone Disease

- Adequate bone biopsy; both cortex and trabeculae present?

- Hyperparathyroid-like picture: incipient or full-blown?

- Increased or diminished bone mass?

- Increased osteoid? Appropriate stains: Goldner, Ladewig, toluidine blue.

- Less fibrosis than in primary HPT? Reticulin stain.

- Initially both hematopoiesis and fat are not affected; later hematopoiesis reduced.

- Subsequently, marrow atrophy and little osseous remodeling: low turnover osteopenia and hypocellularity.

Clinical correlations

- Mainly in patients with chronic renal failure: due to diabetes, hypertension, urologic disorders, unknown. Congenital such as polycystic kidney.
- Three main predisposing factors: anomalies of vitamin D metabolism, hyperparathyroidism and aluminum retention. Hypocalcemia stimulates PTH secretion.
- Muscular weakness, pruritus, vascular calcification.
- History: hematuria, dysuria, nocturia, flank pain.
- Biochemical profile: characteristic abnormalities.
- In children, chronic renal failure leads to growth retardation and skeletal deformities.
- Bone pain and fractures, aseptic necrosis of femoral head.
- Anemia in patients with long-standing disease and/or bone marrow fibrosis.
- Lymphomas may further complicate the situation.
- Deposition of B_2 microglobulin in walls of arteries, 'dialysis amyloidosis'.

Bibliography

Adams N.D., Carrera G.F., Johnson R.P. *et al.* (1982) Calcium-oxalate-crystal-induced bone disease. *Amer J Kidney*, **1**, 294.

Andress D.L., Maloney N.A., Coburn J.W. *et al.* (1987) Osteomalacia and aplastic bone disease in aluminium-related osteodystrophy. *J Clin Endocrinol Metab.*, **65**, 11.

Andress D.L., Maloney N.A., Endres D.B., Sherrard D.J. (1986) Aluminium-associated bone disease in chronic renal failure: high prevalence in a long-term dialysis population. *J Bone Mineral Res.*, **1**, 391.

Andress D.L., Nebeker H.G., Ott S.M. (1987) Bone histologic response to long-term

treatment with desferrioxamine for aluminium-related bone disease. *Kidney Int.*, **31**, 1344.

Andress D.L., Pandian M.R., Endres D.B., Kopp J.B. (1989) Plasma insulin-like growth factors and bone formation in uremic hyperparathyroidism. *Kidney Int.*, **36**, 471.

Boyce B.F., Fell G.S., Elder H.Y. (1982) Hypercalcaemic osteomalacia due to aluminium toxicity. *Lancet*,**ii**, 1009.

Burnell J.M., Teubner E., Wergedal J.E., Sherrard D.J. (1974) Bone crystal maturation in renal osteodystrophy in humans. *J Clin Invest.*, **53**, 52.

Carroll R.N.P., Williams E.D., Aung T. *et al.* (1973) The effects of renal transplantation on renal osteodystrophy. *Proc Europ Dialysis Transpl Assoc.*, **10**, 446.

Casey T.T., Stome W.J., DiRaimondo C.R. *et al.* (1986) Tumoral amyloidosis of bone of beta-2-microglobulin origin in association with long-term hemodialysis: a new type of amyloid disease. *Hum Pathol.*, **17**, 731.

Cassidy M.J.D., Owen J.P., Ellis H.A. (1985) Renal osteodystrophy and metastatic calcification on long-term continuous ambulatory peritoneal dialysis. *Quart J Med.*, **54**, 29.

Chan Y., Furlong T.J., Cornish C.J., Posen S. (1985) Dialysis osteodystrophy. A study involving 94 patients. *Medicine*, **64**, 296.

Coburn J.W., Slatopolsky E. (1991) The renal osteodystrophies. In Brenner and Rector (eds), *The Kidney*, 4th edn. Philadelphia: W.B. Saunders, pp. 2057.

Connor M.O., Garrett P., Dockery M. *et al.* (1986) Aluminium-related bone disease: correlation between symptoms, osteoid volume, and aluminium staining. *J Clin Pathol.*, **86**, 168.

Cotran R.S., Kumar V., Robbins S.L., Schoen F.J. (eds) (1994) The kidney. In *Robbins Pathologic Basis of Disease*, 5th edn. Philadelphia: W.B. Saunders, pp. 927–89.

Cundy T.F., Humphreys S., Watkins P.J., Parsons V. (1990) Hyperparathyroid bone disease in diabetic renal failure. *Diabetes Res.*, **14**, 191.

Damjanov I., Linder J. (eds) (1996) Kidney. In *Anderson's Pathology*, 10th edn. Mosby, pp. 2073–137.

Editorials (1991) Dialysis amyloidosis. *Lancet*, **338**, 349.

Gejyo F., Yamada T., Odani S. (1985) A new form of amyloid protein associated with chronic hemodialysis was identified as β2-microglobulin. *Biochem Biophys Res Comm.*, **129**, 701.

Harris P.C., Ward C.J., Peral B., Hughes J. (1995) Autosomal dominant polycystic kidney disease: molecular analysis. *Hum Mol Genet.*, **4**, 1745–9.

Harris P.C., Ward C.J., Peral B., Hughes J. (1995) Polycystic kidney disease. 1: Identification and analysis of the primary defect. *J Am Soc Nephrol.*, **6** (4), 1125–33.

Heath D.A. (1991) Primary hyperparathyroidism and renal osteodystrophy. *Curr Opin Rheumat.*, **3**, 490.

Henry H.L., Norman A.W. (1992) Metabolism of vitamin D. In Coe and Favus (eds), *Disorders of Bone and Mineral Metabolism*. New York: Raven Press, pp. 149–93.

Hutchinson A.J., Freemont A.J., Lumb G.A., Gokal R. (1991) Renal osteodystrophy in CAPD. *Adv Perit Dial.*, **7**, 237.

Kleinman K.S., Coburn J.W. (1989) Amyloid syndromes associated with hemodialysis. *Kidney Int.*, **25**, 567.

Linke R.P., Nathrath W.B.J., Eulitz M. (1986) Classification of amyloid syndromes from tissue sections using antibodies against various amyloid fibril proteins: report of 142 cases. In G.G. Glenner, E.F. Osserman, E.P. Benditt, E. Calkins, A.S. Cohen, D. Zucker-Franklin (eds), *Amyloidosis*. London: Plenum.

Llack F. (1991) Renal bone disease. *Transplant Proc.*, **23**, 1818.

Malluche H.H., Faugere M.C. (1989) Renal osteodystrohpy. *N Engl J Med.*, **321**, 317.

McCarthy J.T., Kumar R. (1990) Renal osteodystrophy. *Endocrinol Metabol Clin N Amer.*, **19** (1), 65.

McCarthy J.T., Milliner D.S., Kurtz S.B. *et al.* (1986) Interpretation of serum aluminium values in dialysis patients. *Amer J Clin Pathol.*, **86**, 629.

Rebel A., Malkani K. (1974) Fine structure of mast cells in iliac crest biopsies during renal osteodystrophy. *Pathol Biol.*, **22**, 221.

Sherrard D.J. (1986) Aluminium and renal osteodystrophy. *Semin Nephrol.*, **6**, 5.

Slatopolsky E., Coburn J.W. (1990) Renal osteodystrophy. In Avioli and Krane (eds), *Metabolic Bone Disease*. Philadelphia: W.B. Saunders, pp. 452.

Vandevyer F.L., Visser W.J., Haese P.C., DeBroe M.E. (1990) Iron overload and bone disease in chronic dialysis patients. *Nephrol Dial Transplant.*, **5**, 781.

Wendelaar Bonga S.E., Pang P.K.T. (1991) Control of calcium regulating hormones in the vertebrates: parathyroid hormone, calcitonin, prolactin. And stanniocalcin. *Int Rev Cytol.*, **128**, 139–213.

11 Paget's disease of bone

Pathogenesis

Paget's disease (previously called osteitis deformans) is triggered by structurally and functionally abnormal osteoclasts, whose unrestrained activity then stimulates the osteoblasts so that greatly increased overall remodeling results, with an overgrowth of disorganised bone formation. Though also occurring in young adults, it is commonest in middle and old age and is slowly progressive, causing bone pain, skeletal deformities, pathological fractures and neurological problems. A slow viral infection has been held responsible because of the presence of virus-like particles in the osteoclasts, positive antiviral reactions in the serum of patients with Paget's disease and presence of mRNA of some viruses in the bone cells. The incidence of Paget's disease is high – an estimated 4–5% of the general population in some countries (more men than women), and moreover other conditions, especially those affecting the older age groups, may also occur in patients with Paget's disease.

Characteristic histologic features

The disease manifests as a uni- or multifocal skeletal disorder characterised by rapid turnover, most readily visualised by bone scintigraphy, though about 12% of patients without pelvic involvement on scans had positive bone biopsies. Histologically large, multinucleated osteoclasts often with intranuclear and cytoplasmic inclusions are typical of the disease (Figures 11.1–11.4). They are hyperplastic as well as hypertrophic. Their size may reach many times that of normal osteoclasts. The

number of nuclei per cell also varies greatly – as many as 100 per cell have been counted (Figure 11.4). Initially, there is a marked increase in bone resorption, possibly due to raised secretion of IL-6; osteolytic lesions are produced (Figures 11.5 and 11.6). These evoke a compensatory osteoblastic reaction leading to uneven deposition of osteoid. This process is accompanied by vascular hyperplasia and fibrosis (Figure 11.7), which together with the enlarged trabeculae encroach on the marrow cavities and thereby cause a reduction in hematopoietic tissue (Table 11.1, Figures 11.8 and 11.9), and the anemia frequently observed in these patients. Both cortical and cancellous bone are involved (Fig.11.10–11.13), and the final result is structurally altered and abnormal bone, which is unable to withstand mechanical stress and therefore gives rise to the typical deformities in severely affected patients, especially of the cranium and the long bones of the limbs. In early lesions the osteoclastic activities and the overall picture may resemble that of primary hyperparathyroidism. The osteoblasts and osteocytes show no morphological abnormalities, though the bone produced is both woven and lamellar and has the mosaic pattern pathognomonic for Paget's disease (Figures 11.10–11.11). The mosaic pattern is due to cement lines of the newly formed bone which is randomly deposited by the osteoblasts to fill the cavities left by the osteoclasts. There is generally a focal involvement of the pelvis, vertebrae, femur, skull, tibia, clavicles and ribs, in decreasing order of frequency. Bone marrow biopsies are indicated both to establish the diagnosis and to monitor the effects of therapy. The osteoclasts are located

11.1–11.3 Osteoclast erosion of bone typical of Paget's disease of bone.

11.1 (left) BMBS plastic, Giemsa, osteoclast tunneling into bone.

11.2 (right) BMBS plastic, Gomori, showing typical multinucleated osteoclast in erosion cavity; note also osteoblasts, right, and fibrosis with blood vessels.

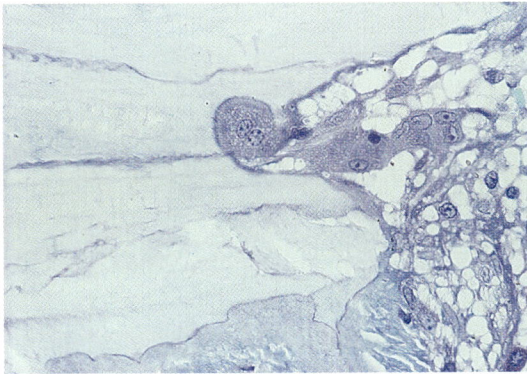

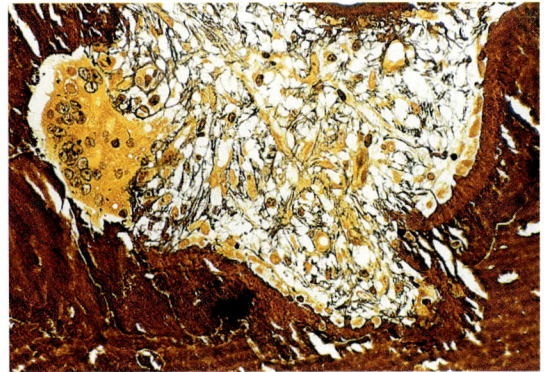

11.3 BMBS plastic, Giemsa, showing multinucleated osteoclasts; somewhat pleomorphic nuclei, some with large nucleoli. Note irregular cement lines in bone.

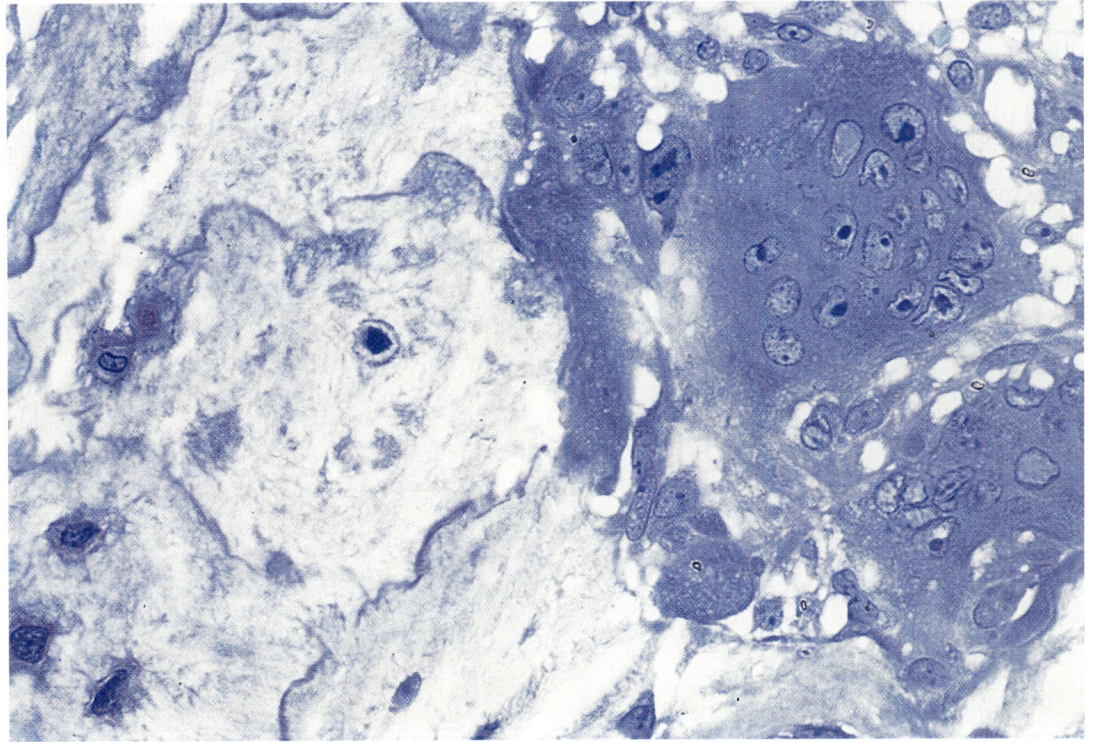

11.4 (left) Frequency of types of osteoclasts in iliac crest biopsies of patients with Paget's disease (n = 100).

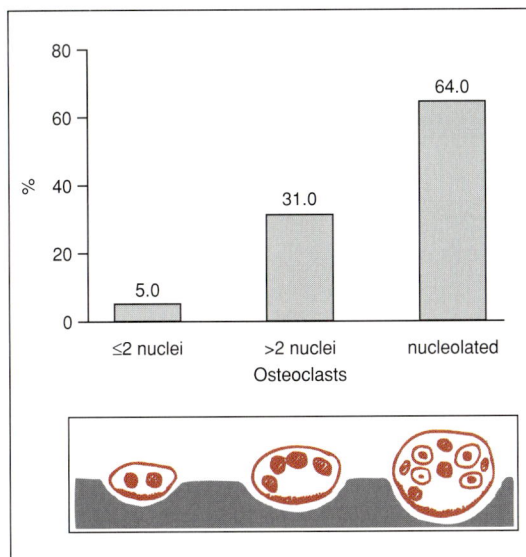

11.5 (right) BMBS plastic, Giemsa, showing erosion of trabecula.

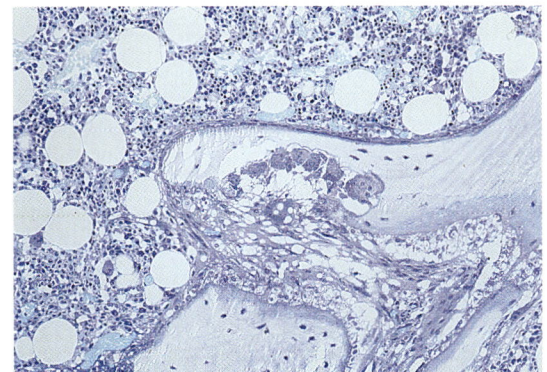

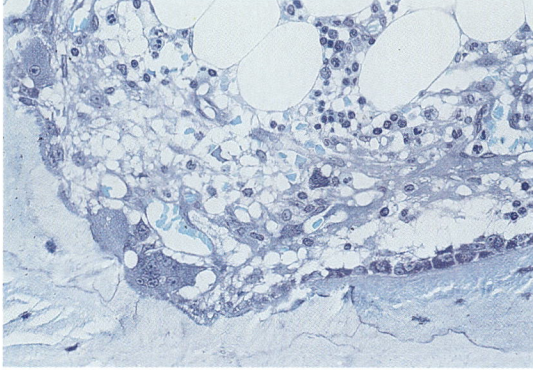

11.6 (left) BMBS plastic, Giemsa, illustrating side-by-side remodeling – erosion, left, formation, right.

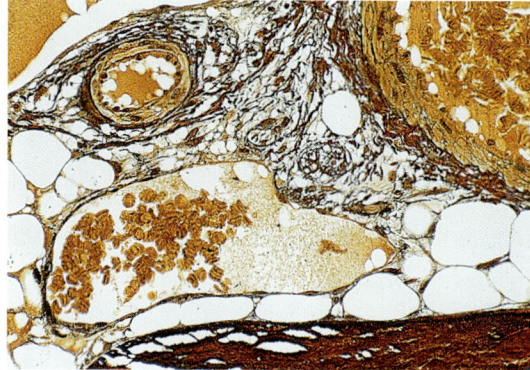

11.7 (right) BMBS plastic, Gomori, prominent blood vessels typical of Paget's disease near foci of remodeling.

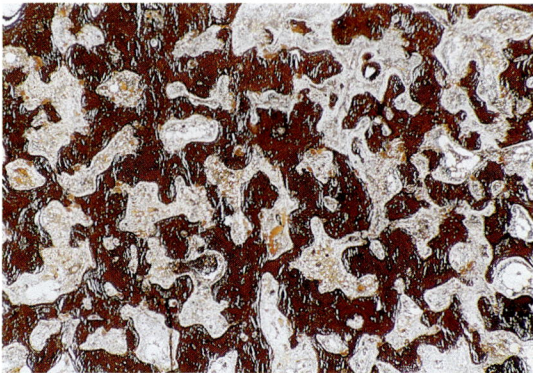

11.8 (left) BMBS plastic, Gomori, obliteration of normal trabecular structure, great increase in trabecular bone volume, remodeling still evident.

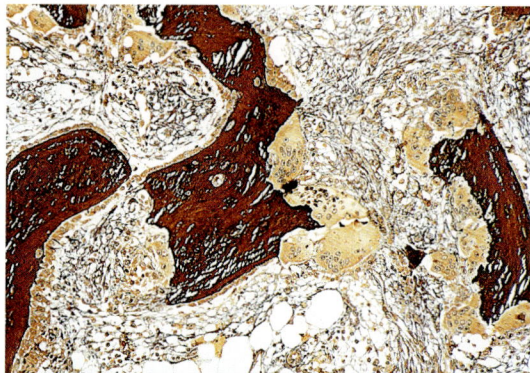

11.9 (right) As for Figure 11.8, higher magnification to show osteoclastic remodeling and fibrosis.

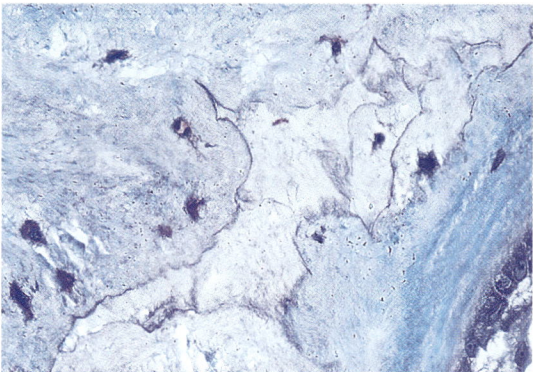

11.10 (left) BMBS plastic, Giemsa, cortical bone with mosaic pattern.

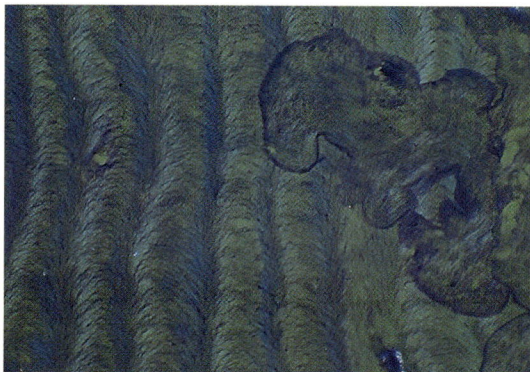

11.11 (right) As for Figure 11.10, cortical bone showing lamellae, left, filled erosion cavity outlined by cement lines, right.

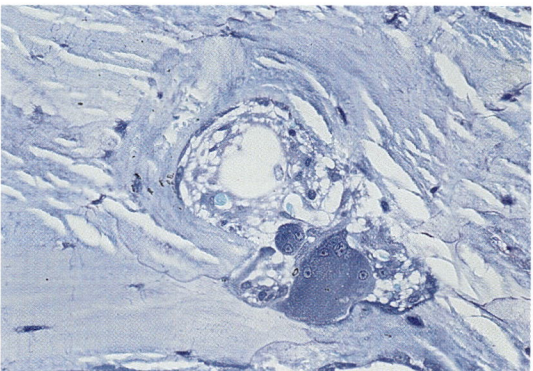

11.12 (left) As for Figure 11.11, cortical bone showing Haversian canal with osteoclastic remodeling.

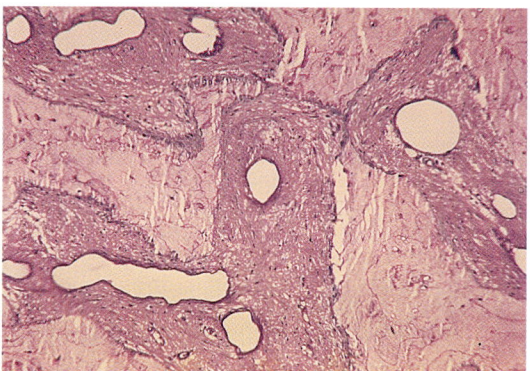

11.13 (right) BMB section paraffin, H&E, showing mosaic bone and marrow replaced by dense connective tissue, no remodeling and no hematopoiesis.

TABLE 11.1 Histomorphometry of iliac crest biopsies in patients with Paget's disease ($n = 100$)

Parameters	Units	Paget's disease	Normal
Spongiosa	%TV	42	22
Osteoid	%TV	3	1
Fibrosis	%TV	12	0
Hematopoiesis	%TV	17	47
Fatty tissue	%TV	18	27
Sinusoids	%TV	5	3
Osteoclasts	%TV	2	0
Osteoclasts	per mm² B.Ar.	4	1
Osteoblasts	per mm² B.Ar.	6	2
Mast cells	per mm² M.Ar.	14	3
Arteries	per mm² M.Ar.	1.2	0.4
Arterioles	per mm² M.Ar.	6.5	1.3
Capillaries	per mm² M.Ar.	48	18
Sinusoids	per mm² M.Ar.	53	34

TV, tissue volume; BV, bone volume; MV, marrow volume; B.Ar, bone area (2D); M.Ar, marrow area (2D).

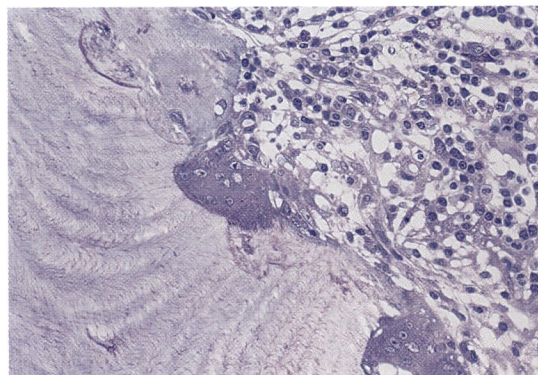

11.14 BMBS plastic, Giemsa, showing Paget's disease and lymphocytic infiltration in a patient with CLL.

in deep erosion cavities or in the vascular connective tissue adjacent to them. They resorb bone in a disorganised fashion, thus forming the mosaic or jigsaw pattern of bone after the cavities have been filled by the osteoblasts, and the cement lines remain to mark their boundaries (Figure 11.13). Part of the newly formed matrix is irregular 'woven' rather than linear lamellar bone. The bone marrow adjacent to the areas of active remodeling is frequently replaced by fibrous, vascular connective tissue with variable quantities and types of infiltrating cells, plasma and mast cells, lymphocytes and macrophages. In cases with additional disorders, these may also be found in the bone biopsy (Figure 11.14), in this case CLL.

Evolution of disease

Repeated waves of resorption and formation are eventually followed by the chronic or burnt-out phase, leaving sclerotic trabecular bone with abnormal structure but with high fragility, enclosing small marrow cavities filled with fibrotic tissue. This progression does not always occur evenly and various bones may be in different phases at any one time. Rarely, osteosarcoma may develop in one of the affected bones. In the generalised form of the disease the incidence of benign and malignant tumors has been estimated at 10%, though overall it is <1%. Most of the malignant tumors are osteosarcomas occurring most frequently in the pelvis.

Check list: Paget's Disease of Bone

- Cortex present, thick, thin, porous?
- Cancellous bone network present, altered, mosaic pattern?
- Volume of bone present: normal range increased, decreased?
- Remodeling: present, osteoclasts normal or abnormal, multinucleated – few, many; erosion cavities, osteoblasts present – few, many? In doubtful cases, immunohistology cytokeratin, EMA, S100, LCA, etc., to rule out other pathological processes.
- Balanced formation and resorption?
- Normal mineralisation?
- Paratrabecular fibrosis, alterations of blood vessels?
- Hematopoiesis: quantity, topography?
- Fat: normal proportion, increased, reduced?
- Iron quantity.

Example
Bone biopsy 3 × 30 mm. Biopsy showing stout cortical and trabecular bone with altered architecture and mosaic pattern of cement lines. Erosion cavities containing large multinucleated osteoclasts, many foci of osteoblastic remodeling with osteoid seams, paratrabecular fibrosis with blood vessels and infiltration of lymphocytes, plasma and mast cells. Hematopoiesis reduced (fat cells increased) but all maturational stages present.

Storage iron not increased. No infiltrations present. Summary: biopsy showing cortical and trabecular bone structure and remodeling and multinucleated osteoclasts indicative of Paget's disease of bone. Overall reduction in hematopoiesis. Diagnosis: Paget's disease of bone.

Clinical correlations

- Condition frequently asymptomatic; fortuitous discovery.
- Raised serum alkaline phosphatase, lytic or sclerotic or mixed foci on X-ray; hot spots on scan; osteocalcin not increased; urinary hydroxyproline and pyridinoline crosslinks are increased.
- Mono- or polyostotic involvement, X-ray, scan, CT, MRI.
- Bone deformity and enlargement present, 'hat too small', deafness.
- Pain, often strong, if lesion is in back (vertebrae), hip or long bones.
- Spinal cord symptoms due to pressure on nerves and blood vessels.
- Cardiac failure.
- Transformation to osteosarcoma (rare).
- Therapy – previously calcitonin. Today bisphosphonates that inhibit osteoclasts and resorption and later formation, due to 'coupling' of the two processes; newly formed bone is lamellar, symptoms are generally relieved.
- Monitor by levels of alkaline phosphatase in blood, urinary hydroxyproline and pyridinoline crosslinks; bone biopsy.

Bibliography

Freydinger J., Duling J., McDonald L. (1963) Sarcoma complicating Paget's disease of bone. *Arch Pathol.*, **75**, 496.

Guyer P.B. (1981) Paget's disease of bone. The anatomical distribution. *Metab Bone Dis Rel Res.*, **4**, 239.

Hailbach H., Farrell C., Dittrich F.J. (1985) Neoplasms arising in Paget's disease of bone: a study of 82 cases. *Amer J Clin Pathol.*, **83**, 594

Hamdy R.C. (1981) *Paget's Disease of Bone: Assessment and Management.* New York: Praeger.

Krane S.M. (1977) Paget's disease of bone. *Clin Orthop.*, **127**, 24.

Merkow R.L., Lane J.M. (1990) Paget's disease of bone. *Endocrinol Metab Clin N Amer.*, **19 (1)**, 177.

Meunier P.J., Coindre J.M., Edouard C.M., Arlot M.E. (1980) Bone histomorphometry in Paget's disease. Quantitative and dynamic analysis of pagetic and non pagetic bone tissue. *Arthritis Rheum.*, **23**, 1095.

Rebel A., Malkani K., Basle M., Bregeon C. (1987) The classic osteoclast ultrastructure in Paget's disease. *Clin Orthop.*, **217**, 4.

Roodman G.D. (1995) Osteoclast function in Paget's disease and multiple myeloma. *Bone,* **17 (2)**, 57S–61S,

Singer F.R. (1980) Paget's disease of bone: a slow virus infection? *Calcif Tissue Int.*, **31**, 185.

Siris E.S. (1990) Paget's disease of bone. In Favus (ed), *Primer on the Metabolic Bone Diseases and Disorders of Mineral Metabolism.*

Kelseyville: American Society for Bone and Mineral Research. pp. 253–9.

Wick M.R., Siegal G.P., Unni G.P. (1981) Sarcomas of bone complicating osteitis deformans (Paget's disease): fifty years' experience. *Amer J Surg. Pathol.*, **5**, 47.

Yates A.J.P. (1988) Paget's disease of bone. *Clin Endocrinol.*, **2 (1)**, 267.

Ziegler R., Holz G., Rotzler B., Minne H. (1985) Paget's disease of bone in West Germany. Prevalence and distribution. *Clin Orthop Rel Res.*, **194**, 199.

12 Miscellaneous bone disorders

This chapter deals very briefly with only a few conditions that may affect the bones of the pelvis, though primarily occurring in other skeletal areas, e.g. the long bones, but which may be found in iliac crest biopsies.

Gorham's disease (vanishing or disappearing bone disease, phantom bone, massive osteolysis)

This is a rare disorder where whole bones disappear; the cause is unknown The disease is possibly due to immune or other activation of osteoclasts, whose unbalanced activity is responsible for the vanishing bone. The first case of 'a boneless arm' was reported in 1838. The disorder affects mainly young adults. No genetic, metabolic or endocrine abnormalities have so far been identified. It may affect one or more bones and often occurs in the pelvic region as well as in long bones, ribs, vertebrae and other bones. Involvement of critical areas such as thorax and spine lead to severe complications (Figure 12.1). Histologic examination of affected sites shows marked osteoclastic resorption (Figures 12.2 and 12.3); though the osteoclasts appear morphologically normal. The resorption lacunae and sites of the vanished bone are filled by fibrous, vascularised connective tissue containing inflammatory cells. Adjacent to the lytic lesions, bone is covered by osteoid seams, with or without osteoblasts. The rate of progression is unpredictable, treatment (surgical excision and bone grafts) may be followed by recurrence; spontaneous remission has been reported.

Fibrous dysplasia

This is a fibro-osseous abnormality of the skeleton, possibly a developmental disorder of the mesenchyme of bone tissue. Bone and marrow are replaced by fibrous tissue in which bone may develop subsequently (Figures 12.4–12.7). Commonly involved skeletal sites include pelvis, long bones, ribs and facial bones. There are three main categories: (1) monostotic variant, (2) polyostotic type, which may be unilateral with a segmented distribution of the lesions, and (3) the McCune–Albright syndrome: multiple bone lesions, skin pigmentations and endocrine abnormalities. These include thyrotoxicosis, Cushing's disease, acromegaly, hyperprolactinemia, hyperthyroidism, rickets and osteomalacia. The differential diagnosis includes bone cysts, Paget's disease and primary hyperparathyroidism.

The fibrous dysplasia appears to commence in the marrow spaces and spreads to encroach on both cortical and trabecular bone (Figure 12.7). The lesions range in size from a few millimeters to large areas, causing distortion of the normal contour of the bone involved. The fibrous tissue consists of spindle-shaped fibroblasts and fibers arranged in whorls with foci of woven bone, osteoblasts, osteoclasts and occasional cysts and islands of cartilage. Malignant transformation is rare, occurring in <1% of the cases.

Osteosarcoma

This is the most common primary malignant tumor of bone (excluding hematopoietic

12.1 Involvement of skeletal sites in Gorham's vanishing bone disease. Data compiled from a review of the literature, each dot represents one involved site reported.

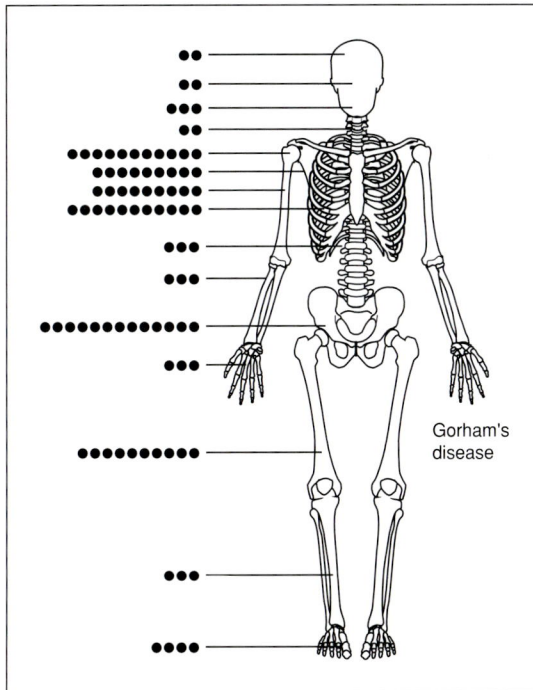

Gorham's disease

tumors); it is of mesenchymal origin and produces bone matrix. In young people most osteosarcomas occur in the long bones, especially of the leg; in adults, long and flat bones may equally be involved, including the pelvic bones. More than 12 different subtypes have been described, of which the most common is the primary, solitary intramedullary subtype which produces a bony matrix. The incidence of osteosarcoma shows two peaks: in the second decade and in the fifth and sixth decades of life when it may develop in a pre-existing lesion such as Paget's disease of bone. The malignant cells in osteosarcoma are alkaline-phosphatase positive.

Cytogenetics

Alterations of chromosome 9 have been reported, involving deletion of genes with tumor suppressor activity.

12.2 and 12.3 Osteoclastic remodeling in Gorham's disease.
12.2 (left) BMBS plastic, Giemsa, osteoclasts in cortical bone, left, on endosteal surface, upper right, and osteoblasts below osteoclast.
12.3 (right) BMBS plastic, Giemsa, osteoclasts on endosteal cortical surface; note blood vessels and developing osteoclasts.

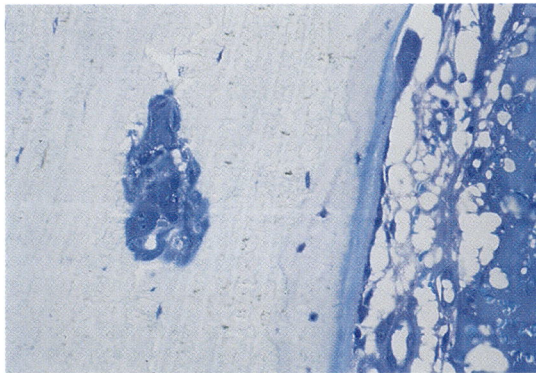

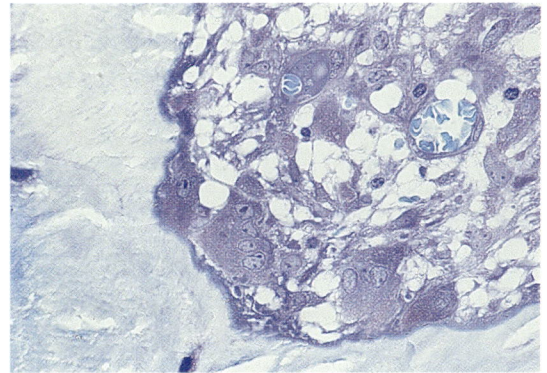

12.4–12.7 Examples of fibrous dysplasia.
12.4 (left) BMBS plastic, toluidine blue, erosion of both cortical and trabecular bone and replacement of marrow by dense fibrous tissue.
12.5 (right) BMBS plastic, Gomori, showing little bone, osteoblastic remodeling and fibrosis.

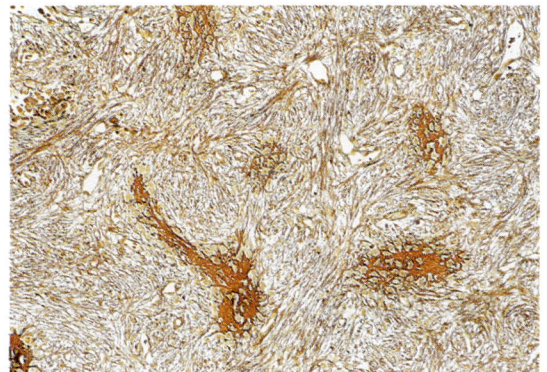

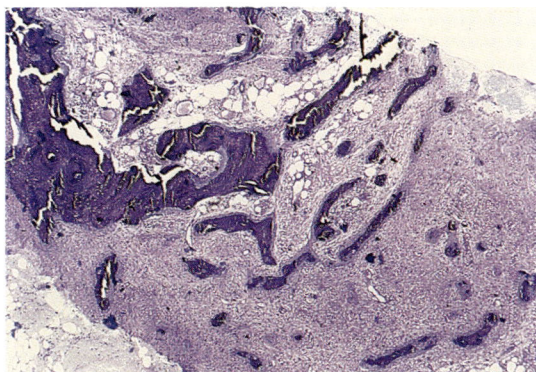

Chondrosarcoma

These tumors commonly arise in the central parts of the skeleton, including the pelvic bones. Chondrosarcoma is the second most common cancer of bone after osteosarcoma, and in about half of the cases the pelvic bones may be involved. When centrally located, the chondrosarcoma may spread within the marrow cavities (Figures 12.8–12.10) replacing the normal tissues by cartilaginous-like masses. The aspect of the cells in these masses is important for diagnosis (which may be difficult). The cells are not arranged in columns and their nuclei may be hyperchromatic, multiple, contain many lobes or have bizarre shapes, and many mitotic figures may be seen. Ossification may take place, and when it does it starts in the cartilage. Some chondrosarcomas may also contain myxomatous areas. Chondro- and fibrosarcomas are both alkaline-phosphatase negative.

Cytogenetics

Abnormalities of chromosome 9 t(9;22) (q22;q12) have been reported; two putative suppressor genes, mapped to this region, have been shown to be deleted in various malignancies and in chrondrosarcoma indicating their possible involvement in the development of chondrosarcomas. Other complex cytogenetic alterations have been reported in individual cases.

Fibrosarcoma and malignant fibrous histiocytoma

These are fibroblastic sarcomas of bone that produce collagen that usually develop in the

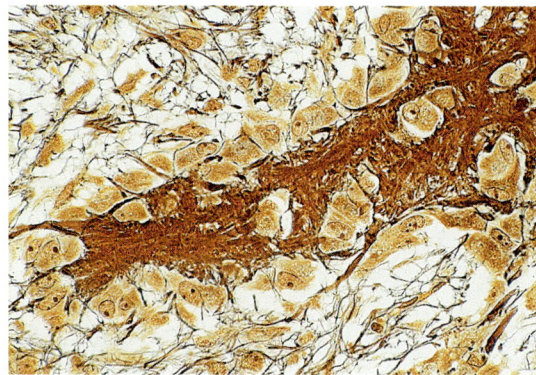

12.6 As for Figure 12.5, showing mainly osteoblasts around the bone and between the fibers.

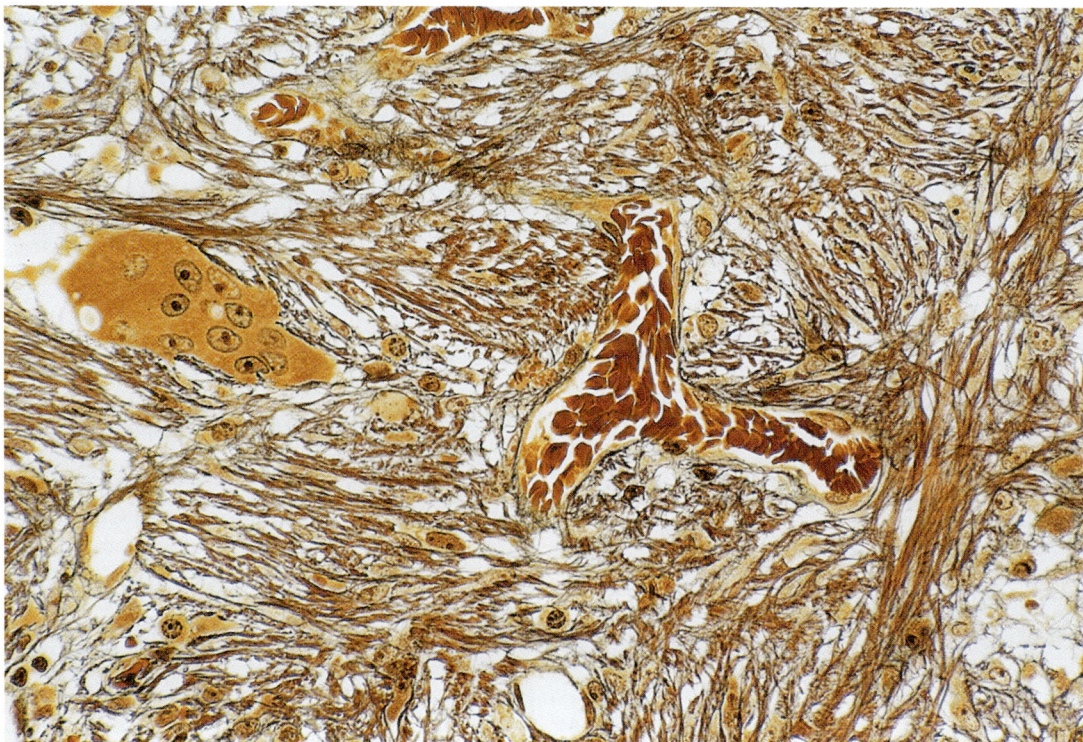

12.7 As for Figure 12.5, higher magnification; note large osteoclast, left, and dense fibrosis, right.

12.8–12.10 Examples of chondrosarcoma.
12.8 (left) BMBS plastic, Giemsa, with atypical cartilage cells.

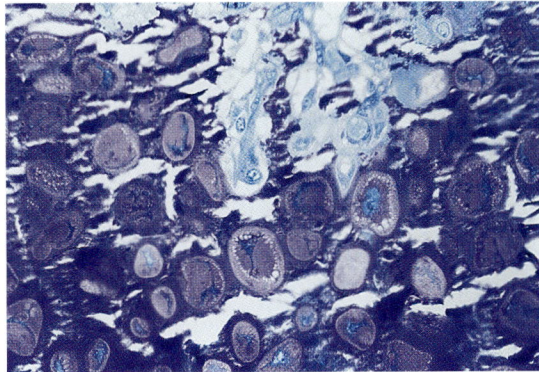

12.9 (right) BMBS plastic, Ladewig, showing multinucleated polymorphic chondroblasts.

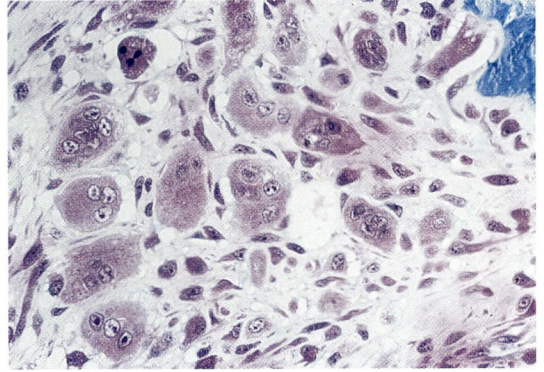

12.10 BMBS plastic, Gomori, with chondroblasts and fibrosis.

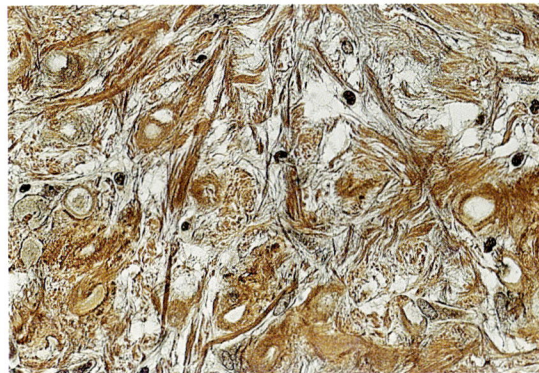

metaphyses of the long bones and in the flat bones of the pelvis. The malignant fibroblasts may be arranged in a pattern (herring-bone type) and produce variable amounts of collagen. Fibrous histiocytoma consists of spindle-shaped fibroblasts and multi-nucleated giant cells.

Ewing's sarcoma

This is a primary tumor of bone of small, round cells, with little cytoplasm but positive for glycogen, slightly larger than lymphocytes. The tumor arises in the medullary cavity, has little stroma and consists of sheets of monomorphic cells often with necrosis and hemorrhage. The presence of pseudo-rosettes (circular arrangement of the cells) is considered indicative of neural differentiation. Ewing's sarcoma is currently thought to have a primitive neural phenotype.

The differential diagnosis includes lymphoma, rhabdomyosarcoma, neuroblastoma and small cell carcinoma of the lung. The diagnosis is supported by cytogenetic analysis that reveals the t(11:22)(q24;q12) chromosomal translocation. Ewing's sarcoma arises in the diaphysis of the long bones, especially the femur and the flat bones of the pelvis.

Giant cell tumor of bone

Giant cell tumor of bone is also called osteoclastoma because it consists of multi-nucleated osteoclast-like giant cells and is interspersed with mononuclear stromal cells, with distinct cell membranes, but it apparently grows in a syncytium. Reactive features include necrosis, hemorrhage, deposition of hemosiderin, and reactive fibrosis and new bone formation. The nuclei of the mononuclear stromal cells and those of the multi-nucleated giant cells appear identical. Though affecting primarily the long bones, any bone may be involved, including the pelvis; most tumors are solitary. Though histologically benign, a small number (<4%) may metastasise to the lung, possibly as emboli after surgery. Sarcomatous degeneration is rare.

Myelogenous osteopathies

Alterations in trabecular bone have been observed in all hematologic malignancies as well as in non-neoplastic alterations of bone marrow cellularity and possibly vascularity (Tables 12.1 and 12.2). These are considered in the appropriate chapters.

TABLE 12.1 Myelogenous osteodysplasia (MOD)

Conditions	No. of patients	MOD (%)
Osteomyelosclerosis	350	100
Multiple myeloma (MM)	710	70
Hodgkin's disease (HD)	130	61
Myelofibrosis	620	50
Aplastic anemia	155	40
Chronic myeloid leukemia (CML)	710	40
Polycythemia vera (PV)	800	25
Malignant lymphomas (ML)	1255	20
Acute leukemias (AL)	895	10
*Congenital hemolytic conditions		
*Storage diseases		

* Only few cases in these groups examined; all had some degree of osteodysplasia.

TABLE 12.2 Bone changes in skeletal X-rays and in iliac crest biopsies in hematological malignancies

Parameters	Units	PV	CML	AL	ML	HD	MM
Patients	n	210	190	200	510	85	300
Skeletal X-ray							
Normal	%	72	69	89	72	84	32
Porotic	%	22	27	3	23	10	24
Lytic	%	2	4	6	4	4	44
Sclerotic	%	4	0	2	1	2	2
Bone biopsy							
Bone structure							
Normal	%	69	60	63	65	72	52
Porotic	%	27	37	23	28	19	44
Sclerotic	%	4	3	4	7	9	4
Bone remodeling							
Increased	%	15	8	3	4	53	80

Check list: Miscellaneous Bone Disorders

- Adequate biopsy?
- Presence of cortex?
- Trabecular network intact?
- Partial resorption of cancellous bone?
- Osteoclastic activity by morphologically normal osteoclasts? On immunohistology (I.H.) osteoclasts positive for acid phosphatase and tartrate-resistant acid phosphatase (TRAP).
- Adjacent to lytic lesions – osteoid seams, stains for osteoid?
- Within the lesions – fibrous tissue containing blood vessels and inflammatory cells? On I.H. blood vessels stain with Factor VIII-related antigen and the fibrous tissue with vimentin; reticulin stain.
- Reduction in amount of trabecular bone?
- State of hematopoiesis, inflammatory reactions? On I.H. stain for LCA, B and T cells, many T cells present. CD68 for monocytes, macrophages on I.H.

Clinical correlations

- Diagnosis usually made on clinical grounds, characteristic for each disorder.
- Radiology and imaging in Gorham's vanishing bone disease.
- Fibrous dysplasia: radiology, dermatology and endocrinology. Radiology may show change in shape or outline of involved bone, monostotic more common than polyostotic, especially skull and long bones. Sarcomatous degeneration rare, <1%.
- Osteo- and chondrosarcomas: patient's age, location of lesion, radiology and results of imagining techniques indicate the diagnosis which is confirmed by surgery and biopsy.

Bibliography

Abel M., Smith G. (1974) The case of the disappearing pelvis. *Radiology*, **111**, 105.

Abrahams J., Ganick D., Gilbert E., Wolfson J. (1980) Massive osteolytis in an infant. *Amer J Radiol.*, **135**, 1084.

Adelman H.M., Wallach P.M., Flannery M.T. (1991) Ewing's sarcoma of the ilium presenting as unilateral sacroilitis. *J Rheumatol.*, **18** (7), 1109–11.

Cannon S.R. (1986) Massive osteolytis: a review of seven cases. *J Bone Jt Surg.*, **68B**, 24.

De Lure F., Campanacci L. (1995) Clinical and radiographic progression of fibrous dysplasia: cystic change or sarcoma? Description of a clinical case and review of the literature. *Chir Organi Mov.*, **80** (1), 85–9.

DeGeorge A.M. (1975) Albright's syndrome: is it coming of age? *J Pediatr.*, **87**, 1018.

Dickson G.R., Hamilton A., Hayes D. *et al.* (1990) An investigation of vanishing bone disease. *Bone*, **11**, 205.

Editorial (1971) Fibrous dysplasia of bone. *Br. Med J.*, **1**, 685.

Geigl D., Seidel L., Marmor A. (1981) Gorham's disease of the clavicle with bilateral pleural effusions. *Chest*, **79**, 242.

Gibson M.J. Middlemiss J.H. (1971) Fibrous dysplasia of bone. *Br. J. Radiol.*, **44**, 1.

Gorham L.W., Stout A.P. (1955) Massive osteolytis (acute spontaneous absorption of bone, phantom bone, disappearing bone): its relation to menangiomatosis. *J Bone Jt Surg.*, **37A**, 985.

Gorham L.W., Wright A.W., Schultz H.H., Maxon F.C. (1954) Disappearing bones: a rare form of massive osteolysis. *Am. J. Med.* **17**, 674.

Grabias S.L., Campbell C.J. (1977) Fibrous dysplasia. *Orthop Clin N Amer.*, **8**, 771.

Haddad J.G. (1988) Estrogen receptors in bone in a patient with polyostotic fibrous dysplasia (McCune-Albright Syndrome) *New Eng J Med.*, **319**, 421.

Hahn S.B., Lee S.B., Kim D.H. (1991) Albright's syndrome with hypophosphatemic rickets and hyperthyroidism: a case report. *Yonsei Med.*, **32**, 179.

Hemingway A., Leuny A., Lavender J. (1983) Familial vanishing limbs: four generations of idiopathic multicentric osteolysis. *Clin Radiol.*, **34**, 585.

Jagasia A.A., Block J.A., Diaz M.O. *et al.* (1996) Partial deletions of the CDKN2 and MTS2 putative tumor suppressor genes in a myxoid chonrosarcoma. *Cancer Lett.*, **105** (1), 77–90.

Johnson N.A. (1990) Musculoskeletal problems in hemoglobinopathy. *Orthop Clin N Amer.*, **21** (1), 191.

Kaplan F.S., Fallon M.D., Boden S.D. *et al.* (1988) Estrogen receptors in bone in a patient with polyostotic fibrous dysplasia (McCune-Albright Syndrome). *New Engl J Med.*, **319**, 421.

Kumar B., Murphy W.A., Whyte M.P. (1981) Progressive diaphyseal dysplasia (Engelman disease): scintigraphic-radiographic-clinical correlations. *Radiology*, **140**, 87.

Lopez-Gines C., Carda-Batalla C., Lopez-Terrada L., Llombart-Bosch A. (1996) Presence of double minutes and monosomy 17p in xenografted human osteosarcomas. *Cancer Genet Cytogenet.*, **90** (1), 57–62.

Miller C.W., Aslo A., Campbell M.J. *et al.* (1996) Alterations of the p15, p16 and p18 genes in osteosarcoma. *Cancer Genet Cytogenet.*, **86** (2), 136–42.

Pedicelli G., Mattia P., Zorzoli A. *et al.* (1984) Gorham-syndrome. *Amer J Med.*, **252**, 1449.

Sear H.R. (1948) Engelman's disease. *Br. J Radiol.*, **21**, 236.

Smith R. (1987) Fibrous dysplasia. In Weatherall, Ledingham and Warrell (eds), *Oxford Textbook of Medicine*. Oxford: Oxford University Press, pp. 17–33.

Swarts S.J., Neff J.R., Johansson S.L., Bridge J.A. (1996) Cytogenetic analysis of dedifferentiated chondrosarcoma. *Cancer Genet Cytogenet.*, **89** (1), 49–51.

13 Necrosis, fractures, grafts and healing in bone

Non-traumatic primary necrosis

Non-traumatic bone death is called idiopathic (primary) necrosis. The most common site is the femoral head due to deprivation of its blood supply. Obstruction of blood vessels by thromboembolism, fat embolism or other causes results in skeletal infarction. Other weight-bearing bones may likewise be affected. Osteonecrosis (Figures 13.1–13.3) in non-weight bearing skeletal sites is frequently clinically silent and painless. Avascular necrosis belongs to the 'aseptic' variants of osteonecrosis and four groups are distinguished: (1) traumatic, (2) marrow compartment syndrome, (3) small vessel occlusion and (4) idiopathic.

Necrosis of bone marrow and bone due to interruption of blood flow starts by disruption of sinusoids and small blood vessels, followed by extravation of erythrocytes, degeneration of hematopoietic and fat cells, and death of bone cells, including osteocytes. Repair begins with ingrowth from adjacent healthy tissue of blood vessels, fibroblasts and macrophages which remove the necrotic debris (Figure 13.4) and reconstitute the marrow stroma with, in addition, formation of woven bone and lamellar bone (Figures 13.5 and 13.6). Necrotic bone is partially removed by osteoclasts. The exact etiology is clarified only in rare cases. A summary of conditions in which necrosis of bone has been reported is given in Table 13.1. Initially, MRI is useful in detecting sites of osteonecrosis; subsequently bone scans reveal skeletal reconstitution, while radiographs only pick up areas of osteoporosis, and of osteosclerosis later on in the process of repair.

Traumatic bone fracture and healing
(Table 13.2)

Major fractures caused by trauma to bone result in extensive tissue injury with displacement, hemorrhage and clot formation, which is an integral part of the unique and complex healing process. Minor breaks or cracks (microfractures) occur chiefly in weight-bearing bones, especially the vertebrae and usually after reduction in the amount and the architecture of trabecular bone, as in osteoporosis.

The sequence of events in normal fracture healing has been divided into three phases:

1. Inflammatory phase: injury followed by degeneration, an intensive inflammatory reaction, hematoma organisation, phagocytosis and intracellular lysosomal breakdown of the ingested debris.

2. Reparative phase characterised by formation of callus – a complex tissue consisting of fibrous, cartilaginous and osseous elements derived from mesenchymal cells. With further proliferation of blood vessels the soft, fibrous callus is converted to hard, bony callus by mineralisation of osteoid and by enchondral ossification.

3. Remodeling phase, during which the woven bone is slowly converted to lamellar bone and then regains its original shape and strength.

113

TABLE 13.1 Osteonecrosis

Idiopathic
Trauma
Corticosteroid administration
Infections and chronic inflammations
Vascular disorders
Radiation therapy
Gaucher's disease
Sickle cell and other anemias
Coagulation disorders
Alcohol abuse
Tumors: primary and metastatic

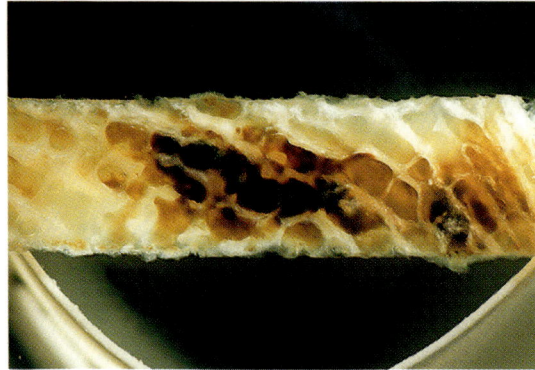

13.1–13.4 Manifestations of necrosis in bone marrow and bone.

13.1 Bone biopsy plastic, surface of trimmed block showing areas of necrosis (dark color) in center and right of biopsy, cause unknown, possibly vascular.

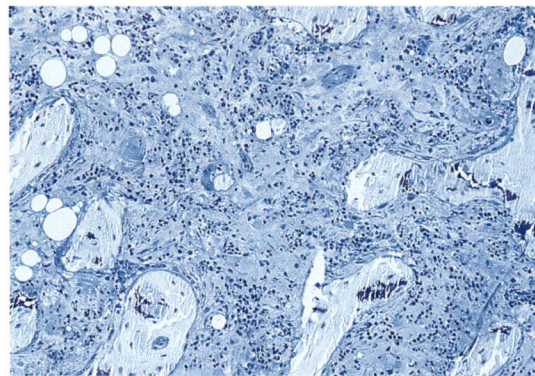

13.2 BMBS plastic, Giemsa, showing areas of necrotic cells, case of bone marrow metastases.

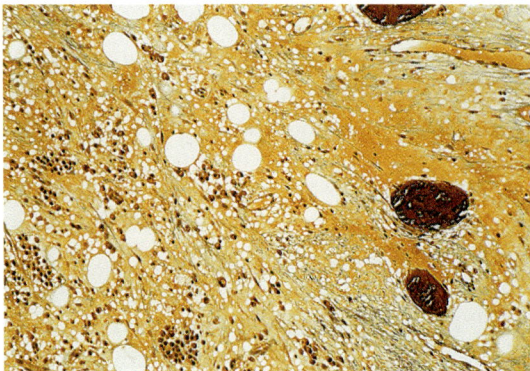

13.3 (left) BMBS plastic, Gomori, showing hemorrhage and necrosis, post-chemotherapy.

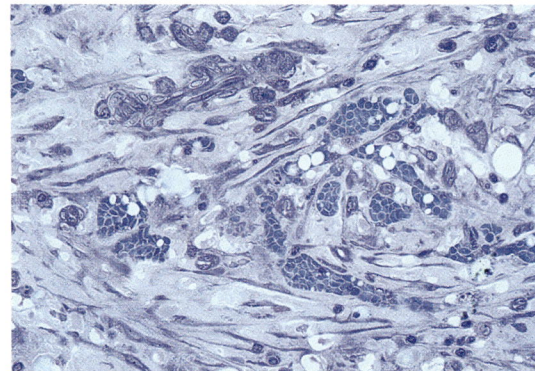

13.4 (right) BMBS plastic, Giemsa, showing removal of necrotic tissue and ingrowth of blood vessels, also macrophages, lymphocytes and plasma cells.

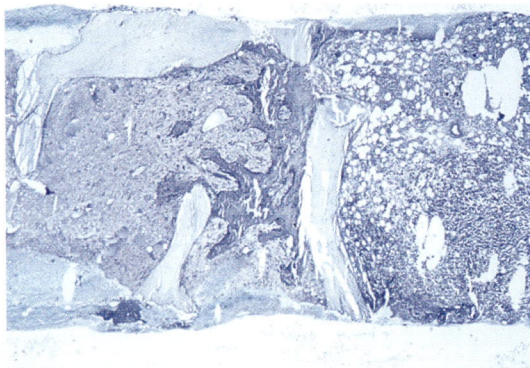

13.5 and 13.6 Repair.
13.5 (left) Plastic, Giemsa, low-power, marrow replaced by connective tissue, left, and new bone, left of center.

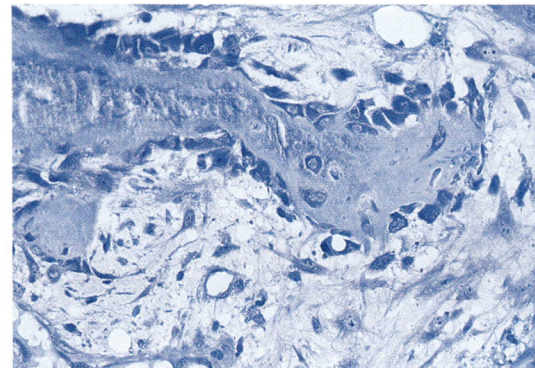

13.6 (right) As for Figure 13.5, higher magnification to show osteoblastic new bone formation on remains of old trabecula.

114

TABLE 13.2 Causes of ischemic necrosis of bone

Hematologic
DIC
Leukemias – especially fast growing acute
Haemoglobinopathies, e.g. sickle cell disease
Storage disease, e.g. Gaucher's disease

Endocrine/metabolic
Drugs: steroid therapy, cytotoxic therapy
Cushing's disease
Diabetes
Osteomalacia
Ethanol abuse

Miscellaneous
Trauma
Irradiation
Burns
Hemodialysis
Collagen vascular disorders
Transplantations
Idiopathic
Vascular obstruction, embolism
Metastatic bone disease

Gastrointestinal
Renal
Infections

The roles of transforming growth factor β (TGFβ) and other bone morphogenic proteins, have recently been emphasised in the regulation of fracture healing. In addition, mast cells are consistently found on or near the trabecular bone surface during both resorption and formation of bone, suggesting their participation in both processes.

Site of bone biopsy

The stages of repair described above may be observed in sequential bone biopsies taken from the same site within a relatively short period. The 'hole' may be 3–4 mm wide and 3–6 cm long. In addition, pieces of ilium may be removed for use as grafts in reconstructive surgery, so that correct interpretation of the histologic findings is essential.

Pathological fractures

These may rarely occur in the pelvis, although the femur, vertebrae and distal radius are the commonest sites. The main factors that are associated with fracture risk are given in Table 13.3.

A pathological fracture is defined as one that occurs after minor trauma or during normal physical activity, and many osseous and extraosseous factors contribute, while the fracture site is influenced by age, sex and the nature of the patient's disease.

Osseous disorders associated with fractures

Owing to the disorganised lamellar architecture, bones affected by Paget's disease are structurally weak, despite an increased mineral content. Likewise, the thickness of bones in fluorosis contributes to their fragility due to the defective mineralisation (osteomalacia).

Alterations of trabecular architecture – decrease in numbers of ossicles and in their connections, as well as attenuation of the trabecular network, contribute to fracture risk. These defects commonly occur in age-related osteoporosis.

Metastases from carcinomas, primary bone tumors and multiple myeloma, all cause osteolyses with collapse and fracture of bone. Many other developmental, metabolic, inflammatory, neoplastic, genetic, nutritional and iatrogenic disorders increase bone fragility and lead to a high fracture risk.

Bone grafts and substitutes

Bone grafts are second in frequency only to grafts of blood products. Grafts are used to accelerate osteogenesis between adjacent bones, and to bridge and fill cavities, gaps or defects in bone (Figure 13.7), for example after curettage, resection or biopsies.

TABLE 13.3 Factors that may increase fracture risk

Age and sex

Propensity to fall
Weight
Balance
Sensory capacity
Cognitive impairment
Gait
Neurological and psychiatric disorders
Foot problems
Genetic factors?
Environmental factors (uneven surfaces)

Capacity to resist trauma
Fat and muscle mass
Muscle conditioning
Speed of reflexes
Physical activity

Increased bone fragility
Osteoporosis
Localised osteopenia
Undermineralisation
Osteolytic lesions
Osteosclerotic lesions
Unbalanced bone
    remodeling

Drugs
Alcohol
Sedatives
Antihypertensives

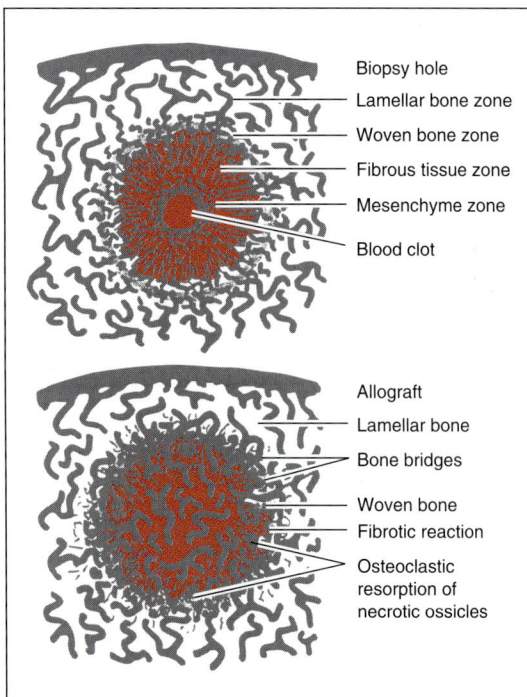

Biopsy hole
Lamellar bone zone
Woven bone zone
Fibrous tissue zone
Mesenchyme zone
Blood clot

Allograft
Lamellar bone
Bone bridges
Woven bone
Fibrotic reaction
Osteoclastic resorption of necrotic ossicles

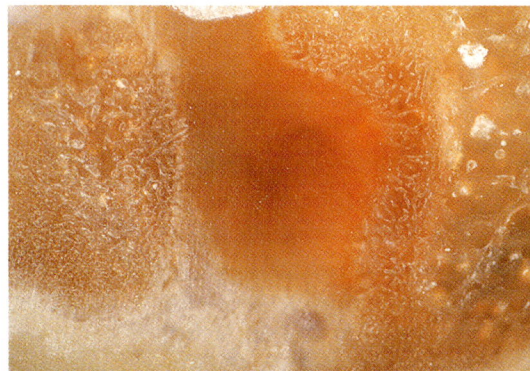

13.7 (left) Sequence of bone repair of biopsy hole and of integration of bone allograft.

13.8 (right) Hole in bone filled with blood clot.

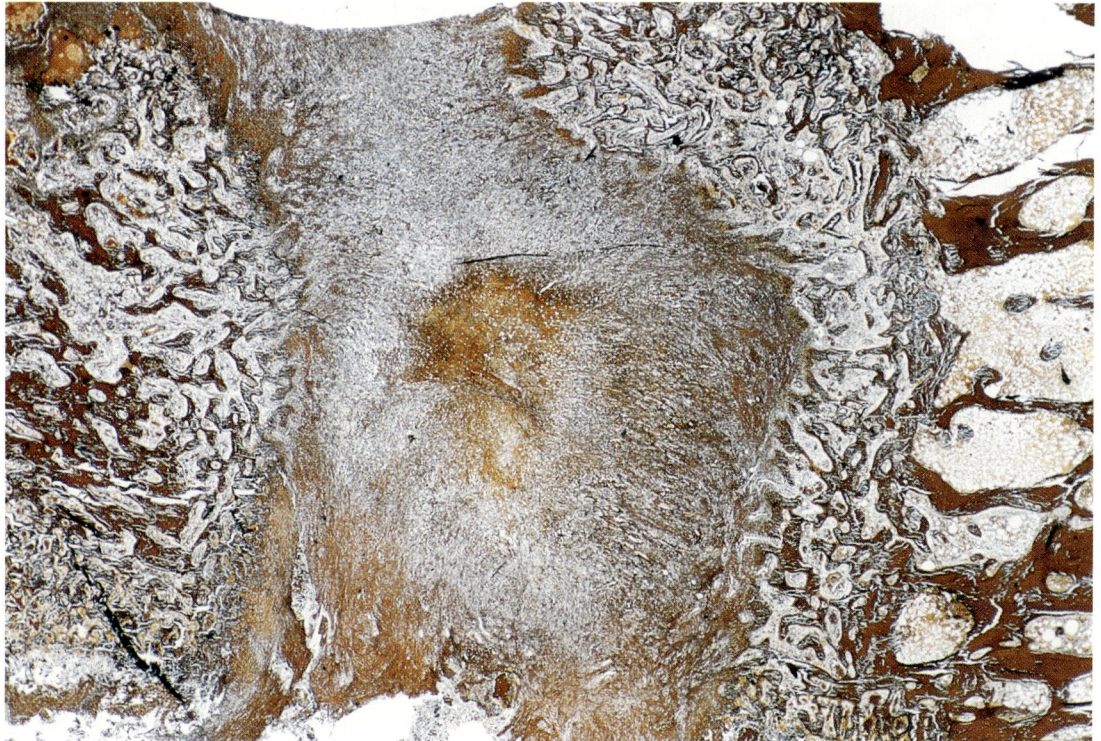

13.9 Connective tissue moving into blood clot from the edges of the hole.

13.10 (left) Different integration of two types of coralline hydroxyapatite substitutes.

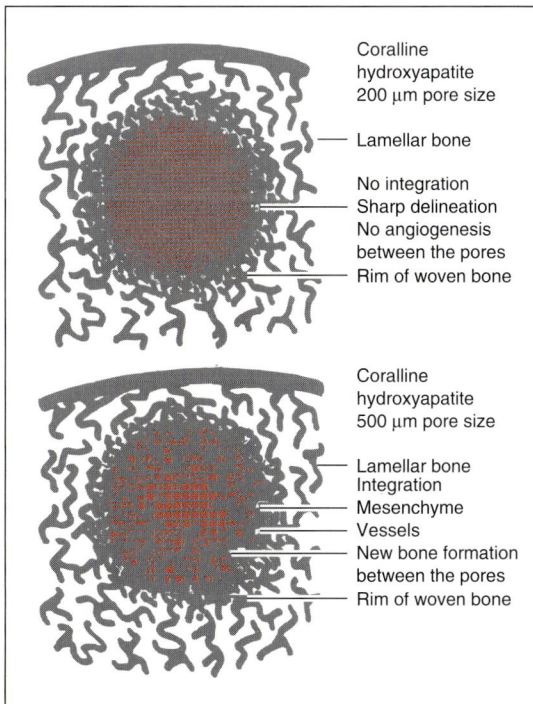

Coralline hydroxyapatite 200 μm pore size

— Lamellar bone

No integration
Sharp delineation
No angiogenesis between the pores
Rim of woven bone

Coralline hydroxyapatite 500 μm pore size

Lamellar bone
Integration
Mesenchyme
Vessels
New bone formation between the pores
Rim of woven bone

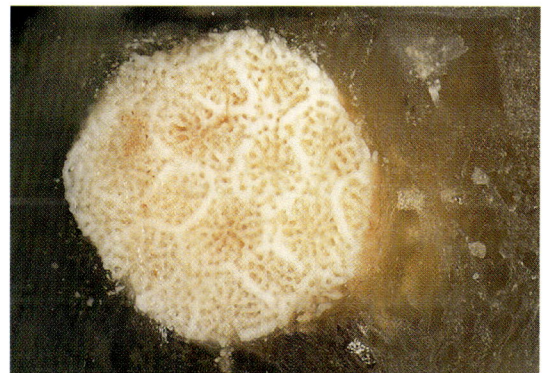

13.11 (right top) Surface of trimmed plastic block showing coralline hydroxyapatite graft (200 μm pore size).

13.12 (right bottom) Section from block shown in Figure 13.11 showing sharp demarcation between transplant (which has dropped out) and surrounding bone.

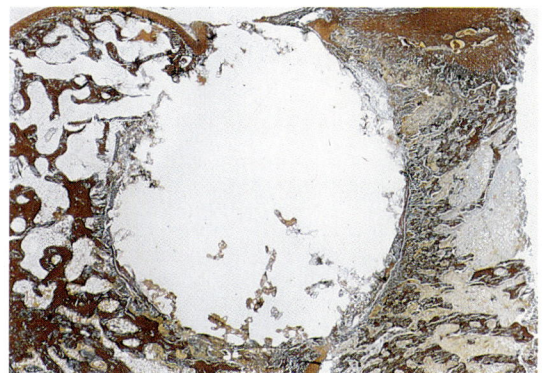

Types of bone grafts

A cancellous autograft consists of a vascularised piece of bone removed from, say, the ilium and transfered to the site of a bone defect. Such a graft in a well-vascularised bed is rapidly incorporated, with production of new bone and resorption of dead bone.

Bone allografts consist of dead tissue and have two main functions: mechanical support and osteoinduction, preceded by an inflammatory reaction evoked by the graft. Deep frozen or heat-treated allografts initially induce osteoinduction by recruitment of mesenchymal cells from the surrounding tissues; these then produce vessels and bone forming cells.

Marine coral, after sterilisation and conversion of calcium carbonate to hydroxyapatite, provides an excellent substitute for bone grafts. It is not rejected by the body (Figures 13.8–13.14).

Stages of graft incorporation

Five stages of bone graft incorporation have been described, though they overlap and merge into a continuum: inflammation, osteoclastic resorption, osteogenesis, revascularisation and remodeling, resulting in a mechanically efficient structure. Cancellous grafts are eventually completely resorbed.

Clinical significance of bone grafts

The significance of bone grafts is highlighted by the establishment of a steadily increasing number of bone banks, analogous to blood banks.

Clinical correlations

- Necrosis in non-weight-bearing bones, e.g. pelvis, is rare and may be asymptomatic.
- Necrosis in weight-bearing bones, e.g. femur, is painful.
- Extensive necrosis leads to bone pain in any bone.
- Necrosis in fast-growing malignancies – acute lymphoblastic leukemia in children and various metastatic tumors in adults – leads to necrosis of bone, bone pain and fever.
- Fractures: evident clinically and radiologically.
- Microfractures: in vertebrae, usually not in pelvis. Accumulation leads to overt fractures.
- Pathological fractures: also not in pelvis but in weight-bearing bones.
- Patient's history, clinical, biochemical and radiologic findings indicate diagnosis in pathologic fractures.
- Incidence of pathologic fractures in malignancies is decreasing (e.g. in multiple myeloma and in metastatic breast cancer) with early administration of osteoclast-inhibiting factors, especially bisphosphonates.
- Increasing use of bone grafts to stimulate fracture repair and bridge gaps.

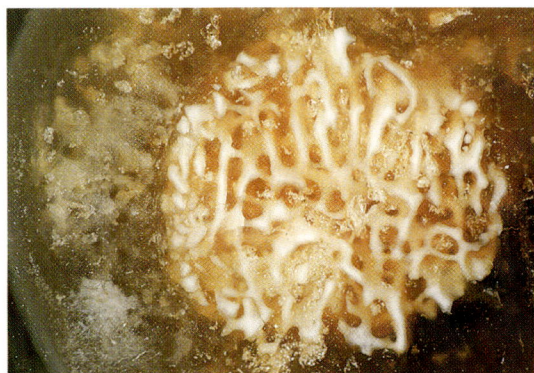

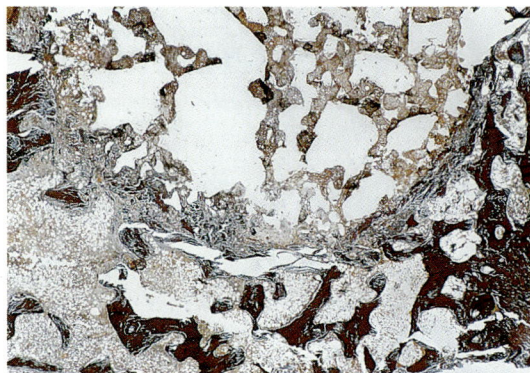

13.13 (left) Surface of trimmed plastic block showing coralline hydroxyapatite graft (500 μm pore size).

13.14 (right) Section from block shown in Figure 13.13; the pores of the graft (which has dropped out) were filled with connective tissue and blood vessels.

Bibliography

Aebi M., Regazzoni P. (1989) *Bone Transplantation*. Berlin: Spinger.

Atrah H.I. (1992) Bone banks: could be held by regional transfusion centres. *Br Med J.*, **304**, 68.

Brand R.A., Rubin C.T. (1990) Fracture healing. In McCollister-Evarts (ed.), *Surgery of the Muscoloskeletal System*. NewYork: Churchill Livingstone, pp. 93.

Burchardt H. (1983) The biology of bone graft repair. *Clin Orthop.*, **174**, 28.

Conrad M.E., Carpenter J.T. (1979) Bone marrow necrosis. *Amer J Hematol.*, **7**, 181.

Delaere O., Orloft S., Autrique J.C. *et al.* (1991) Long term sequelae of pelvis irradiation: histological and microradiographic study of a femoral head. *Clin Rheumatol.*, **10**, 206.

Dodds R.A., Emery R.J., Klenrman L. *et al.* (1990) Selective depression of metabolic activities in cortical osteoblasts at the site of femoral neck fractures. *Bone*, **11**(3), 157.

Duncan J.S., Ramsay L.E. (1984) Widespread bone infarction complicating meningococcal septicaemia and disseminated intravascular coagulation. *Br. Med J.*, **288**, 111.

Dunn P., Shih LY, Liaw S.J., Sun C.F. (1993) Bone marrow necrosis in 38 adult cancer patients. *J Formos Med Assoc*, **92 (12)**, 1107–10.

Editorial (1991) Thiazide diuretics and osteoporosis: time for a clinical trial? *Ann Intern Med.*, **115**, 64.

Editorials (1990) New treatments for osteoporosis. *Lancet*, **335**, 1065.

Editorials (1992) New bone? *Lancet*, **339**, 463.

Eide J. (1982) Bone infracts in bacterial endocarditis. *Human Pathol.*, **13**, 631.

Enneking W.F., Mindell E.R. (1991) Observations on massive retrieved human allografts. *J Bone Jt Surg.*, **73A**, 1123.

Eventov I., Frisch B., Alk D. *et al.* (1989) Bone biopsies and serum vitamin-D levels in patients with hip fracture. *Acta Orthop Scand.*, **60 (4)**, 411.

Eventov I., Frisch B., Cohen Z., Hammel I. (1991) Osteopenia, hematopoiesis, and bone remodelling in iliac crest and femoral biopsies: a prospective study of 102 cases of femoral neck fractures. *Bone*, **12**, 1.

Fleming D.R., Doukas A. (1992) Acute tumor lysis syndrome in hematologic malignancies. *Leuk. Lymph.*, **8 (4–5)**, 315–18.

Friedlander G.E. (1991) Bone allografts: the biological consequences of immunological events (Editorial) *J Bone Jt Surg.*, **73A (8)**, 119.

Goldberg V.M., Stevenson S. (1990) Bone transplantation. In McCollister-Evarts (ed.), *Surgery of the Musculoskeletal System*. New York: Churchill Livingstone, p. 115

Grisso J.A., Kelsey J.L., Strom B.L. *et al.* (1991) Risk factors for falls as a cause of hip fracture in women. *N Engl J Med.*, **324**, 1326.

Gross T.P., Jinnah R.H., Clarke H.J., Cox Q.C. (1991) The biology of bone grafting. *Orthopedics*, **14**, 563.

Harper P.G., Trask C., Souhami R.L. (1984) Avascular necrosis of bone caused by combination chemotherapy without corticosteroids. *Br. Med J.*, **288**, 267.

Hiehle J.F., Kreeland J.B., Dalinka M.K. (1991) Magnetic resonance imaging of the hip with emphasis on avascular necrosis. *Rheum Dis Clin N Amer.*, **17**, 669.

Hughes R.G., Islam A., Lewis S.M., Catowksy D. (1981) Spontaneous remission following bone marrow necrosis in chronic lymphocytic leukaemia. *Clin Lab Haematol.*, **3**, 173.

Ibels L.S., Alfrey A.C., Huffer W.E., Weil R. (1978) Aseptic necrosis of bone following renal transplantation. *Medicine*, **57**, 25.

Joyce M.E., Jingushi S., Bolander M.E. (1990) Transforming growth factor-β in the regulation of fracture repair. *Orthop Clin N Amer.*, **21 (1)**, 199.

Kleerekoper M., Villanueva A.R., Stanciu J. *et al.* (1985) The role of three-dimensional trabecular microstructure in the pathogenesis of vertebral compression fractures. *Calcil. Tissue Int.*, **37**, 594.

Kühne J.H., Bartl R., Hammer C. *et al.* (1993) Moderate heat treatment of bone allografts: Experimental results of osteointegration. *Arch Orthop Trauma Surg.*, **112**, 1.

Mankin H.J. (1992) Non-traumatic necrosis of bone (osteonecrosis) *N Engl J Med.*, **326**, 1473.

Melton L.J. (1988) Epidemiology of fractures. In Riggs and Melton (eds), *Osteoporosis: Etiology, Diagnosis, and Managementa*. New York: Raven Press, p. 133.

Mizuno K., Mineo K., Tachibana T. *et al.* (1990) The osteogenic potential of fracture haematoma. Subperiosteal and intramural transplantation of the haematoma. *J Bone Jt Surg.*, **72B**, 829.

Murphy R.G., Greenberg M.L. (1990) Osteonecrosis in pediatric patients with acute lymphoblastic leukemia. *Cancer*, **65**, 1717–21.

Nolan P.C., Mollan R.A.B., Wilson D.J. (1992) Living bone grafts. Cell culture may overcome the limitations of allografts. *Br Med J.*, **304**, 1520.

Ripamonti U. (1991) The morphogenesis of bone in replicas of porous hydroxyapatite obtained from conversion of calcium carbonate exoskeletons of coral. *J Bone Jt Surg.*, **73A**, 692.

Saito S., Inoue A., Ono K. (1987) Intra-medullary hemorrhage as a possible cause of avascular necrosis of the femoral head. *J Bon Jt Surg.*, **68B**, 346.

Scudla V., Dusek J., Macak J. *et al.* (1989) Bone marrow necrosis in malignant diseases. A report on seven intravitally recognized cases. *Neoplasma*, **36 (5)**, 603–10.

Sissons H., Nuovo M.A., Steiner G.C. (1992) Pathology of osteonecrosis of the femoral head. *Skel Radiol.*, **21**, 229.

Solomon L. (1991) Bone grafts (Editorial) *J Bone Jt Surg.*, **73B**, 706.

Taylor L.J. (1984) Multifocal avascular necrosis after short-term high-dose steroid therapy. *J Bone Jt Surg.*, **66B**, 431.

Terheggen H.G., Lampert F. (1979) Acute bone marrow necrosis caused by streptococcal infection. *Eur J Paed.*, **130**, 53.

Urist M.R., Strates B.S. (1970) Bone formation in implants of partially and wholly demineralized bone matrix. *Clin Orthop.*, **71**, 271.

Vesterby A., Jensen O.M. (1985) Aseptic bone/bone marrow necrosis in leukaemia. *Scand J Haematol.*, **35**, 365.

Ware H.E., Brooks A.P., Toye R., Berney S.I. (1991) Sickle cell disease and silent avascular necrosis of the hip. *J Bone Jt Surg.*, **73B**, 947.

Zizic T.M., Hungerford D.S., Stevens M.B. (1990) Ischemic bone necrosis in systemic lupus erythematosis: the early diagnosis of ischemic necrosis of bone. *Medicine*, **67**, 83.

14 Metastatic bone disease

Metastatic involvement of marrow and bone

Evidence has accumulated that any primary tumor has the ability to spread as soon as it is established and has access to lymphatic or blood vessels.

The sinusoidal system of the red hematopoietic marrow is lined by a thin endothelial layer, has no tight junctions, has a slow perfusion rate but large blood flow thus facilitating passage of tumor cell emboli into the extravascular space, as well as the formation of tumour–cell–platelet thrombi. Moreover, the hematopoietic and stromal cells of the bone marrow probably provide the tumor cells with growth and other factors, including adhesion molecules required for their survival, establishment and expansion. Since bone and bone marrow have no lymphatics, metastatic cells reach the bone marrow via the blood stream, or by contiguous spread. Bone metastases start in the marrow.

Indications for bone biopsies in oncology

Many indications for bone biopsies have now been established in oncology. These include:

1. Part of the initial investigation for staging.
2. Clinical suspicion of metastases.
3. Follow-up and monitoring of therapy.
4. Anemia, weakness and fatigue.
5. Otherwise unexplained pyrexia.
6. Hypercalcemia.
7. Raised alkaline phosphatase levels (osseous).
8. Suspicious areas on X-ray, scan, CT or MRI.
9. And, more recently, investigation of the bone marrow before and after autologous (or allogeneic) bone marrow transplantation; or peripheral blood stem cell transplantation.

In some cases, to investigate the possibility of graft versus host disease, or the possibility of a failed transplant and therefore an empty marrow with pancytopenia, and finally, monitoring of the effects of growth factors: colony-stimulating factors, erythropoietic and others, as well as those of immunosuppressive therapy. Many studies have been published in which detection of metastasis has been based on bone marrow aspirates. This method has the major limitation that there is a large component of peripheral blood, even if taken from the bone marrow sinusoids, the tumor cells detected may be circulating ones and therefore give no indication of whether the bone marrow is involved by established metastases, even small ones. Moreover, some metastases stimulate an almost immediate desmoplastic reaction and therefore will not be aspirated. In one study, tumor cells were detected more frequently in bone marrow aspirates but there was no difference in survival of patients between those with positive or negative aspirates. In contrast, patients with positive bone biopsies had significantly shorter survivals.

Frequently a cytopenia occurs during the course of treatment in oncology and the question arises whether there is therapy-induced hypo- or aplasia or whether there is replacement of the bone marrow by metastases; a bone biopsy will provide the answer in many cases. In addition to these clinical questions, a bone biopsy provides information on the effects of malignancy on the marrow, the bone, on the reserve capacity of the marrow and on tumor–host interactions. Occasionally an emergency may arise if metastases exert pressure on a vital organ – such as spinal cord; and when metastases of an unknown primary tumor are responsible, a bone biopsy may provide tissue for identification of the primary and thereby aid in choice of therapy.

Hypercalcemia of malignant disease

In the hypercalcemia of malignant disease one or more of four mechanisms is involved:

1. Osteolytic lesions of bone associated with widespread metastases as in some cases of metastases of carcinomas of breast, thyroid, lung and in some lymphomas, due to local osteoclast activating factors (OAFs) and to growth factors such as transforming growth factor β (TGFβ).

2. Osteolysis in the absence of demonstrable osseous metastases, but associated with some carcinomas which elaborate sterols related to vitamin D.

3. Osteolysis in the absence of demonstrable bony metastases but associated with tumors which appear to secrete a parathyroid-like hormonal substance: PTH-like peptide, especially tumors of bladder, ovary, kidney and lung.

4. Osteolysis in the absence of demonstrable metastases but in the presence of tumors that secrete some hormonal substance other than PTH or its prohormone forms, for example cancers of the lung, kidney, uterus, pancreas and colon.

Thus the production of hypercalcemia may depend on the involvement of long-range humoral factors produced by the tumor cells, and the direct stimulation of bone resorption by the metastatic deposits in the bones.

Methods of detection of bone metastases

It should be remembered that metastases, especially small ones, may be present in the bones in spite of negative X-rays and radionuclide scans as these reflect the sum of the dynamic processes involved – that is both bone formation and bone resorption. CT and MRI are more sensitive, but are still not routinely available, and CT is toxic as the dose of radiation is greater. In addition, a positive bone scintigraphy is entirely non-specific. Numerous conditions that perturb local bone metabolism will cause a 'hot spot' that represents the localised skeletal response to a fracture, infection and humoral stimulation.

Osteolytic lesions

The lytic component of small metastases as well as early osteolytic foci are not picked up by the X-ray or scan, and when osseous involvement is detected by iliac crest biopsy it is fairly safe to assume that in the majority of cases this will not be an isolated lesion and the cumulative effect of many such foci throughout the skeleton may well affect the serum calcium levels. This applies especially to tumors such as mammary cancers in which both osseous metastases and hypercalcemia frequently occur, but no long-range humoral mechanisms have actually been identified. In these cases the osteolysis is mediated by OAFs produced by the neoplastic cells and it may be significantly reduced by therapy with prostaglandin inhibitors and the bisphosphonates, or combinations of these two agents.

Raised alkaline phosphatase level

A raised osseous alkaline phosphatase level is correlated with the presence and activity of osteoblasts, and is frequently observed in prostatic cancer in men and breast cancer in women when a strong osteoblastic reaction has been evoked. In contrast, there is no clear correlation between the hematological values in the peripheral blood and the size and type of metastases in the bone marrow.

Frequency of bone metastases

The frequency of bone metastases in carcinoma patients reported in the literature varies from 28 to 85%, the wide range presumably reflecting: the primary tumor, stage of disease, method of investigation, thoroughness of search and, in the case of bone biopsies, size of the biopsy core (and possibly single or double biopsies; see Chapter 1), and the quality of the histologic preparation (Table 14.1). Metastases of breast, prostate and lung demonstrate osteotropism, i.e. they possess a unique affinity for bone. But in addition, epidermal growth factors (EGFs) and other factors in the bone marrow constitute chemo-attractants for the tumor cells. Conversely, expression of bone sialoprotein in breast cancer cells is also associated with metastases and a poor prognosis. In breast cancer this correlates with positive steroid receptors, and in prostate cancer with histologic grade. Oat cell carcinoma metastasises to bone more frequently than the other histologic types of bronchial cancers.

Additional factors contributing to predilection for bone are: (1) stimulation of tumor growth by local growth factors and hormones present in bone and marrow, and (2) circulating tumor cells possibly respond to collagen fragments and minerals derived from normal bone resorption which may be chemotatic for the neoplastic cells.

Distribution of skeletal metastases

This reflects closely the distribution of red marrow in the adult. The incidence of involvement of the thoracic and lumbar spine and pelvis (iliac bones) is statistically equal, 70% each, due not only to their anatomical mass, but also to the role of the vertebral venous system in conveying metastases to the bones, especially retrograde flow in Batson's vertebral plexus. Other bones are less frequently affected: ribs 68%; proximal femur 45%; skull 40%; cervical spine 25%; proximal humerous 15%; scapula/clavicle 10%. In addition, an interaction occurs between the cancer cell embolus and the site at which it is arrested – the 'seed and soil' hypothesis of Paget. The complex series of interactions between cancer cells and host tissues has only partly been unraveled, and may be summarised as follows:

TABLE 14.1 Frequency of positive bone biopsies in carcinoma patients

	Patients	Positive biopsies	Percentage
Primary tumor			
Breast	504	211	42
Prostate	255	80	32
Lung	389	56	14
Other	294	48	19
Unknown	283	205	72
Biopsy size			
<60 mm²	1230	357	29
>60 mm²	495	243	49
Total	1725	600	35

Stages of metastatic process
(Figure 14.1)

Some of the regulatory factors have been identified and the process divided into four stages:

1. Invasion of blood or lymph vessels at site of origin, and embolism, single cells or clusters split off into the circulation.
2. Extravation out of the blood stream into the interstitium.
3. Adherence to stromal tissue.
4. Growth with induction of connective tissue and blood vessels.

Biological and clinical aspects of metastases

Resorption of bone near a tumor cell aggregate may aid the development of a metastatic focus, by providing matrix factors which attract tumor cells and promote their growth. Conversely, the rate of new bone formation around a tumor cell aggregate is inversely proportional to its rate of expansion. The numerous factors involved in these complex reactions are beyond the scope of this book, which is concerned mainly with the histologic findings in bone biopsies. There are five aspects of particular significance which may be investigated in bone biopsies:

1. Frequency of involvement, i.e. clinical staging.
2. Tumor cell differentiation, i.e. biological behavior.
3. Mode of spread in the bone marrow, i.e. progression of disease.
4. Stromal reactions, i.e. host response to the presence of metastases.
5. Osseous reactions, i.e. mechanisms and extent of bone destruction and formation.

Mode of spread of metastases
(Figures 14.2–14.13)

Metastases in bone biopsies may be divided into four groups according to the mode of spread:

1. Microcolonies – single cells or very small clusters.
2. Multiple small foci with stromal induction.
3. One or more large masses.

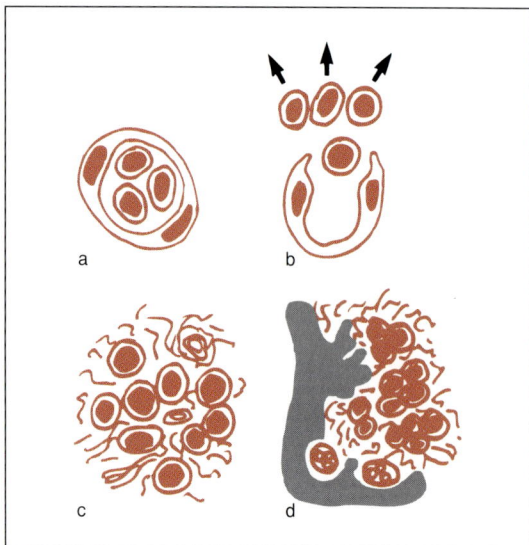

14.1 (left) Stages in metastatic invasion of bone marrow and bone. (a) Circulating tumor cells, (b) tumor cell invasion, (c) micrometastasis, (d) metastatic bone disease.

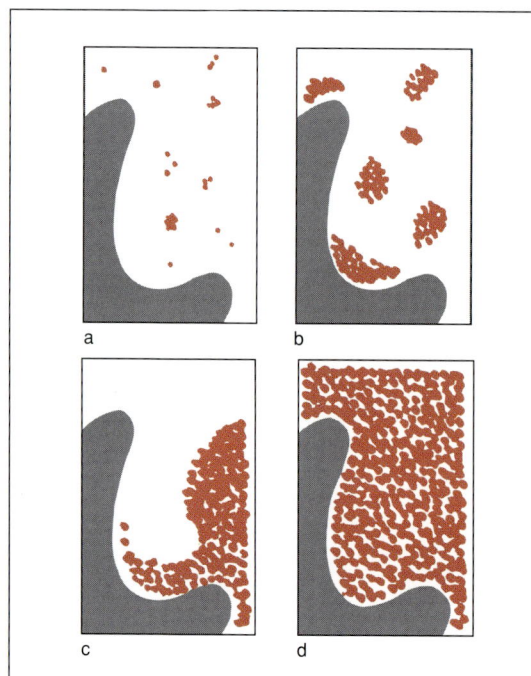

14.2 (right) Histological aspects of bone marrow involvement by metastases: multiple microemboli or colonies (a); multiple extravascular foci (b); large masses (c) and complete replacement of the normal marrow (d).

4. Total replacement of the normal trabecular bone and marrow.

It should be noted that identification of single or small clusters of tumor cells may be difficult in paraffin-embedded material and immunohistology may be required. Various methods have been applied for detection of single tumor cells or micrometastases; however, the significance of their detection as well as the most effective method to apply are points still under investigation. There appears to be some correlation between the type of spread and survival which was less favorable when multiple small foci were present. The degree of tumor cell differentiation (well, moderate or poor) also showed some correlation with survival: well-differentiated metastases with a homogenous aspect indicated a better prognosis than poorly differentiated, heterogeneous metastatic cells.

Bone reactions to the metastases
(Figure 14.14)

Increased osseous remodeling was present in >90% of biopsies with metastases, and though either resorption or formation predominated both were usually present resulting in alteration of trabecular structure. This ranged from large areas devoid of bone to extensive osteosclerosis; often both were found in one biopsy. Overall five patterns were seen: normal 7%, lytic 18%, mixed lytic/sclerotic 38%, sclerotic/lamellar with appositional bone formation and wide trabeculae 10%, and sclerotic/woven with normal trabeculae but woven bone in between 27% (Figures 14.15–14.18). There are two types of osteolytic lesions – one is mediated by osteoclasts and the other appears to be caused by expansion and pressure of the metastases (Figures 14.19–14.25). In

14.3–14.12 Establishment of metastases in bone marrow and bone.
14.3 (left) BMBS paraffin, H&E, showing isolated metastatic cells in the bone marrow.

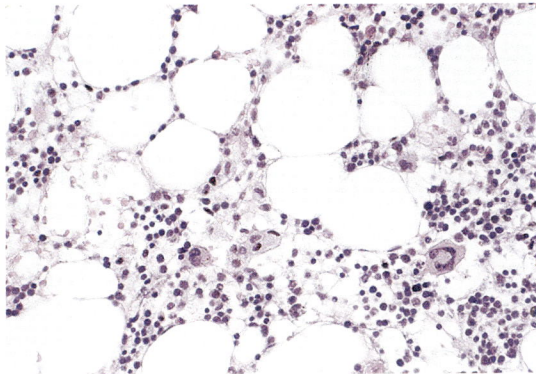

14.4 (right) BMBS paraffin, I.H. cytokeratin: metastatic cells stain positively.

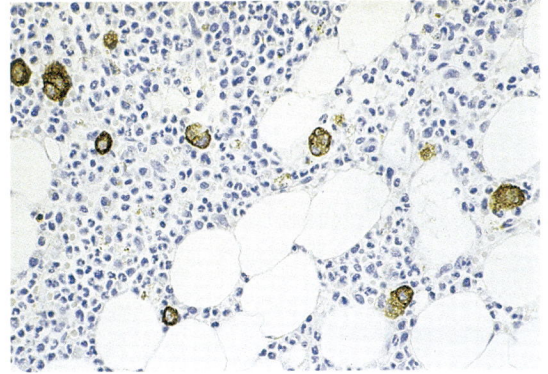

14.5 (left) BMBS plastic, Giemsa, showing clusters of metastatic cells.

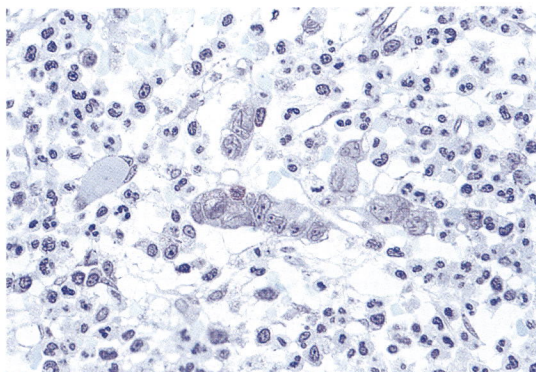

14.6 (right) BMBS plastic, I.H. cytokeratin; metastases stain positively.

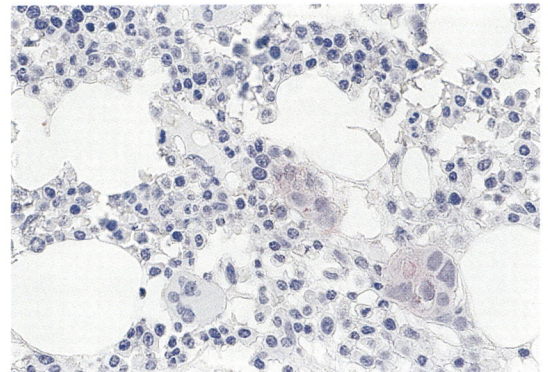

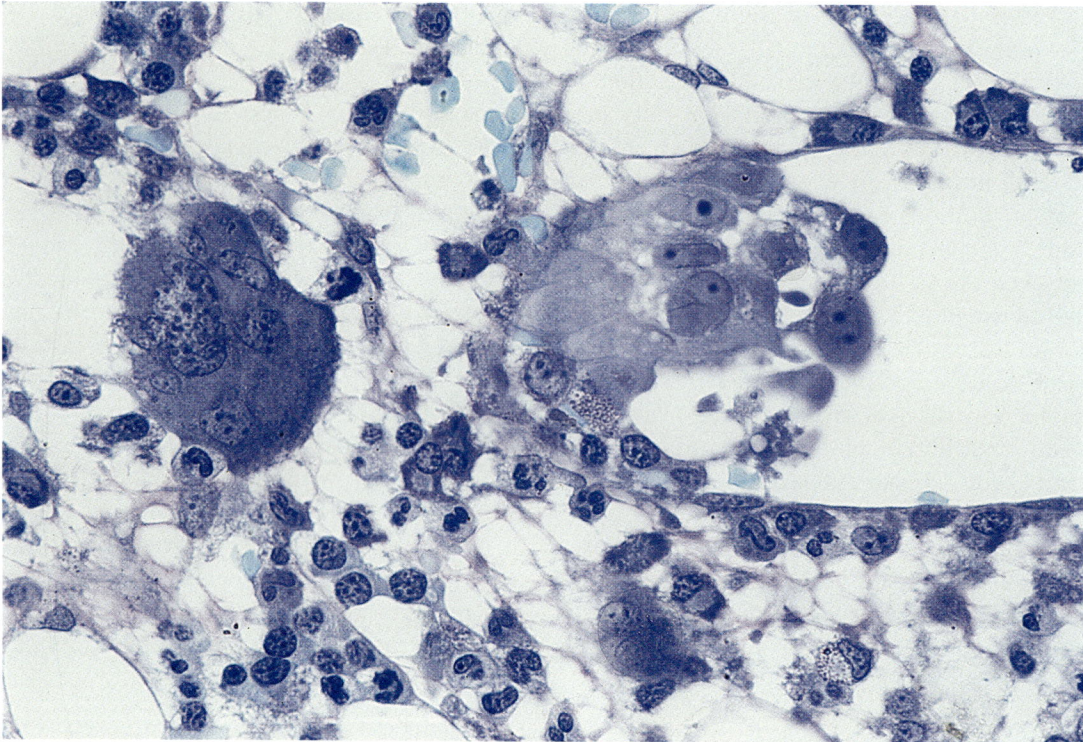

14.7 BMBS plastic, Giemsa: metastases attached to vascular endothelium.

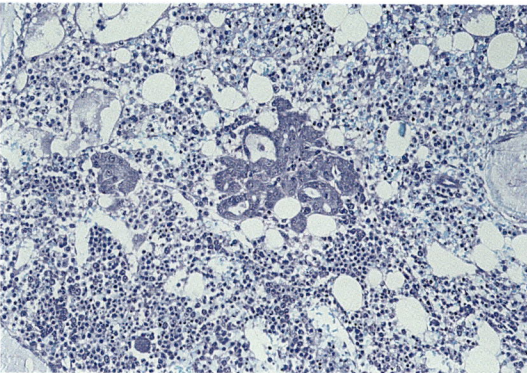

14.8 (left) BMBS plastic, Giemsa: metastases established in the bone marrow, outside the blood vessels.

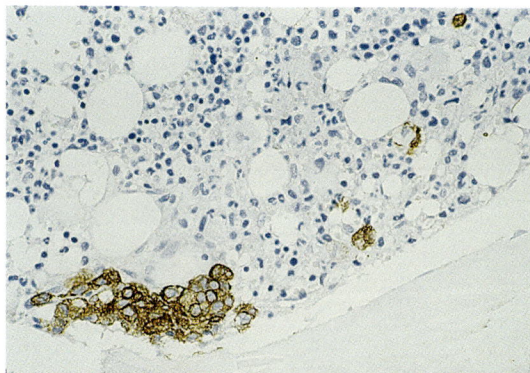

14.9 (right) BMBS paraffin, I.H. Large cluster of metastatic cells in paratrabecular sinus, cytokeratin positive.

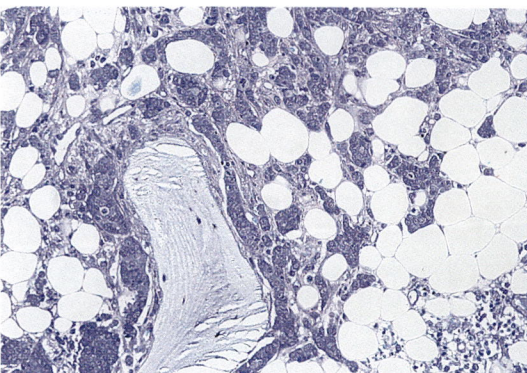

14.10 (left) BMBS plastic, Giemsa, tumor cells in paratrabecular sinus surrounding an ossicle, and in the interstitium.

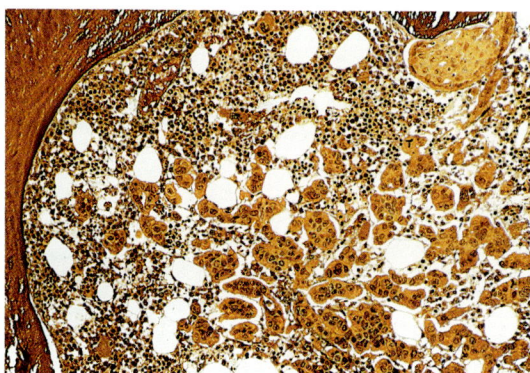

14.11 (right) BMBS plastic, Gomori: metastases spreading in the marrow with little osseous reaction.

14.12 (left top) BMBS plastic, Giemsa, larger groups of metastatic cells, spreading and replacing bone marrow.

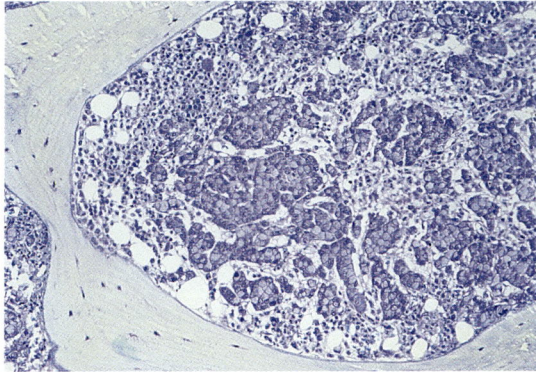

14.13 (left Middle) Establishment of metastasis in the bone marrow: passage of the tumor cells through the sinusoidal endothelium (**a**) intrasinusoidal; (**b**) trans-sinusoidal, and stimulation of host cells to produce the stroma for neoplastic cells (**c**).

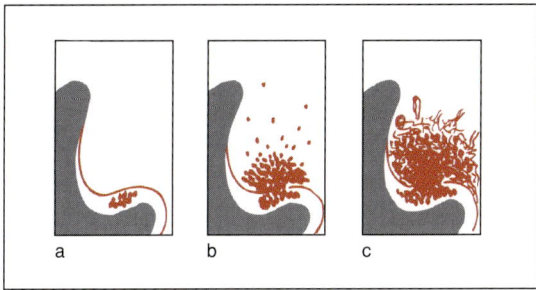

14.14 (right) Osseous reactions to metastases (normal is 7%); (**a**): osteolysis/osteoporosis, 18% (**b**) mixed type, 38% (**c**) osteosclerosis/lamellar bone, 10% (**d**) osteosclerosis/woven bone, 27% (**e**).

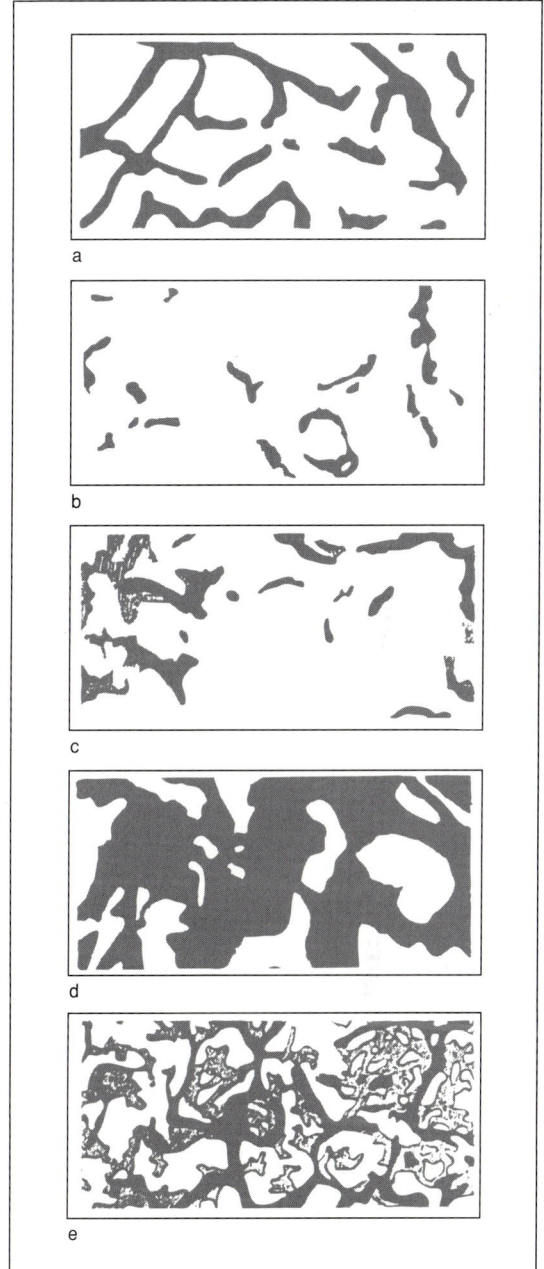

14.15–14.18 Effect of metastases on trabecular bone.

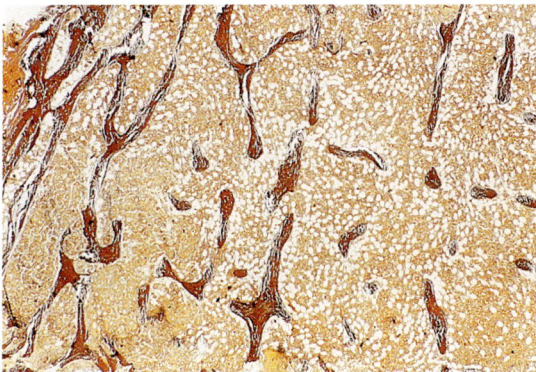

14.15 (left bottom) BMBS plastic, Gomori: primarily osteoporosis.

some cases, e.g. some bronchial cancers and malignant melanoma, only a minimal or no reaction is evoked, which accounts for negative X-rays and scans, in spite of metastatic involvement of the bone marrow.

Stromal reactions to the metastases

In primary tumors, the stromal components have been divided into four main groups:

1. New blood vessels.
2. Inflammatory cells.
3. Connective tissue including matrix components such as fibronectin, collagens, elastins and glycosaminoglycans, as well as fibroblasts and myelofibroblasts.
4. The fibrin–gel matrix which initially traps proteins and water and forms a provisional matrix.

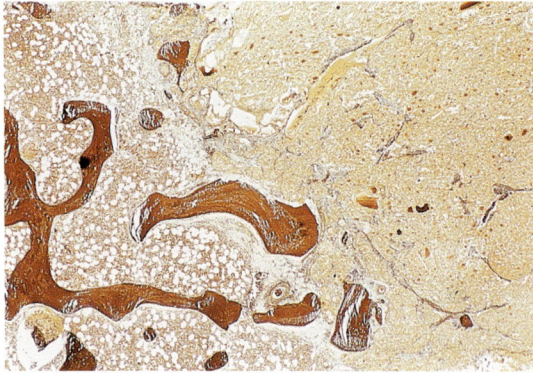

These processes in the formation of the stroma of tumors are similar to those of wound healing. Rarely, metastases in the bone marrow are confined to the vascular system. In all other cases, stimulation of new blood vessels – neo-angiogenesis – occurs at the margins of the metastases. There are often irregular channels with incomplete endothelium, or even lined by tumor cells, and with scanty perivascular tissue. Neo-angiogenesis – the formation of new blood vessels – is stimulated by an

14.16 (left) BMBS plastic, Gomori: primarily osteolytic with erosion of trabecular bone in metastatic area.

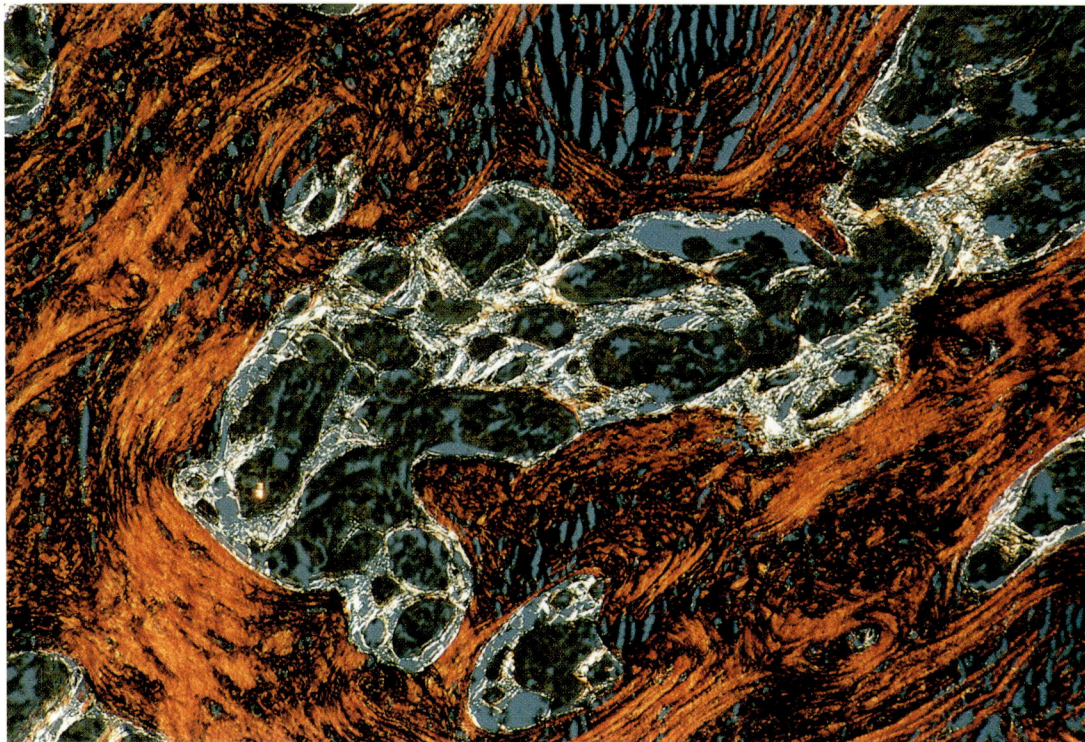

14.17 and 14.18 Osteosclerotic reaction to metastases of cancer of prostate.

14.17 BMBS plastic, Gomori, seen in polarised light showing fibrosis around the tumor cells and osteosclerosis.

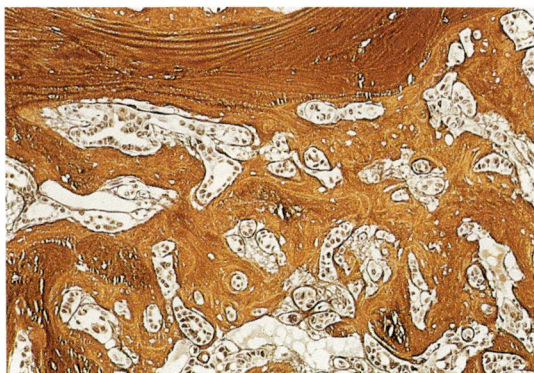

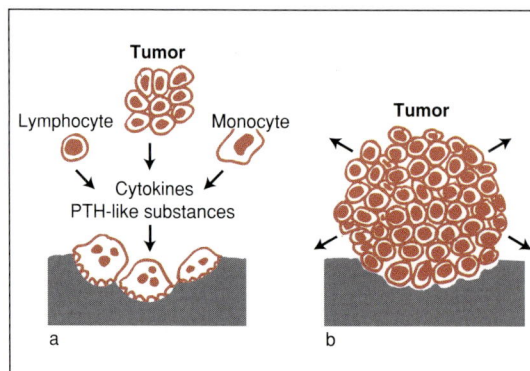

14.18 (left) BMBS plastic, Gomori, showing osteoblastic reaction; note tumor cells inside the bone.
14.19 (right) Two main mechanisms of osteolysis: production of osteoclast activating factors by the tumor cells and host cells (**a**), direct metastatic expansion and pressure on bone (**b**).

128

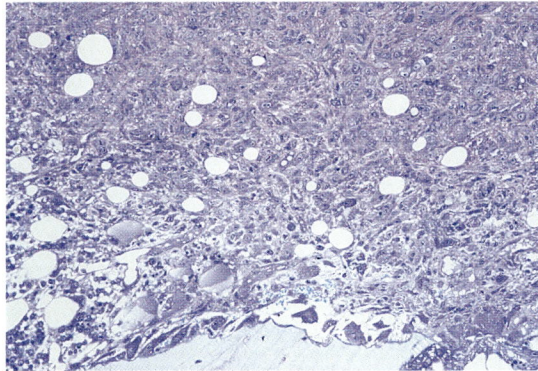

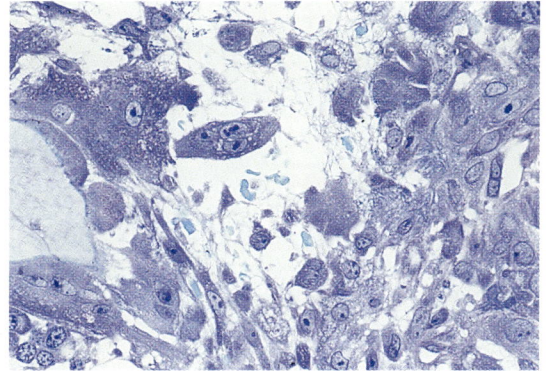

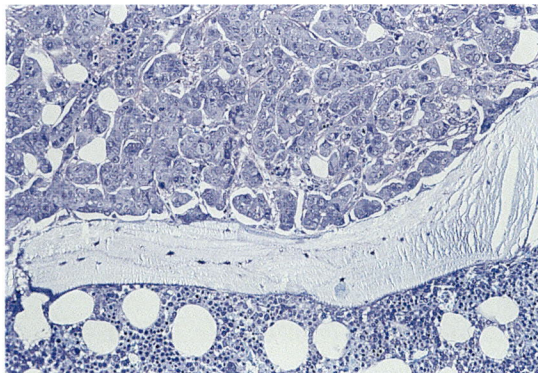

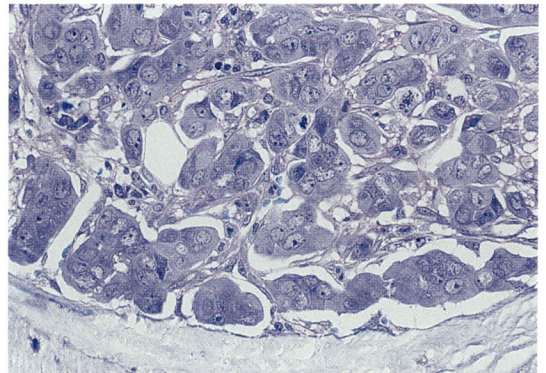

14.20 and 14.21
Osteoclast-mediated bone resorption.
14.20 (left) BMBS plastic, Giemsa, breast cancer metastases, osteolytic lesion. Note row of osteoclasts on trabecular surface, bottom center.
14.21 (right) BMBS plastic, Giemsa, as for Figure 14.20, high magnification to show osteoclasts on and near bone.

14.22 and 14.23 Erosion of bone by tumor cells.
14.22 (left) BMBS plastic, Giemsa. Note tumor cells in direct apposition to bone.
14.23 (right) As for Figure 14.22, tumor cells eroding bone without presence of osteoclasts.

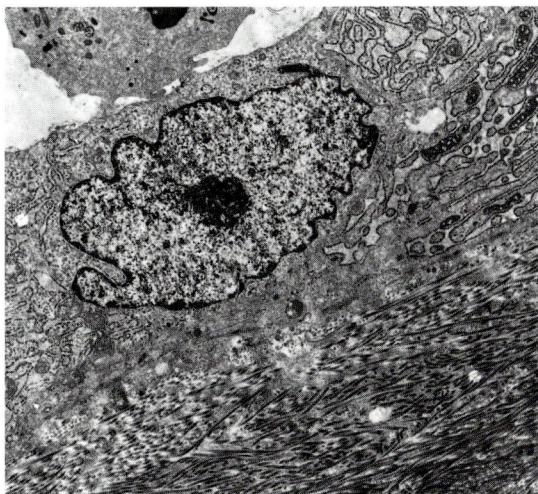

14.24 BMBS, EM, OAF-stimulated osteoclast eroding bone in a case of metastases of breast cancer with osteolytic lesions.

angiogenic factor produced by the tumor cells. This process may now be prevented by antibody-mediated blockade of a receptor on the vessels which results in their apoptosis and consequent tumor cell degeneration and growth inhibition. Fibroblasts and fibers, mast cells, monocytes, lymphocytes, and various other infiltrating cells enter the metastases together with the blood vessels. These in turn produce cytokines and evoke additional stromal reactions (Figures 14.26–14.29).

The stroma of the metastases depends partly on their ability to organise themselves and also on their capacity to produce factors which elicit the host's tissue reactions and these capacities may vary in different parts of the same metastases. Sometimes very small metastases evoke striking angiogenic, osteoblastic or osteoclastic reactions. Other tumor factors may stimulate hematopoiesis or the different cell lines separately, or the tumor cells may be chemotactic for the host tissue's infiltrating cells, such as lymphocytes, monocytes, macrophages and others. Necrosis of bone marrow and of the tumor cells may also be seen especially when the blood supply to the former is interrupted and the rate of multiplication of

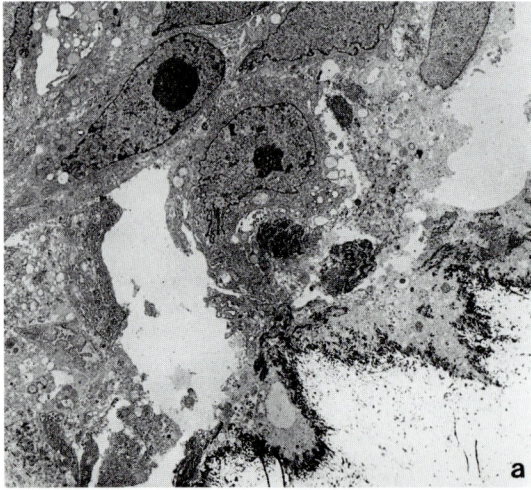

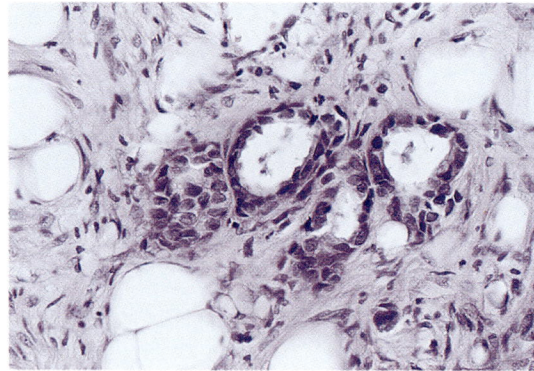

14.25a and b (left) BMBS, EM, aggressive carcinoma cells eroding bone without mediation by osteoclasts. Bone at bottom.

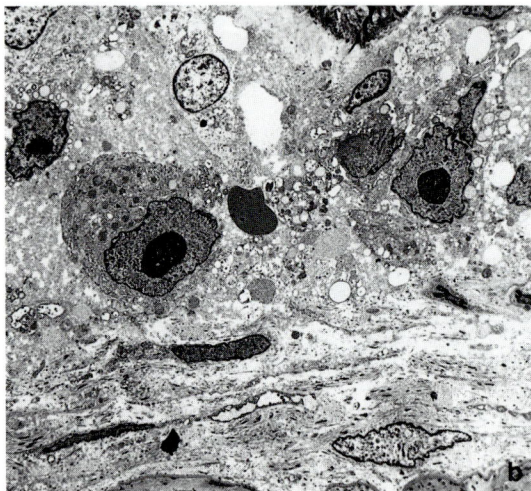

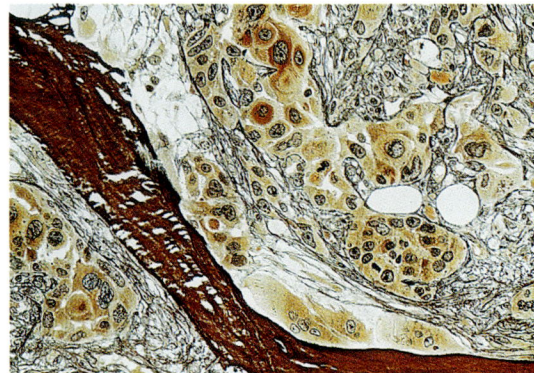

14.26–14.29 Metastases in bone marrow space containing reactive connective tissue, without hematopoiesis.
14.26 (right top) BMBS paraffin, H&E, metastases forming glandular structures within stromal connective tissue.
14.27 (right, second down) BMBS plastic, Gomori, to show extent of fiber content in the stroma supporting the tumor cells. Note osteoclast (left, center) on lower side of the trabecula and cluster of metastases next to it, and on the bone, examples of both types of osteolysis (see also Figure 19).
14.28 BMBS paraffin, I.H., actin-positive stroma.

the latter outstrips the vascular capacity so that extensive bone pain and fever result. Rarely, bone marrow metastases are confined to the vascular system, in which case they consist of masses of tumor cells with little discernible stroma. The following histological types of bone metastases are recognised: solid, adenomatous, scirrhous, squamous, small cell and mixed. Bone marrow metastases, as elsewhere, are composed of parenchyme and stroma in varying proportions. Owing to limitations of space, only metastases of prostate and of breast will be illustrated in detail as examples of the immunohistologic identification of metastatic tumor cells in the bone marrow. Only some of the most commonly applied antibodies are listed here, however. Many more are, of course, available.

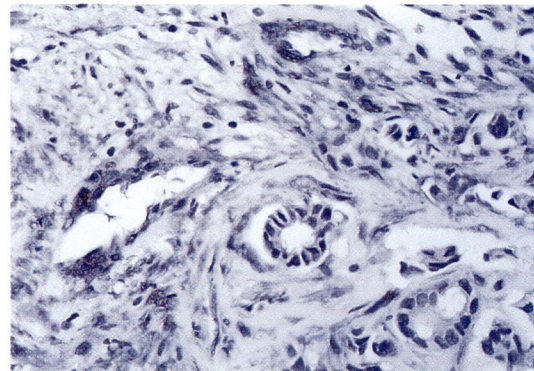

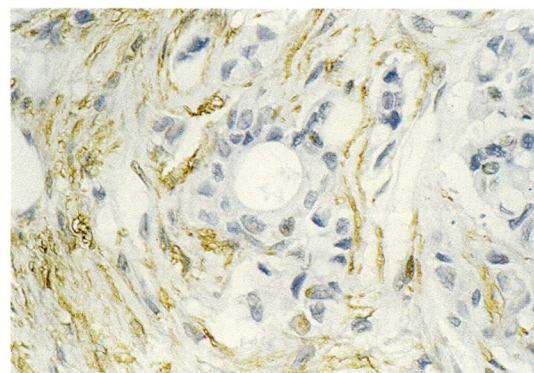

14.29 BMBS paraffin, I.H., vimentin-positive stroma around metastases.

130

Metastases according to tumor of origin

It should be stressed that included in this chapter are only metastases most likely to spread to the bones, especially the iliac crest, or conditions which must be considered in the differential diagnosis. Particularly important in this respect are the so-called 'small cell tumors' whose differential diagnosis, especially in children, includes tumors of bone, for example sarcomas (especially Ewing's, today considered with the neuroectodermal tumors), neuroblastomas, rhabdomyosarcomas, medulloblastomas and retinoblastomas. These are taken into account in the histologic diagnosis of myelomas, leukemias and lymphomas. Tumors of bone are relatively rare; in the USA there are about 1500 new cases a year, while there are about 93,000 of lung and 100,000 new cases of breast cancer annually.

Prostatic cancer

Immunohistology: prostate specific antigen (PSA), prostatic acid phosphatase (PAP), cytokeratin (Figures 14.30–14.36).

Many other diagnostic and prognostic markers are available and have been used in characterisation of the primary prostate tumor.

Cancer of the prostate is now the second most common cancer in Western men. As the life span of the population increases more men are living long enough for prostatic cancer to become clinically significant, to disseminate and thus to increase the contribution made by prostatic cancer to the overall death from malignancies. It has variously been estimated that distant metastases are present at diagnosis in 50–80% of the patients. There are still divergent opinions on the correlation between histology and prognosis, perhaps because the histology of the cells in the primary tumor

14.30–14.33 Bone metastases of prostatic cancer.
14.30 (left) BMBS paraffin, H&E, metastases in stroma with incipient new bone formation on upper trabecular surface, right.

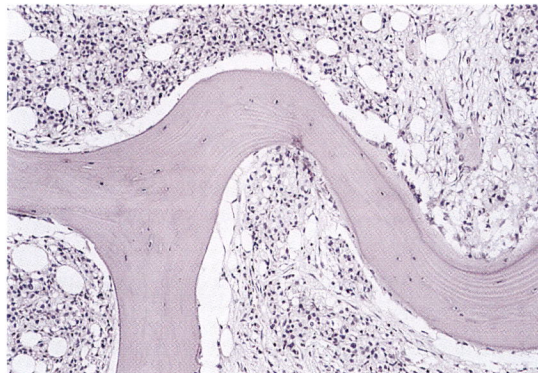

14.31 (right) As for Figure 14.30, I.H., cytokeratin strongly positive in the tumor cells.

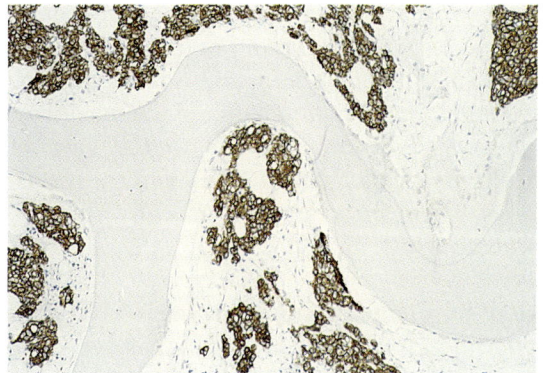

14.32 (left) As for Figure 14.30, I.H., prostatic specific antigen (PSA)-positive in the tumor cells.

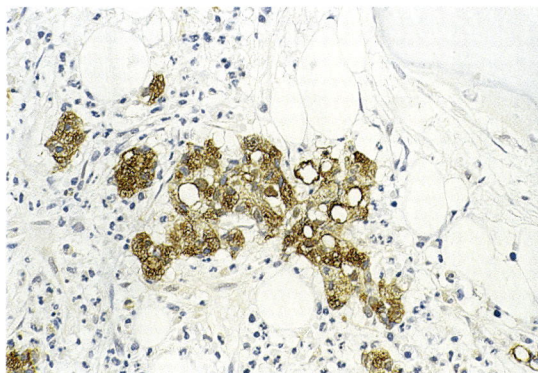

14.33 (right) As for Figure 14.30, I.H., prostatic acid phosphatase (PAP)-positive in the tumor cells.

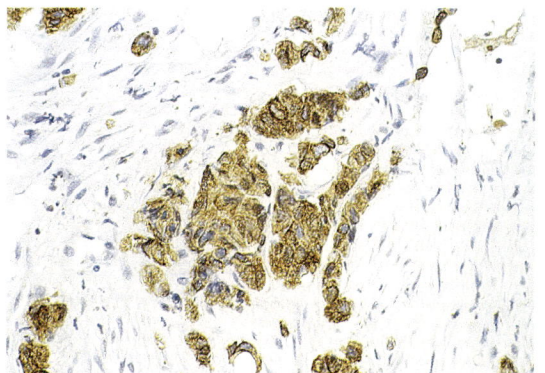

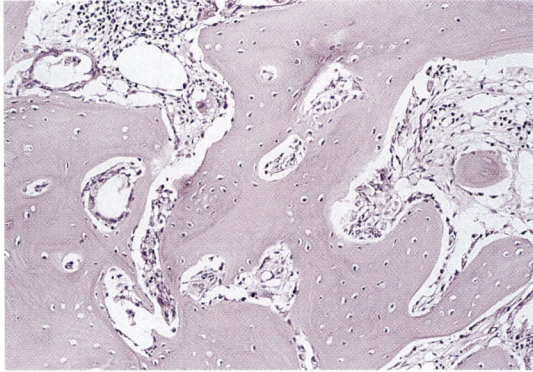

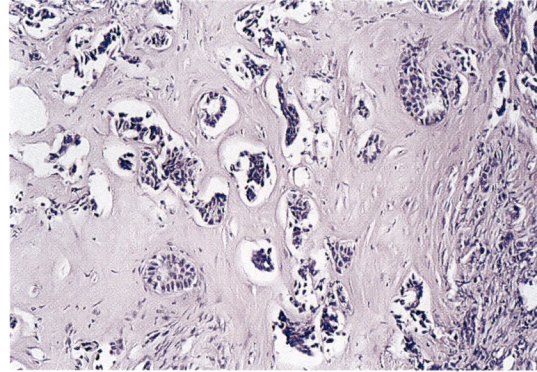

14.34–14.36 BMBS paraffin, H&E, a case of well-differentiated metastases of prostatic carcinoma, with marked osteosclerosis.
14.34 (left) H&E, low power, note metastases in bone.
14.35 (right) H&E, higher magnification showing glandular structures.

does not reflect the potential behavior of the cells at other sites as metastases. However, diagnostic methods are being investigated and developed to predict the aggressiveness of the primary tumor, that is, its metastatic potential. Some of the factors involved are demonstrable by immunohistology and by *in situ* hybridisation. In the future, such investigations could be carried out on both the primary tumor and its metastases to establish a possible correlation, for example, as already done for p53 and its nuclear accumulation in prostatic carcinoma and its metastases; p53 is thought to be essential for the maintenance of the malignant phenotype. Another factor is the rate of replication which may be altered in the metastases when the primary tumor is removed. Consequently, though estimates (more or less accurate) may be made of the speed of replication of the primary, these may have little relevance for its metastases. Moreover there are some indications that the variable natural history of prostatic cancer may be related to the response of the immune system in the individual patients, and to the hormone responsiveness of the tumor. From studies recorded in the literature it appears that bony metastases will develop in 75% of patients with involvement of the pelvic lymph nodes, even if these have been treated by dissection, by external beam radiation or both. The onset is often insidious, and patients may present with advanced disease and symptoms such as anemia resulting from skeletal metastases. Though there is still disagreement concerning the mode of spread and the distribution of

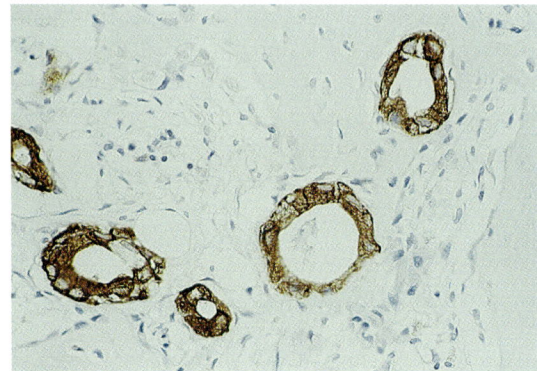

14.36 I.H. cytokeratin-positive, PSA and PAP were also positive, though not illustrated.

osseous metastases, the bones of the pelvis and the lumbar vertebrae are regarded as the most frequent sites for metastases. Both perineural lymphatic spread and dissemination via the vertebral venous plexus have their advocates as possible routes. Willis (1973) maintained that metastatic deposits reach the bones by way of the systemic circulation from secondary deposits in the lung.

Metastases of prostatic cancer in the bones often appear as lobules separated by bands of connective tissue, which may have some kind of glandular structure or present as solid masses of cells. The alveolar type is usually composed of small-to-medium-sized cells, while the medullary type may consist of large anaplastic cells with large, prominent nucleoli. It should be stressed that the appearance of prostatic cancer cells in the bone marrow varies considerably; nevertheless, all the types appear capable of evoking an osteoblastic reaction. In some cases this is so marked that the tumor cells themselves appear to get swallowed up in it. In other cases there may be large areas of necrosis when the expansion of the tumor cells has been intravascular. When a considerable portion of the newly formed bone is not mineralised wide osteoid seams result, so that a picture similar to osteomalacia is produced. The expression of several metastases related genes in the primary tumor has been related to its metastatic potential, particularly those genes involved in angiogenesis, invasion, adhesion and growth.

Cytogenetics

Structural alterations of chromosomes 7 and 10: del(7)(q22) and del(10)(q24). Metastasis suppressor genes have been localised to chromosomes 8, 10, 11 and 17.

Breast cancer

Immunohistology: a panel of antibodies may be required, including cytokeratin, epithelial membrane antigen (EMA), CA125, CEA, CA19-9, BCA225, estrogen and progesterone receptors (Figures 14.37–14.42).

Breast cancer is today the main cause of death from cancer in women in the USA (and many other parts of the world) and about 100,000 new cases are diagnosed each year. Moreover, another important point is that despite all therapeutic advances and earlier detection, the death rate appears to have remained fairly stable over the past several decades and there has been little significant benefit from adjuvant chemotherapy. In addition, autopsy findings have demonstrated a high incidence of skeletal metastases in patients with mammary cancer who died either in the first or the second 5-year period irrespective of the immediate cause of death. Such observations raise a number of important issues: (1) correlation between the histological features of the primary tumor and those of the metastases in the bones; (2) the effect of the more aggressive treatment schedules on early

14.37 and 14.38 BMBS paraffin, a case of bone marrow metastases of mammary carcinoma.
14.37 (left) H&E, metastases in connective tissue stroma.

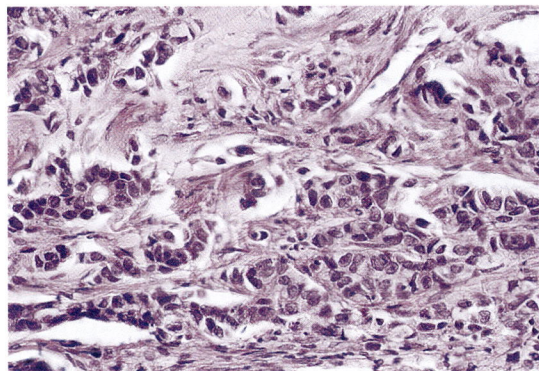

14.38 (right) I.H., tumor cells positive for cytokeratin.

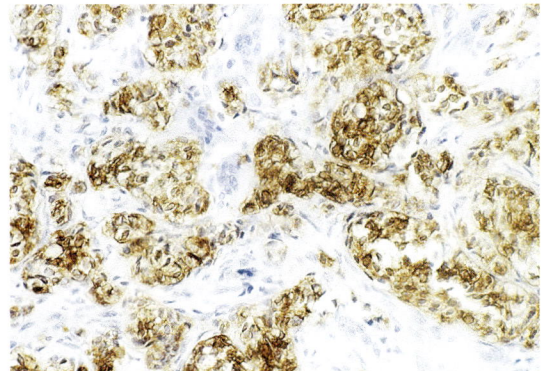

14.39 and 14.41 BMBS paraffin, another case of metastases of breast cancer.
14.39 (left) I.H., epithelial membrane antigen (EMA)-positive.

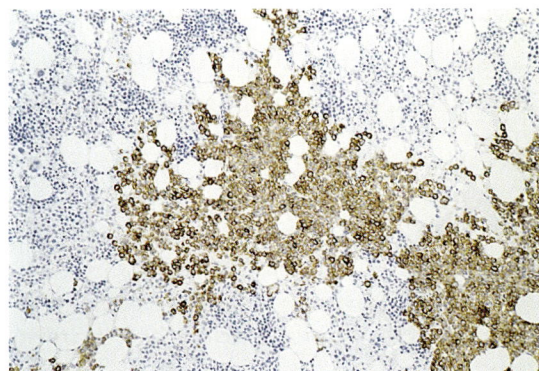

14.40 (right) I.H., progesterone receptor-positive.

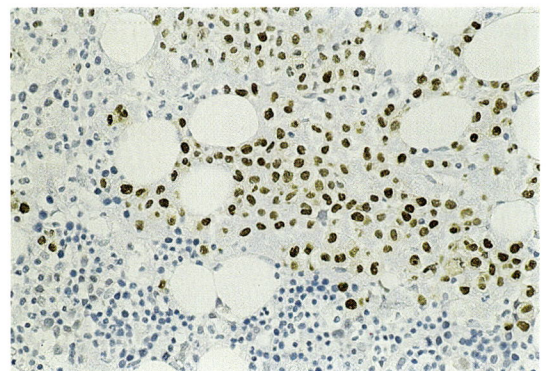

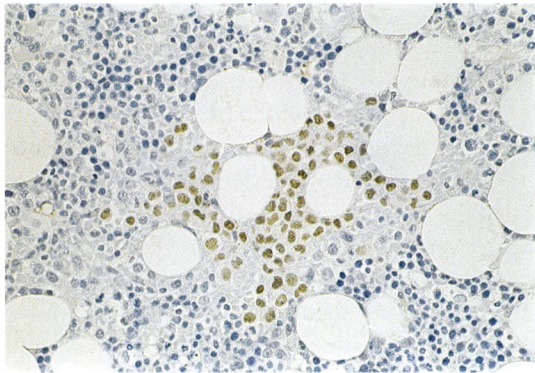

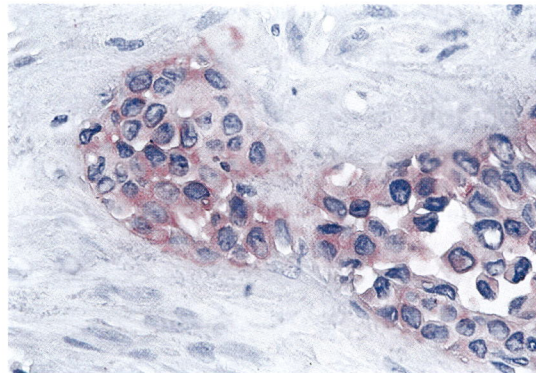

14.41 (left) I.H. for P53, which is also positive in the tumor cells. Estrogen receptors were also positive as were BCA225 and CA19.9, though not illustrated.

14.42 (right) BMBS plastic, I.H., tumor cells of breast cancer positive for cytokeratin.

or late metastatic potential and growth rate; and (3) the problem of late recurrences.

With respect to the histopathology of the primary tumor, the natural history of mammary cancer shows that it encompasses a heterogeneous group of diseases, with variable time courses. Little if any mention is made of this in many clinical trials, though various studies have indicated an association between histological types and probability of recurrence. Certain multicenter trials tend to stratify breast tumors only according to lymph node status and ignore the histopathological nature of the primary neoplasm. Nevertheless, a correlation between the histology of the primary tumor and that of its metastases may well provide information for a better understanding of the histological grade and the malignant potential of the primary growth. This is all the more important as some neoplasias may appear histologically malignant, but be relatively benign from the point of view of their biological behavior. Assessment of the results of therapeutic trials requires precise classification of the primary tumor, and also of the metastases being treated with a view to eradication.

Similar considerations apply to the hormone dependency of human breast cancer: it is not an all or nothing phenomenon, but a spectrum because of the mixture of receptor-positive and -negative cells in various proportions in every tumor. Therefore clinical trials must also incorporate this sort of information into their experimental design. Finally, there is the question of late recurrences. These have

been documented as occurring from several months to over 10–20 years after removal of a primary tumor. This necessitates permanent follow-up at regular intervals of such patients, especially as skeletal metastases may be detected by bone biopsy in the absence of noteworthy changes in the peripheral blood or abnormalities in other tests. These 'dormant' metastases may have been stimulated to grow by perturbation of their environment, i.e. the host tissues, by events such as changes in hormone or immune status, or by surgery, or other major biologic events which upset the balance keeping the metastases in check.

There are no effective tests available today for the early detection of skeletal metastases other than direct examination of the bone marrow. The relative merits of X-rays and skeletal scintigraphy for early detection of breast carcinoma metastases in bone have been investigated in a large series of patients and some investigators concluded that both were unnecessary. Biopsies are considered to be better than serial bone scans to assess the response to chemotherapy in breast cancer.

Cytogenetics

The non-random chromosomal abnormalities reported include aberrations of chromosomes 1, 3, 6, 11, 16 and 17. When correlated with survival, patients without complex karyotypes appeared to have a better prognosis. Moreover, mutations affecting cancer susceptibility genes *BRCA1* and *BRCA2* are responsible for approximately 5–10% of all cases and 45% of inherited cases. *BRCA2* is involved in DNA repair, which also makes the cells with the mutated genes more sensitive to toxic damage, including radiation and chemotherapy.

Pulmonary cancer (Figures 14.43–14.46)

Immunohistology: carcinoembryonic antigen (CEA), cytokeratin, epithelial membrane antigen (EMA) and neuroendocrine markers in small cell carcinoma.

This accounts for about one-third of all cancer deaths. The mortality in women is approximately one-quarter that of men but it is increasing. The association between lung cancer and smoking now appears thoroughly documented from clinical, statistical and experimental aspects. In patients with bronchogenic cancer, histological classification of the primary tumor is required before therapy is initiated. The major groups according to the WHO classification are (1) squamous cell carcinoma, (2) small cell carci-noma, (3) adenocarcinoma, and (4) large cell carcinoma; each of these groups has variants and subtypes. Pulmonary cancer is characterised by early and widespread invasion of the lymphatics and blood vessels and metastases may occur anywhere, especially in the brain and bones, even from small and clinically silent primary tumors. Extracellular matrix-degrading enzymes (urokinase-type plasmino-gen activator, stromelysins and matrilysins) are involved in the transition from lung pre-neoplasia to invasive carcinoma and thus to metastases. Importantly, recent work suggests that these invasion-associated proteases are derived predominantly from non-neoplastic tumor elements, therefore therapy should be targeted against these host factors too. Such host-derived stromal components are also con-stituents of the metastases. Overall about 20% of patients are thought to have positive iliac crest biopsies at diagnosis. In small cell carci-noma, this may rise to 30% if large unilateral

14.43 (left) BMBS plastic, Gomori, metastases of bronchial cancer. Note complete absence of osseous reaction.

14.44 (right) BMBS paraffin, H&E, bone marrow metastasis of unknown primary tumor. Solid mass of tumor cells replacing bone marrow. There was no osseous reaction.

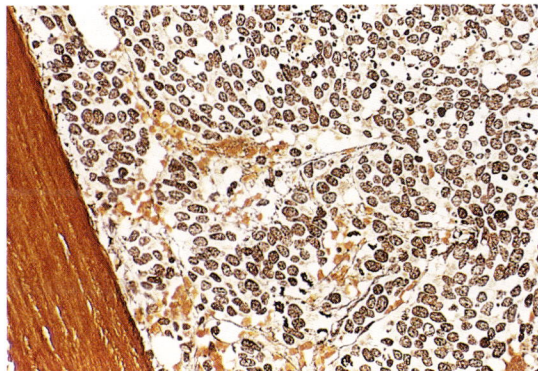

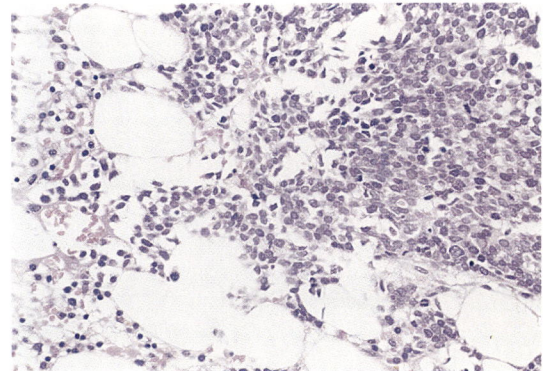

14.45 (left) Same as for Figure 14.44 showing positive reaction with neurospecific enolase.

14.46 (right) Same as for Figure 14.44 showing a reaction with synapto-physin; these reactions suggest an oat cell carci-noma of the lung confirmed on further investigation.

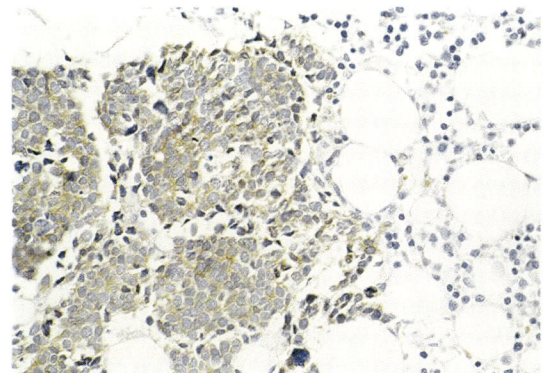

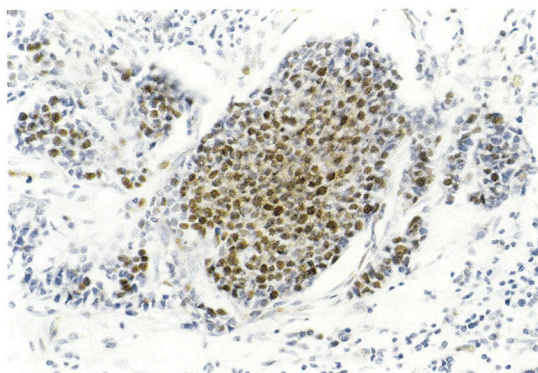

or bilateral biopsies are taken. An incidence of 17–42% has been reported in anaplastic small cell carcinoma. Studies in large series of patients with the other histological groups have not yet been reported. It is useful to employ a combination of markers, for example BCA225+, CEA+, CA125+ and CA19.9 may indicate metastases of pulmonary tumors; in small cell carcinoma, neuroendocrine markers are useful (Figures 14.44–14.46). However, metastases of pulmonary adenoca in the bone marrow positive for both estrogen and progesterone receptors have been described. These markers, therefore, cannot be relied on as discriminating between breast and lung as primary sites in patients with metastases of unknown origin. Non-small cell carcinoma may also be reactive with some lymphoid cell markers.

Cytogenetics

Deletions of chromosomes 3, 7 and 10 have been reported.

Gastrointestinal tumors

Immunohistology: CEA, cytokeratin, EMA (Figures 14.47–14.50).

About 20% of patients with known gastrointestinal tumors have skeletal metastases. Recent studies have shown that metastases of colorectal tumors are also far more frequent than previously suspected – in 29% of patients undergoing apparently curative resection occult hepatic metastases were present at operation and were revealed by computed tomography. Such tumors may also metastasise to the bones. Metastases of tumors of colon may be CEA+, CA19.9+, but BCA225 and CA125 negative. Carcinoid may produce signet-ring-like cells in metastases.

Gastric carcinomas

Variable numbers of numerical and structural changes have been reported: polysomy of chromosomes 2 and 20, rearrangements of chromosomes 1, 3, 7 and 13, as well as 11p13-

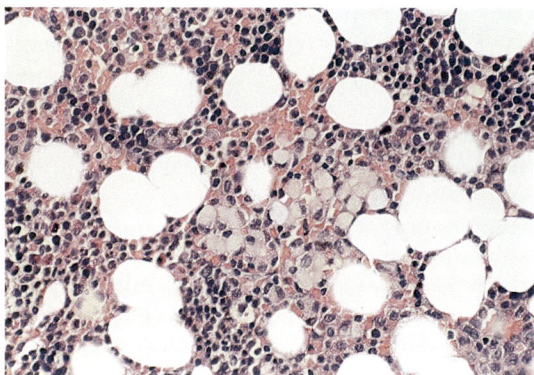

14.47 (left) BMBS paraffin, H&E, metastases of colon cancer.

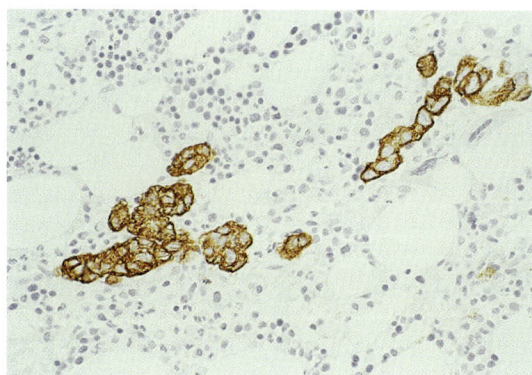

14.48 (right) As for Figure 14.47, I.H., cytokeratin positive.

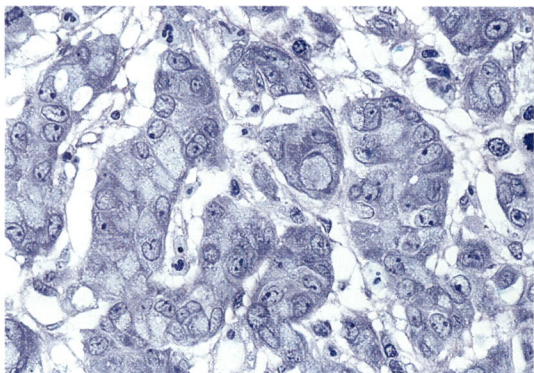

14.49 (left) BMBS plastic, Giemsa, metastases of colon cancer.

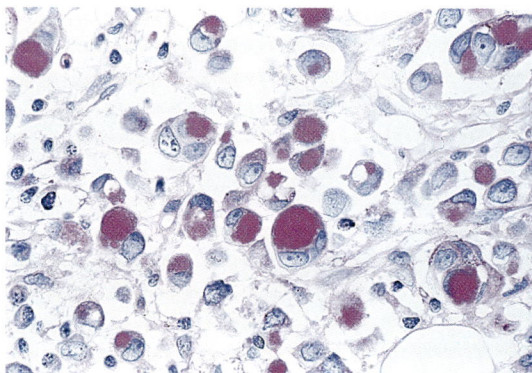

14.50 (right) BMBS plastic, PAS-positive metastatic tumor cells, scattered in bone marrow; case of gastric cancer.

15, and other aberrations. In advanced gastric tumors many other chromosomes are also involved.

Renal tumors

Immunohistology: cytokeratin, EMA, metastases of the genitourinary tract may be CEA, CA19.9 and CA125-positive, while BCA225 is negative.

The incidence of metastases of renal tumors in children is relatively low and males are affected more than females. In adults, metastases of renal carcinoma (hypernephroma) may consist of large, clear cells with a high cytoplasmic to nuclear ratio (Figures 14.51 and 14.52).

Cytogenetics

Loss or rearrangement of 3p has been reported in renal clear cell carcinoma. Other structural changes including translocations t(9;14) and t(X:1).

Malignant melanoma

Immunohistology: HMB45, 0.13, S100, Fontana stain.

Metastases of malignant melanoma may be detected in the bone marrow in a small percentage of the patients (Figure 14.53). There is no difficulty in recognition if the melanotic granules are present; but when there are no or very few granules, immediate identification may not be possible. However, melanoma cells are stained by the stain even when pigmentation is not observed after routine staining of smears and sections. Cells positive in the stain do not reveal blue granules (iron) with the Prussian blue method. Though the pleomorphic character of the melanoma cells makes them easy to identify as a rule, in doubtful cases immunohistology (I.H.) will show a positive reaction with S100 and 013; a positive Fontana stain, and EM will substantiate the diagnosis.

Cytogenetics

Frequent losses of chromosomes 5, 9, 17 and Y; complex structural abnormalities involving chromosomes 1p, 1q, 3p, 9p and 12q, chromosome 6 and trisomy 7.

Ewing's sarcoma

Immunohistology: HBA-71, 0-13, vimentin.

In children this has a high rate (52%) of involvement in iliac crest biopsies.

14.51 and 14.52 Bone marrow metastases of renal carcinoma.

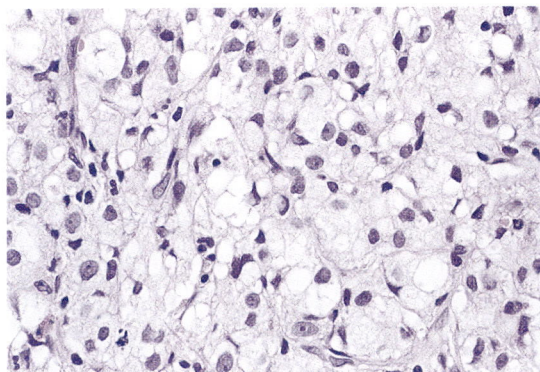

14.51 BMBS paraffin, H&E, showing the typical large 'clear' cells.

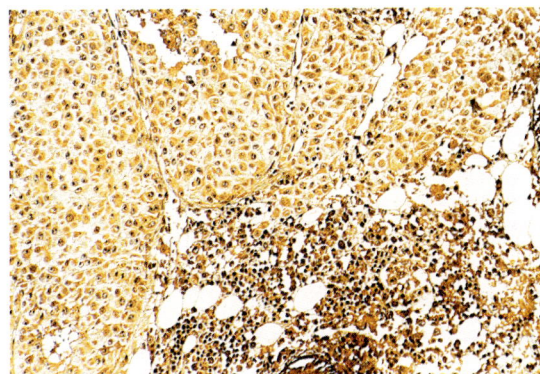

14.52 BMBS plastic, Giemsa similar large 'clear' metastatic cells, with connective tissue and residual hematopoiesis fat cells (left).

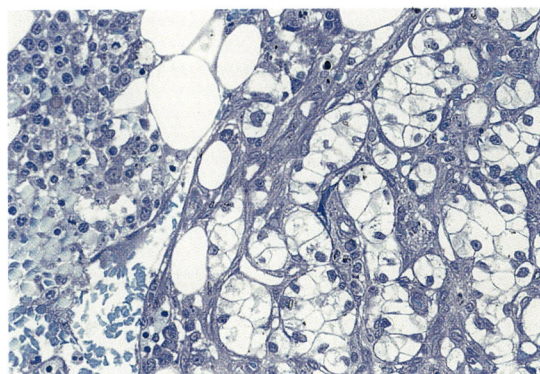

14.53 BMBS plastic, Gomori, malignant melanoma, with massive invasion of bone marrow, without an osseous reaction and a normal bone scan.

Cytogenetics

There is a specific translocation t(11;22) (q24;q12) that can be used as a marker of this tumor. Metastases of Ewing's and the following four groups of tumors are considered in the differential diagnosis of malignant small cell involvement of the bone marrow, especially in children.

Neuroblastomas

Immunohistology: chromogranin, neurofilaments, neuron-specific enolase (NSE).

Secondaries of these tumors may show a rosette-like arrangement of metastatic cells, both in smears and sections.

Cytogenetics

Deletions of chromosome 1, double minute chromosomes and homogeneously staining regions (HSRs) have been described.

Rhabdomyosarcoma

Immunohistology: vimentin, actin, desmin, myoglobin.

Cytogenetics

t(2,13)(q35-37;q14).

Medulloblastomas

Immunohistology: neurofilaments, chromogranin, vimentin.

In some cases, medulloblastomas may metastasise early, and these small-cell undifferentiated tumors may then mimic leukemia. Rarely, dissemination to the skeleton occurs before the intracranial mass is evident. Metastases of hemangiopericytomas (a form of angioblastic meningioma) may also be found in the pelvic bones, among others.

Cytogenetics

The most commonly detected are structural abnormalities of chromosomes 1 and 17, though structural changes in other marrow chromosomes have also been described.

Retinoblastoma

Immunohistology: the cells are positive for neurofilaments and chromogranin.

This occurs as a hereditary and a non-hereditary form.

Cytogenetics

A deletion of 13q14 in 5% has been shown, as well as structural rearrangements of 1 and -13, and i(6)(p).

Ovarian tumors

Immunohistology: cytokeratin.

Skeletal deposits of these tumors may consist of signet-ring-like cells, containing strongly PAS-positive material. A panel of antibodies showing characteristic results may be required, e.g. CA125+, BCA225+, while CEA and CA19.9 are negative.

Cytogenetics

Structural changes of chromosomes 1, 17 and trisomy 12 and t(6;14)(q21;q24).

Metastases of unknown primary tumors

Immunohistology: panel of antibodies, depending on clinical setting.

These are sometimes called ACUP (adenocarcinoma of unknown primary). The histological aspect of the metastases may give an indication of their possible source. Metastases of intestinal origin frequently have the histological features of adenocarcinomas with tubular or acinous structures possibly containing PAS-positive material. A medullary arrangement may be observed in metastases of bronchogenic carcinoma. Prostatic and mammary cancers will have the features described above.

Solid masses of tumor cells sometimes indicate metastases of prostatic carcinoma (though there is a great histological variation in these metastases). A scirrhous type frequently indicates secondaries of mammary carcinoma. Metastases of both prostatic and mammary cancer sometimes produce such a strong osteoblastic reaction that the bone in the biopsy resembles that seen in extreme osteosclerosis, with tiny marrow cavities occupied by connective tissue of variable density in which the tumor cells may not be present, or are unrecognisable.

Where morphology is inadequate, there are now many markers available which provide information on the histogenesis of tumors and metastases, for example Factor VIII-related antigen, which indicates a vascular origin, vimentin for sarcomas, desmin and actin for muscles, chromogranin and neurofilament antigen for tumors of neural origin. Alternatively, a panel of antibodies may be required.

In rare cases, it may be necessary to attempt to identify metastases in the bone marrow in a patient who suffers from two primary tumors, for example, bronchial and mammary cancer. In this case, even estrogen and progesterone receptors are not discriminatory as they may be positive in metastases of adenocarcinoma of both organs; thus, there may be instances in which more sophisticated methods need to be employed.

A fundamental weakness of modern tumor therapy is that it neglects variation in a given tumor population, both in appearance and the properties of the cells. Moreover, such histological diversity characterises the metastases as well as primary tumors. Tumor cell diversity is now amenable to investigation, as is correlation of the features of the primary tumor with those of its metastases. Both of these aspects are important in decisions on therapy.

Moreover, reliable histopathologic markers are under investigation with the aim of their inclusion in cancer evaluation and the results considered in treatment protocols; for example, demonstration of the presence or absence of p27 Klpl. p27 is a cyclin-dependent kinase inhibitor which is reduced or absent in aggressive tumors, consequently its loss may contribute to oncogenesis and tumor progression. Levels of p27 may be checked by a simple and reliable histochemical technique.

Check list: Metastastic Bone Disease

- Adequate to large biopsy (3 × 50 mm or larger)?
- Cortex and cancellous bone present?
- Normal or altered trabecular network?
- Alterations of osseous remodeling?
- Areas of fibrosis or serous atrophy? Reticulin stain, vimentin.
- Single, clusters, groups or masses of metastatic cells in interstitium and/or in sinusoids? Micrometastases?
- Stromal, cellular or osseous reactions?
- Mitotic figures in tumor cells?
- Morphologic type of tumor cells?
- Structure of metastases – glands, secretion?
- Extent of occupation of biopsy by the metastases?
- Identification of organ or origin: by morphology and by immunohistology, e.g. by means of cytokeratin, epithelial membrane antigen (EMA) and the specific antigens for each type of malignancy, where available, or combination of others.
- Host reactions to metastases: atrophy, infiltration, osteolysis and/or osteosclerosis?

Example

Bone biopsy, 3 × 40 and 3 × 30 mm. Periosteal tissues, cortical and trabecular network present. Portions of both pieces show normal trabecular architecture, remodeling and bone marrow, except for small clusters of malignant cells in interstitium and blood vessels. The rest of both pieces show altered sclerotic trabecular structure with mainly osteoblastic remodeling, and marrow cavities filled with large groups of metastases, with some glandular formation within variably dense, vascular connective tissue. On immunohistology, the malignant cells are

Continued

positive with cytokeratin, prostatic acid phosphatase and prostate specific antigen. Diagnosis: bone biopsy showing extensive replacement by metastases of adenocarcinoma of prostatic origin, and osteosclerotic reaction.

Clinical correlations

- Clinical history and site of primary tumor.
- Metastases especially frequent in 'osteotropic' metastatic tumors.
- Biochemical markers in blood and urine – tumor markers, and indicators of bone resorption and formation, osteocalcin, alkaline phosphatase.

- X-ray, bone scan, CT and MRI evidence of location and extent of involvement.
- Type and duration of therapy, and time elapsed since its completion are important for evaluation of patient in follow-up and interpretation of biopsy findings.
- Correlation of characteristics of metastases with those of primary tumor, if and when possible.
- Hypercalcemia: especially in metastases of breast, renal, pulmonary and ovarian tumors (and in MM).
- Hypercalcemia: cardiac, gastrointestinal, renal and neuromuscular dysfunctions.
- Osteoprotection with bisphosphonates? It is important to know when assessing cortical and trabecular bone.

Bibliography

Abeloff M.D.(1987) Paraneoplastic syndromes. *N Engl J Med.*, **317**, 1598.

Adelman H.M., Wallach P.M., Flannery M.T. (1991) Ewing's sarcoma of the ilium presenting as unilateral sacroilitis. *J Rheumatol.*, **18 (7)**, 1109–11.

Akerman M., Dreinhofer K., Rydholm A. *et al.* (1996) Cytogenetic studies on fine-needle aspiration samples from osteosarcoma and Ewing's sarcoma. *Diagn Cytopathol.*, **15 (1)**, 17–22.

Algra P.R., Bloem J.L., Tissing H. *et al.* (1991) Detection of vertebral metastases: comparison between MR imaging and bone scintigraphy. *Radiographics*, **11 (2)**, 219–32.

Amanao Y., Kumazaki T. (1996) Case report: serous atrophy of bone marrow and subcutaneous tissue enhancement associated with recurrent rectal carcinoma: MR appearances. *Comput Med Imaging Graph.*, **20 (3)**, 183–5.

Anderson I.C., Shpall E.J., Leslie D.S. *et al.* (1989) Elimination of malignant clonogenic breast cancer cells from human bone marrow. *Cancer Res.*, **49 (16)**, 4659–64.

Anner R.M., Drewinko B. (1977) Frequency, and significance of bone marrow involvement in metastatic solid tumors. *Cancer*, **39**, 160.

Arden K.C., Anderson M.J., Finckenstein F.G. *et al.* (1996) Detectioon of the t(2;13) chromosomal translocation in alveolar rhabdomyosarcoma using the reverse transcriptase-polymerase chain reaction. *Genes Chromosomes Cancer*, **16 (4)**, 254–60.

Batson O.V. (1940) The function of the vertebral veins and their role in spread of metastases. *Ann Surg.*, **112**, 138.

Bellahcene A., Menard S., Bufalino R. *et al.* (1996) Expression of bone sialoprotein in primary human breast cancer is associated with poor survival. *Int J Cancer*, **69 (4)**, 350–3.

Ben-Eliyahu S., Page G.G., Yirmiya R., Taylor A.N. (1996) Acute alcohol intoxication suppresses natural killer cell activity and promotes tumor metastasis. *Nature Med*, **2 (4)**, 457–61.

Berger U., Bettelheim R., Mansi J.L. *et al.* (1988) The relationship between micrometastases in the bone marrow, histopathologic features of the primary tumor in breast cancer and prognosis. *Am. J Clin Pathol.*, **90**, 1.

Berthold F., Schneider A., Schumacher R., Bosslet K. (1989) Detection of minimal disease in bone marrow of neuroblastoma patients by immunofluorescence. *Pediatr. Hematol. Oncol.*, **6 (2)**, 73–83.

Bijvoet O.L.M., Lipton A. (eds) (1991) *Osteoclast Inhibition in the Management of Malignancy-related Bone Disorders.* Lewiston: Hografe & Huber.

Bitter M.A., Fiorito D., Corkill M.E. *et al.* (1994) Bone marrow involvement by lobular carcinoma of the breast cannot be identified reliably by routine histological examination alone. *Hum Pathol*, **25 (8)**, 781–8.

Bolon I., Devouassoux M., Robert C. *et al.* (1997) Expression of urokinase-type plasminogen activator, stromelysin 1, stromelysin 3, and matrilysin genes in lung carcinomas. *Am J Pathol.*, **150 (5)**, 1619.

Boyce B.F. (1991) Normal bone remodeling and its disruption in metastatic bone disease. In Rubens and Fogelman (eds), *Bone Metastases: Diagnosis and Treatment.* London: Springer.

Bratt O., Anderson H. (1996) Metaphase cytogenetics and DNA flow cytometry with analysis of S-phase fraction in prostate cancer: influence on prognosis. *Urology*, **47 (2)**, 218–24.

Brown R.W., Campagna L.B., Dunn J.K., Cagle P.T. (1997) Immunohistochemical identification of tumor markers in metastatic adenocarcinoma. A diagnostic adjunct in the determination of primary site. *Am J Clin Pathol.*, **107 (1)**, 12–9.

Bundred N.J., Ratcliffe W.A., Walker R.A. *et al.* (1991) Parathyroid hormone related protein and hypercalcemia in breast cancer. *Br. Med J.*, **303**, 1506.

Burtis W.J., Bradt T.G., Orloff J.J. *et al.* (1990) Immunochemical charcterization of circulating parathyroid hormone-related proteins in patients with humoral hypercalcemia of cancer. *N Engl J Med.*, **322**, 1106.

Carter R.L. (1985) Patterns and mechanisms of bone metastases. *J Roy Soc Med.*, **78 (9)**, 2.

Castello A., Coci A., Magrini U. (1992) Paraneoplastic marrow alterations in patients with cancer. *Hematologica*, **77 (5)**, 392–7.

Cervantes M., Glassman A.B. (1996) Breast cancer cytogenetics: a review and proposal for clinical application. *Ann Clin Lab Sci.*, **26 (3)**, 208–14.

Caizavelos C., Bhaitagharya N., Ung Y.C. *et al.* (1997) Decreased levels of cell-cycle inhibitor p27[klpl] protein. Prognostic implications in primary breast cancer. *Nature Medicine*, **3 (2)**, 227.

Cho K.R., Olson J.L., Epstein J.I. (1988) Primitive rhabdomyosarcoma presenting with diffuse bone marrow involvement: an immunohistochemical and ultrastructural study. *Mod Pathol*, **1 (1)**, 23–8.

Clarke M.R., Landreneau R.J., Finkelstein S.D. *et al.* (1997) Extracellular matrix expression in metastasizing and nonmetastasizing adenocarcinomas of the lung. *Human Pathol.*, 54–9.

Clarke N.W., McChire J., George N.J. (1991) Morphometric evidence for bone resorption and replacement in prostate cancer. *Br. J Urol.*, **68**, 74.

Dahiya R., Deng G., Chen K.M. *et al.* (1996) P53 tumor-suppressor gene mutations are mainly localised on exon 7 in human primary and metastatic prostate cancer. *Br J Cancer*, **74 (2)**, 264–8.

Daly H.A., Davison E.V., Pearson A.D. *et al.* (1987) Chromosomes of metastatic retinoblastoma. *Arch. Dis. Child.*, **62 (4)**, 410–1.

Dawson C., Whitfield H. (1996) Urological Malignancy –1: Prostate cancer. *BMJ*, **312**, 1032–4.

Devaney K., Vinh T.N., Sweet D.E. (1993) Small cell osteosarcoma of bone: An immunohistochemical study with differential diagnostic considerations. *Human Pathol.*, **24 (11)**, 1211–25.

Diel I.J., Kaufmann M., Bastert G. (eds) (1994) *Metastatic Bone Disease: Fundamental and Clinical Aspects.* Springer.

Dunn P., Shih LY., Liaw S.J., Sun C.F. (1993) Bone marrow necrosis in 38 adult cancer patients. *J Formos Med Assoc*, **92 (12)**, 1107–10.

Dunphy C.H. (1996) The role of wide-spectrum cytokeratin staining of the bone

marrow cores in patients with ductal carcinoma of the breast. *Mod Pathol*, **9 (10)**, 955–8.

Evans C.W. (1991) *The Metastatic Cell: Behavior and Biochemistry.* London: Chapman & Hall.

Feliu J., Gonzalez-Baron M., Artal A. *et al.* (1991) Bone marrow examination in small cell lung cancer – when is it indicated? *Acta. Oncol.*, **30 (5)**, 587–91.

Fitzmaurice R.J., Johnson P.R., Yin J.A., Freemont A.J. (1991) Rhabdomyosarcoma presenting as 'acute leukemia'. *Histopathology*, **18 (2)**, 173–5.

Franklin W.A., Shpall E.J., Archer P. *et al.* (1996) Immunocytochemical detection of breast cancer cells in marrow and peripheral blood of patients undergoing high dose chemotherapy with autologous stem cell support. *Breast Cancer Res Treat.*, **41 (4)**, 1–13.

Frassica F.J., Sim F.H. (1988) Pathogenesis and Prognosis. In Sim (ed.), *Diagnosis and Management of Metastatic Bone Disease.* New York: Raven.

Frewin R., Henson A., Provan D. (1997) ABC of clinical haematology: Haematological emergencies. *BMJ*, **314**, 1333–6.

Frisch B., Bartl R. (1990) *Atlas of Bone Marrow Pathology.* Dordrecht: Kluwer.

Frisch B., Bartl R., Mahl G., Burkhardt R. (1984) Scope and value of bone marrow biopsies in metastatic cancer. *Invasion Metastasis*, **4 (1)**, 12–30.

Frisch B., Lewis S.M., Burkhardt R., Bartl R. (1985) *Biopsy Pathology of Bone and Bone Marrow.* London: Chapman & Hall.

Galasko C.S.B. (1982) Mechanisms of lytic and blastic metastatic disease of bone. *Clin Orthop.*, **169**, 20.

Giaccone G., Ciuffreda L., Donadio M. *et al.* (1987) Bone marrow evaluation in small cell carcinoma of the lung. *Acta. Oncol.*, **26 (3)**, 185–8.

Giai M., Natoli C., Sismondi P. et al. (1990) Bone marrow micrometastases detected by a monoclonal antibody in patients with breast cancer. Anticancer Res., 10 (1), 119–21.

Gibbons B., Scott D., Hungerford J.L. et al. (1995) Retinoblastoma in association with the chromosome breakage syndromes Fanconi's anemia and Bloom's syndrome: clinical and cytogenetic findings. Clin Genet., 47 (6), 311–17.

Gittes R.F. (1991) Carcinoma of the prostate. N Engl J Med., 324, 236.

Greene G.F., Kitadai Y., Pettaway C.A. et al. (1997) Correlation of metastasis-related gene expression with metastatic potential in human prostate carcinoma cells implanted in nude mice using an in situ messenger RNA hybridization technique. Am J Pathol., 150 (5), 1571–82.

Gussetis E.S., Ebener U., Wehner S., Kornhuber B. (1989) Immunologic identification of undetectable neuroblastoma cells by current cytohistological studies of bone marrow samples. Onkologie, 12 (1), 9–11.

Honn K.V., Aref A., Chen Y.Q. et al. (1996) Prostate cancer: old problems and new approaches. Pathol Oncol Res., 2 (3), 191–211.

Ioachim H.L., Pambuccian S.E., Hekimgil M. et al. (1996) Lymphoid monoclonal antibodies reactive with lung tumors. Am J Surg Pathol., 20 (1), 64–71.

Isaacs J.J. (1997) Molecular markers for prostate cancer metastasis. Am J Pathol., 150 (5), 1511–21.

Jay V., Squire J., Zielenska M. et al. (1995) Molecular and cytogenetic analysis of a cerebellar primitive neuroectodermal tumor with prominent neuronal differentiation: detection of MYCN amplification by differential polymerase chain reaction and Southern blot analysis. Pediatr Pathol Lab Med., 15 (5), 733–44.

Johansson M., Heim S., Mandahl N. et al. (1993) Cytogenetic analysis of six bronchial carcinoids. Cancer Genet Cytogenet., 66 (1), 33–8.

Loda M., Cukor B., Tam S.W. et al. (1997) Increased proteasome-dependent degradation of the cyclin-dependent kinase inhibitor p27 in aggressive colorectal carcinomas. Nature Medicine, 3(2), 222.

Manishen W.J., Sivananthan K., Orr F.W. (1986) Resorbing bone stimulates tumor cell growth: a role for the host micro-environment in bone metastasis. Am. J Pathol., 123, 39.

Mareel M.M., deBaetselier P., VanRoy F.M. (1991) Mechanisms of Invasion and Metastasis. Boca Raton: CRC Press.

Mathieu M.C., Friedman S., Bosq J. et al. (1990) Immunohistochemical staining of bone marrow biopsies for detection of occult metastasis in breast cancer. Breast Cancer Res. Treat., 15 (1), 21–6.

McManus A.P., Gusterson B.A., Pinkerton C.R., Shipley J.M. (1995) Diagnosis of Ewing's sarcoma and related tumors by detection of chromosome 22q12 translocations using fluorescence in situ hybridization on tumor touch imprints. J Pathol., 176 (2), 137–42.

Micheau C., Boussen H., Klijanieko J. et al. (1987), Bone marrow biopsies in patients with undifferentiated carcinoma of the nasopharyngeal type. Cancer, 60 (10), 2459–64.

Morandi S., Manna A., Sabattini E., Porcellini, A. (1996) Rhabdomyosarcoma presenting as acute leukemia. J Pediatr Hematol Oncol, 18 (3), 305–7.

Mosekilde L., Eriksen E.F., Charles P. (1991) Hypercalcemia of malignancy: patho-physiology, diagnosis and treatment. Crit Rev Oncol Hemat., 11, 1.

Moss T.J., Reynolds C.P., Sather H.N. et al. (1991), Prognostic value of immuno-cytologic detection of bone marrow metastases in neuroblastoma. N. Engl. J. Med., 324 (4), 219–26.

Mundy G.R., Martin T.J. (1993) Pathophysiology of skeletal complications of cancer. In Munday and Martin (eds), Physiology and Pharmacology of Bone. Handbook of Experimental Pharmacology, vol. 107, pp. 641–71.

Nabel G.J., Grunfield C. (1996) Calories lost – another mediator of cancer cachexia? Nature Med, 2 (4), 397–9.

Neville A.M. (1990), Functional immunocytopathology and the diagnosis of bone marrow micrometastases. Cytopathology, 1 (4), 223–31.

Nielsen O.S., Munro A.J., Tannock I.F. (1991) Bone metastases: pathophysiology and management policy. J Clin Oncol., 9, 509.

Nussbaum S.R., Gaz R.D., Arnold A. (1990) Hypercalcemia and ectopic secretion of parathyroid hormone by an ovarian carcinoma with rearrangement of the gene for parathyroid hormone. N Engl J Med., 323, 1324.

Oberlin O., Bayle C., Hartmann O. et al. (1995) Incidence of bone marrow involvement in Ewing's sarcoma: value of extensive investigation of the bone marrow. Med pediatr Oncol, 24 (6), 343–6.

Ozisik Y.Y., Meloni A.M., Altungoz O. et al. (1994) Cytogenetic findings in 21 malignant melanomas. Cancer Genet Cytogenet., 77 (1), 69–73.

Pantel K., Izbicki J., Passlick B. et al. (1996) Frequency and prognostic significance of isolated tumor cells in bone marrow of patients with non-small-cell lung cancer without overt metastases. Lancel, 347 (9002), 649–53.

Parfitt A.M. (1995) Bone remodeling, normal and abnormal: a biological basis for the understanding of cancer-related bone disease and its treatment. Can J Oncol., 5 (1), 1–10.

Pasini F., Pelosi G., Ledermann J.A., Cetto G.L. (1994) Detection of small-cell-lung-cancer cells in bone marrow aspirates by monoclonal antibodies NCC-LU-243, NCC-LU 246 and MLuC1. Int J Cancer Suppl, 8, 53–6.

Patanaphan V., Salazar O.M., Risco R. (1988) Breast cancer: metastatic patterns and their prognosis. *S Med J.*, **81**, 1112.

Paterson A.H.G. (1987) Bone metastases in breast cancer, prostate cancer and myeloma. *Bone*, **8**, 17.

Pelkey T.J., Frierson H.F. Jr., Bruns D.E. (1996) Molecular and immunological detection of circulating tumor cells and micrometastases from solid tumors. *Clin Chem*, **42 (9)**, 1369–81.

Perkel V.S., Mohan S., Herring S.J. *et al.* (1990) Human prostatic cancer cells (PC3) elaborate mitogenic activity which selectively stimulates human bone cells. *Cancer Res.*, **50**, 6902.

Rajan R., Vanderslice R., Kapur S. *et al.* (1996) Epidermal growth factor (EGF) promotes chemomigration of a human prostate tumor cell line, and EGF immunoreactive proteins are present at sites of metastasis in the stroma of lymph nodes and medullary bone. *Prostate*, **28 (1)**, 1–9.

Reid M.M., Roald B. (1996) Central review of bone marrow biopsy specimens from patients with neuroblastoma. *J Clin Pathol.*, **49 (8)**, 691–2.

Reid M.M., Wallis J.P., McGuckin A.G. *et al.* (1991) Routine histological compared with immunohistological examination of bone marrow trephine biopsy specimens in disseminated neuroblastoma. *J. Clin. Pathol.*, **44 (6)**, 483–6.

Rufini V., Salvatori M., Saletnich I. *et al.* (1996) Disseminated bone marrow metastases of insular thyroid carcinoma detected by radioiodine whole-body scintigraphy. *J Nucl Med*, **37 (4)**, 633–6.

Saintati L., Bolcato S., Montaldi A. *et al.* (1996) Cytogenetics of pediatric central nervous system. *Cancer Genet Cytogenet.*, **91 (1)**, 13–27.

Schneider B.F., Shashi V., von Kap-herr C., Golden W.L. (1995) Loss of chromosomes 22 and 14 in the malignant progression of meningiomas. A comparative study of fluorescence in situ hybridization (FISH) and standard cytogenetic analysis. *Cancer Genet Cytogenet*, **85 (2)**, 101–4.

Seruca R., Castedo S., Correia C. *et al.* (1993) Cytogenetic findings in eleven gastric carcinomas. *Cancer Genet Cytogenet.*, **68 (1)**, 42–8.

Shpall E.J., Gee A.P., Hogan C. *et al.* (1996) Bone marrow metastases. *Hematol/Oncol Clin N. Am*, **10 (2)**, 321–44.

Singer F.R. (1991) Pathogenesis of hypercalcemia of malignancy. *Semin Oncol.*, **18**, 4.

Smith M.R., Biggar S., Hussain M. (1995) Prostate-specific antigen messenger RNA is expressed in non-prostate cells: implications for detection of micrometastases. *Cancer Res.*, **55 (12)**, 2640–4.

Stahl A., Levy N., Wadzynska T. *et al.* (1994) The genetics of retinoblastoma. *Ann Genet*, **37 (4)**, 172–8.

Steiner G., Sidransky D. (1996) Molecular differential diagnosis of renal carcinoma: from microscopes to microsatellites comment. *Am J Pathol.*, **149 (6)**, 1791–5.

Su J.M., Hsu K.H., Chang H. *et al.* (1996) Expression of estrogen and pogesterone receptors in non-small-cell lung cancer: immunohistochemical study. *Anticancer Res.*, **16 (6B)**, 3803–6.

Turner G.E., Reid M.M. (1993) What is marrow fibrosis after treatment of neuroblastoma? *J Clin Pathol*, **46 (1)**, 61–3.

Unni K.K., Inwards C.Y. (1995) Tumors of the osteoarticular system. In C.D.M. Fletcher (ed.), *Diagnostic Histopathology of Tumors*, vol. 2. Edinburgh: Churchill Livingstone, pp. 1097–159.

Vagner-Capodano A.M., Poitout D. (1994–5) Cytogenetics of bone sarcomas. *Chirurgie*, **120 (13)**, 188–92.

Valgardsdottir R., Steinarsdottir M., Anamthawat-Jonsson K. *et al.* (1996) Molecular genetics and cytogenetics of breast carcinomas: comparison of the two methods. *Cancer Genet Cytogenet*, **92 (1)**, 37–42.

Van den Berg E., Gouw A.S., Oosterhuis J.W. *et al.* (1995) Carcinoid in a horseshoe kidney. Morphology, immunohisto-chemistry, and cytogenetics. *Cancer Genet Cytogenet.*, **84 (2)**, 95–8.

Van der Velde-Zimmermann D., Verdaasdonk M.A., Rademakers L.H. *et al.* (1997) Fibronectin distribution in human bone marrow stroma: matrix assembly and tumor cell adhesion via alpha 5 beta 1 integrin. *Exp Cell Res*, **230 (1)**, 111–20.

Vassilopoulou-Sellin R., McLaughlin P., Hickey R.C. (1992) Diagnosis of thyroid cancer by bone marrow biopsy in a patient with lymphoma and goiter. *Am. J. Med. Sci.*, **304 (6)**, 360–2.

Willis R.A. (1973) *The Spread of Tumors in the Human Body*. London: Butterworths.

Wimalawansa S.J. (ed.) (1995) *Hypercalcemia of Malignancy, Etiology, Pathogenesis and Clinical Management*. Berlin: Springer.

Yadav M., Hopwood V.L., Multani A.S. *et al.* (1996) Non-random primary and secondary chromosomal abnormalities in human gastric cancers. *Anticancer Res.*, **16 (4a)**, 1787–95.

Yates J.R.W. (1996) Medical genetics. *BMJ*, **312**, 2021–5.

Zajicek G. (1987) Long survival with micrometastasis. At least 9% of breast cancer patients carry metastases for more than 10 years. *Cancer J.*, **1**, 381.

Zych J., Polowiec Z., Wiatr E. *et al.* (1993) (Value of bone marrow trephine biopsy in evaluating the extent of small cell lung cancer) *Pneumonol Alergol Pol*, **61 (9–10)**, 474–80.

15 Major aspects of bone marrow biopsy pathology

Cellularity

Since the bone marrow is enclosed in a rigid frame (trabecular and cortical bone) which cannot expand or contract, increases or decreases in the parenchyme, that is the red hematopoietic cells, lead to expansion or contraction of the fatty, yellow marrow. For example, encroachment of hematopoiesis into the shafts of long bones in some hemolytic anemias. However, local and transient increases or decreases may also be balanced by contraction or widening of blood vessels, especially sinusoids.

Bone marrow cellularity, especially in the subcortical areas, is to some extent dependent on age (see Chapter 3).

Proportions of the hematopoietic cell lines

The proportions of the precursors of the cell lines in the bone marrow are directly related to the numbers, utilisation (or activity) and survival of their mature products in the peripheral blood. Increased peripheral utilisation or destruction, for example of platelets or granulocytes, induces increased production in the bone marrow. Conversely, decreased production in the bone marrow will lead to marrow hypocellularity and an increase in fat cells.

Topography: architectural organisation

Changes in proportions of the precursors inevitably leads to alterations in their topography and the architecture of the bone marrow. Moreover, reduction or increase in trabecular bone also influences the localisation of the hematopoietic cell lines.

Stromal reactions: cellular and extracellular

There are many types ranging from acute and chronic inflammatory reactions, with the corresponding infiltrations accompanied by vascular changes, exudations, hemorrhage and varying degrees of fibrosis, to the more localised ones, exemplified by granulomas. It should be remembered that the stroma constitutes the microenvironment (both cells and extracellular matrix), which has a profound influence on the function of the bone marrow (see Chapter 4).

Hematologic disorders at the extremes of life

Hematologic disorders in infants and older individuals have their own manifestations and require special consideration. However, in infants biopsies are rarely performed. In contrast, older individuals frequently undergo biopsies because of a raised sedimentation rate, cytopenia, lymphadenopathy or suspected malignancy – all of which have an increased incidence in the older age group together with alterations in the immune system. These conditions are dealt with in the appropriate chapters.

Malignant infiltrations: two main types

1. Development of neoplastic clones of hematopoietic origin and their occupation of the intertrabecular spaces. These clones are identified by their morphology and immunologic characteristics on immunohistology, as well as by FACS and cytogenetics on nucleated cells of the bone marrow aspirate.

2. Replacement of bone marrow and bone by malignant metastatic cells, characterised whenever possible by immunohistology and the accompanying stromal and osseous reactions.

Histologic evaluation of neoplasias in the bone marrow

Four parameters are considered:

1. The proliferative cell system – basis for subdivisions.

2. The proliferation pattern – additional information for diagnosis and evolution of disease.

3. The tumor cell burden (or load, vol%) – basis for histological staging and supplemental clinical staging system.

4. Stromal reactions – which may influence the evolution of disease as well as the response to therapy of pathological processes in the bone marrow; for differential diagnosis see Table 15.1.

Many bone marrow disorders have an uneven distribution, and this can be demonstrated by magnetic resonance imagining (MRI). Since differences between fatty, fibrotic, normocellular and hypercellular marrow may be detected, MRI may also be helpful in choosing a site for a biopsy, if one taken from the iliac crest proves inconclusive.

TABLE 15.1 Differential diagnosis in lympho- and myeloproliferative diseases

Reactive hyperplasias	Granulomas
Infections	Infections
Immune diseases	Sarcoidosis
Malignancies	Malignancies
Splenic disorders	Drugs
Hepatic disorders	Allergic/immune/rheumatic
Pulmonary disorders	AIDS
Hypertension	Unknown
Hyperplasia of unknown etiology	Fibrosis of bone marrow
Hypo- and aplasias	Metastatic carcinoma
Enzyme deficiencies	Hyperparathyroidism
Storage diseases	Osteoporosis
Eosinophilic syndromes	Osteomalacia
Mastocytosis	
Autoimmune lymphoproliferative disease	

Pathogenic mechanisms of leukemias and lymphomas

Since both lymphocytes and other white blood cells migrate and are carried everywhere by the blood stream, disorders of both are systemic diseases which are genetic as they are passed on by cell division, which itself is no longer properly regulated. These structural changes in the DNA – mutations – are due to translocations, deletions, additions and rearrangements which produce fusion proteins. The products of the oncogenes are involved in proliferation, differentiation and survival of cells. Another mechanism is the loss or inactivation of tumor suppressor genes.

The four major oncogenic changes in the hematologic disorders are: translocations, amplifications, deletions and point mutations, and these produce the oncogenes.

When a translocation occurs, a gene is removed from its normal location to a different one, in which its function is changed, so that it may induce activation of a growth stimulator or inactivation of a suppressor. Deletions likewise may cause uncontrolled cell division if a tumor suppressor gene was located in the deleted segment of a chromosome. If a particular segment of DNA is repeatedly copied, instead of only once, amplifications occur that may lead to uncontrolled cellular division if a stimulation gene is amplified. Looked at under the microscope, amplifications appear as homogeneously staining regions (HSR) in a chromosome, instead of the usual 'bands'. In a point mutation only a few nucleotides in a gene are altered, which may be due to substitution, insertion or deletion. Here again, if a growth regulatory protein is involved, the cell may become malignant. Most oncogenes so far characterised are divided into growth factors, signal transducers and transcriptional activators – and this last group is the most frequent in human leukemias and lymphomas.

Tumor suppressor genes are also of particular significance in human malignancies. Of particular interest is p53, and not only because it is demonstrable by immunohistology. Initially thought to be an oncogene, p53 (a 393-amino acid molecule called P53 because of its molecular weight of about 53,000 daltons) was subsequently recognised as being a tumor suppressor and that p53 mutations (nearly all point mutations) are involved in about half of all human cancers.

The mutated p53 no longer exercises its suppressor or inhibitory effect on cell multiplication. Moreover, p53 is also involved in three other cellular functions: (1) response to damage – instead of arresting progression into S phase and first repairing the damage, as normal cells do (due to this function, p53 is considered the watchdog, or guardian, of genomic integrity), cells with deficient or mutated p53 do not undergo repair but continue DNA replication, which in turn may lead to a higher rate of subsequent mutations; (2) When these damaged cells replicate, amplification of segments of the damaged genome are increased, and among them oncogenes are inevitably present; (3) Though in some cells p53 promotes apoptosis after growth arrest, the deficient or mutated P53 does not. All these factors together confer on a mutated p53 a capacity for accelerating and sustaining tumor development.

Interest in p53 has also focused on its potential role in the regulation of the MDRI (multidrug resistance) gene and its relationship with chemoresistance. In this connection, it is worth noting that a high level of BCL2 expression also correlates with a poor response to chemotherapy because of a decreased susceptibility of the leukemia cells to the apoptosis-inducing effects of the cytotoxic drugs. BCL2, though first characterised in B cell follicular lymphoma, is present in many cells and leads to cellular accumulation by promoting cell survival, as it inhibits most stimuli which induce apoptosis.

The elucidation of these genetic mechanisms has initiated a new era of potential therapy, targeted to the products of the genetic lesions and thereby removing the stimulus for the malignancy without toxicity or damage to other cells in the patient.

Bibliography

Begley C.G., Aplan P.D., Davey M.P. *et al.* (1989), Chromosomal translocation in a human leukemic stem-cell line disrupts the T-cell antigen receptor delta-chain diversity region and results in a previously unreported fusion transcript. *Proc. Natl. Acad. Sci. U.S.A.*, **86 (6)**, 2031–5.

Boehm T., Rabbitts T.H. (1989), A chromosomal basis of lymphoid malignancy in man. *Eur. J. Biochem.*, **185 (1)**, 1–17.

Brito-Babapulle V. (1991) Cytogenetic abnormalities of mature T-cell malignancies. *Leukemic Cell*, **2**, 327–38.

Catovsky D. (ed.) (1991) *The Leukemic Cell*, 2nd edn. Edinburgh: Churchill Livingstone.

Coignet L.J.A., Schuuring E., Kibbelaar R.E. *et al.* (1996) Detection of 11q13 rearrangements in hematologic neoplasias by double-color fluorescence in situ hybridization. *Blood*, **4**, 1512–19.

Cotran, Kumar, Robbins (1994) *Pathologic Basis of Disease*, 5th edn. Philadelphia: W.B. Saunders.

Cuneo A., Boogaerts M., Ferrant A. *et al.* (1995) Cytogenetics of hybrid acute leukemias. *Leuk Lymphoma*, **18 (1)**, 19–23.

Dilly S.A., Jagger C.J. (1990), Bone marrow stromal cell changes in hematological malignancies. *J. Clin. Pathol.*, **43 (11)**, 942–6.

Dono M., Hashimoto S., Fais F. *et al.* (1996) Evidence for progenitors of chronic lympho-cytic leukemia B cells that undergo intraclonal differentiation and diversification. *Blood*, **4**, 1586–94.

Foroni L., Mason P., Luzzatto L. (1991) Immunoglobin and T-cell receptor gene analysis for the investigation of lymphoproliferative disorders. *Leukemic Cell*, **2**, 339–91.

Fuscoe J.C., Setzer R.W., Collard D.D., Moore M.M. (1996) Quantification of t(14;18) in

the lymphocytes of healthy adult humans as a possible biomarker for environmental exposures to carcinogens. *Carcinogenesis*, **17 (5)**, 1013–20.

Gebhart E., Liehr T., Harrer P. *et al.* (1995) Determination by interphase-FISH of the clonality of aberrant karyotypes in human hematopoietic neoplasias. *Leuk Lymphoma*, **17 (3–4)**, 295–302.

Glassman A.B. (1995) Cytogenetics, gene fusions, and cancer. *Ann Clin Lab Sci.*, **5 (25)**, 389–93.

Hodgson S.V., Maher E.R. (1993) A practical guide to human cancer genetics.

Hunger S.P. (1996) Chromosomal translocations involving the ERA gene in acute lymphoblastic leukemia: clinical features and molecular pathogenesis. *Blood*, **4**, 1211–24.

Inokuchi K., Miyake K., Takahashi H. *et al.* (1996) DCC protein expression in hematopoietic cell populations and its relation to leukemogenesis. *J Clin Invest*, **97 (3)**, 852–7.

Janossy G., Campana D. (1991) Monoclonal antibodies in the diagnosis of acute leukemia. *Leukemic Cell*, **2**, 168–95.

Joos S., Otaño-Joos M.I., Ziegler S. *et al.* (1996) Primary mediastinal (thymic) B-cell lymphoma is characterized by gains of chromosomal material including 9p and amplification of the REL gene. *Blood*, **4**, 1571–8.

Jotterand-Bellomo M., Parlier V., Muhlematter D. *et al.* (1992) Three new cases of chromosome 3 rearrangements in bands q21 and q26 with abnormal thrombopoiesis bring further evidence to the existence of a 3q21q26 syndrome. *Cancer Genet. Cytogenet.*, **59 (2)**, 138–60.

Kasprzyk A., Mehta A.B., Secker-Walker L.M. (1995) Single-cell trisomy in hematologic

malignancy. Random change or tip of the iceberg? *Cancer Genet Cytogenet*, **85 (1)**, 37–42.

Knuutila S. (1997) Review: Lineage specificity in haematological neoplasms. *Br J Haematol.*, **96**, 2–11.

Le Beau M.M. (1990) Chromosomal abnormalities in hematologic malignant diseases. *Prog. Clin. Biol. Res.*, **340B**, 325–35.

Lewis J.P., Tanke H.J., Raap A.K. *et al.* (1993) Somatic pairing of centromeres and short arms of chromosome 15 in the hematopoietic and lymphoid system. *Hum. Genet.*, **92 (6)**, 577–82.

Maio M., Pinto A., Carbone A. *et al.* (1990) Differential expression of CD54/intercellular adhesion molecule-1 in myeloid leukemias and in lymphoproliferative disorders. *Blood*, **76 (4)**, 783–90.

Marie J.P., Zittou R., Sikic B.I. (1991) Multidrug resistance (mdr1) gene expression in adult acute leukemias: correlations with treatment outcome and in vitro drug sensitivity. *Blood*, **78**, 586.

Melo J.V. (1996) Overview: The molecular biology of chronic myeloid leukaemia. *Leukemia*, **10**, 751–6.

Merkel D.E., Dressler L.G., McGuire W.L. (1987) Flow cytometry, cellular DNA content, and prognosis in human malignancy. *J Clin Oncol.*, **5**, 1690–1703.

Michalova K., Lemez P., Bartsch O. *et al.* (1996) Derivative (6) t (1; 6) (q22; p21) revealed in bone marrow cells by FISH 9 months before diagnosis of acute T-lymphoblastic leukemia. *Cancer Genet Cytogenet.*, **86 (2)**, 131–5.

Mitelman F. (ed.) (1995) *An International System for Human Cytogenetic Nomenclature.* Basel: Karger.

Mollnes T.E., Harboe M. (1996) Clinical immunology. *BMJ*, **312**, 1465–9.

Orfao A., Ruiz-Arguelles A., Lacombe F. *et al.* (1995) Flow cytometry: its applications in hematology. *Haematologica*, **80 (1)**, 69–81.

Ott G., Kalla J., Ott M.M. *et al.* (1997) Blastoid variants of mantle cell lymphoma: frequent bcl-1 rearrangements at the major translocation cluster region and tetraploid chromosome clones. *Blood*, **89 (4)**, 1421–29.

Rasko I., Downes C.S. (1995) *Genes in Medicine: Molecular Biology and Human Genetic Disorders*. London: Chapman & Hall.

Robinson J.P. (ed.) (1993) *Handbook of Flow Cytometry Methods*. Chichester: John Wiley.

Sadamori N., Amagasaki T., Nakamura H. *et al.* (1990) Appearance time of leukemic cells with t(8; 21) in bone marrow. *Cancer Genet. Cytogenet.*, **50 (1)**, 149–52.

Savill J. (1997) Role of molecular cell biology in understanding disease. *BMJ*, **314**, 203–8.

Shippey C.A., Layton M., Secker-Walker L.M. (1990) Leukemia characterized by multiple sub-clones with unbalanced translocations involving different telomeric segments: case report and review of the literature. *Genes Chromosom. Cancer.*, **2 (1)**, 14–17.

Showe L.C., Croce C.M. (1987) The role of chromosomal translocations in B- and T-cell neoplasia. *Annu. Rev. Immunol.*, **5**, 253–77.

Sneller M.C., Wang J., Dale J.K. *et al.* (1997) Clinical, immunologic, and genetic features of an autoimmune lymphoproliferative syndrome associated with abnormal lymphocyte apoptosis. *Blood*, **89 (4)**, 1341–8.

Steiner R.M., Mitchell D.G., Rao V.M., Schweitzer M.E. (1993) Magnetic resonance imaging of diffuse bone marrow disease. *Radiol Clin North Am*, **31 (2)**, 383–409.

Verhoef G.E.G., Boogaerts M.A. (1996) Cytogenetics and its prognostic value in myelodysplastic syndromes. *Acta Haematol*, **95**, 95–101.

Weh H.J., Seeger D., Junge I., Hossfeld D.K. (1996) Trisomy 8 preceding diagnosis of acute nonlymphocytic leukemia by 2 years in a patient with multiple myeloma without cytological evidence of myelodysplasia. *Ann Hematol*, **72 (2)**, 81–2.

Williams D. (1991) Cytogenetics of acute leukemia. *Leukemic Cell*, **2**, 288–326.

Yates J.R.W. (1996) Medical genetics. *BMJ*, **312**, 2021–5.

16 Hypoplasias and aplasias of the bone marrow

General aspects of cytopenias not due to neoplastic disorders

Cytopenia refers to a decrease (or decreases) in the levels of any of the formed elements of the peripheral blood. The cause(s) may be due to decreased or ineffective production, increased peripheral utilisation, destruction or loss without an adequate compensatory increase in production, or a combination of these mechanisms. Therefore, the cause may be in the bone marrow, the periphery or both. The numerous extrinsic causes range from deficiency of essential factors for hematopoiesis, such as vitamins and iron, to toxic substances also ranging from radiation and chemotherapy, to other drugs and alcohol, microcirculatory defects, endocrine dysfunction, viral infections from hepatitis to AIDS, and other infections including tuberculosis and typhoid fever, chronic diseases, immunologic conditions with inhibition of hematopoiesis as well as replacement of the bone marrow in neoplastic infiltrations, which include the myelo- and lymphoproliferative disorders. In addition, aplastic anemia may also precede other hematologic disorders, for example acute leukemia and hairy cell leukemia. Most patients with cytopenias will already have had (before bone marrow biopsy) a thorough hematologic, biochemical and clinical investigation that generally will have indicated the diagnosis or at least reduced the possibilities. Details of the above and other possible causes of cytopenias can be found in textbooks of hematology. Here, conditions are included in which a bone biopsy may provide diagnostic or supplementary information.

Cytopenias are divided into congenital and acquired, and may involve defects in proliferation, i.e. production, in maturation and differentiation, and in survival.

Aplastic anemia(s) (AA)

This term refers to a reduction in the formed elements of the peripheral blood due to reduced production in the bone marrow – hence hypo or aplastic anemia. Though called aplastic anemia these conditions are characterised by reductions in red cells, white cells and platelets in the peripheral blood, i.e., pancytopenia, together with hypocellularity of the bone marrow. The familial or congenital aplastic anemias are usually of early onset, while the acquired (of unknown etiology) are generally of late onset. The congenital disorders include Fanconi's anemia, dyskeratosis congenita, Shwachman–Diamond syndrome, Tar syndrome and familial aplastic anemia. Some of these conditions are associated with a greater risk of developing myelodysplasia, leukemia or other tumors, for example patients with Fanconi's anemia, which is characterised by a DNA repair defect. Bone marrow cells of Fanconi's anemia proliferate slowly and resist cell division and separation, so that they accumulate in the G_2 phase of the cycle. Abnormalities typical of Fanconi's anemia –

149

chromosome breaks, gaps, rearrangements, chromatid interchanges and endoreduplication become more apparent when the cells are cultured with certain chemicals, including oxidants (Figure 16.1). The gene mutated in Fanconi's anemia has been localised to chromosome 9.

In the secondary aplasias a potential cause is identified, such as exposure to agents known to inflict bone marrow damage, often depending on the extent and duration of exposure. A small proportion of patients develop aplasia after exposure to substances that are quite innocuous to the majority of people. Generally, the cause cannot be determined from examination of the bone marrow aspirate or biopsy. Primary and secondary aplasias are hypocellular, with decreased precursors in the bone marrow and corresponding increases in fat cells. For a reliable assessment of bone marrow cellularity a biopsy of $2-3 \times 20-30\,mm$ excluding the cortex is required. The types of bone marrow hypoplasia are illustrated in Figure 16.2.

Bone marrow histology

Attempts at aspiration in many cases may result only in a 'dry tap'. A biopsy is required to rule out many of the conditions that may underlie peripheral cytopenias as well as to estimate the extent of the hypo- or aplasia, the stromal reactions and other presumably reactive elements such as lymphocytic aggregates and nodules, increased interstitial lymphocytes and mast cells, and perivascular and interstitial plasma cells, macrophages, lipomacrophages, as well as hemosiderin or iron-laden histiocytes. Hemophagocytosis may also be evident. The amount of hematopoiesis is drastically reduced. Histologically, islands of erythropoiesis ('hot spots') close to sinusoids may be found showing maturation arrest, and possibly mitotic figures and dyserythropoiesis. The residual hematopoietic tissue may show signs of dysplasia and left shift. Immature myeloid cells and an occasional megakaryocyte will also be found. Clusters of megakaryocytes are not typical of aplastic

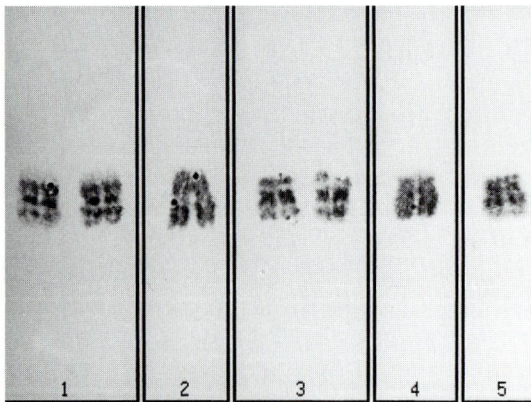

16.1 (left) Fanconi anemia. Partial karyotype (chromosomes 1–5) illustrating 'stickiness' of chromosomes.

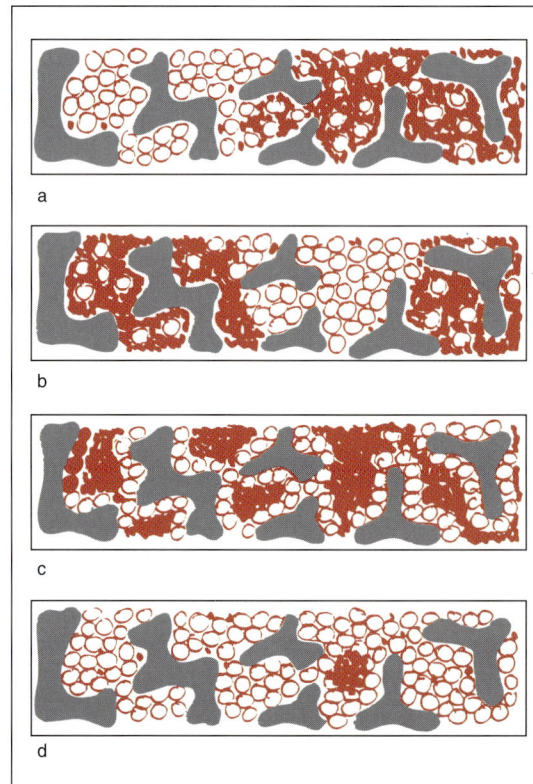

16.2 (right) Types of marrow hypoplasia (atrophy). (a) Subcortical, (b) patchy, (c) endosteal (incipient osteoporosis), (d) total (aplastic anemia).

conditions. Owing to the hematopoietic hypoplasia (Figures 16.3–16.5), lymphocytes, mast and plasma cells, macrophages, and other histiocytes may be prominent. The bone marrow cellularity may be down to 5–10% or less of the normal age-related values. In long-standing hypoplasias there is trabecular osteopenia, probably due to atrophy of nutrient blood vessels (Figures 16.6 and 16.7). The cause of the cytopenia usually can not be identified on bone marrow histology nor are there typical histologic features which indicate a good or a poor prognosis. However, patients with marked hypo or aplasia due to starvation (for example, anorexia nervosa or gastric pathology) will usually have restitution of marrow function after resumption of normal nutrition. In early cases, the bone marrow picture is characterised by interstitial edema, necrotic cells and capillaries and the presence of lipomacrophages. Likewise, normal hematopoiesis is usually also restored after radiotherapy.

Bone marrow histology in patients with unexplained cytopenias may be very variable when the condition is not due to bone marrow aplasia (Table 16.1). Some possible causes such as metastatic replacement or radio- and chemotherapy are not included, as these will be suspected beforehand. Though aplastic anemia is generally regarded as a disease of hematopoietic precursor cells, some cases are

16.3 BMBS plastic, Gomori, low magnification showing extensive replacement by fat cells.

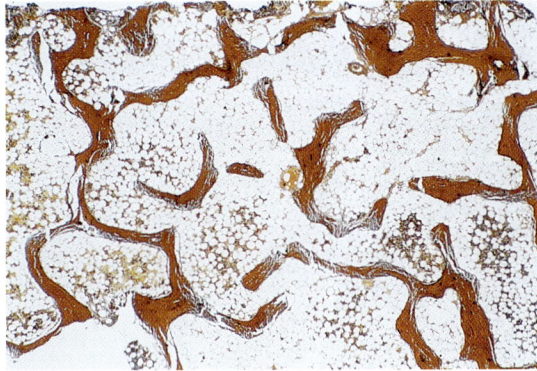

16.4–16.6 Aplastic anemia – atrophic marrow with hot spots.
16.4 (left) BMBS paraffin, H&E, low power illustrating hypoplasia and osteopenia.

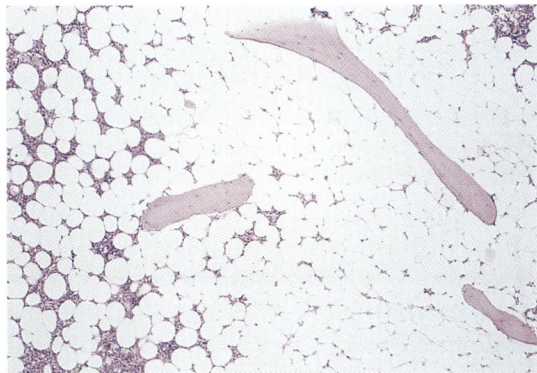

16.5 (right) BMBS paraffin, H&E, marrow space with some hematopoiesis.

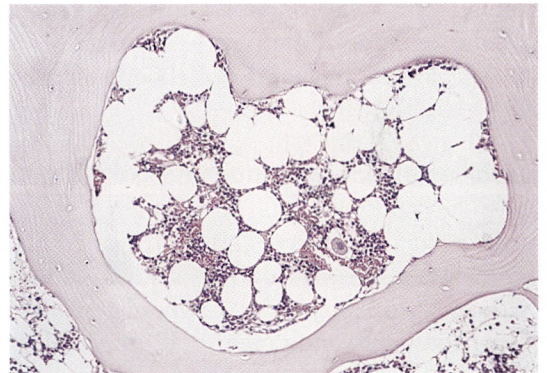

16.6 (left) BMBS paraffin, H&E, empty marrow.

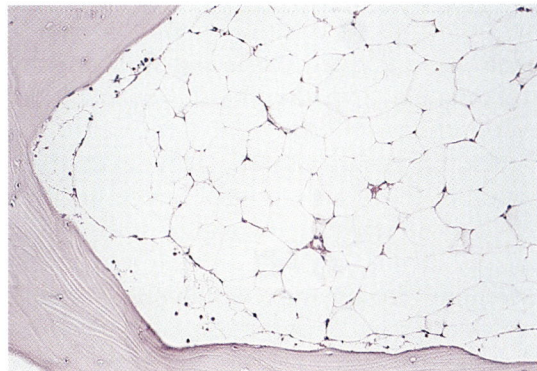

16.7 (right) BMBS plastic, Gomori, in polarised light, fibers around blood vessels, but few in hypocellular marrow.

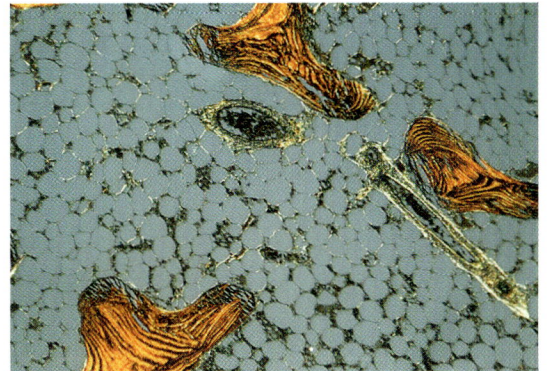

TABLE 16.1 Cytopenia and bone marrow pathology

Bone marrow histology	Number	Percentage of total
Refractory anemia	141	32
Aplastic anemia	60	14
Malignant lymphomas (non-Hodgkin)	58	13
Acute leukemia	50	11
Hairy cell leukemia	45	10
Agnogenic myeloid metaplasia	40	9
Hodgkin's disease	14	3
Multiple myeloma	10	2
Preleukaemia (sequential biopsies)	5	1
Systemic mastocytosis	4	1
Malignant histiocytosis	3	1
Angioimmunoblastic lymphadenopathy	2	1

apparently due to failure of the microenvironment and/or defects in the microcirculation, and others to imbalances of regulatory mechanisms. However, these cannot be recognised by routine histologic methods. Some cases of aplastic anemia represent clonal bone marrow stem cell disorders.

The hypoplastic phases of various preleukemic conditions and other neoplastic conditions, such as hypoplastic MDS, acute leukemia and myeloma, are dealt with in the appropriate chapters. The histologic distinction between aplastic anemia and hypoplastic MDS may be difficult, and demonstration of CD34, QBEND10-positive cells by immunohistology may be helpful because of the larger component of early myeloid precursors in MDS.

Pure red cell aplasia and bone marrow histology

This may be acute or chronic, which may be congenital – such as the Blackfan–Diamond syndrome – or acquired, with selective inhibition of erythropoiesis. On low magnification the marrow shows no striking alterations. There may be patchy replacement by fat cells together with areas of normal cellularity which, on closer inspection, contain no erythropoietic islands but only an isolated erythroid precursor or two. There are iron deposits in the stromal cells, aggregates of lymphoid cells (and in many cases 'hematogones' in children; these are cells of lymphoid origin with a high nucleo-cytoplasmic ratio), macrophages containing cellular debris, mast cells and plasma cells, as well as megakaryocytes and granulopoiesis of normal aspect (Figures 16.8–16.11). Pure red cell aplasia has been ascribed to many different causes and has also been reported in lymphoproliferative and myeloproliferative disorders, in addition to other conditions with an immunologic background such as cold hemaglutinin disease or cases with an obscure etiology. Red cell aplasia has been associated with thymoma, with systemic lupus erythematosus and with primary autoimmune hypothyroidism. In addition, excess of certain subsets of T cells has been shown to interfere with the terminal differentiation of erythroid and granulocytic progenitors. Certain transient erythroblastopenias and aplastic anemias of childhood may follow viral infections. The aplastic crisis in children with sickle cell anemia has recently been shown to be associated with parvovirus infection. A few

16.8–16.11 Bone biopsy aspects of pure red cell aplasia (PRCA).

16.8 (left) BMBS plastic, Giemsa, showing bone marrow without erythroid islands.

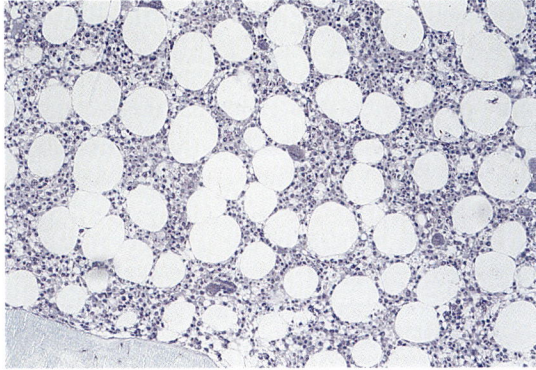

16.9 (right) As for Figure 16.8, lymphocytic aggregate in PRCA.

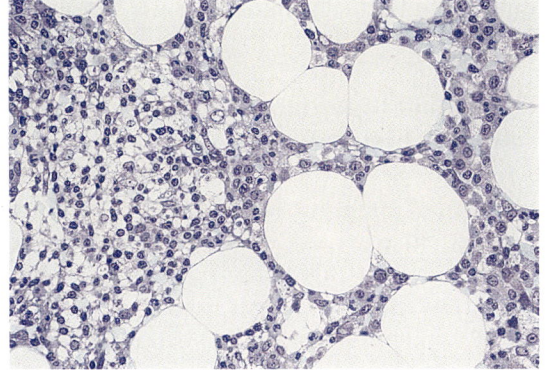

16.10 (left) BMBS paraffin, I.H., T cells in PRCA.

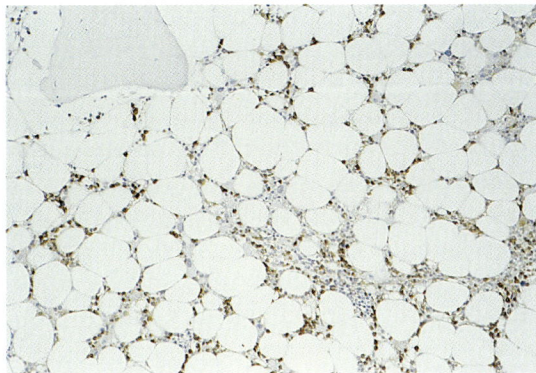

16.11 (right) As for Figure 16.10, stain for iron – accumulation of iron (blue) in macrophages and stromal cells.

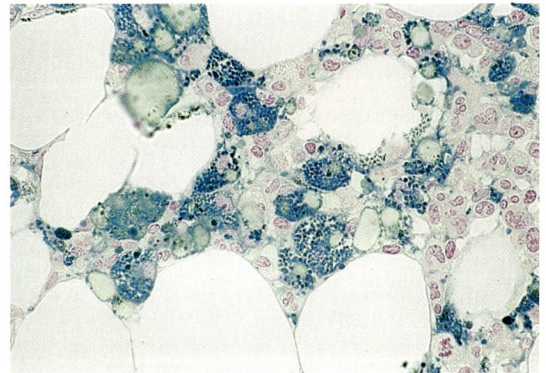

large atypical erythroblasts with nuclear inclusions may be found in the bone marrow.

Selective depression of erythropoiesis also occurs in chronic renal disorders and in patients on hemodialysis inadequate levels of erythropoietin have been implicated. Several other factors have also been suggested including inhibition by aluminum in the latter group. Improvement of the anemia may be achieved by administration of chelating agents to eliminate the aluminum.

In summary, many bone biopsies are taken because of an unexplained anemia; together, infections and iron deficiency are the causative factors in nearly half of these cases, and the rest are due to miscellaneous etiologies such as hemolysis, vitamin deficiencies, bleeding, aplastic anemias, myelodysplastic syndromes and other malignancies or chronic disorders.

Anemia of chronic disease and bone marrow histology

This is due to a number of factors including impaired response by the bone marrow and defects in the metabolism of iron, manifest in reduced erythroid iron while bone marrow storage iron is increased. Among the conditions in which this type of anemia occurs are: chronic infections, chronic inflammatory non-infectious states, malignancies, chronic renal and hepatic disorders. Iron-containing cells in the bone marrow are usually increased. Anemias in many conditions may also be due partly to a reduced erythropoietin response. These include: infections and inflammatory conditions, malignancies, renal diseases and endocrine deficiency states. In hepatic and rheumatic diseases, the peripheral cytopenia may be accompanied by a cellular bone marrow, often showing maturation arrest or left shift. However, in cases of hepatic disease due to alcohol abuse, the marrow may be hypocellular, with the presence of dys-erythropoiesis and sideroblasts, due not only to the alcohol, but also to inadequate diet and therefore nutritional defects: vitamins, iron, proteins. Finally, it is worth stressing that the underlying cause of an iron deficiency anemia may be an occult malignancy such as colonic cancer.

Granulocytopenia and bone marrow histology

Few studies on bone marrow biopsy have been reported in this condition, especially in the acute phase. In this phase bone marrow histology is variable; it ranges from hypocellularity with extensive edema and extravasation of erythrocytes from the disrupted sinusoids to a reduction in myeloid precursors and/or maturation inhibition, while the other cell lines are not apparently affected (Figures 16.12–16.14). When there is little or no reduction in the numbers of myeloid precursors, or even an apparent increase, together with profound maturation inhibition, the bone marrow picture may resemble that seen in promyelocytic leukemia due to the presence of the early precursors and the absence of the later maturational stages. In acute toxic conditions, hematopoiesis may be completely absent, the walls of the blood vessels appear damaged, and there is widespread precipitation of fibrinoid material. Neutropenia, together with a cellular bone marrow, is seen in autoimmune states such as rheumatoid arthritis, Felty's syndrome (arthritis, splenomegaly and leukopenia) and certain types of lymphoma. Human cyclic neutropenia is probably due to abnormal regulation of production and granulocyte precursors are decreased. In addition to the known causes of acquired neutropenia, pure white cell aplasia (agranulocytosis) may occur as a consequence of antibody-mediated autoimmune inhibition of granulopoiesis or T-lymphocyte-mediated granulopoietic failure. Selective neutropenia also occurs in systemic mastocytosis and other hematological malignancies, in hypersplenism, in autoimmune disorders, e.g. SLE and Felty's syndrome, and may be drug-induced.

Extensive necrosis of the bone marrow with profound granulocytopenia may occur after drug-induced bone marrow cytotoxicity. On bone marrow histology there is an extensive necrosis occupying the intertrabecular spaces with small areas of residual hematopoiesis infiltrated by lymphocytes and plasma cells; macrophages and lipomacrophages may be prominent (see Chapter 31). The term 'myelokathexis' is used for a rare constitutional anomaly in which there is hyperplasia and marked dysplasia of the granulocytic series, leading to granulocytopenia. However, the most common causes of acquired neutropenia are increased utilisation or destruction, particularly frequent in infections (including AIDS).

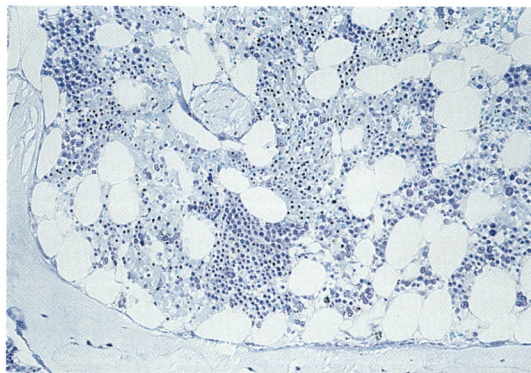

16.12 BMBS, plastic, Giemsa, case of agranulocytosis; note the lack of granulocytic cells.

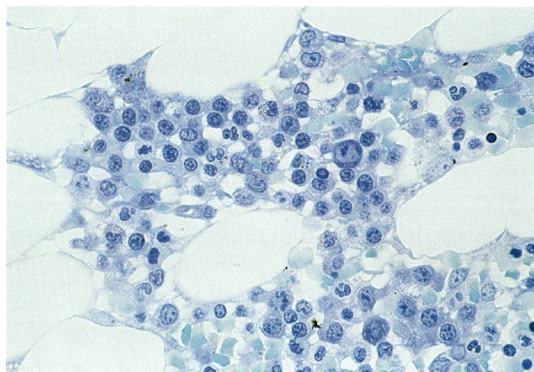

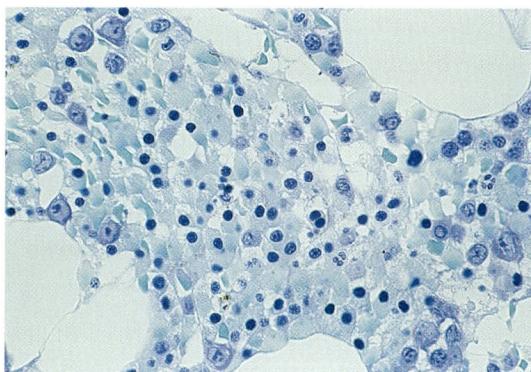

16.13 (left) As for Figure 16.12, higher magnification showing only a few myeloid precursors.

16.14 (right) As for Figure 16.13, large erythroid island but isolated myeloid cells only.

A bone biopsy is unlikely to be taken in most of the congenital anomalies of the granulocytic series, therefore these are not included here. Morphologic abnormalities of the granulocytic series are also a feature of many of the acquired conditions, such as vitamin deficiencies, immune deficiency states, infections, drugs, and after bone marrow transplantation. These morphologic abnormalities may be more prominent in peripheral blood smears than in bone marrow sections.

Thrombocytopenia and bone marrow histology

Quantitative variations in numbers of megakaryocytes occur in a large number of conditions (Table 16.2). Disorders with a decrease in megakaryocytes in the bone marrow will generally entail a lesser or greater degree of thrombocytopenia – in these cases, a failure of production. Three main mechanisms are distinguished: defective production, accelerated loss or utilisation and abnormal distribution, especially in splenomegaly. As with the other cytopenias, they may be classified into primary and secondary. The primary group includes constitutional and congenital thrombocytopenia (e.g. Tar syndrome due to greatly reduced numbers of megakaryocytes) and some cases of idiopathic thrombocytopenic purpura (ITP) (Figures 16.15 and 16.16). In the constitutional types the marrow is cellular with virtual absence of megakaryocytes. Thrombocytopenia, together with genetic hemachromatosis, has been described, as well as sex-linked thrombocytopenias in the Wiskott–Aldridge syndrome and its variants. Such cases are also characterised by reduced numbers of megakaryocytes in the bone marrow. Rare cases of ITP have been reported in which there was an absence of morphologically recognisable megakaryocytes and their precursors from the bone marrow, due to the presence of an antibody cytotoxic to antigens on platelets and megakaryocyte precursor cells. This is in contrast with most cases of ITP due to IgG antibodies directed primarily against platelet antigens, but which are also able to react with marrow megakaryocytes. However, in these conditions the number of megakarytocytes may be normal immediately after an onset, or greatly increased (up to 4.8-fold) in the chronic stage. On bone marrow histology, there is a preponderance of young megakaryocytes which are smaller, with less convoluted nuclei; but some larger ones are also present.

TABLE 16.2 Thrombocytopenia

Production decreased	Utilisation increased
Congenital	DIC in infections, in malignancies
Fanconi	Hemolytic syndrome
Tar	Uremic syndrome
May–Heglin	TTP
Wiskott–Aldrich	HELLP syndrome
X-linked	Immune disorders
Acquired	Drugs
Toxins	SLE
Infections	Allo-immunisation
Malignancies	ITP
	Lymphoproliferative disorders

When a reduction in platelets is due to cytotoxic agents and is part of an aplastic condition, the picture is that of an aplastic anemia with reduction in megakaryocytes. Thrombocytopenia may be a presenting symptom of a preleukemic condition (described in the section on myelodysplastic syndromes). The thrombocytopenia that occasionally occurs after drugs such as nalidixic acid is not accompanied by a reduction of bone marrow megakaryocytes. The same holds true for the reduction in platelets seen in some cases of hypothermia because of sequestration in the liver and spleen. Bone marrow megakaryocytes are within the normal range.

Splenomegaly and bone marrow histology

Splenomegaly due to causes other than neoplasias such as vascular disease may also be accompanied by thrombocytopenia (megakaryocytes are not decreased). Alcoholic liver disease is frequently associated with cytopenias, and in many such cases the bone marrow

histology shows marked hypoplasia. In contrast, small or even micromegakaryocytes may be found in the normo- or cellular bone marrows of patients with hepatic cirrhosis due to other (non-hematological) causes. Sea-blue histiocytes and foamy macrophages may be found in the bone marrow in thrombocytopenias, and it has been suggested that they develop due to phagocytosis of platelets. Thrombocytopenia may be found in almost any type of autoimmune disease; mega-

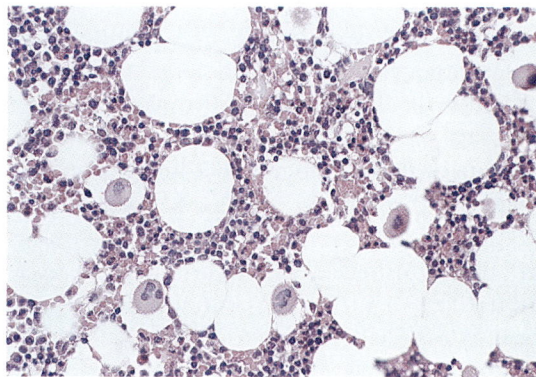

16.15 and 16 Bone biopsy in case of ITP.

16.15 BMBS paraffin, H&E, megakaryocytes prominent. Many appear morphologically within normal limits.

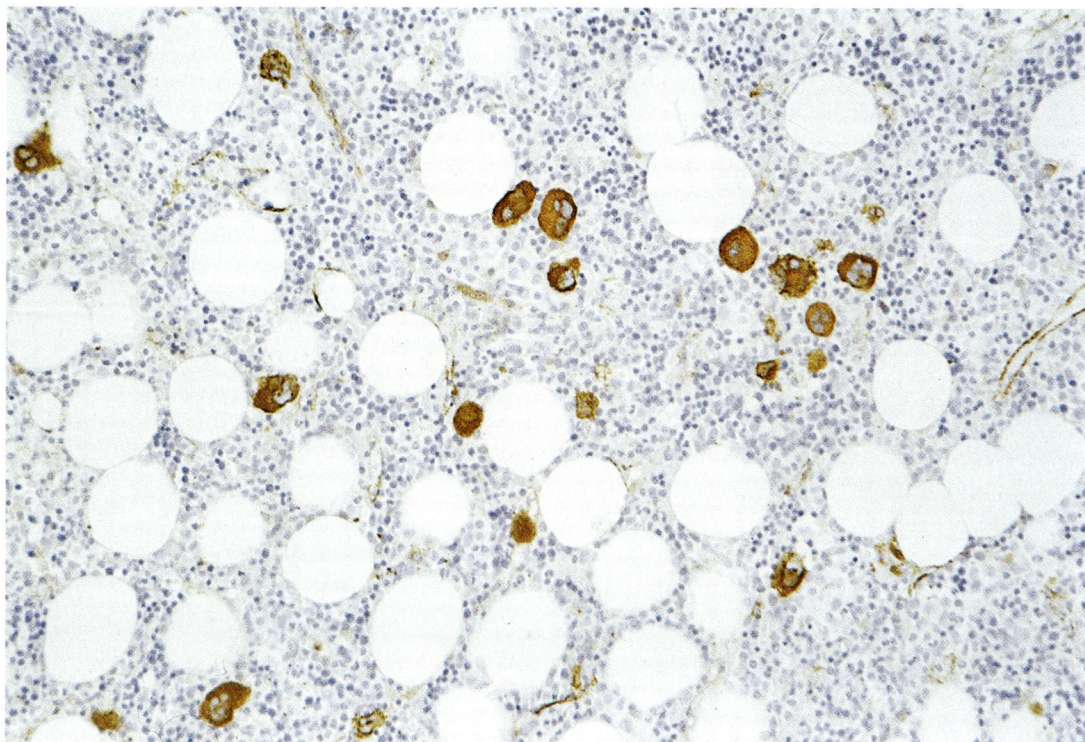

16.16 As for Figure 16.5, I.H. with Factor VIII-related antigen highlights the megakaryocytes including the small ones.

karyocytes in the bone marrow are normal or increased (with the exceptions mentioned above). In thrombotic thrombocytopenic purpura (TTP) the bone marrow architecture is essentially normal, megakaryocytes are within the normal range or increased and clumps of platelets may be found in small arterioles in the bone marrow, coating the plaques of fibrinoid necrosis in the blood vessel walls.

Additional causes of thrombocytopenia

Thrombocytopenia in the myelo- and lymphoproliferative disorders and the myelodysplastic syndromes is considered in the appropriate sections. The bone marrow changes due to chemotherapy and radiotherapy are dealt with in Chapter 31.

Increased platelet utilisation, in contrast with destruction by immune mechanism, occurs in disseminated intravascular coagulation (DIC), hemolytic uremic syndrome and septicemia. Secondary autoimmune thrombocytopenia may be associated with diseases such as collagen disorders, lymphoproliferative disorders, some solid tumors, viral infections (Figures 16.17–16.19) (HIV, hepatitis A), post-transfusion and hyperthyroidism. In these cases, bone marrow megakaryocytes are usually increased with left shift and immature forms with hypolobulated nuclei are present. The megakaryocytes are dispersed throughout the bone marrow with no (or only a few small) clusters. So called 'naked megakaryocytic nuclei' are also found, especially in some viral infections (such as AIDS). However, on electron microscopy, most such nuclei are not pyknotic, are able to synthesize DNA and are surrounded by narrow rims of cytoplasm.

It should be stressed that not only a reduction in the platelet count can lead to bleeding but also abnormalities in platelet function. Some commonly used drugs have this effect, such as aspirin, other non-steroidal anti-inflammatory agents, a long list of antibiotics belonging to the penicillin group, and volume expanders such as dextran, heparin and fibrinolytic agents.

Pancytopenias with hypercellular bone marrow, for example, refractory anemias characterised by marrow hypercellularity and peripheral cytopenia(s), are due to anomalies of maturation, leading to accumulation of precursors. These conditions are dealt with in Chapter 20. Cytopenias due to replacement of the bone marrow, as in myelo- and lymphoproliferative disorders, bone marrow

16.17–16.19 BMBS plastic, Giemsa of 44-year-old patient with hepatitis, chronic drug abuse and pancytopenia; HIV-negative.

16.17 Low magnification showing hypocellular marrow with dysplasia, and high turnover osteopenia.

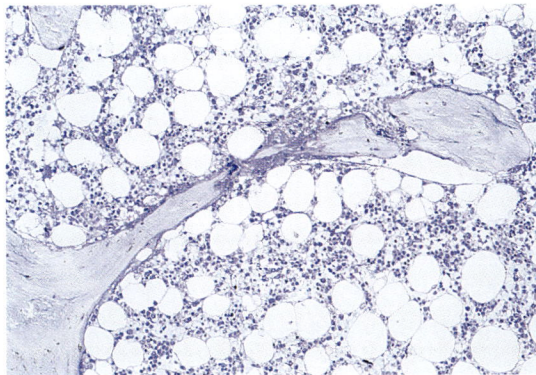

16.18 (left) As for Figure 16.17, higher magnification showing transection of ossicle and mast cells at trabecular edge.

16.19 (right) As for Figure 16.18 illustrating hematopoiesis with dysplastic features; note atypical megakaryocytes.

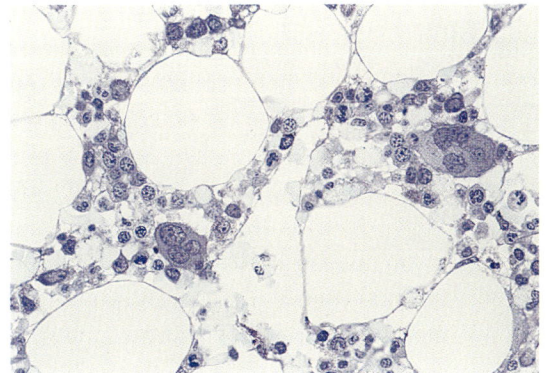
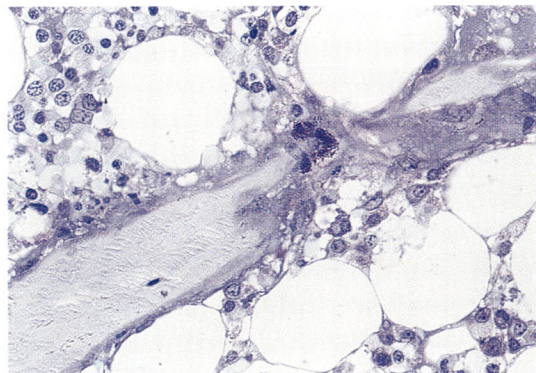

metastases, infections especially with granulomas, and as a consequence of cytotoxic drugs and radiation, are dealt with in the appropriate chapters.

Check list: Hypoplasias and Aplasias in Bone Marrow

- Adequate biopsy: must be 25–30 mm after exclusion of cortical and subcortical area.
- Biopsy must not have been taken from irradiated area (e.g. in Hodgkin's disease).
- Previous cytotoxic therapy must be excluded.
- Bone: evidence of alterations of: bone mass and bone architecture, bone mineralisation, bone remodeling?
- Hypoplasia secondary to bone pathology?
- Pathologic infiltration replacing marrow?
- Cellularity: ratio of hematopoiesis to fat cells?
- All three cell lines equally decreased? Immunohistology (I.H.) Factor VIII – few megakaryocytes.
- Distribution of residual hematopoiesis, 'hot spots'? I.H. erythroid, myeloid antigens, CD34 (QBENDIO).
- Stromal changes present?
- Degree of inflammatory reaction? On I.H. most lymphocytes stain with T cell marker, CD68-positive cells may be relatively prominent.
- Correlation of histologic findings with peripheral blood values?

Clinical correlations

Anemia

- Micro-normo-macrocytic erythrocytes indicates direction of investigation.
- Time of onset and duration of symptoms.
- Dizziness, headache, tinnitus, decreased ability to concentrate.
- Moderate tachycardia, angina pectoris, retinal hemorrhage, peripheral edema.

Peripheral anemia, bi- or tricytopenia

- Often insidious onset, increasing weakness, fatigue, pallor.
- Infections, fever, bleeding.
- No indication in peripheral blood count and blood film of underlying bone marrow pathology.
- No known cause: cytotoxic drugs, radiotherapy must be excluded.
- Frequently dry tap or insignificant material on aspiration.
- Bone biopsy to rule out secondary cytopenias.
- Aplasia may follow episodes of fever and/or viral infections.

Anemia of chronic disease

- Clinical evidence of chronic disease.
- Biochemical evidence of chronic disease
- Blood count: normochromic, normocytic.

Pure red aplasia

- Chronic or acute: patient's history decisive.
- Precipitating cause should be evident clinically: autoimmune diseases, lymphoproliferative disorders, viral infections, T cell subsets.
- Chronic renal disorders, possibly inadequate production of erythropoietin.

Granulocytopenia

- Neutropenia known to occur in various clinical conditions, such as autoimmune states, Felty's syndrome, mastocytosis.
- As a consequence of cytotoxic therapy.
- In acute infections: due to extensive utilisation.

Thrombocytopenias

- A decrease in platelets occurs in many and varied clinical conditions.
- A specific cause is frequently demonstrable.
- Important to establish whether megakaryocytes are normal, increased or decreased.
- Platelet function tests – if sufficient platelets are present to do so.
- Important to establish trend in platelet numbers: increasing, stable or decreasing, to initiate appropriate tests and treatment.

Bibliography

Ackland S.P., Bur M.E., Adler S.S. *et al.* (1988) White blood cell aplasia associated with thymoma. *Am J Clin Pathol*, **89 (2)**, 260–3.

Alter B.P., Scalise A., McCombs J., Najfeld V. (1993) Clonal chromosomal abnormalities in Fanconi's anemia: what do they really mean? *Br. J Haematol.*, **85 (3)**, 627–30.

Alter B.P., Knobloch M.E., Weinberg R.S. (1991) Erythropoiesis in Fanconi's anemia. *Blood*, **78 (3)**, 602–8.

Antin J.H., Smith B.R., Holmes W., Rosenthal D.S. (1988) Phase I/II study of recombinant human granulocyte-macrophage colony-stimulating factor in aplastic anemia and myelodysplastic syndrome. *Blood*, **72 (2)**, 705–13.

Auerbach A., Allen R. (1991) Leukemia and preleukemia in Fanconi anemia patients. *Cancer Genet Cytogenet.*, **51**, 1.

Ballon D., Jakubowski A., Gabrilove J. *et al.* (1991) In vivo measurements of bone marrow cellularity using volume-localized proton NMR spectroscopy. *Magn. Reson. Med.*, **19 (1)**, 85–95.

Barriga F.J., Legues M.E., Bertin P. (1996) Selective engraftment of the granulocyte compartment after allogeneic bone marrow transplantation in a patient with severe aplastic anemia. *J Pediatr Hematol Oncol*, **18 (2)**, 216–17.

Berger R., Le Coniat M., Schaison G. (1993) Chromosome abnormalities in bone marrow of Fanconi anemia patients. *Cancer Genet Cytogenet.*, **65 (1)**, 47–50.

Bichile S.K. (1989) Diagnosis of iron deficiency. *J Assoc Physicians India*, **37 (11)**, 681–2.

Bonilla M.A., Gillio A.P., Ruggeiro M. *et al.* (1989) Effects of recombinant human granulocyte colony-stimulating factor on neutropenia in patients with congenital agranulocytosis. *N Engl J Med*, **320 (24)**, 1574–80.

Brown K.E., Young N.S. (1995) Parvovirus B19 infection and hematopoiesis. *Blood Rev.*, 9 (3), 176–82.

Buhr T., Georgii A. (1995) The histological picture of anemia in bone marrow biopsies. *Pathologe*, **16 (1)**, 46–52.

Butturini A., Gale R., Verlander P. *et al.* (1994) Hematologic abnormalities in Fanconi anemia: an International Fanconi Registry Study. *Blood*, **84**, 1650.

Cohen H., Walker H., Delhanty J.D. *et al.* (1991). Congentical spherocytosis, B19 parvovirus infection and inherited interstitial deletion of the short arm of chromosome 8. *Br. J. Hematol.*, **78 (2)**, 251–7.

Demiroglu H., Ozcebe Ol., Ozdemir L. *et al.* (1994) Pancytopenia with hypocellular bone marrow due to miliary tuberculosis: an unusual presentation. *Acta Haematol*, **91 (1)**, 49–51.

Diamond T., Pojer R., Steil D. *et al.* (1991) Does iron affect osteoblast function? Studies in vitro and in patients with chronic liver disease. *Calcif Tissue Int.*, **48**, 373.

Drachtman R., Weinblatt M., Sitarz A. *et al.* (1990) Marrow hypoplasia associated with congenital neurologic anomalies in two siblings. *Acta. Pediatr. Scand.*, **79 (10)**, 990–3.

el Khatib Y., Gidali J., Feher I. *et al.* (1991) Growth kinetics and blast-colony forming cell binding capacity of aplastic anaemic stromal cells. *Med. Oncol. Tumor. Pharmacother.*, **8 (4)**, 281–5.

Feng C.S., Ng M.H., Szeto R.S., Li E.K. (1991) Bone marrow findings in lupus patients with pancytopenia. *Pathology*, **23 (1)**, 5–7.

Frewin R., Henson A., Provan D. (1997) ABC of clinical haematology: haematological emergencies. *BMJ*, **314**, 1333–6.

Gibbons B., Scott D., Hungerford J.L. *et al.* (1995) Retinoblastoma in association with

the chromosome breakage syndromes Fanconi's anaemia and Bloom's syndrome: clinical and cytogenetic findings. *Clin Genet.*, **47 (6)**, 311–17.

Hall J.G. (1987) Thrombocytopenia and absent radius (TAR) syndrome. *J Med Genet.*, **I24**, 79–83.

Hamill R.L., Woods J.C., Cook B.A. (1991) Congenital atransferrinemia. a case report and review of the literature. *Am. J. Clin. Pathol.*, **96 (2)**, 215–18.

Hanada T., Koike K., Hirano C. *et al.* (1989) Childhood transient erythroblastopenia complicated by thrombocytopenia and neutropenia. *Eur J Hematol*, **42 (1)**, 77–80.

Heegard E.D., Hornsleth A. (1995) Parvovirus: the expanding spectrum of disease. Review article. *Acta Paediatr*, **84**, 109–17.

Ikushima Y., Kobayashi H., Imaishi K. *et al.* (1990) Ritodrine-induced agranulocytosis. *Arch. Gynecol. Obstet.*, **248 (1)**, 53–4.

Imbert M., Scoazec J.Y., Mary J.Y. *et al.* (1989) Adult patients presenting with pancytopenia: a reappraisal of underlying pathology and diagnostic procedures in 213 cases. *Hematol Pathol*, **3 (4)**, 159–67.

Juliusson G., Hast R., Ljungman P. *et al.* (1991) Simultaneously presenting aplastic anemia and Hodgkin's disease successfully treated with allogeneic bone marrow transplantation. *Eur. J. Hematol.*, **46 (5)**, 314–16.

Keisu M., Heit W., Lambertenghi-Deliliers G. *et al.* (1990) Transient pancytopenia. A report from the International Agranulocytosis and Aplastic Study. *Blut*, **61 (4)**, 240–4.

Kiely P.D., McGuckin C.P., Collins D.A. *et al.* (1995) Erythrocyte aplasia and systemic lupus erythematosus. *Lupus*, **4 (5)**, 407–11.

Lomuto M., Carotenuto M., Amini M. (1987) Sweet's syndrome and hemopoietic dysplasia. *G Ital Dermatol Venerol.*, **122 (3)**, 131–4.

Lu J.C., Lin M.T. (1989) Paroxysmal nocturnal hemoglobinuria: report of one case. *Acta Pediatr. Sin.*, **30 (5)**, 323–5.

Maarek O., Jonvueaux P., LeConiat M. *et al.* (1996) Fanconi anemia and bone marrow clonal chromosomal abnormalities. *Leukemia*, **10**, 1700.

Marsh J.C., Chang J., Testa N.G. *et al.* (1990) The hematopoietic defect in aplastic anemia assessed by long-term marrow culture. *Blood*, **76 (9)**, 1748–57.

Marsh J.C., Chang J., Testa N.G. *et al.* (1991) In vitro assessment of marrow 'stem cell' and stromal cell function in aplastic anemia. *Br. J. Hematol.*, **78 (2)**, 258–67.

Marsh J.C., Willa A.J., Hows J.M. *et al.* (1992) 'Stem cell' origin of the hematopoietic defect in dyskeratosis congenita. *Blood*, **79 (12)**, 3138–44.

Mathieson P.W., O'Neill J.H., Durrant S.T. *et al.* (1990) Antibody-mediated pure neutrophil aplasia, recurrent myasthenia gravis and previous thymoma: case report and literature review. *Q J Med*, **74 (273)**, 57–61.

Mathew C. (1997) Recent advances in the genetics of Fanconi anaemia. *J. Med. Genet.*, **34 (1)**, S25.

Mehta B.C., Pandya B.G. (1989) Bone marrow iron in nutritional anemias. *J Assoc Physicians India*, **37 (11)**, 687–8.

Mijovic A., Rolovic Z., Novak A. *et al.* (1989) Chronic myeloid leukemia associated with pure red cells aplasia and terminating in promyelocytic transformation. *Am. J. Hematol.*, **31 (2)**, 128–30.

Mikhailova N., Sessaraego M., Fugazza G. *et al.* (1996) Cytogenetic abnormalities in patients with severe aplastic anemia. *Haematologica*, **81 (5)**, 418–22.

Najean Y., Lecompte T. (1989) Chronic pure thrombocytopenia in elderly patients. An aspect of the myelodysplastic syndrome. *Cancer*, **64 (12)**, 2506–10.

Nakakuma H., Nagakura S., Iwamoto N. *et al.* (1995) Paroxysmal nocturnal hemoglobinuria clone in bone marrow of patients with pancytopenia. *Blood*, **85 (5)**, 1371–6.

Nakao S., Harada M., Kondo K. *et al.* (1991) Reversible bone marrow hypoplasia induced by alcohol. *Am. J. Hematol.*, **37 (2)**, 120–3.

Newland A.C., Evans T.G.J.R. (1997) ABC of clinical haematology: Haematological disorders at the extremes of life. *BMJ*, **314**, 1262–5.

Novitzky N., Jacobs P. (1991) Marrow stem cell and stroma cell function in aplastic anaemia (letter). *Br. J. Hematol.*, **79 (3)**, 530–1.

Ohta S., Shimada M., Katsura T. *et al.* (1987) Unusual inclusions in mature polymorpho-nuclear neutrophils of cyclic neutropenia. *Am J Pediatr Hematol Oncol*, **9 (3)**, 197–9.

Orazi A., Albitar M., Heerema N.A. *et al.* (1997) Hypoplastic myelodysplastic syndromes can be distinguished from acquired aplastic anemia by CD34 and PCNA immunostaining of bone marrow biopsy specimens. *Am J Clin Pathol*, **107 (3)**, 261–4.

Picker L.J., Furst A., Robinson S.H., Kadin M.E. (1987) Immunoarchitecture of the bone marrow in neutropenia: increased HNK-1 + cells define a subset of neutropenic patients. *Am J Hematol*, **25 (1)**, 29–41.

Pisciotta A.V. (1990) Drug-induced agranulocytosis. peripheral destruction of polymorphonuclear leukocytes and their marrow precursors. *Blood Rev.*, **4 (4)**, 226–37.

Plebani A., Cantu-Rajnoldi A., Collo G. *et al.* (1988) Myelokathexis associated with multiple congenital malformations:

immunological study on phagocytic cells and lymphocytes. *Eur. J. Hematol.*, **40 (1)**, 12–17.

Rosenthal N.S., Farhi D.C. (1989) Bone marrow findings in connective tissue disease. *Am J Clin Pathol*, **92 (5)**, 650–4.

Sardeo G., Gaion F., Artusi T. *et al.* (1987) Aplastic anemia and myelodysplasia: a not-always-easy distinction. *Minerva Med.*, **78 (20)**, 1519–22.

Shimuzu H., Sawada K., Katano N. *et al.* (1990) Intramedullary neutrophil phagocytosis by histiocytes in autoimmune neutropenia of infancy. *Acta Hematol.*, **84 (4)**, 201–3.

Sood R., Roy S., Kaushik P. (1997) Typhoid fever with severe pancytopenia. *Postgrad Med J*, **73 (855)**, 41–2.

Soutar R.L., Birnie D.H., Bennett B. (1993) Parvovirus B19 induced red cell aplasia in myelofibrosis. *Br. J. Hematol.*, **85 (3)**, 623–4.

Till S.H., Grundman M.J. (1997) Prevalence of concomitant disease in patients with iron deficiency anaemia. *BMJ*, **314**, 206–8.

Tong J., Bacigalupo A., Piaggio G. *et al.* (1989) Effect of antilymphocyte globulin (ALG) on bone marrow T/non-T cells from aplastic anaemia patients and normal controls. *Br. J Haematol*, **73 (4)**, 546–50.

Tong J., Bacigalupo A., Piaggio G. *et al.* (1991) Severe aplastic anemia (SAA): response to cyclosporin A (CyA) in vivo and in vitro. *Eur. J. Hematol.*, **46 (4)**, 212–16.

Trimble M.S., Glynn M.F., Brain M.C. (1991) Amegakaryocytic thrombocytopenia of 4 years duration: successful treatment with antithymocyte globulin. *Am. J. Hematol.*, **37 (2)**, 126–7.

Tsai P.H., Arkin S., Lipton J.M. (1989) An intrinsic progenitor defect in Diamond–Blackfan anemia. *Br. J. Hematol.*, **73 (1)**, 112–20.

Vadhan-Raj S., Buescher S., Broxmeyer H.E. *et al.* (1988) Stimulation of myelopoiesis in patients with aplastic anemia by recombinant human granulocyte-macrophage colony-stimulating factor. *N. Engl. J. Med.*, **319** (25), 1628–34.

Van Kamp H., Smit J.W., Ven den Berg E. *et al.* (1994) Myelodysplasia following paroxysmal nocturnal haemoglobinuria: evidence for the emergence of a separate clone. *Br. J Haematol.*, **87** (2), 399–400.

Vansteenkiste J.F., Boogaerts M.A. (1989) Adult respiratory distress syndrome in neutropenic leukemia. *Blut*, **58** (6), 287–90.

Vashi P., Patel B., Musson P. *et al.* (1987) Corticosteroid-responsive pure red cell aplasia in chronic lymphatic leukemia. *Am. J. Hematol.*, **26** (3), 279–84.

Vreugdenhil G., Lowenberg B., van Eijk H.G., Swaak A.J. (1990) Anemia of chronic disease in rheumatoid arthritis. Raised serum interleukin-6 (IL-6) levels and effects of IL-6 and anti-IL-6 on in vitro erythropoiesis. *Rheumatol Int.*, **10** (3), 127–30.

Walsh C.E., Liu J.M., Anderson S.M. *et al.* (1992) A trial of recombinant human interleukin-1 in patients with severe refractory aplastic anaemia. *Br. J. Hematol.*, **80** (1), 106–10.

Weatherall D.J. (1997) ABC of clinical haematology: The hereditary anaemias. *BMJ*, **314**, 492–6.

Wetzler M., Talpaz M., Kleinerman E.S. *et al.* (1990) A new familial immunodeficiency charcterized by severe neutropenia, a defective marrow release mechanism, and hypogammaglobulinemia. *Am J Med*, **89** (5), 663–72.

Young N.S. (1992) The problem of clonality in aplastic anaemia: Dr. Dameshek's riddle restated. *Blood*, **79**, 1385–92.

17 Hyperplasias of the bone marrow

Erythrocytosis and bone marrow histology

Erythrocytosis or secondary polycythemia (raised red blood cell mass), without leucocytosis or thrombocytosis, may occur when erythropoiesis is stimulated by raised levels of erythropoietin. This occurs as a result of abnormal mutant hemoglobins with increased oxygen affinity and also in acquired conditions in which erythrocytosis occurs as a result of 'appropriate' stimuli such as high altitude, pulmonary or cardiovascular disease; or 'inappropriate' stimuli when excess erythropoietin production is due to non-physiologic causes such as renal carcinoma, cerebellar adenomas and uterine myelomas. The causes of an increase in erythropoiesis are listed in Table 17.1. The diagnosis of the cause of the erythrocytosis is made by appropriate clinical investigation; the appearance of the bone marrow is similar irrespective of cause: normal architectural pattern, normocellular to increased cellularity with numerous foci of erythropoiesis exhibiting all maturational stages (Figures 17.1–17.3). In some cases, the parenchyme-to-fat ratio may be unaltered, or exceptionally even increased. In the absence of iron deficiency, iron stores are not depleted and there is normal reticulin. There may be a discrepancy between the erythrocytosis in the peripheral blood and the apparent activity in the bone marrow – an expression of its reserve capacity and the efficiency and speed with which it can compensate. Chronic erythroid hyperplasia may be accompanied by accelerated bone turnover.

An elevated blood count is also seen in relative polycythemia (also referred to as 'pseudo' or 'stress' polycythemia or erythrocytosis). This is due to a reduced plasma volume. The red cell mass is not increased and the bone marrow is normal.

Familial erythrocytosis

This may be a type of secondary erythrocytosis due to a hemoglobin defect or possibly an early phase of polycythemia vera (PV) (Figure 17.4). Other possible mechanisms include a defect in the regulation of erythropoietin production so that the level is high, or greater sensitivity of the precursors to normal levels of erythropoietin.

Neonatal erythrocytosis is not considered here as biopsies are usually not required.

Leucocytosis and bone marrow histology

Leukemoid reaction

This term refers to peripheral blood values and pictures resembling those seen in certain leukemias, notably CML (Figures 17.5 and 17.6). Such reactions may be elicited by numerous conditions, including infections, bacterial and viral, inflammatory diseases, necroses, allergic reactions, hemolytic anemias, burns, drugs, cytokines, hormones, toxins and neoplasms. Characteristically, and most frequently, there is a leucocytosis involving the neutrophilic granulocytes with a shift to the left, though other cell lines may also be implicated. Thus, eosinophils are involved in parasitic (Figure 17.7), allergic and dermatologic conditions, in connective tissue diseases,

17.1 and 2 BMBS plastic, Giemsa, erythroid hyperplasia, low and high magnification.
17.1 (left) Note hypercellular bone marrow with decrease in fat cells, and increase in erythropoiesis.

17.2 (right) Erythroid islands near sinusoids.

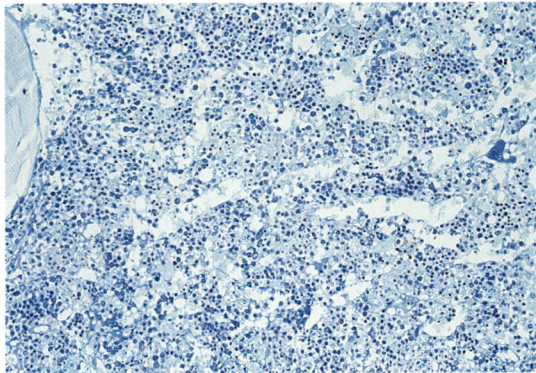

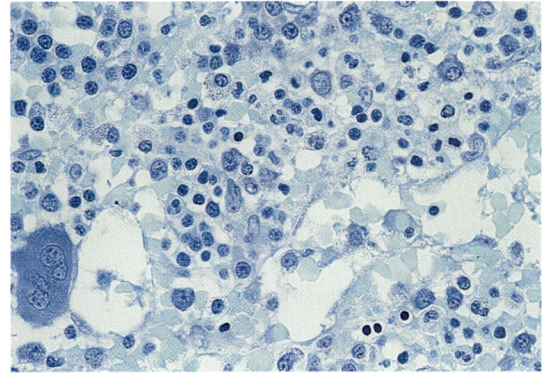

17.3 (left) Histogram, flow cytometry of nucleated cells of bone marrow aspirate. From left to right: red, control; gray, CD2; green, CD20; brown, CD33; blue, CD41; dark green, glycophorin, showing large population (57%) of erythroid cells.
17.4 (right) BMBS plastic, Giemsa, relative erythroid hyperplasia in somewhat hypocellular bone marrow; note dilated sinusoids, case of familial erythrocytosis.

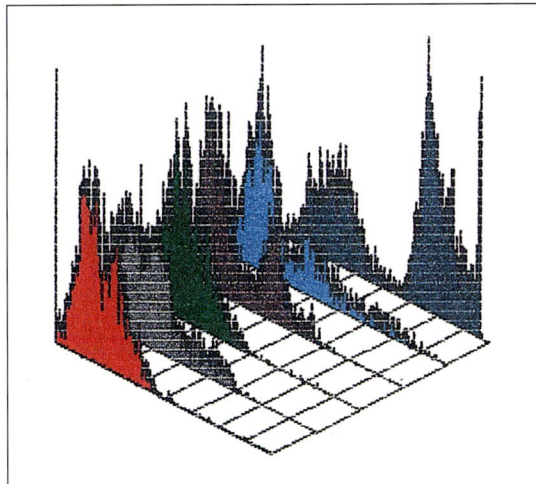

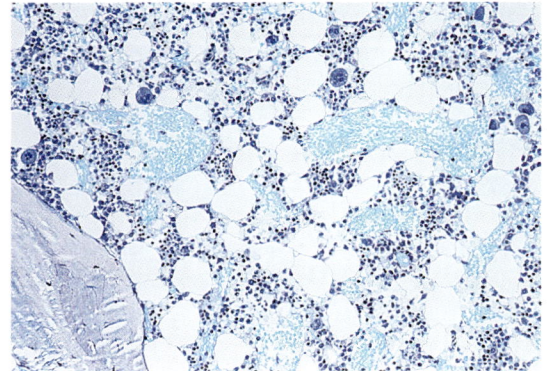

17.5 & 6 Leukemoid reaction in case of infection.
17.5 (left) BMBS plastic, Giemsa, low power, precursors at trabecular edge, progressive maturation towards central intertrabecular area.

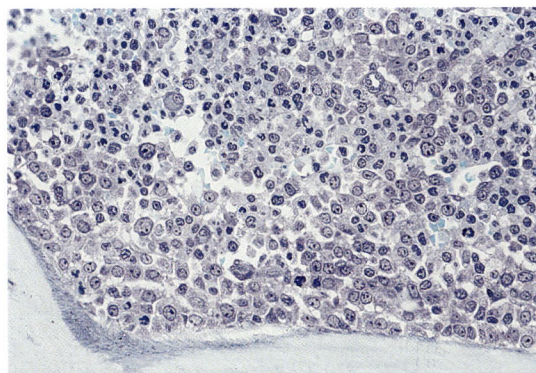

17.6 (right) As for Figure 17.5, myeloid cells are mainly neutrophilic.

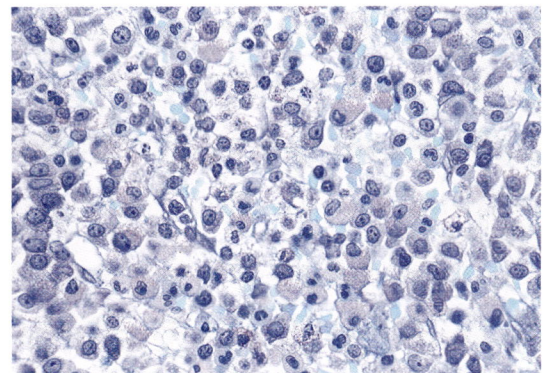

in systemic mastocytosis and drug reactions; lymphocytes in whooping cough, chicken pox and infectious mononucleosis, and monocytes in some granulomatous disorders. Marked lymphocytosis suggesting chronic lymphocytic leukemia has been observed in hyposplenism.

Eosinophilia has been described in lymphoblastic leukemias and lymphomas, in Hodgkin's disease and in some cases of early myeloproliferative disorders, or preceding a myeloproliferative disorder for variable periods (Tables 17.2 and 17.3).

TABLE 17.1 Conditions with quantitative changes in erythropoiesis

Decreased	Increased	Neoplastic (increased)
Congenital	Congenital	MPD
Thymomas	CDAs	PV
Pure red cell aplasia	Hemoglobinopathies	CML
Aplastic crisis (PNH, etc.)	Hemorrhage	MF/OMS
Aplastic anemia	Hemolysis	Erythroid malignancies
Infections	Megaloblastic anaemias	Preleukemias
Chronic diseases	Iron deficiencies	
SLE	Secondary erythrocytosis	
Renal	Refractory anemias	
Malignancies (preleukemia hypoplastic phase)	Sideroblastic anemias	
Unknown		

CDA, congenital dyserythropoietic anemias; CML, chronic myeloid leukemia; HD, Hodgkin's disease; IT, idiopathic (essential) thrombocythemia; ITP; idiopathic thrombocytopenic purpura; LPD, lymphoproliferative disorders; MF/OMS, myelofibrosis/osteomyelosclerosis; MPD, myeloproliferative disorders; PV, polycythemia vera; TTP, thrombotic thrombocytopenia purpura.

The histological differentiation between a leukemoid reaction and CML in the bone marrow alone may not be possible. The same holds for eosinophilic CML and a marked eosinophilic reaction or the hypereosinophilic syndrome. However, in the reactive conditions overall cellularity is increased proportionately. In bacterial sepsis, granulocytic precursors may replace the fat completely, with numerous polymorphonuclear leucocytes scattered throughout the marrow. Macrophages with crystalloid inclusions are rare but Charcot–Leyden crystal-containing cells may be found whenever there is eosinophilic hyperplasia; perivascular plasmacytosis may be pronounced, granulocytic hyperplasia is perivascular and intertrabecular rather than the marked paratrabecular localisation seen in CML. Megakaryocyte numbers vary. There may be hyperplasia but with no atypical features, and micromegakaryocytes are absent. Mild increase in reticulin fibers and granulomas may be seen. When the peripheral blood counts are very high the bone marrow picture

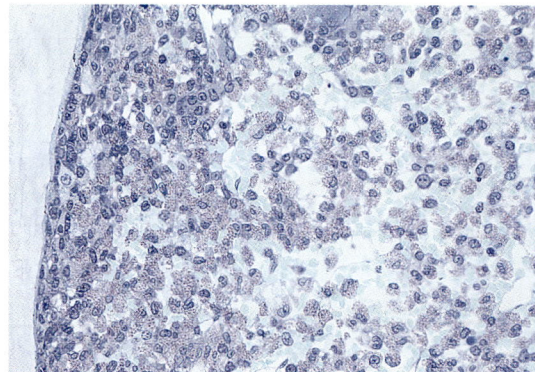

17.7 BMBS plastic, Giemsa, mainly eosinophilic precursors; case of parasitic infection.

may resemble that of promyelocytic leukemia. In leukemoid reactions hyperplasia involves mainly the neutrophilic and eosinophilic lines (Figures 17.6 and 17.7) while in CML basophils are also involved, as reflected by the increased basophil count in the peripheral blood (see Chapter 22).

In infectious mononucleosis the marrow is hypercellular with increases in all hematopoietic elements as well as reticular cells; granu-

TABLE 17.2 Conditions with quantitative changes in granulopoiesis

Decreased	Increased	Neoplastic (increased)
Congenital	Congenital	MPD
Aplastic anemia	Infections	PV
Drugs/radiation	Inflammations	IT
Infections	Trauma	CML
	Metabolic	MF/OMS
	Hypersensitivity	Acute leukemias
	Hypersplenism	Preleukemias
	Post-therapy	
	Malignancies	

TABLE 17.3 Causes of eosinophilia

Allergic disorders (bronchial asthma, etc.)
Skin diseases (psoriasis, eczema, pemphigus)
Parasitic infections (toxoplasmosis, amoebiasis)
Loeffler's syndrome and other pulmonary
  disorders
Primary hypereosinophilic syndrome
'Tropical' eosinophilia
Infections
Myelo- and lymphoproliferative disorders
Malignancies (especially with metastases,
  necrosis)
Post-radiation
Immune and collagen diseases: vasculitis,
  rheumatoid arthritis
Hodgkin's disease
Mastocytosis

lomas may also be present. Hypercellularity with an increase in histiocytes showing erythrophagocytosis is also seen in Kawasaki's disease.

Thrombocytosis and bone marrow histology

An elevated platelet count may occur as a temporary phenomenon post-splenectomy, in acute or chronic inflammations, after hemorrhage, in iron deficiency and after operations. It is also seen in patients with Hodgkin's disease, malignant lymphomas and carcinomas; in the latter it may represent a non-specific proliferative response to tissue necrosis as well as resulting from stimulation by specific factors (Table 17.4). In these secondary thrombocytoses the bone marrow shows a normal architectural pattern, with normal-to-increased cellularity (depending on the etiology), and an increase in megakaryocytes (Figures 17.8 and 17.9), but without the marked polymorphism, atypia, clustering and presence of pyknotic forms which characterise neoplastic megakaryocyte proliferations, except in occasional cases with very severe infections. It should be stressed that very high platelet counts ($>10^{12}$/litre) in reactive conditions may be

---

TABLE 17.4 Conditions with quantitative changes in megakaryopoiesis

Decreased	Increased	Neoplastic (increased)
Congenital	ITP	MPD
Aplastic anaemia	(TTP)	PV
Megaloblastic anemia		Megakaryocytic myelosis
Drugs/radiation	Hemolysis	IT
LPD	Hemorrhage	CML
Other neoplasias	Hypersplenism	MF/OMS
	LPD	Preleukemias
	HD	
	Malignancies	

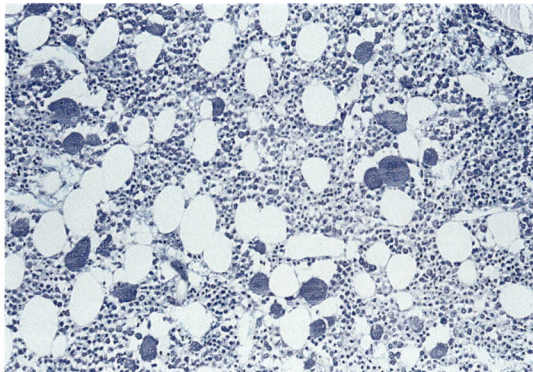

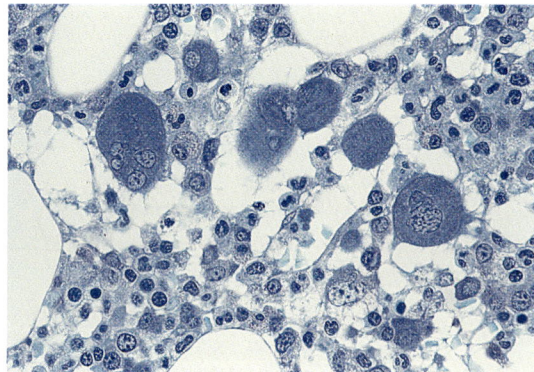

17.8 (left) BMBS plastic, Giemsa, megakaryocytic hyperplasia in case of bone marrow metastases, not shown.

17.9 (right) BMBS plastic, Giemsa, in case of HD without bone marrow involvement.

found in the absence of striking megakaryocytic hyperplasia or hypertrophy in the bone marrow. Localised megakaryocytic increases may be found in the vicinity of metastases in the bone marrow, between granulomas and between nodules or sheets of lymphoid cells in lymphomas (Figure 17.10).

Lymphocytosis and bone marrow histology

The normal bone marrow has few B lymphocytes but more T lymphocytes, and these are increased in numerous reactive conditions (Figure 17.10). Polyclonal blood lymphocytosis is likely to be reactive rather than neoplastic, as in some cigarette smokers. Malignant thymoma may also be accompanied by lymphocytosis. Lymphocytosis may also occur in disorders of the immune system (see Chapter 25), viral and other infections. In many of these a bone biopsy is unlikely to be performed, and if there is an increase in lymphocytes it will be polyclonal, more T than B cells.

Plasmacytosis and bone marrow histology

Plasmacytosis in the bone marrow (reactive plasmacytosis) may occur in numerous conditions, especially those involving antigenic stimulation, allergic and autoimmune states

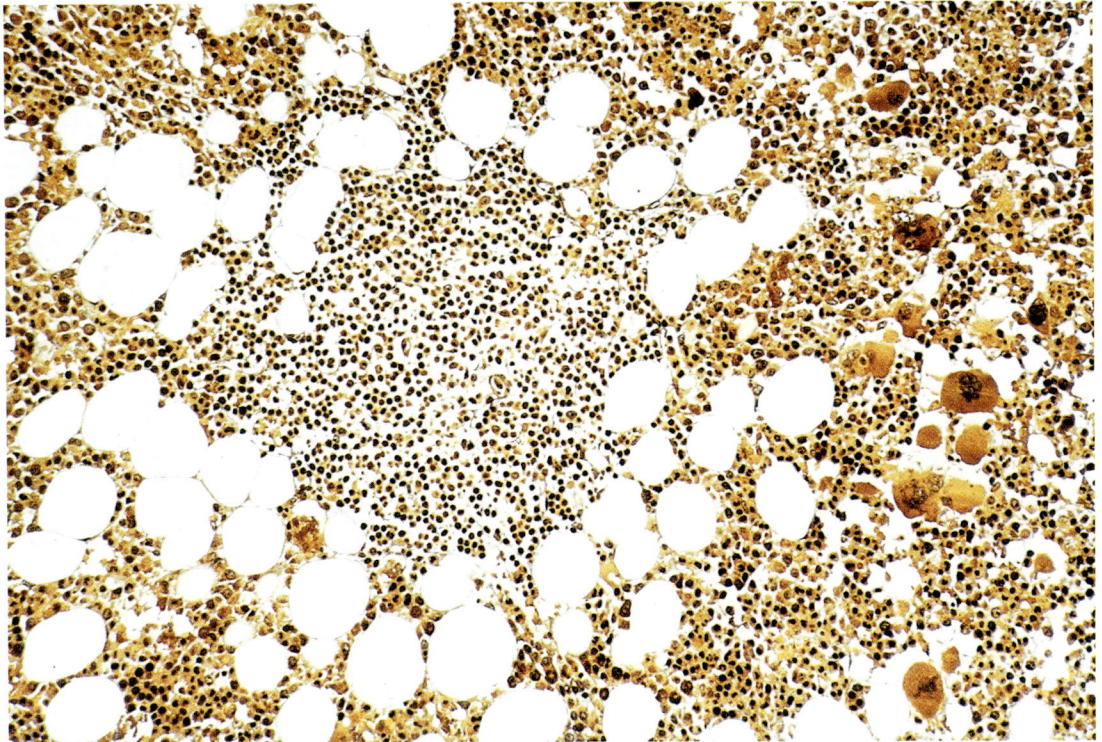

17.10 BMBS plastic, Gomori, lymphocytic aggregate and reactive megakaryocytosis, right, in patient with autoimmune hemolysis.

17.11 (left) BMBS plastic, Giemsa, perivascular and interstitial plasmacytosis in case of renal disease.

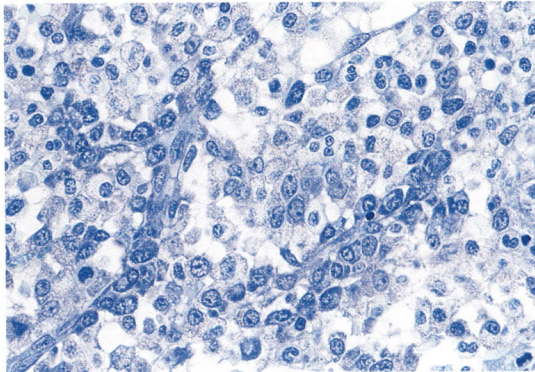

17.12 (right) BMBS paraffin, plasma cells reactive with lambda antibody; a similar result was obtained with the kappa antibody.

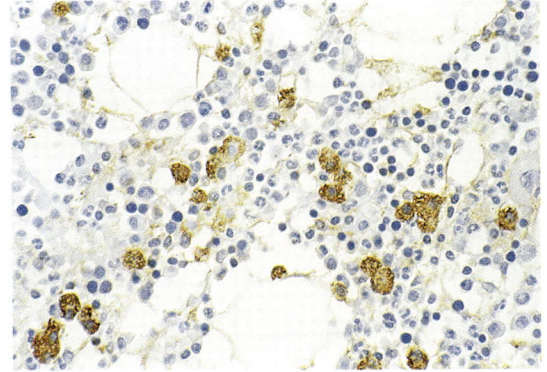

and as an accompanying phenomenon of immunoproliferations elsewhere, for example in immunoproliferative disease of the small intestine (Figures 17.11–17.14). Bone marrow plasmacytosis also occurs in leukemoid reactions and in the presence of other malignancies. In these cases the plasma cells are dispersed throughout the marrow and are clustered around capillaries. In doubtful cases, the presence or absence of light-chain restriction can be demonstrated by antibodies to kappa and lambda light chains (Figures 17.12–17.14).

In the event of a monoclonal proliferation, mainly one – either kappa or lambda – will be positive, while only a few plasma cells will react with the other.

Monocytosis and bone marrow histology

Monocytes migrate from the peripheral blood to the tissues, where they mature to form part of the mononuclear phagocyte and immunoregulatory effector system (MPIRE).

Monocytes in the bone marrow may be increased in chronic infections, lymphomas, autoimmune disorders, splenectomy, various cancers and hematopoietic and hemolytic disorders. The monocytic/histiocytic cells in these conditions are now considered as part of the MPIRE system.

Monocytes/histiocytes resembling 'storage' cells occur in many different conditions associated with high rates of cell turnover and ineffective hematopoiesis. In many of these conditions macrophages packed with cellular debris and hemosiderin are also conspicuous (Figure 17.15). In infections (especially viral) associated with hemophagocytic syndrome, T cells and monocytes–histiocytes are also increased, often considerably.

Increased mast cells in the bone marrow

Increases in mast cells in the bone marrow may occur in allergic and autoimmune conditions, hypoplastic anemias (both relative and absolute increases), lymphoproliferative disorders, as in lymphoplasmacytoid malignant lymphomas and in hairy cell leukemia, vascular diseases, osteoporosis and other osseous disorders, myelodysplasias and preleukemias; and in myelofibrosis. Mast cells are also found in the neighborhood of metastatic carcinoma, and are greatly increased in mastocytosis, both in the interstitial tissue, and in the so-called 'mast cell granulomas' – perivascular, paratrabecular and interstitial (Figure 17.16).

Leukoerythroblastosis and bone marrow histology

A leukoerythroblastic blood picture is characteristic of myelofibrosis, especially that associated with a myeloproliferative disorder. However, other bone marrow abnormalities may also be responsible, including severe infections, hemolytic anemias,

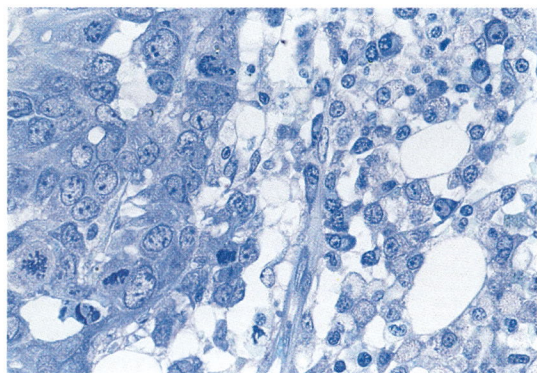

17.13 (left) BMBS plastic, Giemsa, plasmacytosis near metastasis, left.

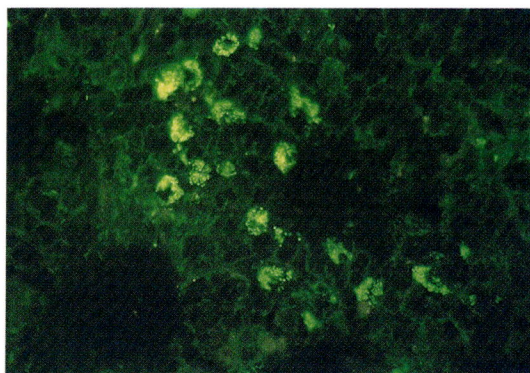

17.14 (right) BMB frozen section incubated with kappa antigen; immunofluorescence, similar result obtained with lambda.

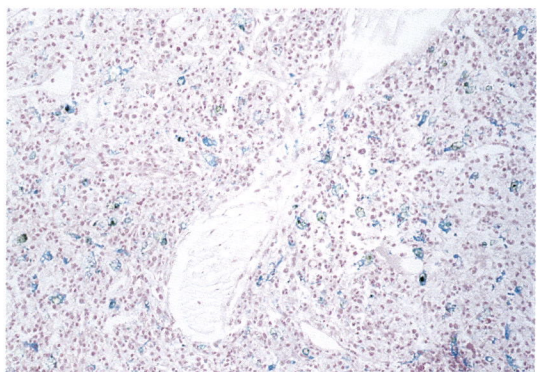

17.15 (left) BMBS plastic, stain for iron shows increase in macrophages.

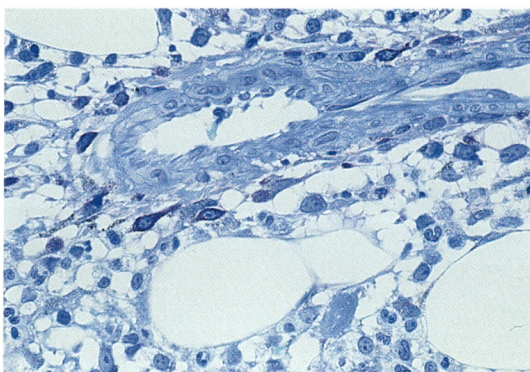

17.16 (right) BMBS plastic, Giemsa, showing perivascular mast cells.

17.17 (left) BMBS plastic, Giemsa, patient had a leucoerythroblastic blood picture and was thought to have myelofibrosis, but was found to have pre-terminal Kaposi.

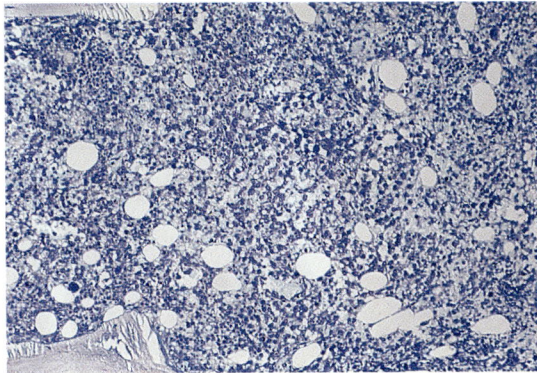

17.18 (right) BMBS plastic, Gomori, this patient also had a leucoerythroblastic blood picture and was presumed to have myelofibrosis; however, metastases of malignant meningioma were found.

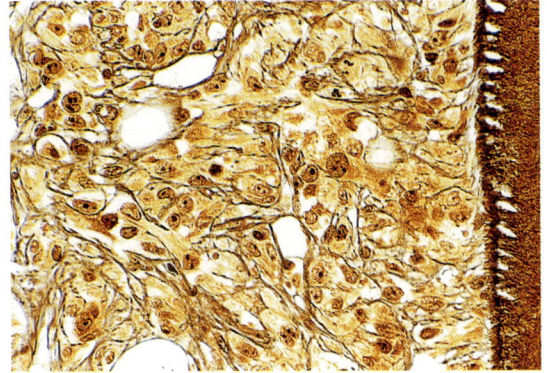

fractures, marrow infiltrations – granulomas and metastases, osseous disorders such as osteoporosis and Paget's disease of bone, Gaucher's disease and amyloidosis. Occasionally diffuse metastatic involvement with a fibrotic reaction may also be responsible for a leukoerythroblastic peripheral blood picture (Figures 17.7 and 17.18).

Check list: Hyperplasias of the Bone Marrow

- Adequate biopsy: to rule out hypoplastic areas alternating with hyperplastic ones.
- Overall reduction in fat cells?
- Hyperplasia of one or more cell lines? Immunohistology (I.H.) for identification and estimation of extent, e.g. glycophorin and hemoglobin for red cell series, Factor VIII for megakaryocytes, myeloperoxidase, and in flow cytometry CD13, CD33, CD34 for granulocytic series, LCA for lymphocytes with B and T cell markers, CD68 for monocytic series.
- Topography of hyperplastic cell line(s)?
- Correlation with peripheral blood values?
- Correlation with other clinical parameters – fever, infection, neoplasias, drugs and other factors.
- Indication for cause? If so, what?

Clinical correlations

- Differentiation between benign, premalignant and malignant conditions must be established.
- Erythrocytosis: cardiovascular and pulmonary conditions to be ruled out.
- Erythrocytosis in malignancies such as renal carcinomas and/or other tumors to be investigated.
- Plasma volume and red cell mass determination to rule out 'pseudo' erythrocytosis.
- If none of the above – rare causes such as familial conditions to be considered.

Leukemoid reactions

- Causative factor(s) are usually detected by appropriate clinical, biochemical, bacteriological and viral tests.
- Fever, malaise and weakness often present.
- LAP is high in reactive states
- Transient – leucocytosis subsides with treatment and elimination of the cause.
- Different cell lines stimulated by different agents, e.g. eosinophilia in parasitic conditions, thus indicating direction of clinical investigation.

Thrombocytosis

- Associated clinical conditions: infections, inflammations, surgery, tissue damage, malignancies, blood loss, post-splenectomy, rebound after chemotherapy.

Continued

169

- Thrombocytosis may indicate or support a particular diagnosis.
- Therapy of the causative condition reduces the platelet count.
- Aspirin for prevention of complications usually not required.

Monocytosis
- Peripheral monocytosis may indicate direction of investigation, e.g. autoimmune or preleukemic condition, MDS.
- Considered part of the MPIRE system response to various stimuli.
- In infections, especially viral, possibly associated with hemophagocytic syndrome.

Eosinophilia
- Often accidental findings.
- Parasitic and fungal infections.
- Allergic and hypersensitivity reactions.
- In malignancies: HD, some lymphomas, carcinomas, myeloproliferative disorders.
- In cutaneous, pulmonary and immune disorders.

Leukoerythroblastic blood picture
- Decreased peripheral blood values.
- Possibly splenomegaly.
- Any pathologic process with accompanying bone marrow fibrosis.

Bibliography

Bennet O.M., Namnyak S.S. (1990) Bone and joint manifestations of sickle cell anaemia. *J Bone Jt Surg.*, **72B**, 494.

Bewig B., Wacker H.H., Parwaresch M.R. *et al.* (1993), Eosinophilia as the leading symptom of highly malignant enteropathy-associated T-cell lymphoma. *Z. Gastroenterol.*, **31 (11)**, 666–70.

D'Angelo G., Mattaini R., Cosini I., Zanco M.D. (1990) Acquired idiopathic sideroblastic anemia with cyclic hypereosinophilia of unclear significance. A case report. *Minerva Med*, **81 (5)**, 433–7.

Furukawa T., Narita M., Sakaue M. *et al.* (1997) Primary familial polycythaemia associated with a novel point mutation in the erythropoietin receptor. *Br. J. Haematol*, **99**, 222–7.

Horiike S., Misawa S., Nishada K. *et al.* (1989), Myelodysplastic syndrome preceding acute myelomonocytic leukemia with dysplastic marrow eosinophilia and inv (16). *Acta Hematol.*, **82 (3)**, 161–4.

Horny H.P., Wehrmann M., Griesser H. *et al.* (1993) Investigation of bone marrow lymphocyte subsets in normal, reactive, and neoplastic states using paraffin-embedded biopsy specimens. *Am J Clin Pathol*, **99 (2)**, 142–9.

Keefer M.J., Solanki D.L. (1988), Dyserythropoiesis and erythroblast-phagocytosis preceding pure red cell aplasia. *Am. J. Hematol.* **27 (2)**, 132–5.

Kitamura H., Kodama F., Odagiri S. *et al.* (1989), Granulocytosis associated with malignant neoplasms: a clinicopathologic study and demonstration of colony-stimulating activity in tumor extracts. *Hum. Pathol.*, **20 (9)**, 878–85.

Mankad V.N., Williams J.P., Harpen M.D. *et al.* (1990) Magnetic resonance imaging of bone marrow in sickle cell disease: clinical hematologic and pathologic correlations. *Blood*, **75 (1)**, 274–83.

Menke D.M., Greipp P.R., Colon-Otero G. *et al.* (1994) Bone marrow aspirate immunofluorescent and bone marrow biopsy immunoperoxidase staining of plasma cells in histologically occult plasma cell proliferative marrow disorders. *Arch Pathol Lab Med*, **118 (8)**, 811–14.

Miranda R.N., Esparza A.R., Sambandam S., Medeiros L.J. (1994) Systemic mast cell disease presenting with peripheral blood eosinophilia. *Hum Pathol*, **25 (7)**, 727–30.

Schichishima T., Terasawa T., Uchida T., Kariyone S. (1989) Complement sensitivity of erythroblasts and erythropoietic precursors in paroxysmal nocturnal hemoglobinuria (PNH) *Br J Haematol*, **72 (4)**, 578–83.

Stefanini M., Claustro J.C., Motos R.A., Bendigo L.L. (1991), Blood and bone marrow eosinophilia in malignant tumors. Role and nature of blood and tissue eosinophil colony-stimulating factor (s) in two patients. *Cancer*, **68 (3)**, 543–8.

18 Qualitative abnormalities of erythropoiesis

Dyserythropoiesis: definition and general aspects

This incorporates both morphological and kinetic aspects of erythropoiesis, and recognises the fact that even when erythroblasts are functionally abnormal some survive and mature, and so reach the circulation, though they are abnormal and their descendent erythrocytes are likely to have a shortened life span. Thus, dyserythropoiesis includes both quantitative and qualitative anomalies of erythropoiesis. A certain degree of morphological dyserythropoiesis may be seen whenever hyperplasia (or perhaps accelerated production) occurs, but this is transitory, lasting only until equilibrium has been re-established, and as such might be considered 'physiological dyserythropoiesis'.

Two broad categories of pathological dyserythropoiesis are recognised: congenital and acquired. Included in the first are the congenital dyserythropoietic anemias (CDA), i.e. CDA I, II (Hempas), III, IV and their variants; as well as red cell membrane defects and red cell enzyme defects, for example glucose 6-phosphate dehydrogenase (G6PD) deficiency, in which the red cells are particularly sensitive to various drugs, ingestion of which cause episodes of hemolysis; the thalassemic syndromes and other hemoglobinopathies; congenital sideroblastic anemias, and others. Of these, the inherited diseases of hemoglobin – the hemoglobinopathies – are the most impor-

tant. Bone marrow biopsies are rarely performed in these conditions as they are usually diagnosed by biochemical and hematological tests. Consequently they will not be considered here. They are characterised by hyperplastic and ineffective erythropoiesis with a hemolytic component of variable magnitude, and associated disturbances in iron metabolism, and possibly relative folic acid or vitamin B_{12} deficiency. Frequently the trabecular bone is affected by the hyperplastic marrow so that varying degrees of osteodystrophy and osteomalacia result.

The second category, i.e. the acquired, embraces a wide range of conditions including nutritional deficiencies (e.g. B_{12}, folate, iron), the myelodysplastic syndromes, hematological malignancies involving the red cell series directly, and those which affect erythropoiesis by altering the microenvironment.

Congenital dyserythropoietic anemias

The diagnosis is usually made by smears of aspirates of bone marrow and by electron microscopy (Figures 18.1–18.3), by means of which and in conjunction with other biochemical and hematological investigations the CDA types and their variants are distinguished. The patients have varying degrees of anemia, with red cell anomalies: anisocytosis and poikilocytosis on the peripheral blood smears. Bone marrow biopsy sections show a hyper-

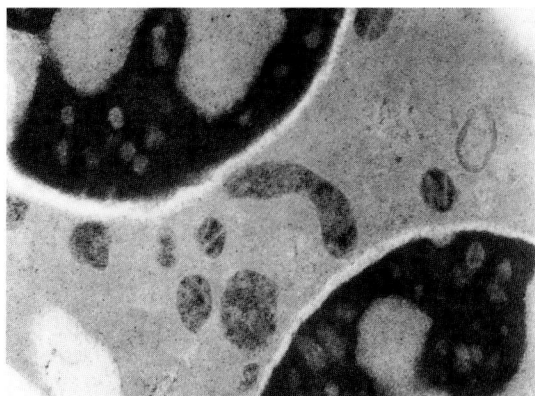

18.1 (left) BMBS, EM, part of binucleate erythroblast with typical nuclear chromatin and iron in mitochondria, CDA.

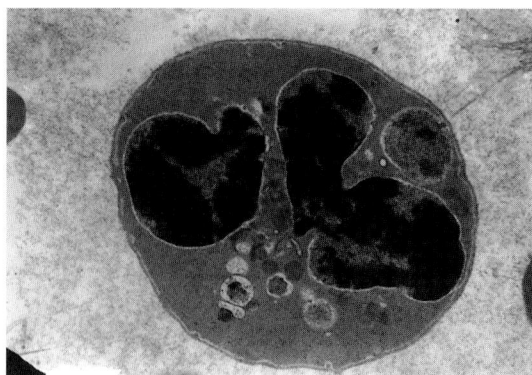

18.2 (right) BMBS, EM, binucleate erythroblast with peripheral double membrane, CDA.

18.3 BMBS, EM, normoblast extruding its nucleus together with organelles such as iron-laden mitochondria.

cellular marrow with an extreme degree of erythropoietic hyperplasia and corresponding reduction in fat cells. At high magnification some characteristic nuclear aberrations are seen even in the light microscope although their detailed structure requires electron microscopy. These include binuclearity, multinuclearity, internuclear bridges, and nuclear budding, fragmentation and degeneration (karyorrhexis), and a variety of atypical mitotic figures. Cytoplasmic abnormalities include vacuolation, basophilic stippling, and iron-containing granules (ringed sideroblasts also occur) and intercellular cytoplasmic connections. Not all erythroid precursors are affected so that apparently normal ones are seen alongside the dyserythropoietic cells.

The CDAs have a characteristic bone marrow morphology:

CDA I. Megaloblastic with binucleate erythroblasts and chromatin bridging.

CDA II (Hempas). Normoblastic, binucleate erythroblasts, positive acid hemolysis test.

CDA III. Giant multinuclear erythroblasts.

CDA IV. Normoblastic, binuclear erythroblasts, negative acid hemolysis test.

Macrophages with engulfed erythroblasts and nuclear debris are prominent; in some cases of CDA II Gaucher-like histiocytes have been observed in the bone marrow. As in most situations with augmented and ineffective erythroid turnover, iron stores are increased and deposits are found (in severe cases) in reticular, endothelial and endosteal cells and, if transfusion overload occurs, even in

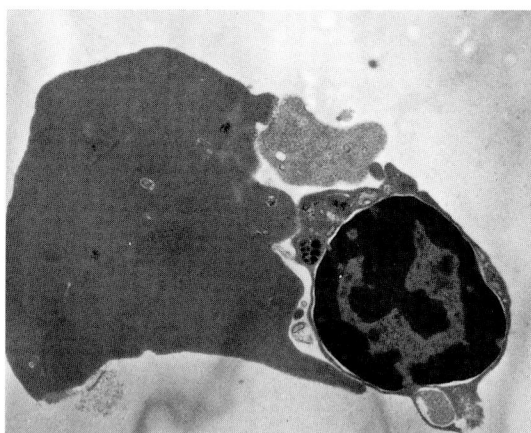

the osteoid seams. In long-standing cases, the trabecular bone is osteopenic with increased osteoid, and normal or increased bone turnover.

Porphyrias

These comprise a group of disorders classified as either erythropoietic or hepatic according to the site of occurrence of the metabolic defect. The bone marrow shows erythroblastic hyperplasia. There may be a dimorphic population, with the presence of macroblasts due (possibly) to folate deficiency, because of increased requirement and consumption and therefore a relative lack. The pathological population of erythroid precursors exhibits marked dyserythropoietic features.

Megaloblastic (and megaloblastoid) erythropoiesis

This is due to deficiency of B$_{12}$ or folic acid, or both (levels in serum), and similar morphological changes are observed whatever the cause, such as increased requirements, defective absorption, insufficient supply, lack of intrinsic factor, effects of drugs, such as anticonvulsants, some oral contraceptives, antitubercular drugs, large doses of other antibiotic agents and vitamin C deficiency (Tables 18.1 and 18.2). The erythroid precursors are larger than normal, with large nuclei that have a much finer chromatin pattern than erythroblasts undergoing normoblastic maturation, and there are proportionally many more immature erythroid cells than late forms (Figures 18.4–18.6). At first glance at low magnification, the bone marrow may resemble that seen in acute leukemia (Figures 18.7 and 18.8). Other dyserythropoietic features such as

TABLE 18.1 Folic acid and vitamin B$_{12}$ deficiencies

Folic Acid	B$_{12}$
Inadequate supply	Congenital conditions
Dietary lack	Inadequate supply
Alcoholism	Malabsorption
Malabsorption	Intrinsic factor deficiency
Sprue	Autoimmune deficiency
Malignancy	Gastric surgery
Crohn's disease	Pancreatic insufficiency
Destruction hemolysis	Small intestinal absorption defects
Increased requirement hemolysis	Crohn's disease
Dermatologic conditions	Sprue
Metabolic inhibition	Malignancy
Drugs	Ileal resection
Vitamin C deficiency	Infections
Alcohol	

18.4 (left) BMBS plastic, Giemsa, showing relative erythroid hyperplasia; note clusters of early erythroblasts, lower center.

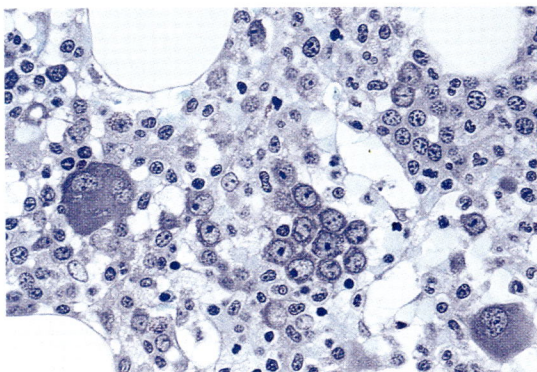

18.5 (right) BMBS plastic, Giemsa, showing maturation arrest and increase in erythroid precursors.

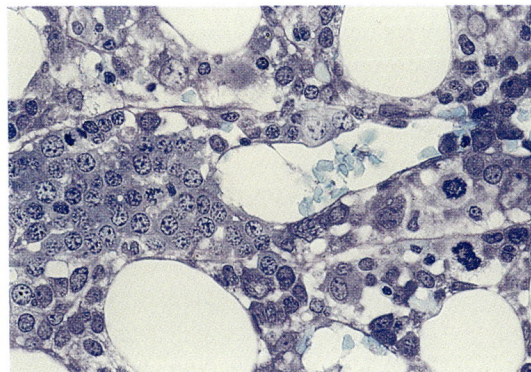

TABLE 18.2 Megaloblastic or mega-loblastoid maturation

1. Defective DNA synthesis (acquired)
   Deficiency of vitamin B_{12} and/or folate
   Dietary GI tract anomalies
   Increased demand drugs
2. Accelerated hematopoiesis due to:
   Hemolysis
   Hemorrhage
3. Congenital anomalies of erythropoiesis
4. Of uncertain origin
   Acquired sideroblastic anemia
   Myelodysplastic symdromes
   Accompanying other malignancies
5. Neoplastic alterations
   Myeloproliferative disorders

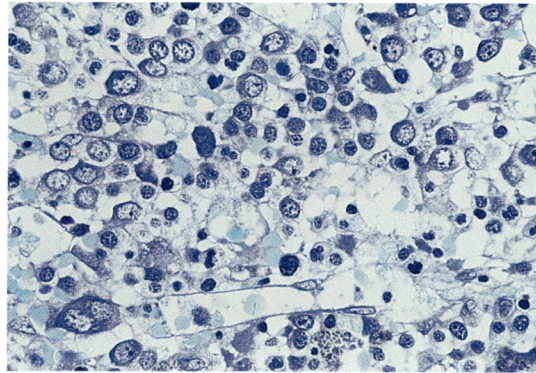

18.6 BMBS plastic, Giemsa, megaloblastoid erythropoiesis, showing large erythroid island with maturation arrest, acute hemolysis.

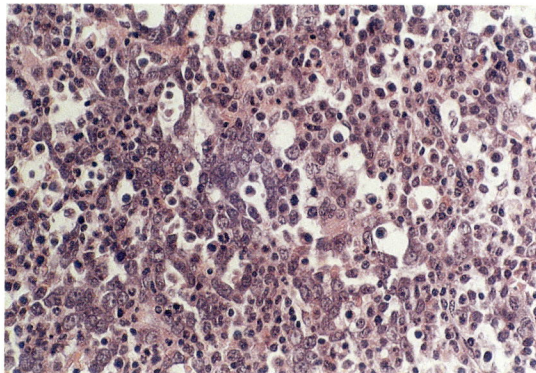

18.7 BMBS paraffin, H&E, hypercellular bone marrow of patient with B_{12} deficiency. Note numerous immature cells.

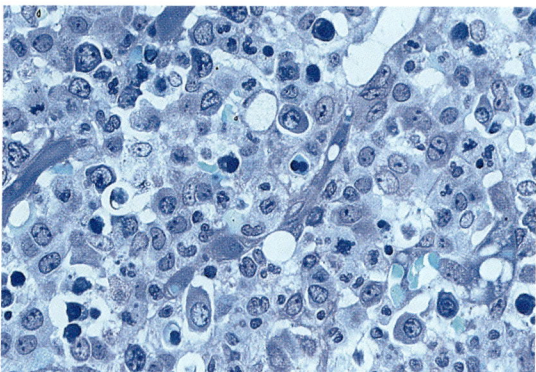

18.8 BMBS plastic, Giemsa, as for Figure 18.7 at higher magnification. The bone marrow resembles that of an acute leukemia.

irregularly shaped nuclei, Howell–Jolly bodies and karyorrhexis are also present. In addition, the other cell lines also show disturbed maturation such as giant bands (metamyelocytes) in the neutrophilic series, hypersegmented polymorphs and multinucleate megakaryocytes. Part of this hyperplastic hematopoiesis is ineffective as many of the cells undergo apoptosis and are phagocytosed in the bone marrow. There is increased iron in the stromal cells unless iron deficiency is also present. The bone marrow is frequently hypercellular with reduction in fat cells. Conditions with hyperplastic erythropoiesis are listed in Tables 18.1 and 18.2. Folic acid deficiency is of particular significance due to the consequent induction of chromosome breaks and the associated increased risk of malignant transformation.

Paroxysmal Nocturnal Hemoglobinuria (PNH)

This is of special interest. The increased sensitivity of erythrocytes to complement-mediated lysis is due to a membrane defect which has also been found in granulocytes, platelets and in colony-forming units, suggesting that PNH results from a change at the level of the pluripotent stem cells. The bone marrow is usually hyperplastic (Figure 18.9), but hypoplasia may occur, and even an 'aplastic crisis', in which there is a transient failure of red cell production, in addition to the shortened survival.

18.9 (left) BMBS plastic, Giemsa, showing erythroid hyperplasia, all maturational stages present, though there is maturation arrest, PNH.

18.10 (right) BMBS plastic, Giemsa, marked erythroid hyperplasia at all maturational stages, case of hemolysis.

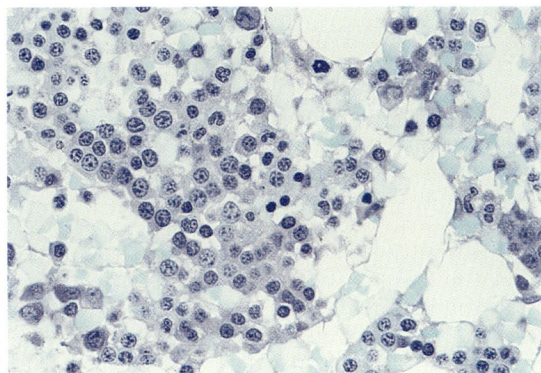

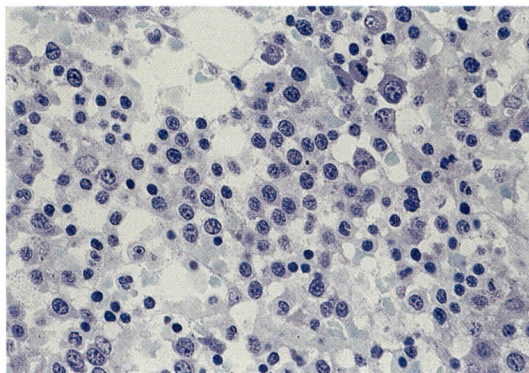

Hemolytic anemias

Bone biopsies are generally not of much diagnostic significance (Figures 18.6 and 18.10). The congenital hemolytic anemias are due to inborn errors of erythrocyte metabolic enzymes, defects in red cell membrane function and unstable abnormal hemoglobins. These defects result in red blood cells (RBCs) unable to meet the normal challenges in the circulation. The characteristic feature to be seen in a biopsy is erythroid hyperplasia. In contrast, in acquired hemolytic anemias biopsies may help in the differential diagnosis, especially when involvement by malignant conditions is a contributing factor. Abnormal antibodies, together with proliferation of the reticuloendothelial system with augmented phagocytosis, may also be involved in the hemolytic episodes in these cases. A number of conditions are associated with autoimmune hemolytic anemias. They include: infections (both viral and bacterial) rheumatic disorders and autoimmune disorders, immunodeficiency states and various malignancies.

Crises in hemolytic conditions may be precipitated by infections, especially those of the upper respiratory tract. Some aplastic crises in hemolytic anemias have recently been ascribed to a parvovirus. In severe hemolysis, the bone marrow fat cells are replaced by hyperplastic normoblastic erythropoiesis with a predominance of early erythroblasts; many mitotic figures are seen as well as macrophages with nuclear remains. These are also found in other situations, such as the aplastic crisis of PNH in which erythropoietic activity is reduced. Increased erythropoiesis due to hemorrhage is also characterised by an imbalance in favor of immature erythroblasts, perhaps due to accelerated passage and release into the circulation. In addition, there is a concomitant increase in megakaryocytes, due to loss and increased utilisation of platelets. In chronic hemolytic anemias, extension of hematopoiesis into shafts of the long bones and even into the liver and spleen may occur. Intravascular hemolysis may be caused by mismatched transfusions, thermal burns, snake bites, infections, mechanical heart valves and PNH.

Episodes of hemolysis may lead to an iron-deficiency anemia. There is possibly an increased risk of MDS and even acute leukemia when bone marrow hypocellularity predominates.

Drugs and hemolysis

Various drugs may be associated with hemolysis, especially when there is a pre-existing condition such as G6PD deficiency. The drugs include various antibiotics and antimalarials; in some cases an immune mechanism may be responsible (quinidine, streptomycin).

Iron deficiency

Iron deficiency is still very prevalent throughout the world, especially in children (measured by iron studies: SI, TIBC, serum, ferritin levels) (Table 18.3). The bone marrow shows hyper-

TABLE 18.3 Conditions with quantitative changes in iron stores

Decreased	Increased
Deficiencies	Congenital hemoglobinopathies
Diet	Sideroblastic anemia
Vegetarians	Congenital dyserythropoietic anemias
Utilization	Hemochromatosis
Pregnancy	Acquired sideroblastic anemias
Lactation	Chronic diseases
Loss	Collagen
Hemorrhage	Renal
Varices	Storage diseases
Diaphragmatic hernia	In older age groups
Parasites	Erythroid malignancies
Malignancies	Myelofibrosis/osteomyelosclerosis
Polycythemia vera	Other malignancies
	Hemosiderosis
	Transfusion overload

plasia of the erythroid series, the cells are small, there are many late forms with pale cytoplasm due to insufficient hemoglobinisation, and the cytoplasmic edges are ragged. There is a considerable degree of ineffective erythropoiesis, with intramedullary destruction. In some cases of marked iron deficiency the marrow may even be hypocellular. Some of the common causes of iron deficiency include defective nutrition, hemolysis, chronic disorders such as renal impairment, and congenital hypotransferrinemia.

Sideroblastosis

Anemias with a sideroblastic component may occur in alcoholics, megaloblastic anemias, inflammatory diseases, hematological malignancies, myelodysplastic syndromes and miscellaneous other conditions (Tables 18.4 and 18.5). Paradoxically, many conditions with anemias are also associated with an increase in

TABLE 18.4 Sideroblastic erythropoiesis

Hereditary	Enzyme deficiencies
Acquired	'Idiopathic'
	Drugs
	Alcohol abuse
	Connective tissue diseases
	Inflammatory diseases
	Hematological malignancies
	Other malignancies

TABLE 18.5 Anemias with a sideroblastic component

May occur in:
- Alcohol abuse
- Megaloblastic anemias
- Inflammatory diseases
- Myelodysplastic syndromes
- Myeloproliferative disease
- Erythroleukemia
- Lymphoproliferative disease
- Vitamin deficiencies
- Drugs
- Heavy metals
- Carcinomas

iron stores in the bone marrow; for example, refractory anemias in the MDS.

Hemosiderosis

This is defined as accumulation of iron in cells of the reticuloendothelial system, especially the liver. When this is extensive, it leads eventually to fibrosis in the affected tissues. In iron overload, iron may be found in macrophages and reticular cells, in sinus endothelial cells, in endosteal cells, and even deposited in osteoid on the surface of the trabecular bone; and in osteocytic lacunae (Figure 18.11). After staining with Prussian blue (or any other iron stain) iron present in cells appears as a pale cytoplasmic 'wash' and as fine-to-coarse clumps in intracellular granules. When considerable hemosiderin is present it will also be seen as brownish-yellow intracellular deposits in the Giemsa stain. Bone marrow iron stores are better assessed in sections than in smears of aspirates, which may not contain sufficient stromal elements to be representative.

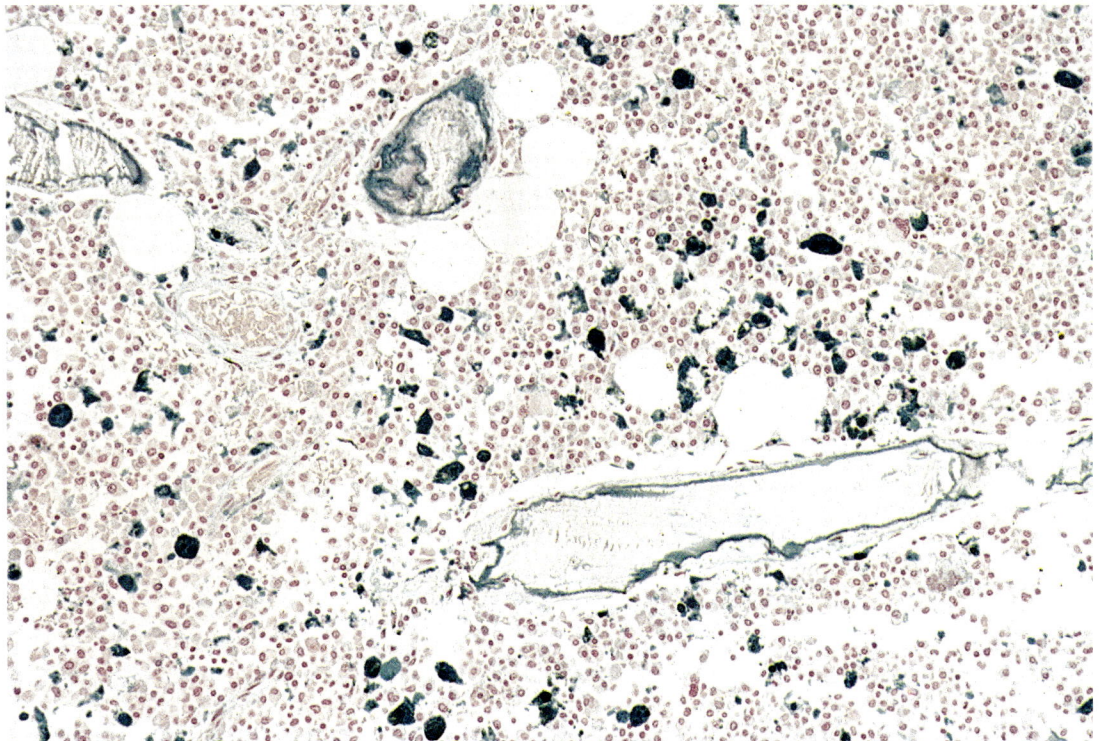

18.11 BMBS plastic, stain for iron, case of hemosiderosis. Note iron deposition around the trabeculae, as well as in stromal cells.

Hemosiderosis is usually due to transfusion overload in hereditary conditions such as thalassemias, sickle cell disease, spherocytosis, red cell enzyme deficiencies or in acquired conditions such as aplastic anemia and myelofibrosis (Table 18.3). Transfusional iron overload is less frequent today because of the administration of chelating agents that bind and remove excess iron via the kidneys.

Hemochromatosis

This may occur as a familial (or primary, or idiopathic) entity, or in association with a variety of hepatic disorders (secondary), and in congenital transferrin deficiency. In the primary form there may be less deposition of hemosiderin in the cells of the reticuloendothelial system. However, osteoporosis and even collapse of a vertebral body have been noted, usually ascribed to ascorbic acid deficiency, which in turn is secondary to the oxidative effects of the body iron. Another mechanism, and possibly a more direct one, is the inhibitory effect on osteoblasts due to the deposition of iron in endosteal cells and osteoid seams. The diagnosis of hemochromatosis is made by measuring serum iron concentration, total iron-binding capacity and transferrin saturation.

Recent studies have shown that determination of the erythrocyte ferritin content is a useful non-invasive test to distinguish hemochromatosis from alcoholic liver disease with iron overload.

Check list: Qualitative Abnormalities of Erythropoiesis

- Adequate biopsy.
- Hyperplastic erythropoiesis with dysplastic features?
- Ineffective erythropoiesis?
- Increased phagocytosis? On immunohistology (I.H.): CD68, lysozyme, alpha 1 antitrypsin, alpha 1 antichemotrypsin.

- Other cell lines not affected (except in conditions such as B_{12} deficiency).
- In absence of iron deficiency, storage iron is increased. In iron deficiency, stores are depleted.
- Storage iron and sideroblasts are readily seen (if necessary under oil) in sections of undecalcified biopsies stained with any of the widely used stains for iron.

Clinical correlations

- Congenital anomalies and porphyrias: marked dyserythropoiesis.
- Usually diagnosed early.
- Transfusion overload if no chelating agents given.
- Sideroblastosis: may be first manifestation of an MDS or acute leukemia.
- Manifestation of alcohol abuse.
- Hereditary sideroblastosis in early adulthood, pyridoxine responsive.
- Hemochromatosis: many asymptomatic.
- Eventually dysfunction of heart, liver, pancreas, endocrine glands and joints.
- Known erythropoietic anomaly.
- Correlation with peripheral blood values and other clinical and biochemical parameters, for example: B_{12} and/or folic acid deficiency.

Iron deficiency anemia

- Microcytic hypochromic.
- Accelerated RBC breakdown.
- Abnormalities of iron mobilisation and delivery.
- Low serum iron and transferrin levels.

Bibliography

Barton J.C., Bertoli L.F. (1996) Hemochromatosis: the genetic disorder of the twenty-first century. *Nature Med*, **2 (4)**, 394–6.

Blount B.C., Ames B.N. (1995) DNA damage in folate deficiency. *Baillères Clinical Haematology*, **8 (3)**, 461–78.

Budde R., Hellerich U. (1995) Alcoholic dyshaematopoiesis: morphological features of alcohol-induced bone marrow damage in biopsy sections compared with aspiration smears. *Acta Haematol*, **94 (2)**, 74–7.

Ciba Foundation Symposium 37 (new series) (1976) *Congential Disorders of Erythropoiesis*. Amsterdam: Elsevier/Excerpta Medica.

Koury M.J., Horne D.W., Brown Z.A. *et al.* (1997) Apoptosis of late-stage erythroblasts in megaloblastic anemia: association with DNA damage and macrocyte production. *Blood*, **89 (12)**, 4617–23.

Simon S.R., Branda R.F., Tindle B.F., Burns S.L. (1988) Copper deficiency and sideroblastic anemia associated with zinc ingestion. *Am. J. Hematol.*, **28 (3)**, 181–3.

Wickramasinghe S.N. (1995) Morphology, biology and biochemistry of cobalamin and folate-deficient bone marrow cells. *Baillères Clinical Haematology*, **8 (3)**, 441–59.

19 Stromal reactions and inflammations in the bone marrow

General aspects

Stromal reactions in the bone marrow may accompany cytopenias. These reactions are also seen especially in the bone marrows of patients who suffer from various underlying clinical conditions such as infections, sarcoidosis, diseases of collagen, Hodgkin's disease, malignant lymphomas and carcinomas, all without bone marrow involvement in the biopsy. However, in many patients with cytopenias no etiology or concomitant disease is discovered, in spite of intensive investigation. Bacterial and chemical toxins, and radiation may all damage the components of the bone marrow stroma. The capillaries and sinusoids are especially vulnerable and are liable to disruption, so that the intra- and extravascular compartments are no longer clearly separated.

The anemia associated with chronic disorders occurs in infections including bacterial and fungal; in chronic inflammatory, non-infectious conditions; in malignant diseases; and in chronic hepatic and renal disorders. The anemia in many of these conditions is thought to be due to impaired marrow response and defective iron metabolism. Investigation of bone marrow biopsies may reveal infections in unusual situations, such as, for example,

Mycobacterium avium in AIDS (Figure 19.1), Donovan bodies in Kala-Azar (Figure 19.2), Coxiella Burnetti in Q fever, and the causative organism in leprosy.

Stromal reactions and bone marrow histology

In severe cases there is disintegration of the sinusoids and degeneration of the walls of the small blood vessels – the larger ones are only affected when the noxae are overwhelming. In addition, such consequences may ensue as a result of allergic and autoimmune states. In chronic inflammatory conditions hemato-poiesis and fat cells are decreased and their place is taken by reticulin and collagen fibers, fibroblasts and capillaries, macrophages and other infiltrating cells. Macrophages with phagocytosed material, cells and cellular debris, may be prominent and range from few to many. In long-standing chronic conditions there is a reduction in trabecular bone volume (osteopenia). Various toxins, including minerals, may also affect the trabecular bone; for example, aluminum poisoning in renal dialysis patients. Non-specific histological changes in the bone marrow may be roughly classified into one acute and four chronic types (Figure 19.3).

19.1 (left) BMBS, Ziehl–Nielsen stain positive in macrophages in biopsy of an HIV-positive patient; well-defined granulomas were not found.

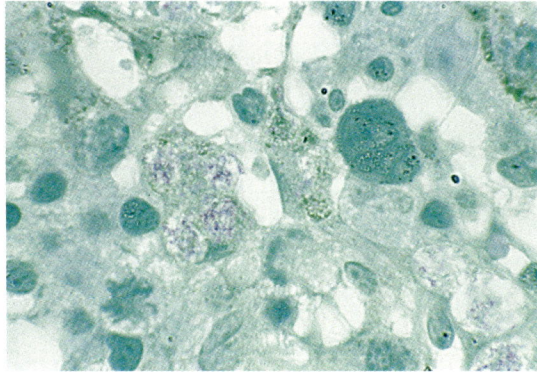

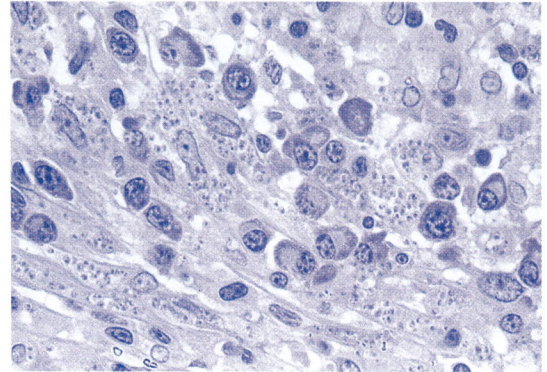

19.2 (right) BMBS, Giemsa, illustrating Donovan bodies in a patient with massive splenomegaly and pancytopenia.

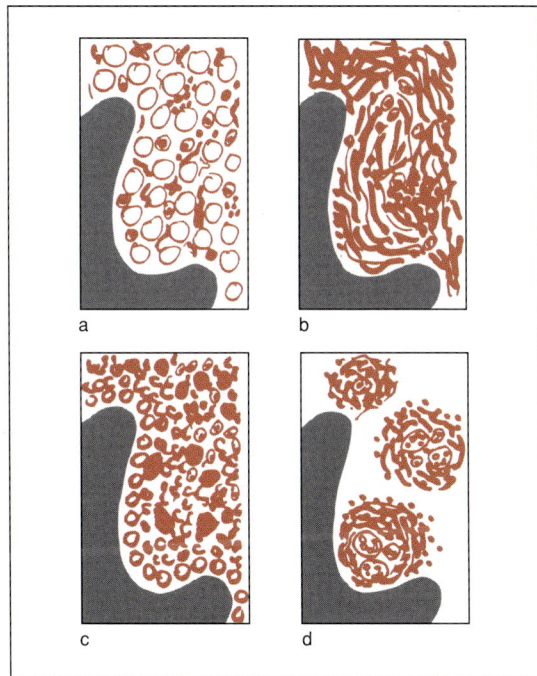

19.3 Schematic representation of bone marrow in chronic inflammations. (a) Atrophic, (b) fibrotic, (c) proliferative, (d) granulomatous.

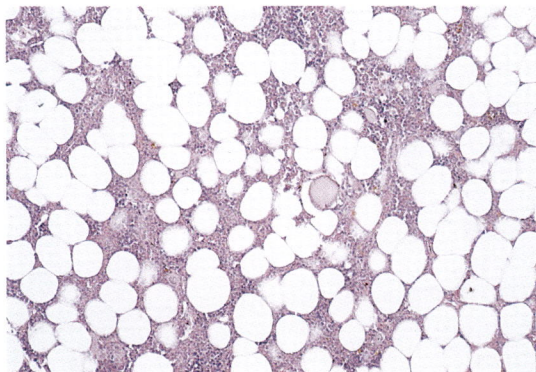

19.4 BMBS paraffin, H&E, exudative myelitis.

Types of inflammatory reactions

1. Acute inflammation, 'exudative' or 'necrotic' types: considerable residual hematopoiesis though necrosis of hematopoietic cells and capillaries is present, as well as edema, and there may be an increase in mature granulocytes. Necrosis of bone marrow may be caused by chemotherapy with or without addition of steroids (Figures 19.4–19.7).

2. Chronic inflammation, 'atrophic type': little hematopoiesis remains; there is edema, infiltration with lymphocytes, plasma cells, and mast cells, macrophages and lipomacrophages. The 'atrophic' type is also referred to as gelatinous transformation, serous atrophy or exudative myelitis. Such changes in the bone marrow may be found in a large variety of diseases including chronic infections, malignancies and poor nutrition. The marrow is hypocellular and fat cells are also reduced (Figures 19.8 and 19.9).

3. Chronic inflammation, 'fibrotic type': hematopoiesis and fat reduction, increase in reticulin (sclerosing myelitis) and development of collagen fibers, plasmacytosis, interstitial edema, variable infiltration with lymphocytes and mast cells, and possibly osteoblastic new bone formation (Figures 19.10–19.15).

4. Chronic inflammation, 'proliferative or leukemoid type': normocellular to hypercellular marrow, but with increases in plasma and mast cells, lymphocytes and granulocytes, and megakaryocytes: all, some or only one of these

181

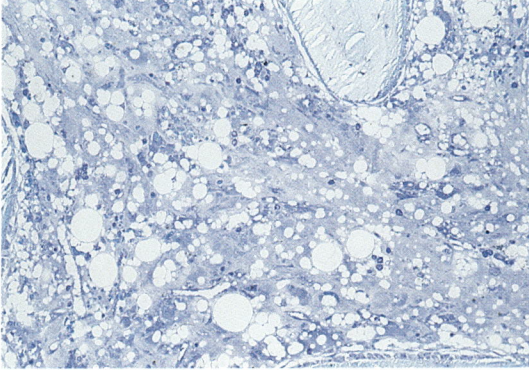

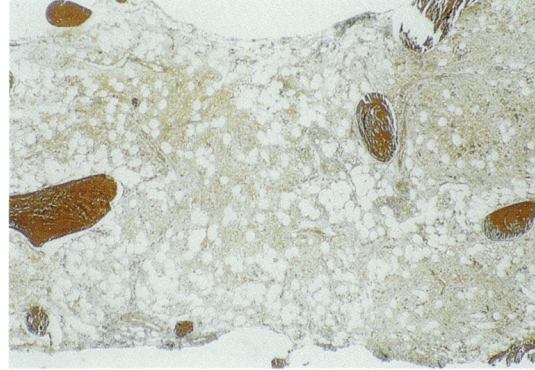

19.5 (left) BMBS plastic, Giemsa, exudative myelitis with necrosis, cause unknown.

19.6 (right) As for Figure 19.5, Gomori, low power to show extent of bone marrow affected. Hypoplasia, exudation, necrosis and incipient fibrosis.

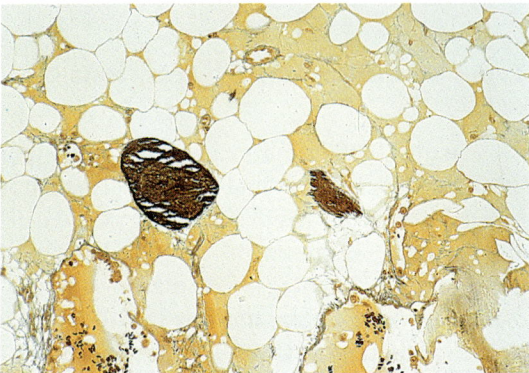

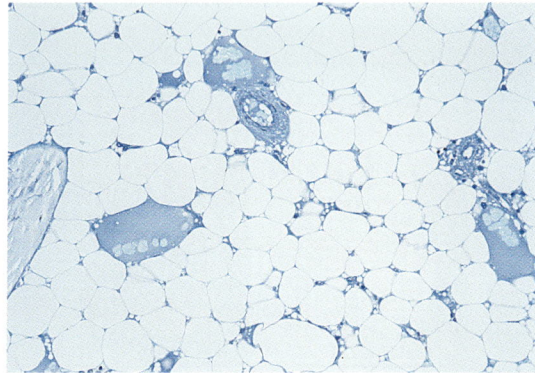

19.7 (left) High power of Figure 19.6 to show serous atrophy.

19.8 and 19.9 BMBS plastic showing atrophic fatty marrow.
19.8 (right) Giemsa, from a biopsy of an HIV-positive patient.

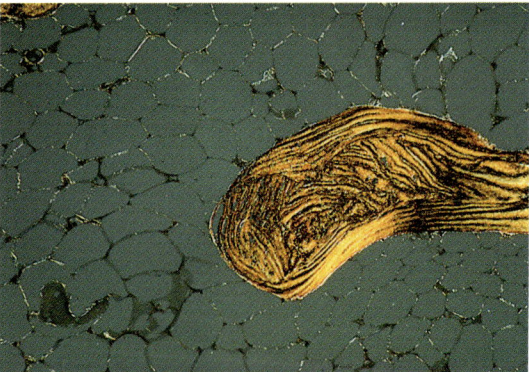

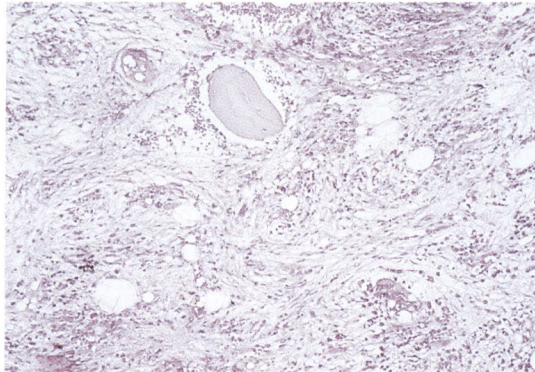

19.9 (left) Gomori in polarised light showing little increase in reticular fibers.

19.10–19.15 Fibrotic reactions.
19.10 (right) BMBS paraffin, H&E, extensive fibrosis with some residual hematopoiesis.

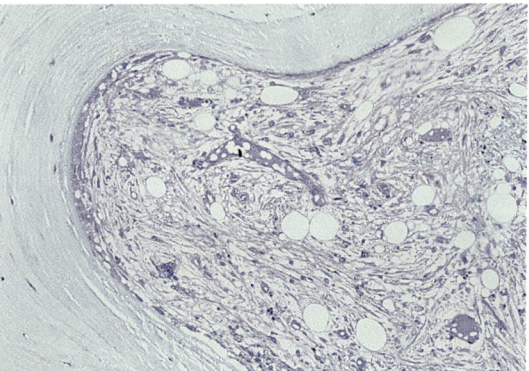

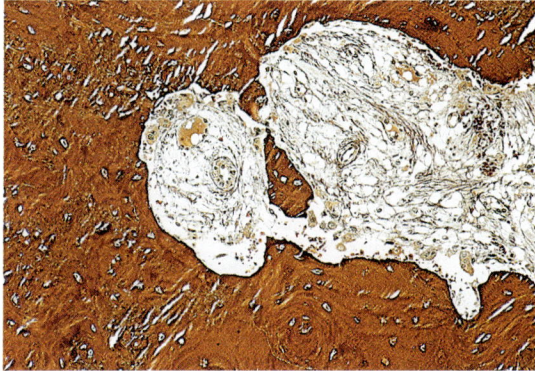

19.11 and 19.12 BMBS plastic, chronic fibrosis with inflammatory cells.
19.11 (left) Giemsa, note blood vessels, plasma cells and lymphocytes.

19.12 (right) Gomori, note thick and thin fibers, and osteoblastic and osteoclastic remodeling.

182

19.13 (left) As for Figure 19.12 seen in polarised light showing increase in fibers. Compare with Figure 19.9.

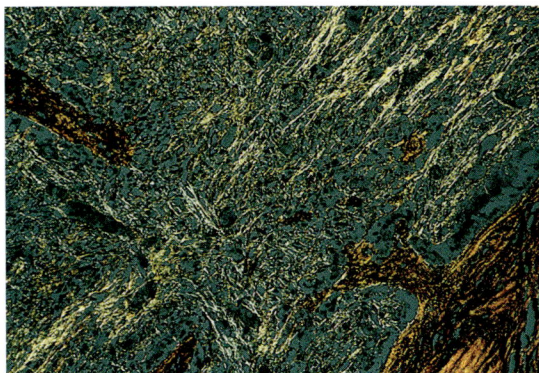

19.14 (right) BMBS plastic, Giemsa, fibrosis (as all previous examples) in absence of megakaryocytes.

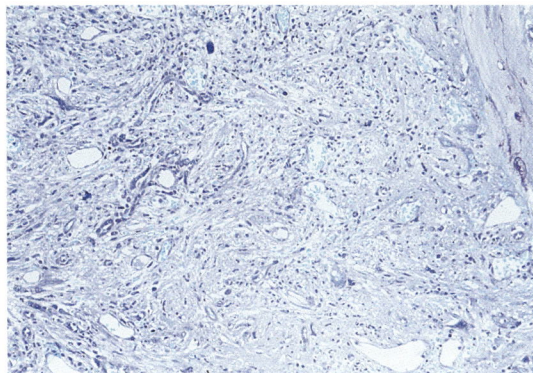

19.15 BMBS plastic, Giemsa, showing fibrotic bone marrow with reactive new bone formation.

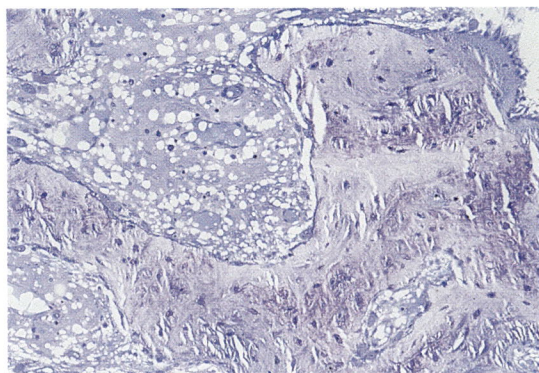

19.16–19.18 Leukemoid reactions and megakaryocytosis.

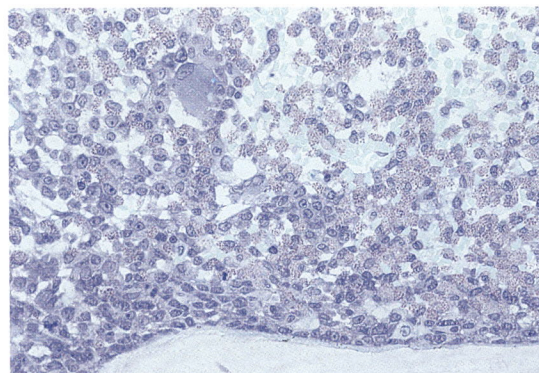

19.16 BMBS plastic, Giemsa, showing eosinophilic hyperplasia in patient with persistent eosinophilia of unclarified etiology.

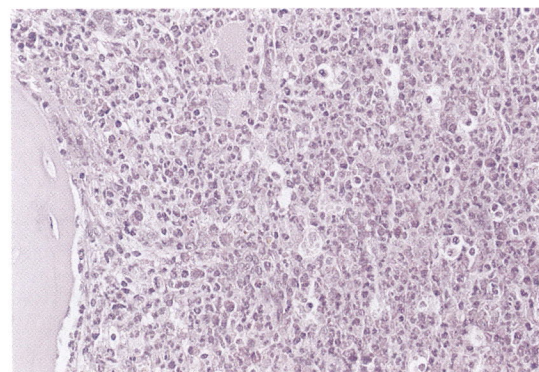

19.17 BMBS paraffin, H&E, mixed myeloid hyperplasia in a patient with persistent low grade fever, cause unknown.

may be involved to a greater or lesser degree (Figures 19.16–19.18).

5. Chronic inflammation, 'granulomatous type': characterised by the presence of giant cell granulomas or lipid granulomas, or epithelioid cell granulomas (with or without accumulation of lymphocytes) (Figures 19.19–19.24). Granuloma is applied to a special pattern of chronic inflammation, granulomas usually being nodular aggregates of inflammatory cells, consisting mainly of modified macrophages also called epithelioid cells, because of their shape. Coalescence or fusion of macrophages gives rise to the multinucleated giant (Langhan's) cells whose nuclei often form a ring at the periphery of the cell mass. The giant cells may reach 300 µm in diameter with numerous (>30) nuclei. The inclusion bodies (Schauman's, asteroid or residual bodies) in giant cells are the non-specific products of metabolism and secretion in various stages of breakdown. Other cells such as fibroblasts, plasma cells, lymphocytes and neutrophils may be found in and around a granuloma.

The types of reaction seen in groups 1–5 have already been dealt with above. With reference to granulomas, it should be stressed that they are not unusual in the bone marrow and may be found in hypocellular, normocellular or hypercellular marrow. Granuloma formation occurs in response to numerous agents including mycobacterium, fungi, toxoplasma, histoplasma, malignant lymphomas and multiple myeloma, Hodgkin's disease, regional ileitis, sarcoidosis, as a reaction to non-hematologic neoplasias in patients with primary

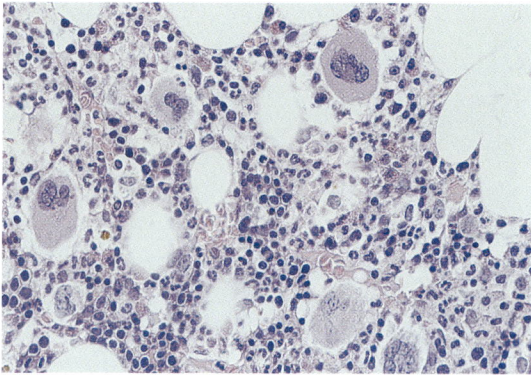

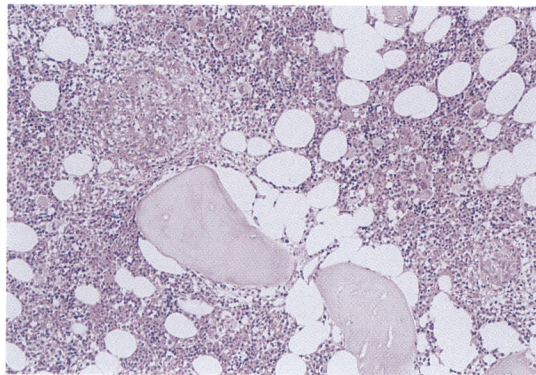

19.18 (left) BMBS paraffin, H&E, megakaryocytic hyperplasia, cause not clarified.

19.19–19.24 Granulomas in the bone marrow in cases of sarcoidosis.

19.19 (right) BMBS paraffin, H&E, low magnification showing paratrabecular granuloma, upper left, and smaller granuloma, lower right.

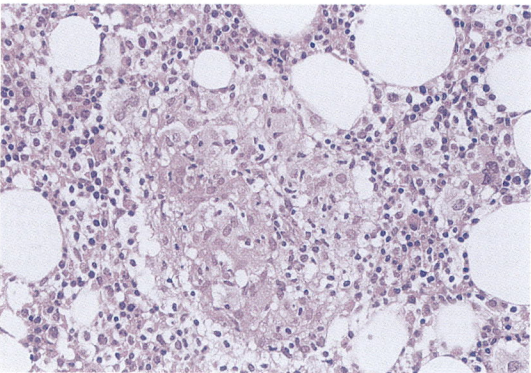

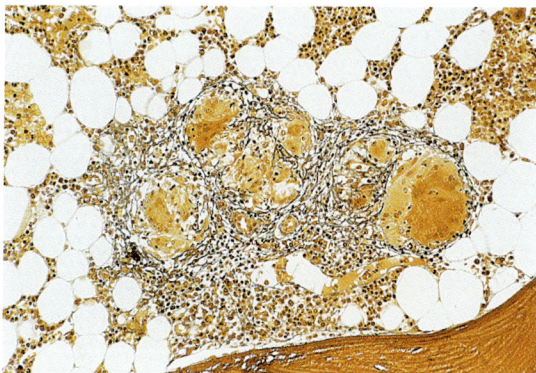

19.20 (left) Higher magnification of Figure 19.19 showing granuloma with mainly epithelioid cells and lymphocytes.

19.21 (right) BMBS plastic, Gomori, illustrating paratrabecular granuloma with epithelioid cells, giant cells, fibers, blood vessels and lymphocytes.

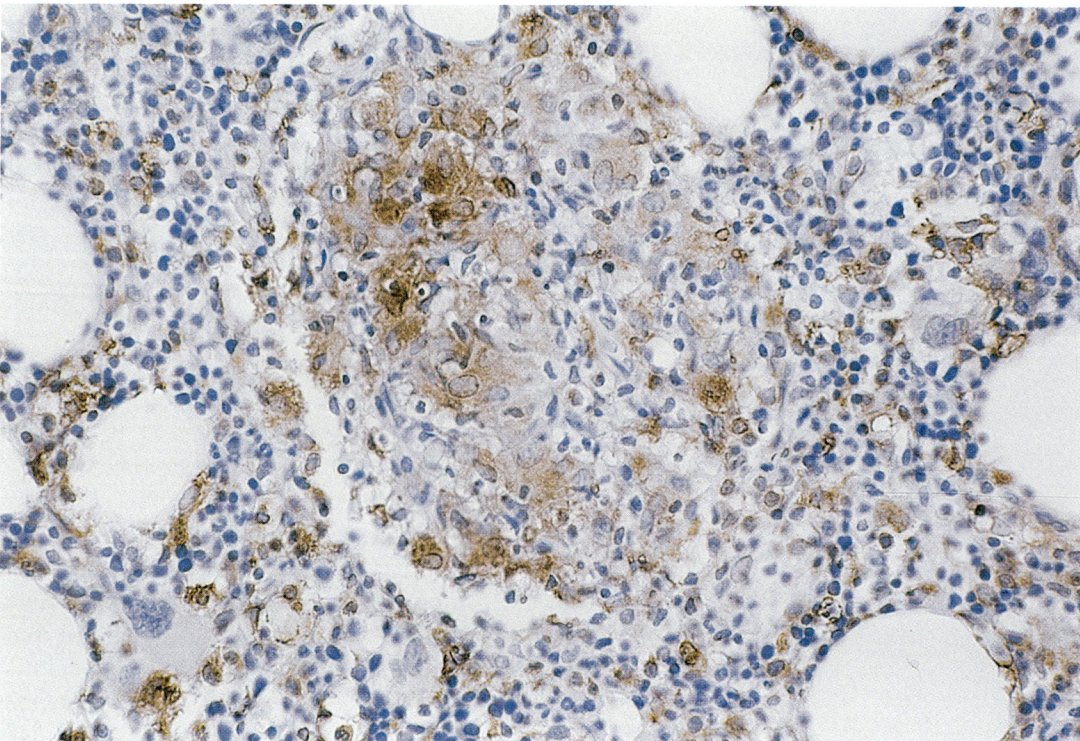

19.22 BMBS paraffin, I.H., CD68, note positive cells in and around the granuloma.

19.23 (left) As for Figure 19.22, I.H., CD68-positive in multinucleated giant cell in the marrow, as well as in many other cells.

19.24 (right) As for Figure 19.22, I.H., T-lymphocytes in stroma around a granuloma.

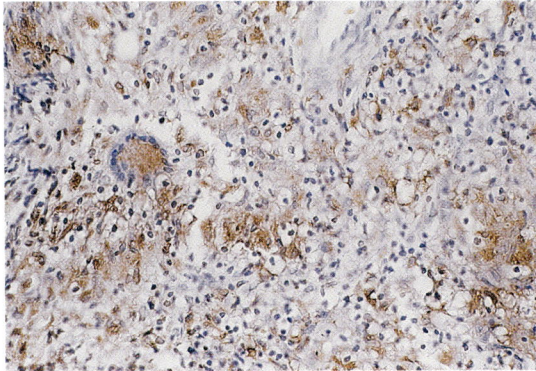
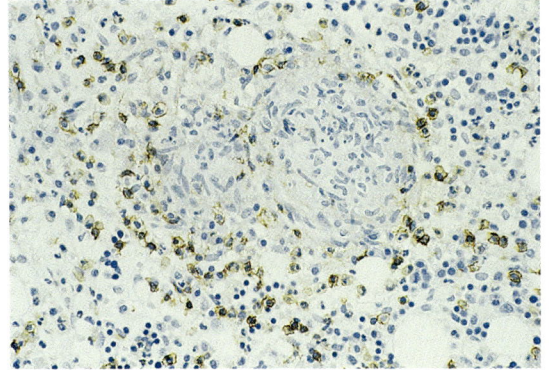

19.25–19.30 Granulomas in bone marrow in a patient with tuberculosis.

19.25 BMBS paraffin, H&E, large paratrabecular granuloma in lypocellular marrow.

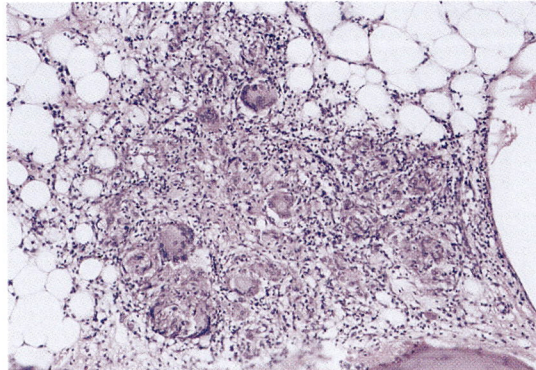

TABLE 19.1 Granulomas in bone marrow biopsies (*n* = 156)

Conditions	% of total
Unknown	22
Systemic mastocytosis	21
Hodgkin's disease	14
Malignant lymphomas	10
Tuberculosis	9
Sarcoidosis	8
Infections	5
Cancers	5
Collagen diseases	4
Polycythemia vera	2

19.26 BMBS paraffin, H&E, higher magnification of Figure 19.25: multinucleated giant cell, epithelioid cells and lymphocytes.

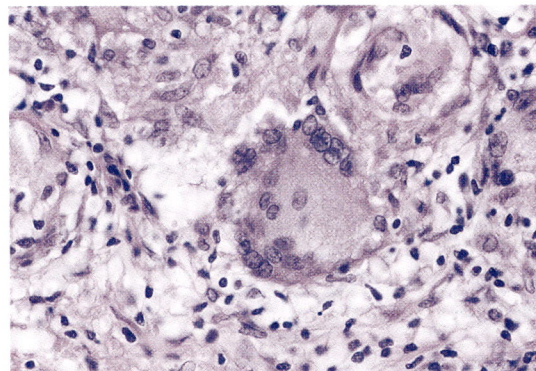

biliary cirrhosis, Q fever, infectious mononucleosis, immune disorders, as a reaction to drugs and in association with mitochondrial antibodies (Table 19.1). Granulomas come in various sizes and of variable composition: they may be large or small, inter- or paratrabecular, single or multiple, consist of isolated giant cells or giant cells and lymphocytes, plasma cells, histiocytes, epithelioid cells, eosinophils, mast cells and capillaries, fibroblasts, and fibers, in varying proportions. The description of granulomas in the bone marrow in tuberculosis serves as an example (Figures 19.25–19.30). Flow cytometry of the nucleated cells of the bone marrow aspirate from the same patient is shown in Figure 19.31.

Lipid granulomas

These consist of lipid-laden macrophages and there may be a small aggregate, or large accu-

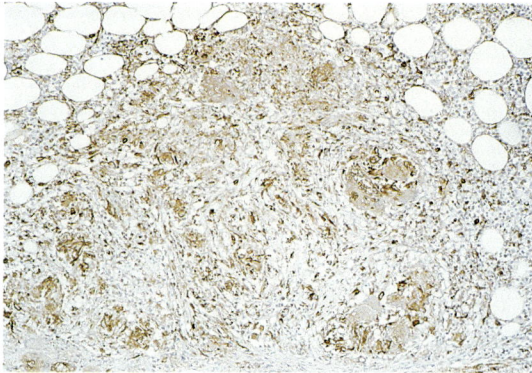

19.27 (left) BMBS paraffin, Vimentin, many cells in and around the granuloma are positive.

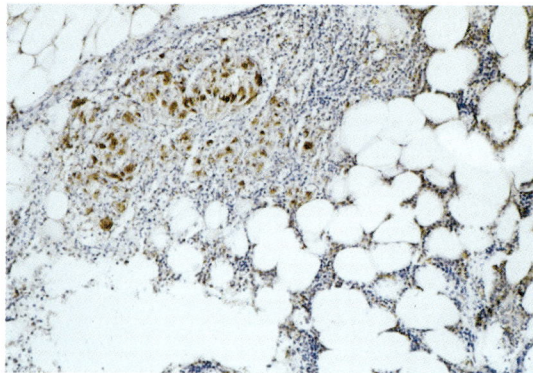

19.28 (right) BMBS, paraffin, CD68, the giant cells and monocytes are strongly positive.

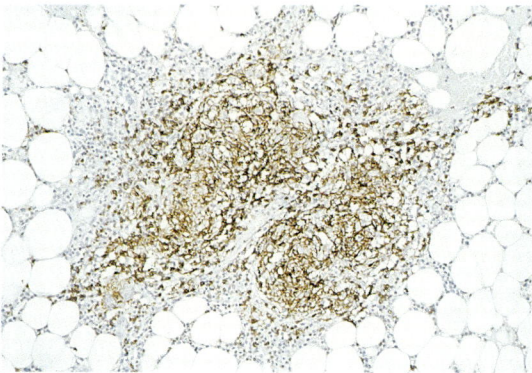

19.29 (left) BMBS, paraffin, T cells, most of the lymphocytes in the granuloma as well as some in the surrounding marrow are positive.

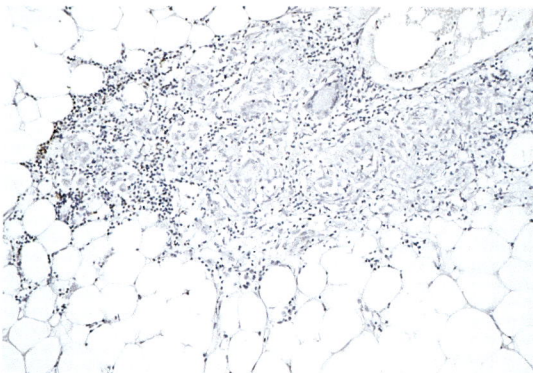

19.30 (right) BMBS, paraffin, B cells, only isolated cells show reactivity.

mulations. Lymphocytes, plasma cells and eosinophils, occasional giant cells, epithelioid cells and fibroblasts may be associated with lipid granulomas. These are usually an incidental finding in BMBs and are not of clinical significance.

Sarcoidosis

About 30% of patients with sarcoidosis have characteristic granulomas in their bone marrow biopsies. They are composed of epithelioid cells and giant cells surrounded by lymphocytes, together with fibers and amorphous eosinophilic material; rarely, Schauman or asteroid bodies are found. The giant cells may reach 300 μm in diameter and contain 30 or so nuclei; the cytoplasm contains inclusion bodies which are the non-specific end-products of the cells' activities. Necrosis is not usually observed, in contrast with granulomas in the bone marrow in tuberculosis

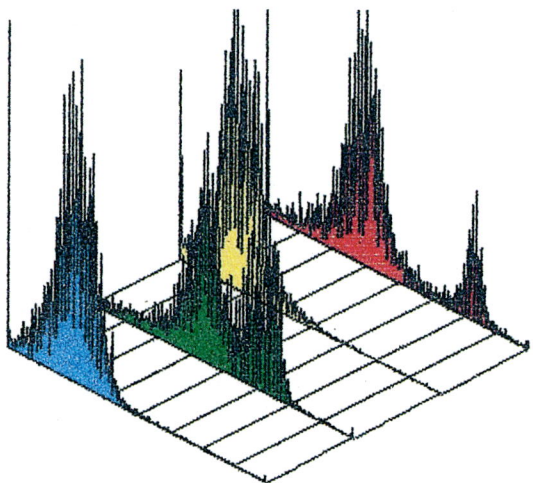

19.31 Histogram of flow cytometry of nucleated cells of bone marrow aspirate, from left: blue, control; green, T cells (CD2) 40%; yellow, B cells (CD20) 4%; red, monocytes (CD14) 19%.

which are otherwise similar to those in sarcoidosis. Increased osteoclastic bone resorption may cause hypercalcemia in sarcoidosis.

Osteomyelitis

This may result from hematogenous spread of organisms, which then settle in the bone marrow. The organisms may gain entrance from contamination of fractures, from surgical operations or from other more unobtrusive (or even completely unnoticed) bruises, cuts and inflammatory lesions. Sites most frequently involved are: long bones, vertebrae, skull, hand and foot, or any bone involved in a fracture. Diabetic patients with foot ulcers may be especially prone to osteomyelitis. The typical lesion in the bone marrow is necrosis (in acute cases) of both marrow and bone, accompanied by an intense reaction of polymorphonuclear leucocytes. This phase is sometimes called suppurative destructive necrosis. Subsequently, there is the phase of reactive reparative response, especially osteoblastic activity, which may eventually give rise to a dense sclerosis (Figures 19.12 and 19.13) (Garré's sclerosing osteomyelitis), due to fibrous and bony repair of the destructive lesions. Many agents and conditions may cause fibrosis in the bone marrow, (see chapter 23).

In summary, the reactive changes include granulocytic hyperplasia and left shift, megakaryocytic hyperplasia, reduction in erythropoiesis and increased plasma cells, lymphocytes, macrophages, and increased sinusoids and patchy fibrosis.

It should be remembered that the bone marrow as the source of reactive cells has the capacity to react promptly and strongly to stimuli; that many such reactions are transitory (as are the stimuli which evoke them) and are followed by complete regeneration and restoration of the normal aspect of the bone marrow. To give but one example: in anorexia nervosa the pancytopenia is due to hypoplasia and exudative myelitis, serous or gelatinous atrophy which are completely reversible on resumption of normal nutrition. However, other cases of exudative myelitis, morphologically similar but due to different causes, may terminate in myelofibrosis or even complete aplasia if repair of the damaged stroma is not effected. Though few data are available, it appears that the nature of the etiologic agent and possibly its persistence, influence the eventual outcome.

Recent developments in inflammatory reactions

In the field of inflammations and inflammatory reactions, molecular techniques have also revolutionised understanding of cell and tissue function especially with respect to intercellular communication by cytokines (messenger molecules); moreover, identification of molecules which regulate cell adhesion (CAMs), motility as well as proliferation (growth) survival and death (apoptosis), is leading to their utilisation as therapeutic agents, as well as more effective vaccines. Their application in immunohistology is already contributing to more comprehensive interpretation in histopathology, e.g. CAMs in multiple myeloma and passage of leucocytes through endothelium, and cytokines in inflammatory conditions and autoimmune diseases, many of which affect the bone marrow. Cytokines, produced by leucocytes and fibroblasts and many other cells, are protein messengers that mediate immune and inflammatory responses. They bind to receptors on target cells, and may stimulate release of other cytokines. The type of inflammatory response is a function of the balance between pro- and anti-inflammatory cytokines. Cytokines participate in regulation of cell proliferation, cell death and cell killing.

Gelatinous transformation or serous atrophy

When this occurs small or large areas of the bone marrow are replaced by an acellular, amorphic gelatinous substance. As mentioned above, this may occur in anorexia nervosa or any other condition associated with poor nutrition, cachexia due to debilitating disease, chronic loss as in coeliac disease, in various infections including AIDS, hypothyroidism and toxic bone marrow damage.

Bone marrow necrosis

This may be found in the acute phase after thrombosis of a vessel, as ischemic necrosis of bone in systemic lupus, in infections such as bacterial endocarditis, Q fever, streptococcal infections, other severe toxic and inflammatory states, rapidly growing leukemias and lymphomas, and in the vicinity of expanding metastases. Necrosis in the bone marrow has also been observed in sickle cell disease: obstruction of vessels leads to ischemia and necrosis of hematopoietic tissue. Fat embolism has also been implicated. When extensive, bone marrow necrosis causes bone pain (see Chapter 13).

Blood vessels in cytopenias

Marrow atrophy (hypoplasia, fatty atrophy, replacement of the hematopoietic tissue by fat cells) may occur whenever pathologic alterations affect the blood vessels, such as in arteriosclerosis, thrombosis and vasculitis. Such changes may also be found in diabetes accompanied by hypoplasia and osteopenia in the affected areas (Figure 19.32). Giant cell arteritis has also been detected by bone biopsy.

Amyloidosis – interstitial and vascular

Amyloid, a fibrillar material, is deposited extracellularly and is found first in the walls of the small blood vessels. Four main types of amyloid fibril protein have been recognised:

1. AL: immunoglobulin light chains.
2. AA: acute phase reactant serum amyloid H.
3. AF: pre-albumin (hereditary-familial amyloidosis)
4. β_2M: beta-2 microglobulin, hemodialysis-associated amyloidosis.

The second is the classic type of secondary amyloidosis that may develop in some chronic inflammatory diseases and in cancers. The first occurs in about 15% of patients with multiple myeloma or other plasma cell dyscrasia, as well as in some cases of so-called primary amyloidosis in which no predisposing cause is found. There are also rare forms of genetically determined amyloidosis. Systemic AA-type amyloidosis with renal involvement is a major complication of familial Mediterranean fever (FMF), and there is a high rate of involvement (80%) in the bone marrow.

Vascular amyloidosis has been described in the bone marrow in many and various conditions, mostly chronic, and though interstitial amyloidosis also occurs in the bone marrow, it is rare (Figures 19.33–19.39). Amyloid is readily observed in Giemsa-stained sections, though other stains such as Congo red are often applied for confirmation. It appears as a homogeneous blue deposit, usually localised in the arterial walls. Extensive studies have shown that amyloid fibrils are formed by proteolysis of delta chains at acid pH. Light chains are not processed by monocytes. Deposits of amyloid in the walls of blood vessels are as readily

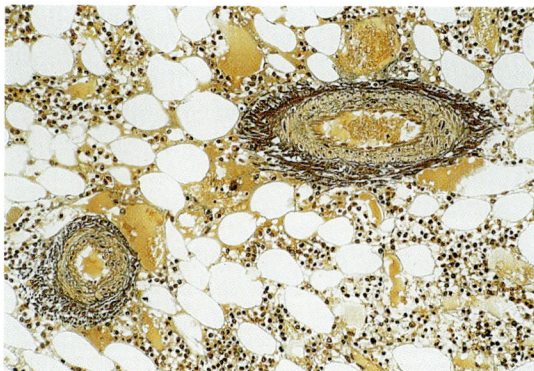

19.32 BMBS plastic, Gomori, sclerosis of vessel walls in long-standing diabetes mellitus.

19.33–19.38 Aspects of amyloidosis.

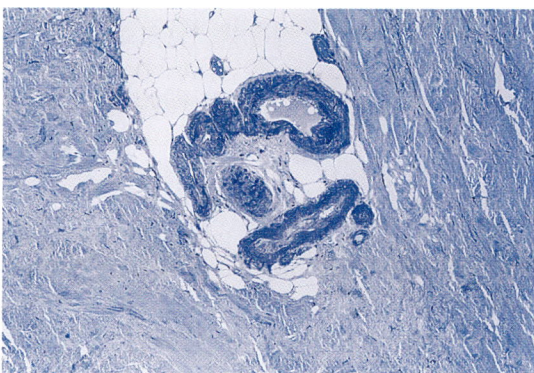

19.33 BMBS plastic, Giemsa, blood vessels in periosteum with deposition of amorphous material in their walls.

19.34 (left) As for Figure 19.33, PAS stain.

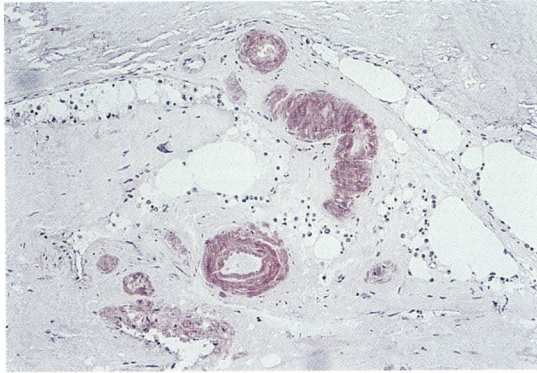

19.35 (right) As for Figure 19.33, Congo red stain in polarised area, left.

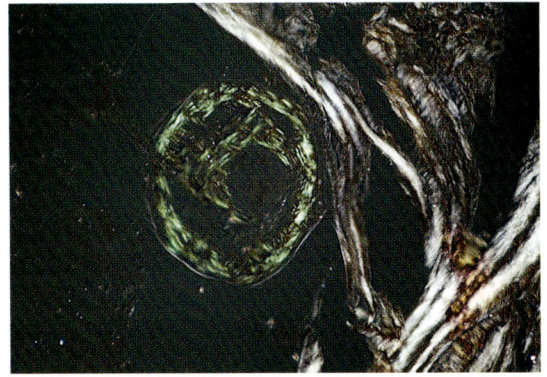

19.36 (left) BMBS plastic, Giemsa, blood vessel wall with amyloid in the bone marrow.

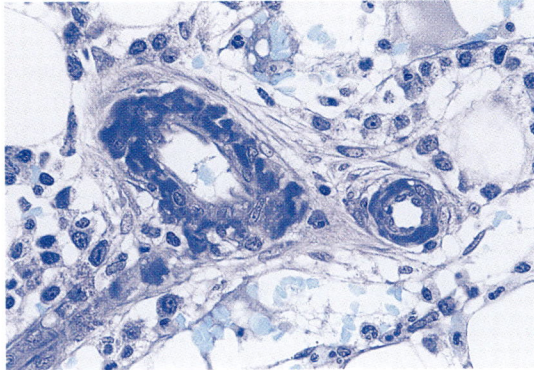

19.37 (right) BMBS paraffin, Congo red stain, showing interstitial deposition of amorphous, pink-stained material.

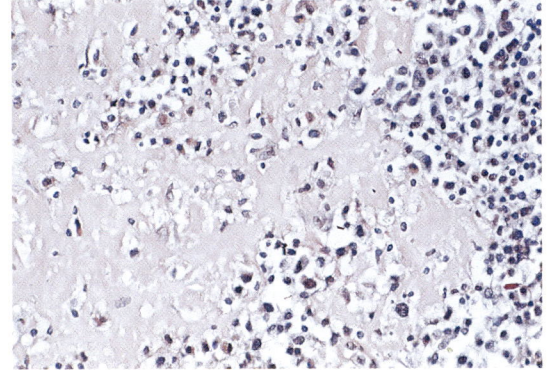

19.38 (left) As for Figure 19.37, interstitial material stained with methyl violet.

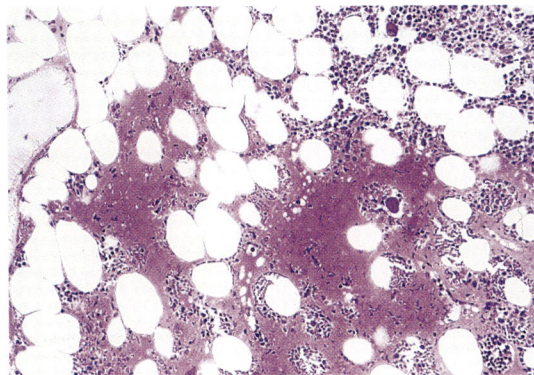

19.39 (right) BMBS plastic, Giemsa, interstitial material stained dark blue showing fluorescence in polarised light after staining with Congo red.

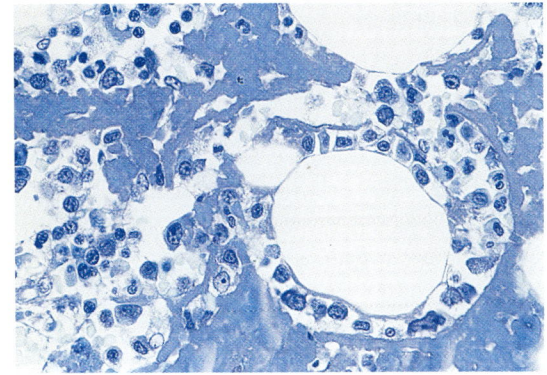

detected in the bone marrow of patients with vascular amyloidosis, as in biopsies of the rectal mucosa (Table 19.2). Interstitial amyloidosis, on the other hand, is infrequent in the bone marrow. Both have deleterious effects on hematopoiesis and the stroma, and lead to hypoplasia and osteopenia.

In summary, amyloidosis may be associated with a variety of conditions, from multiple myeloma and other lymphoproliferative disorders to long-standing infections, rheumatic disorders, cancers, congenital and familial conditions, and with aging, as in Alzheimer's disease.

TABLE 19.2 Frequency of organ involvement by amyloidosis according to results of biopsies. Note high rate of involvement in iliac crest biopsies (85 patients investigated in our series)

Biopsy	Frequency (%)
Kidney	87–100
Liver	50–96
Spleen	100
Rectum	64–96
Bone	*78*
Muscle	75–80
Gingiva	27–100
Subcutaneous fat	42–75
Skin	77–87

Check list: Stromal Reactions and Inflammations in Bone Marrow

- Adequate biopsy to rule out underlying conditions.
- Stains to rule out infectious organisms.
- Reduction in hematopoiesis – which lines are affected?
- Increase in fibers: reticulin and collagenous? Stains for both required.
- Inflammatory reactions, type: acute or chronic, hyperplastic or atrophic, granulomas or infiltrating? Immunohistology (I.H.): LCA, kappa, lambda, CD68, PAS.
- Trabecular bone structure – osteopenia, osteosclerosis?

- Gelatinous or serous atrophy of marrow?
- Necrosis of marrow?
- State of blood vessels? (Factor VIII-related antigen, actin, CD34 on I.H.)
- Amyloidosis: interstitial or vascular? Giemsa, methyl-violet, Congo red.
- Check also periosteal blood vessels for amyloidosis.

Clinical correlations

Osteomyelitis and granulomas

- Three pathways of infection: hematogenous; entry by surgical or other trauma; spread from contiguous site.
- Usual organisms are bacteria; can be virus including AIDS.
- Initially fever, chills, malaise, pain.
- Overlying tissue red, warm, swollen.
- Lytic lesion on X-ray after 30–50% of bone destroyed.
- Sarcoidosis and tuberculosis: may cause hypercalcemia.
- Other organisms, e.g. Leishmaniasis, may evoke bone marrow granulomas without giant cells: fever, splenomegaly, cytopenias.

Amyloidosis

- Nephrotic syndrome, congestive heart failure.
- Fatigue, dyspnea.
- Neuropathy: syncope.
- Weight loss.
- Men : women = 2 : 1; median age 73 years.

Bibliography

Akbar A.N., Salmon M. (1997) Cellular environments and apoptosis: tissue microenvironments control activated T-cell death. *Immunol Today*, **18**, 72–6.

Alexandre C., Chappard D., Vergnon J.M. *et al.* (1987) The bone in non-corticoid-treated sarcoidosis. A histomorphometric study. *Rev. Rhum. Mal. Osteoartic.*, **54** (2), 159–62.

Apperley J.F., Dowding C., Hibbin J. *et al.* (1989) The effect of cytomegalovirus on hemopoiesis: in vitro evidence for selective infection of marrow stromal cells. *Exp. Hematol.*, **17** (1), 38–45.

Axelsson U., Hallen A., Rausig A. (1970) Amyloidosis of bone. Report of 2 cases. *J Bone Joint Surg.*, **528**, 717.

Baurmann H., Schwarz T.F., Oertel J. *et al.* (1992) Acute parvovirus B19 infection mimicking myelodysplastic syndrome of the bone marrow. *Ann. Hematol.*, **64 (1)**, 43–5.

Bhargava B.A., Farhl D.C. (1988) Bone marrow granulomas: clinicopathologic findings in 72 cases and review of the literature. *Hematol Pathol.*, **2**, 43.

Bodem C.R., Hamory B.H., Taylor H.M., Kleopfer L. (1983) Granulomatous bone marrow disease. A review of the literature and clinicopathologic analysis of 58 cases. *Medicine*, **62 (6)**, 372.

Boll K.L., Jurik A.G. (1990) Sternal osteomyelitis in drug addicts. *J Bone Joint Surg.*, **72B**, 328.

Brouland J.P., Audouin J., Hofman P. *et al.* (1996) Bone marrow involvement by disseminated toxoplasmosis in acquired immunodeficiency syndrome: the value of bone marrow trephine biopsy and immunohistochemistry for the diagnosis. *Hum Pathol*, **27 (3)**, 302–6.

Casey T.T., Stome W.J., DiRaimondo C.R. *et al.* (1986) Tumoral amyloidosis of bone of beta-2-microglobulin origin in association with long-term hemodialysis: a new type of amyloid disease. *Hum Pathol.*, **17**, 731.

Ciaudo M., Doco-Lecompte T., Guettier C. *et al.* (1994) Revisited indications for bone marrow examinations in HIV-infected patients. *Eur J Haematol*, **53 (3)**, 168–74.

Cohen A.S. (1985) Amyloidosis. In McCarthy (ed), *Arthritis and Allied Conditions: A Textbook of Rheumatology*, vol. 10. Philadelphia: Lea & Febiger, p. 1109.

Demiroglu H., Ozcebe Ol., Ozdemir L. *et al.* (1994) Pancytopenia with hypocellular bone marrow due to miliary tuberculosis: an unusual presentation. *Acta Haematol*, **91 (1)**, 49–51.

Dittel B.N., LeBien T.W. (1995) Reduced expression of vascular cell adhesion molecule-1 on bone marrow stromal cells isolated from marrow transplant recipients correlates with a reduced capacity to support human B lymphopoiesis in vitro. *Blood*, **86 (7)**, 2833–41.

Eid A., Carion W., Nystrom J.S. (1996) Differential diagnoses of bone marrow granuloma. *West J Med*, **164 (6)**, 510–15.

Elema J.D., Atmosoerodjo-Briggs J.E. (1984) Langerhans' cells and macrophages in eosinophilic granuloma: an enzyme-histochemical, enzyme-cytochemical, and ultrastructural study. *Cancer*, **54**, 2174.

Epps C.H., Bryant D.D., Coles M.J.M., Castro O. (1991) Osteomyelitis in patients who have sickle-cell disease. *J Bone Joint Surg.*, **73A**, 1281.

Fiala M., Colodro I., Talbert W. *et al.* (1987) Bone marrow granulomas in mononucleosis. *Postgrad. Med. J.*, **63 (738)**, 277–9.

Frisch B., Bartl R. (1990) *Atlas of Bone Marrow Pathology.* Dordrecht: Kluwer Academic.

Frisch B., Bartl R., Goebel F.D. (1989) Bone marrow manifestations in the acquired immune deficiency syndrome (AIDS) A study of 40 patients and review of the literature. *Hematol Rev.*, **3**, 177.

Frisch B., Lewis S.M., Burkhardt R., Bartl R. (1985) *Biopsy Pathology of Bone and Marrow.* London: Chapman & Hall.

Gahr M., Jendrossek V., Peters A.M. *et al.* (1991) Sea blue histiocytes in the bone marrow of variant chronic granulomatous disease with residual monocyte NADPH-oxidase activity. *Br. J. Hematol.*, **78 (2)**, 278–80.

Gardner H. (1961) Bone lesions in primary systemic amyloidosis. A report of a case. *Br J Radiol.*, **34**, 778.

Gillespie W.J., Allardyce R.A. (1990) Mechanisms of bone degradation in infections: a review of current hypothesis. *Orthop.*, **13**, 407.

Gimble, J.M. (1990) The function of adipocytes in the bone marrow stroma. *New Biol.*, **2 (4)**, 304–12.

Ifrah N., Saint-Andre J.P., de Gentile L. *et al.* (1989) Gelatinous transformation of the bone marrow: manifestation of an acute leukemia? *Acta. Hematol.*, **82 (3)**, 165–8.

Ishihara T., Takahashi M., Koga M. *et al.* (1991) Amyloid fibril formation in the rough endoplasmic reticulum of plasma cells from a patient with localized A lambda amyloidosis. *Lab. Invest.*, **64 (2)**, 265–71.

Karcher D.S. (1993) Clinically unsuspected Hodgkin disease presenting initially in the bone marrow of patients infected with the human immunodeficiency virus. *Cancer*, **71 (4)**, 1235–8.

Krause J.R. (1977) Value of bone marrow biopsy in the diagnosis of amyloidosis. *South Med J.*, **70**, 1072.

Kyle R.A., Bayrd E.D. (1975) Amyloidosis: review of 236 cases. *Medicine*, **54**, 271.

Levy T.M., Blundell E., Slade R. *et al.* (1993) Diagnosis of sarcoidosis by bone marrow trephine biopsy. *Br J Haematol*, **84 (1)**, 179–81.

Mollnes T.E., Harboe M. (1996) Clinical immunology. *BMJ*, **312**, 1465–9.

Montemurro L., Fraioli P., Rizzato G. (1991) Bone loss in untreated longstanding sarcoidosis. *Sarcoidosis*, **8**, 29.

Muller-Hermelink H.K., Baumann I. (1990) Function and pathology of bone marrow stromal cells. *Verh. Dtsch. Ges. Pathol.*, **74**, 93–105.

Mundy G.R. (1991) Inflammatory mediators and the destruction of bone. *J Peridont Res.*, **26**, 213.

Pepys M.B. (1987) Amyloidosis. In Weatherall, Ledingham and Warrell (eds),

Oxford Textbook of Medicine. Oxford: Oxford University Press, pp. 9–145.

Piazza I., Giunta G. (1991) Lytic bone lesions and polyarthritis associated with acne fulminans. *Br J Rheumat.*, **30**, 387.

Reddehase M.J., Dreher-Stumpp L., Angele P. *et al.* (1992) Hematopoietic stem cell deficiency resulting from cytomegalovirus infection of bone marrow stroma. *Ann. Hematol.*, **64 (Suppl. P)**, A125–7.

Rees R.C. (1992) Cytokines as biological response modifiers. *J Clin Pathol.*, **45**, 93.

Riley U.B., Crawford S., Barrett S.P., Abdalla S.H. (1995) Detection of mycobacteria in bone marrow biopsy specimens taken to investigate pyrexia of unknown origin. *J Clin Pathol*, **48 (8)**, 706–9.

Rodriguez J.N., Dieguez J.C., Moreno M.V. *et al.* (1996) Usefulness of bone marrow examination in patients with advance HIV infection. *Rev Clin Esp*, **196 (4)**, 213–6.

Savill J. (1997) Role of molecular cell biology in understanding disease. *BMJ*, **314**, 203–8.

Sponseller P.D., Malech H.L., McCarthy E.F. *et al.* (1991) Skeletal involvement in children who have chronic granulomatous disease. *J Bone Joint Surg.*, **73A**, 37.

Subbarao K., Jacobson H.G. (1986) Amyloidosis and plasma cell dyscrasias of the musculoskeletal system. *Semin Roentgenol.*, **21**, 139.

Sungur C., Sungur A., Ruacan S. *et al.* (1993) Diagnostic value of bone marrow biopsy in patients with renal disease secondary to familial Mediterranean fever. *Kidney Int*, **44 (4)**, 834–6.

Tavassoli M. (1987) Structural alterations of marrow during inflammation. *Blood-cells*, **13 (1–2)**, 251–61.

Turner G.E., Reid M.M. (1993) What is marrow fibrosis after treatment of neuroblastoma? *J Clin Pathol*, **46 (1)**, 61–3.

Wiley E.L., Perry A., Nightingale S.D., Lawrence J. (1994) Detection of Mycobacterium avium-intracellulare complex in bone marrow specimens of patients with acquired immunodeficiency syndrome. *Am J Clin Pathol*, **101 (4)**, 446–51.

Working Party of the British Committee for Standards in Haematology, Clinical Haematology Task Force (1996) Guidelines for the prevention and treatment of infection in patients with an absent or dysfunctional spleen. *BMJ*, **312**, 430–4.

Wu S.S., Brady K., Anderson J.J. *et al.* (1991) The predictive value of bone marrow morphologic characteristics and immunostaining in primary (AL) amyloidosis. *Am J Clin. Pathol.*, **96 (1)**, 95–9

20 Myelodysplastic syndromes (MDS)

Synonyms, definition and occurrence

Some of the designations previously applied to what are now known as the MDS include: preleukemia, hematopoietic or dysmyelopoietic, or dyshematopoietic disorders, smoldering leukemia, refractory anemia and others.

General aspects and pathogenesis

MDS refers to a heterogeneous group of disorders having in common progressive (often fatal) cytopenia(s) together with ineffective hematopoiesis in the bone marrow. The MDS are stem cell disorders, though they are considered to be preleukemic conditions. They include the idiopathic acquired (primary) syndromes and secondary conditions. Most patients have anemia with or without another cytopenia. In both types of MDS there are alterations in proliferation, development and structure of both hematopoietic and stromal elements in the bone marrow. Recent evidence suggests that the MDS result from neoplastic transformation at the level of a pluripotent stem cell, which is capable of differentiation for variable periods. But the inherent defect results in some degree of morphological (that is, dysplasia) and functional abnormality in erythroid, granulocytic or megakaryocytic cell lines, generally in all three. However, it is thought that initially normal hematopoiesis coexists with the abnormal clone. Eventually the ability to differentiate is lost, normal hematopoiesis is suppressed and acute leukemia ensues. Frequently, however, the patient may succumb to other intercurrent diseases which may be directly related to the MDS, such as infections or bleeding, or may be unrelated, such as renal or intestinal or cardiac disorders.

Primary MDS

The primary MDS (i.e. the idiopathic-acquired MDS) represent early phases of stem cell aberrations that may precede acute or chronic myeloproliferative disorders, while the secondary MDS constitute the hematopoietic consequences of exogenous agents. Recommendations for a morphological, immunological and cytogenetic working classification of the primary and therapy-related myelodysplastic disorders have recently been published, as well as the diagnostic problems that frequently arise (see Bibliography).

The MDS occur mainly in people >50–60 years of age, but have also been observed in children, though rarely. It should be stated that dysplasia in the bone marrow, myelodysplasia, is not synonymous with MDS. Hematopoietic dysplasia (myelodysplasia) may occur in many conditions due to many different causes, and these are quite distinct from MDS (Table 20.1). For example, myelodysplasia may occur in malignancies (solid tumors), infections, rheumatic and other autoimmune disorders, endocrine and after certain drugs (see below); as well as in the residual hematopoiesis between areas of involvement in lymphoproliferative disorders and Hodgkin's disease, for example.

TABLE 20.1 Myelodysplastic syndromes: differential diagnosis of bone marrow histology

Pernicious anemia	Cytotoxic dysplasias
Malignancies elsewhere	Other acquired hypoplasias
Congenital hypoplasias	Leukemoid reactions
Rheumatic conditions	Malignant lymphomas
Other chronic disorders	Hodgkin's disease
Hemolytic conditions	Myeloproliferative disorders

MDS in children

This chapter deals mainly with MDS in adults, though it has recently been suggested that the same criteria could be applied to children. MDS is rare in childhood – one population-based study reported an incidence of 4 per million children. Moreover, it has been suggested that about one-third of the children who develop MDS have a genetic disorder that predisposes them to it, such as constitutional chromosomal disorders, immune deficiency syndromes, and DNA deficiency repair syndromes. In most cases the FAB (French American British) criteria are applied to blood and bone marrow aspirate smears.

The differential diagnosis in children comprises a fairly extensive list of heterogeneous conditions including genetic (CDAs), deficiency states (vitamins or iron), viral, leukemias (CMPDs) and toxic drug reactions. The diagnosis requires morphologic, enzymic, phenotypic, cytogenetic, molecular and possibly cell culture analyses. The difficulties inherent in the diagnosis of pre-leukemic disorders in children have recently been outlined in a comprehensive study (see Bibliography).

FAB classification of MDS

The FAB cooperative study group classified the MDS into five subtypes, which have prognostic significance (Table 20.2). One of the main criteria for these subdivisions was the percentage of blasts in the peripheral blood and in smears of the bone marrow aspirates. The FAB subtypes of the MDS are: refractory anemia (RA), acquired idiopathic sideroblastic anemia (AISA) or refractory anemia with ringed sideroblasts (RARS), refractory anemia with excess of blasts (RAEB), refractory anemia with excess of blasts in transformation (RAEBT) and chronic myelomonocytic leukemia (CMML). To these five subtypes three have been added: CMML in transformation (CMMLt), unclassifiable (MDS-U) and MDS with fibrosis, possibly a variant of MDS or MPD.

Dysplastic features of the three cell lines in the bone marrow may be summarised as follows:

Erythroid series
Multinuclearity, abnormal nuclear shape and decreased nuclear density, cytoplasmic abnormalities and ringed sideroblasts.

Granulocytic series
Changes of nuclear shapes, ring-shaped nuclei, clumped chromatin and larger, often fewer, granules.

Megakaryocytic series
Micromegakaryocytes, large mononuclear megakaryocytes, and cells with multiple small, often peripheral, nuclei.

TABLE 20.2 Myelodysplastic syndromes: cytologic classification

FAB	Subtypes: Bone Marrow Histology
RA Refractory anemia	Mainly erythroid series: dyserythropoiesis with megaloblastoid/tic features and some sideroblasts. Hypercellular marrow with erythroid hyperplasia
RARS Refractory anemia with ringed sideroblasts	Hypercellular marrow with erythroid hyperplasia >15% ringed sideroblasts and increase in iron stores. The other cell lines may also show dysplastic features.
RAEB Refractory anemia with excess of blasts	In most cases, hypercellular bone marrow, the rest normo- or hypocellular, myeloid hyperplasia, left shift and ALIP, atypical megakaryocytes and mild dyserythropoiesis present, possibly some increase in reticular fibers.
RAEBt Refractory anemia with excess of blasts in transformation	Hypercellular marrow with immature precursors and a uniform or focal distribution of blasts. Variable numbers of atypical megakaryocytes and some degree of fibrosis, erythropoiesis reduced (possibly with Auer rods).
CMML Chronic myelomonocytic leukemia	As in RAEB with in addition more monocytes, ALIP more pronounced, fibrosis and dysplastic megakaryocytes.
CMMLt Chronic myelomonocytic leukemia in transformation	As for CMML but more blasts present (possibly with Auer rods).
MDS unclassifiable	Hypercellular bone marrow with panhyperplasia and dysplasia of myeloid, erythroid and megakaryocytic cell lines, left shift with >5% blasts
MDS with fibrosis	Difficult to classify, may be variant of MDS or of MPD

There are many other features, more readily observed in aspirate smears.

The boundaries between these subtypes of MDS are not sharp; there is considerable overlap between them, and many unanswered questions remain concerning the biological and pathological relationships between the groups. Moreover, there is some overlap between MDS, aplastic anemia, some forms of acute leukemia and other myeloproliferative disorders, so that diagnosis, classification and decisions concerning therapy can be very difficult (see below). One of the drawbacks of the FAB classification, since it is based on peripheral blood and bone marrow aspirates, is that it cannot take into account the stromal changes which may alter the microenvironment required for normal hematopoiesis, particularly the cell–matrix interactions and the adhesion molecules involved in them. In addition, the proportion of the different cell lines morphologically affected or increased is reflected more accurately in bone biopsy sections than in smears of aspirates, especially when there is an increase in reticular fibers, which may prevent aspiration of cells from the marrow. Moreover, because of the ineffective hematopoiesis, there may not be a good correlation between the precursors in the bone marrow and their products in the peripheral blood. One important example is provided by megakaryocytes in sideroblastic anemia: there is frequently no correlation between the platelet count in peripheral blood and the number of megakaryocytes in the bone marrow. In addition, a recent study of 121 patients with refractory anemia showed no correlation between the FAB subgroups and cytogenetic findings. Therefore, one must recognise the importance of correlating the histopathological and immunohistological information with all the other clinical and laboratory results.

Marrow architecture and cellularity

From the point of view of bone marrow histology, one must take into account the histopathological definition of dysplasia: 'dysplasia comprises a loss in the regularity of the individual cells as well as a loss in their architectural orientation.' Thus myelodysplasia (i.e. dysplasia in the bone marrow) is characterised by alterations in the growth, maturation, organisation and structure of the hematopoietic tissue including the stromal compartment. Marrow cellularity is more reliably assessed in sections than in aspirate smears. The bone marrow may be hypercellular (the majority), normocellular or hypocellular (Figures 20.1 and 20.2). Some bone marrow sections may present alternating fatty and cellular areas. The paradox of a hypercellular bone marrow and a peripheral cytopenia has been, at least partially, explained by investigation of apoptosis or programmed cell death (PCD) in MDS. It has been demonstrated that the high proliferative rate is cancelled out by an equally or greater rate of PCD. Even marrow cells in S phase as well as stromal cells were undergoing PCD. Consequently the cytopenias are due to ineffective hematopoiesis as the majority of the cells produced do not reach the blood stream. One of the most important histological parameters in MDS is the architectural disorganisation: myeloid precursors (clusters of three to five or more myeloblasts and promyelocytes) in the central intertrabecular areas (abnormal localisation of immature precursors, or ALIP), erythrons and megakaryocytes at the trabecular surface (Figures 20.3–20.11). In addition,

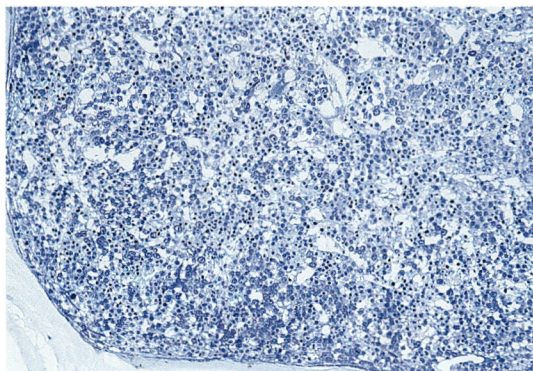

20.1 BMBS plastic, Giemsa, showing hypercellular bone marrow with replacement of fat cells. MDS, refractory anemia, with hyperplastic erythropoiesis, megaloblastoid.

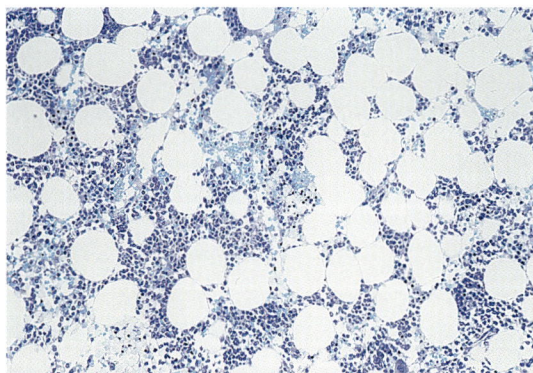

20.2 BMBS plastic, Giemsa, hypocellular bone marrow, fat cells increased; note preponderance of immature cells.

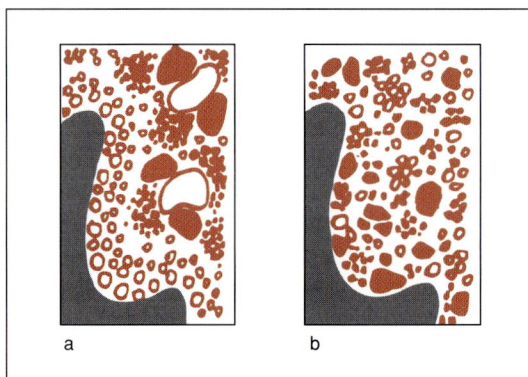

20.3 Representation of architectural disorganisation in MDS: (a) normal architecture of the bone marrow, with granulopoietic precursors at endosteal surface, erythrons and megakaryocytes around the central sinusoids. (b) In MDS there is topographic disorganisation, with precursors of the three cell lines found in all marrow regions. There is no stromal organisation.

20.4 (left) BMBS paraffin, H&E showing cellular marrow in MDS.

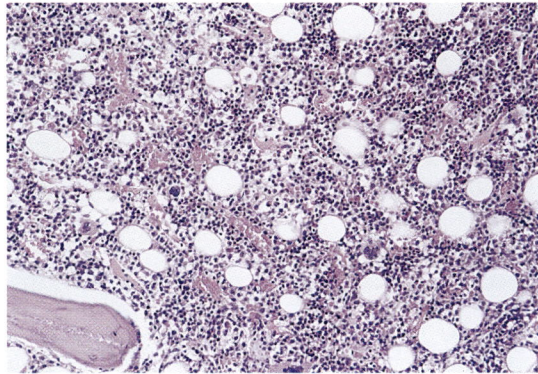

20.5 (right) As for Figure 20.4, I.H., low power myeloid antigen.

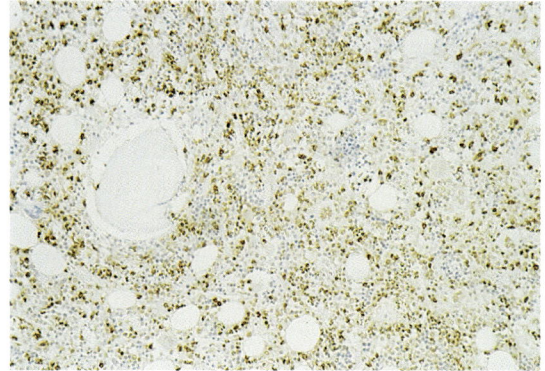

20.6 (left) As for Figure 20.5, higher magnification, myeloperoxidase showing myeloid precursors scattered throughout the marrow.

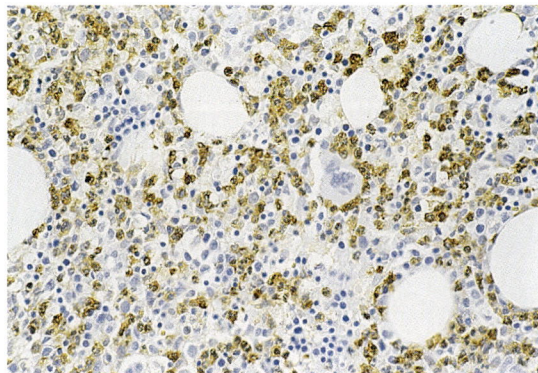

20.7 (right) As for Figure 20.6, I.H., CD68 to identify the monocytic population.

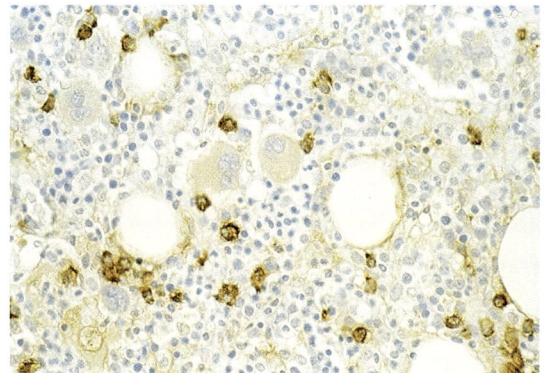

20.8 As for Figure 20.6, I.H., Factor VIII-related antigen variably sized megakaryocytes are stained.

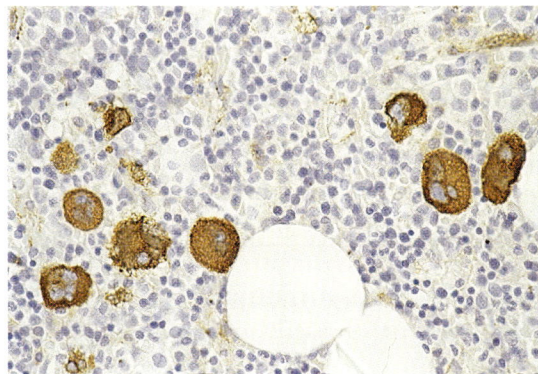

20.9–11 Examples of disorganisation of the bone marrow architecture in MDS.

20.9 BMBS plastic, Giemsa, showing erythroid island, left, and myeloid precursors, right, near trabecula, bottom.

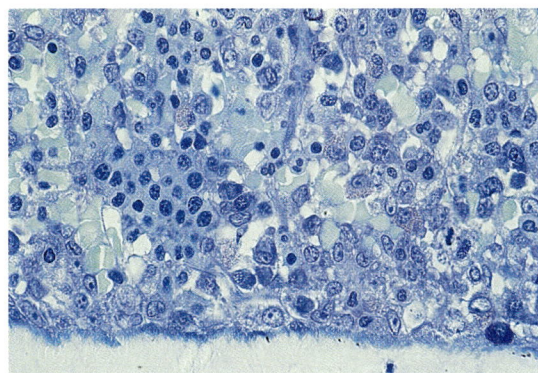

biopsy sections are required for recognition of alterations in the stromal compartment, i.e. of the microenviroment (often more prominent in hypocellular bone marrow): areas of edema, ectatic sinusoids, perivascular and interstitial fibrosis, inflammatory reactions, plasmacytosis, increased mast cells, macrophages often containing cellular debris and hemosiderin, lymphocytosis and lymphoid nodules; aggregates of blasts, not just clusters as in ALIP, may also be found (Figures 20.12–20.14). In this context it is of interest that various immunological changes have been documented in MDS. However, compared with controls, no abnormalities of T cells or T cell subsets were found in MDS; but there appeared to be an association with a poor prognosis in patients with increased numbers of B cells (>3%).

Histology of MDS

The histological criteria in MDS may be summarised as follows: (1) cellularity of the bone marrow, (2) architectural disorganisation,

197

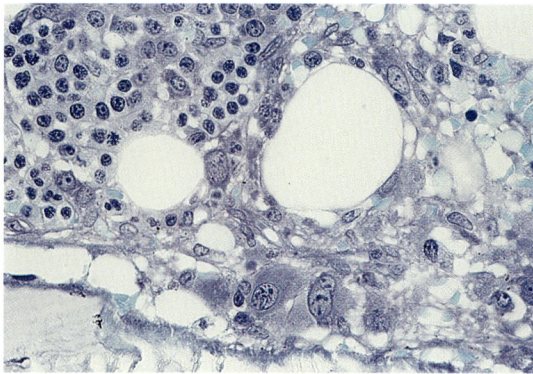

20.10 (left) As for Figure 20.9, megakaryocytes at trabecular surface.

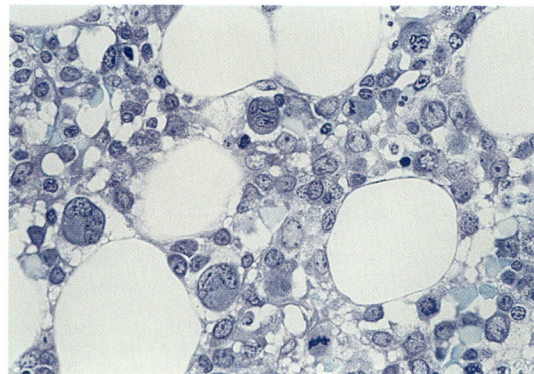

20.11 (right) As for Figure 20.9, immature myeloid cells and dysplastic megakaryocytes dispersed in intertrabecular space.

(3) stromal reactions, (4) predominant cell line(s), (5) cellular abnormalities, and (6) ineffective hematopoiesis. With respect to cellular abnormalities, some of the dysplastic features are: megaloblastoid erythropoiesis with maturation arrest and nuclear irregularities (Figure 20.15); and PAS and cytoplasmic inclusions and ringed sideroblasts (which may also be observed in sections (Figure 20.16). Megakaryocytes may have hypolobulated or small and separated nuclei and micromegakaryocytes are present. Granulopoiesis may be characterised by decreased granulation and alterations in nuclear shape and condensation of chromatin, and hyposegmentation. Iron stores may be increased and variable numbers of sideroblasts (ringed or otherwise) may be present, as well as macrophages with cellular debris.

Histologic subtypes (Table 20.3)

On the basis of the histological criteria listed above, biopsies could be divided into seven MDS categories: (1) sideroblastic (Figures 20.17–20.20), (2) megaloblastoid, (3) inflammatory, (4) fibrotic, (5) hypocellular, (6) proliferative, and (7) blastic.

Chronic myelomonocytic leukemia – CMML – being by definition a leukemia, does not, strictly speaking, belong in the group of myelodysplastic syndromes regarded as pre-leukemic conditions (at least, not overtly leukemic) (Figures 20.21–20.24). Chronic myelomonocytic leukemia may also follow a myelodysplastic syndrome such as refractory anemia. Correlation of the histological types of

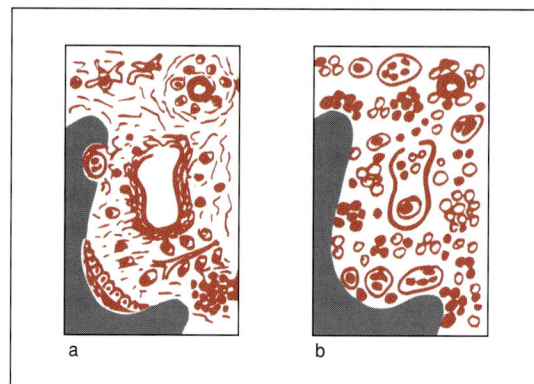

MDS with the FAB classification is given in Table 20.3. The presence of ALIP in the bone biopsy sections constitutes both a diagnostic and prognostic factor, though this is not universally accepted. Moreover, sometimes larger aggregates of blasts may be found, and these are not reflected in the counts of the peripheral blood or of the bone marrow aspirate. Nevertheless, they are a warning signal for the imminent transformation to an acute leukemia. Some authors have described three patterns of blast cell infiltration in the bone marrow: diffuse, cluster and large aggregates; and RAEBt patients accounted for only half of the patients with 'large' aggregates. About half of the patients with clusters had fibrosis, and in these cases leukemic transformation did not occur; in contrast with cases with large aggregates, most of whom transformed. The number of immature cells in bone biopsy sections can be estimated after immunostaining with CD34, (QBENDIO), which can also be used for

20.12 Representation of stroma changes in MDS and their consequences for hematopoiesis. (a) Ectatic, partly disrupted sinusoid and sclerotic wall surrounded by fibrosis, edema, extravasation of erythrocytes and some lymphocytes, plasma cells and mast cells (center); perivascular plasmacytosis and lymphoid nodule (below); iron-loaded macrophages, hemophagocytosis and vasculitis (above); and increased osseous remodeling (trabecula). (b) Ineffective hematopoiesis as a consequence of the disturbed microenvironment: intravascular precursors (center), loss of architectural orientation of the three cell lines with immature erythrons, micromegakaryocytes and multinucleated megakaryocytes in the paratrabecular area (below) and myeloid precursors in clusters and diffusely distributed.

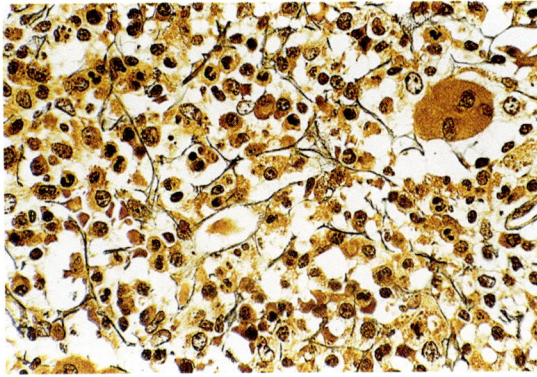

20.13 BMBS plastic, Gomori, cellular marrow with increased reticular fibers.

20.14 (left) BMBS paraffin, H&E, cellular bone marrow with lymphocytic aggregate, bottom center.

20.15 (right) BMBS plastic, Giemsa, megaloblastoid MDS – refractory anemia.

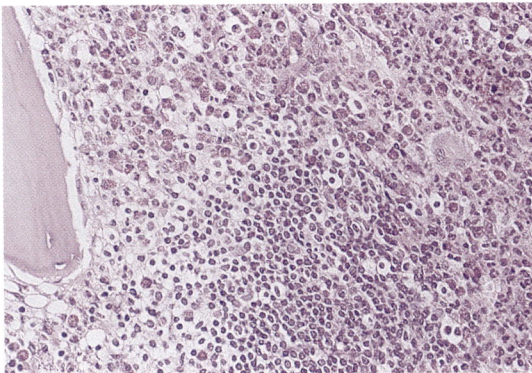

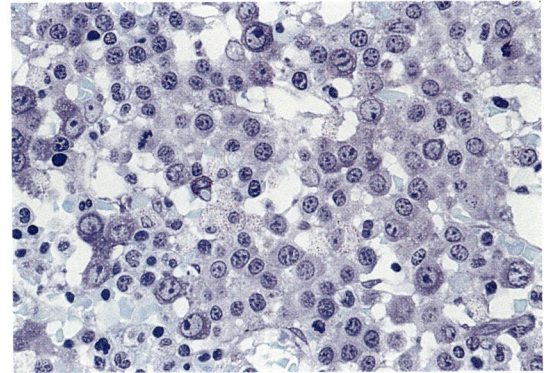

demonstration of incipient transformation (though this is not generally accepted, perhaps because of technical difficulties with the antibody). This approach is also applicable to therapy-related MDS. Hemophagocytosis has been observed in the terminal stages of MDS as in some lymphoproliferative disorders.

5q- syndrome

This occurs in elderly patients, usually females, with macrocytic anemia, mild leucopenia and

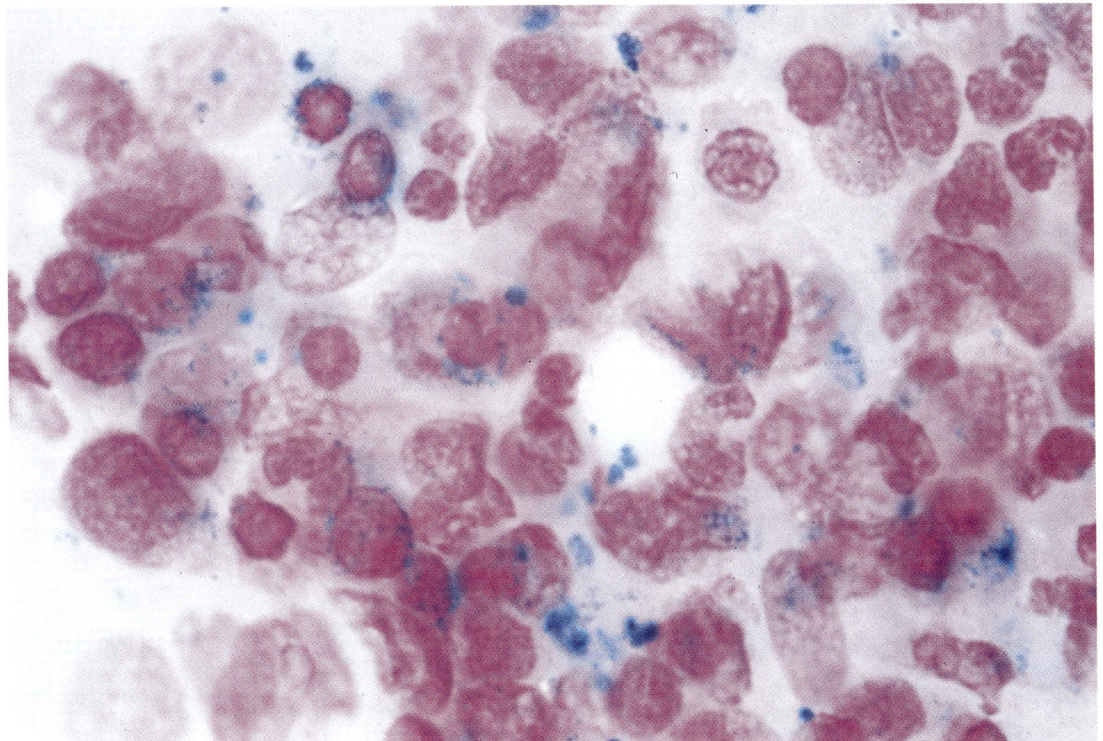

20.16 Bone marrow aspirate smear, iron stain showing increased iron and sideroblasts – sideroblastic MDS.

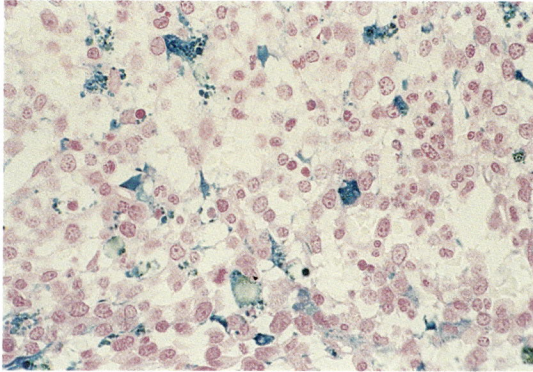

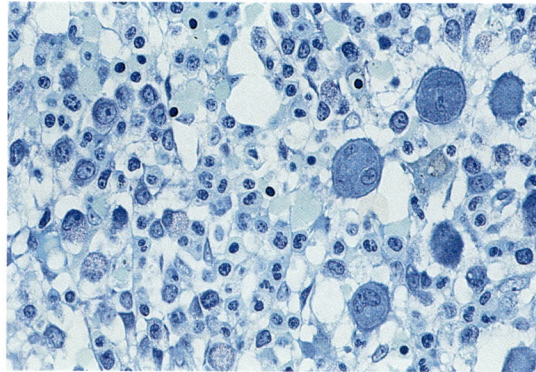

20.17 (left) BMBS plastic, iron stain, sideroblastic MDS, showing increased iron in bone marrow.

20.18 (right) As for Figure 20.17, Giemsa, showing erythroid and megakaryocytic hyperplasia including atypical megakaryocytes.

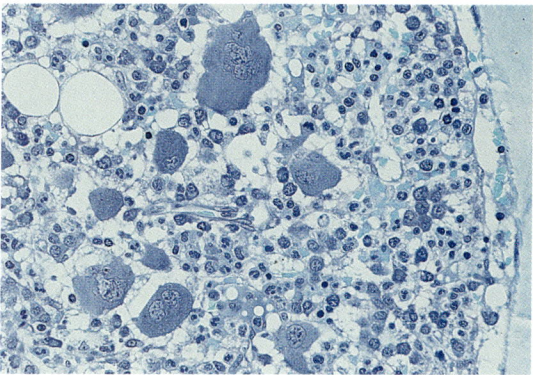

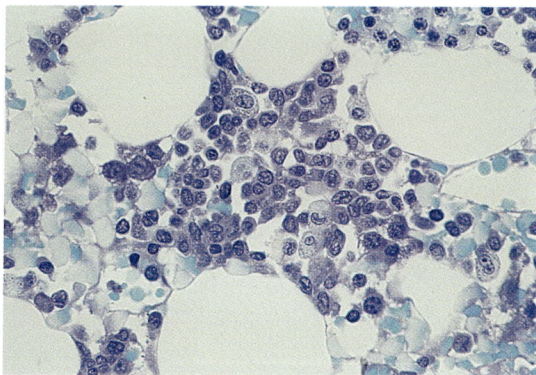

20.19 (left) As for Figure 20.17, different area, illustrating range of megakaryocytic size and morphology in MDS.

20.20 (right) As for Figure 20.17, ALIP (abnormal localisation of immature precursors) in central bone marrow areas in MDS.

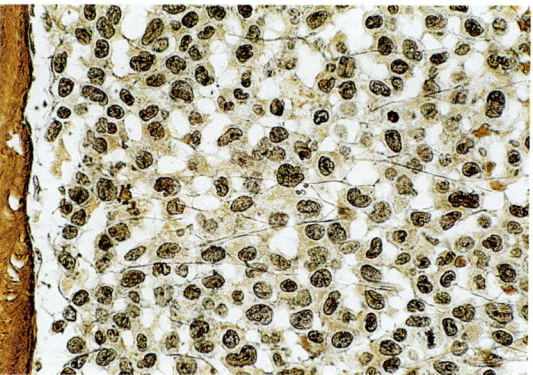

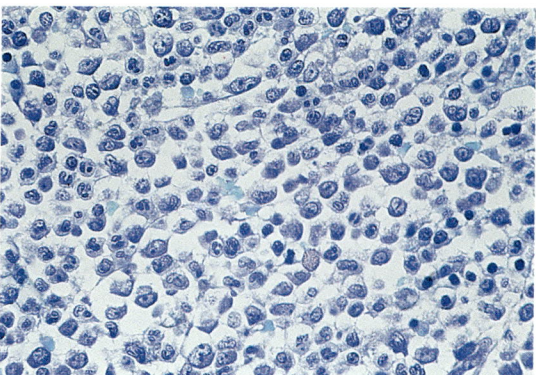

20.21–20.24 Examples of bone marrow histology in CMML.
20.21 (left) BMBS plastic, Gomori, showing myelo- and monocytic precursors at trebecular surface extending into central area.
20.22 (right) BMBS plastic, Giemsa, also case of CMML but with lesser monocytic component, central bone marrow area.
20.23 (left) As for Figure 20.22, high magnification showing cytologic features of the monocytes.

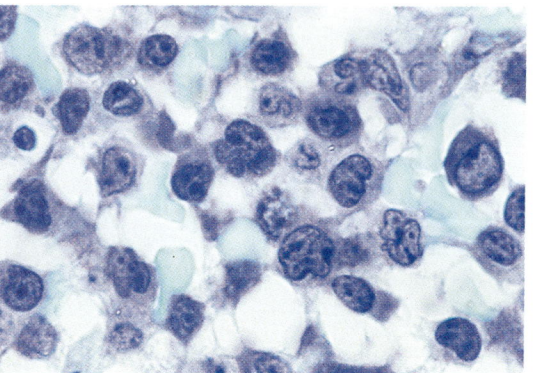

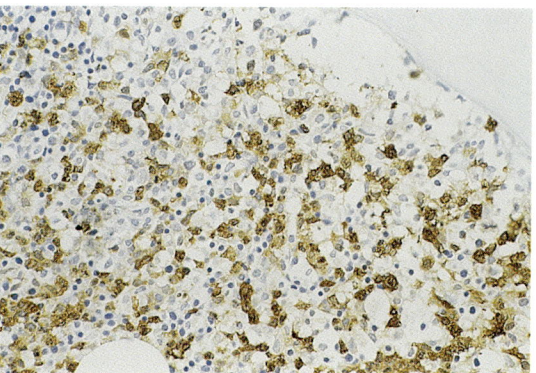

20.24 (right) BMBS paraffin, I.H., CD68-positive in monocytes.

thrombocytosis. There are <20% blasts in the bone marrow. This is no longer considered a separate entity and most cases are now classified as refractory anemias. It should be noted that 5q- is a common cytogenetic abnormality in the MDS (Fig 20.25–20.27).

Evolution of disease (Figure 20.28, Tables 20.4 and 20.5)

Many patients die as a consequence of the complications of the cytopenias; in others, concurrent disorders such as cardiovascular diseases may be present at diagnosis, or may

be detected subsequently, for example in immunologic disorders. Some patients develop aplastic anemia, in others the MDS evolve into acute or smoldering leukemias, myelofibrosis, or other chronic myeloproliferative disorders. As pointed out previously, when criteria for MDS and another MPD overlap, the initial diagnosis may be tentative and a definitive diagnosis is only established subsequently with disease progression. Many retrospective and prospective studies have shown that the subgroups of the MDS have different rates of conversion to overt leukemia. When MDS occurs

---

TABLE 20.3 Correlation of the FAB classification with the histological subtypes

AL	MDS	MDS
Biopsy + imprints	FAB classification	Marrow biopsy (subtypes)
		MDS sideroblastic 19%
	RAS	MDS megaloblastoid 13%
	RA	MDS inflammatory 10%
	RAEB	MDS fibrotic 6%
	RAEBt	MDS hypocellular 15%
	CMML	MDS proliferative 22%
		MDS blastic 15%

20.25 (left) Karyotype of patient with MDS: 46XY, del (5) (q); +8.

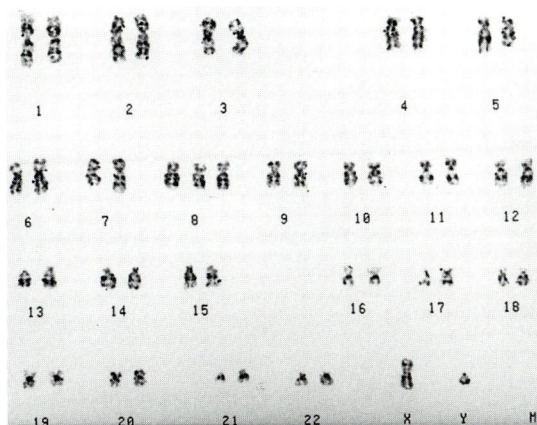

20.26 (right) Single-color FISH using a centromeric probe for chromosome 8. The arrow points to a nucleus with three signals indicating trisomy 8. Case of MDS.

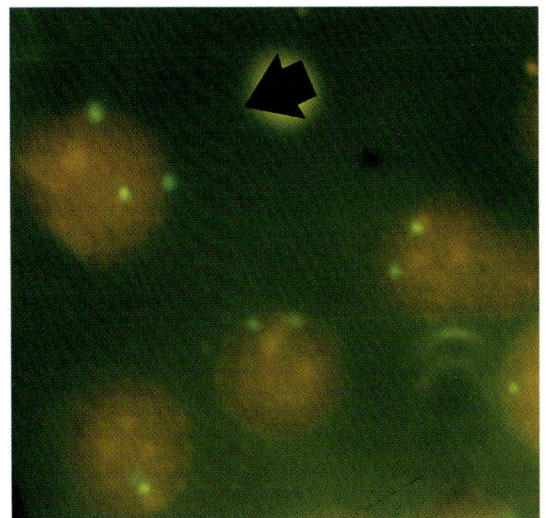

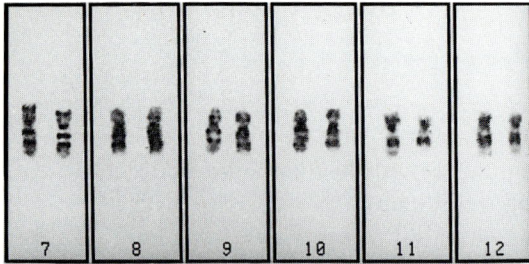

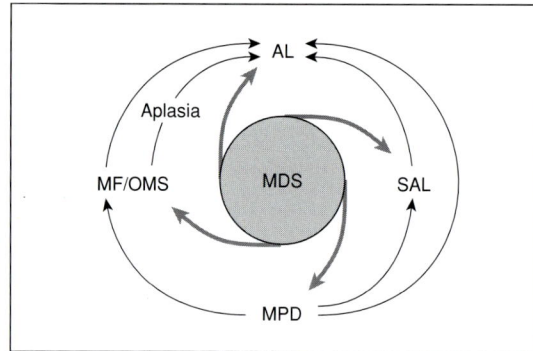

TABLE 20.4 Correlation between initial histology and subsequent course*

Subsequent diagnosis	Suspected acute leukemia (n = 6)	Suspected myeloproliferation (n = 54)	Sideroblastosis (n = 62)	Dysplastic maturation (n = 64)
Initial diagnosis unchanged to date	1	33	25	37
Sideroblastic anemia	–	5	23	1
Myeloproliferation excluded	–	2	8	–
MPD	–	11	–	–
Smoldering leukemia	5	1	3	11
Acute leukemia	–	2	3	15

Sequential biopsies taken within 6–24 months of initial biopsy.

TABLE 20.5 Comparison of the FAB with histologic classification and evaluation of MDS

AL, SAL, CMPD Biopsy + aspirate		MDS-FAB Periph. blood + aspirate		MDS Biopsy + aspirate	
		RARS	18%	MDS sideroblastic	19%, 62m
AL, SAL	←	RAEB-t	8%	MDS blastic	15%, 9m
CMPD, SAL	←	RAEB	24%	MDS proliferative	22%, 31m
CMPD, MF, Ery. L	←	RA	35%	MDS megaloblastoid	13%, 56m
				MDS hypoplastic	15%, 26m
				MDS fibrotic	6%, 29m
				MDS inflammatory	10%, 42m
CMML	⇒	CMML 15%		–	

m, median survival (months) from time of initial diagnosis.

in a patient known to have a malignant solid tumor, or a second malignancy is subsequently discovered in a patient with MDS, the question arises about whether it is a simultaneous (metachronous) condition or a paraneoplastic syndrome. One study that addressed this question has shown that a second malignancy occurred at 2.9 times the expected rate in a group of 138 patients with MDS.

Differential diagnosis of MDS

Many of the histological characteristics of MDS, singly or in a combination, may also be found in other conditions, for example hypoplastic MDS and aplastic anemia or hypocellular acute leukemia. Hence the bone marrow histology is evaluated in the framework of the clinical picture as a whole: patient's age, history, physical examination and results of all the other investigations (e.g. hematological, cytogenetic, biochemical and imaging techniques). Moreover, difficulties and even discrepancies in the diagnosis of the MDS may occur due to: (1) discordance between different bone marrow regions, e.g. sternal aspiration and iliac crest biopsy, (2) temporal variability when comparing sequential bone marrow examinations, (3) overlapping of categories of the MDS as well as with other MPDs, acute leukemias and aplastic

anemias, and (4) previously undetected additional conditions (e.g. metastases in the bone marrow) which may induce myelodysplasia.

Additional myelodysplasias

MDS with fibrosis
Though some authors consider this as a separate entity, it is also included here as many cases of MDS have some degree of increase in reticular fibers (see above). When there is considerable fibrosis, the differential diagnosis will have to be broadened to include other entities such as the chronic MPD and AMF, as well as acute leukemia (Figure 20.29).

Post-leukemic MDS
This is occasionally seen in patients after chemotherapy for acute leukemia, in whom complete restoration of hematopoiesis is not achieved. This condition has also been called 'clonal remission' to indicate stimulation of maturation of the neoplastic clone, rather than re-establishment of normal hematopoiesis. Other forms of clonal remission have also been postulated, i.e. when one aggressive clone has been eliminated, other aggressive clones eventually arise and develop.

Paraneoplastic MDS
Patients with solid tumors sometimes develop MDS. If therapy has not yet been given, the possibility of a metachronous disorder must be considered. Alternatively, the solid tumor may be responsible for production of cytokines; for example, erythropoietin by kidney tumors, or granulocyte stimulating factors by pulmonary neoplasias.

Classification of MDS and future perspectives

Classification, especially histopathological, is an ongoing process, and is constantly revised as new information becomes available. Therefore, it should be stressed that classification based on purely morphological criteria will undoubtedly be modified in the near future. This applies to the FAB classification, based on peripheral blood findings and on smears of aspirates as well as to bone marrow histology

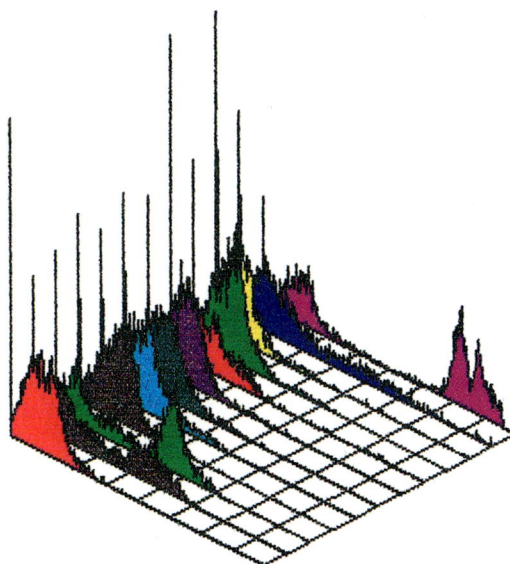

20.29 Flow cytometry of 34-year-old male patient with pancytopenia, showing MDS with fibrosis on histology, with erythroid and megakaryocytic hyperplasia, lymphocytosis and hemophagocytosis. Left to right: red, control; brown, CD7 37%; green CD2 40%; brown, CD19 1%; blue, CD20 6%; dark green, CD10 3%; purple, CD13 3%; red, CD14 4%; green, CD33 3%; yellow, CD34 2%; dark blue, CD41 23%; red, glycophorin 57%. The bone marrow fibrosis undoubtedly influenced the composition of the population of cells in the bone marrow aspirate.

(see Preface and Chapter 2). Classifications of the malignant lymphomas have been, and still are being supplemented and modified by the results of immunological phenotyping. This has not yet been done for MDS, though similar classifications including morphologic, immunologic and cytogenetic characteristics have been proposed but not yet widely accepted. A recently proposed scoring system for evaluating prognosis in MDS includes cytogenetic, morphologic and clinical data in the expectation that this should prove useful for design and analysis of therapeutic trials in the future. At the last international workshop on MDS (April 1997), a method which combines morphology, immunophenotyping and cytogenetics was proposed and was carried out on cells spread on a microscope slide. It is called the MAC technique. However, it is also subject to some of the limitations listed above. In addition, immunological studies of the bone marrow microenvironment, stromal components and of the local regulatory cells and other factors, including adhesion molecules, should contribute to a more precise classification of these disorders in the future as well as a deeper understanding of their etiologies and patterns of evolution.

Secondary myelodysplastic syndromes

Occurrence and predisposing factors

These are also known as therapy-induced myelodysplasias (tMDS) and secondary leukemias which have developed (in most cases after years) in patients previously treated with cytotoxic therapy for a wide range of primary neoplasms. Secondary malignancies also develop due to exposure to other toxic agents. The secondary malignancies that may occur in such patients include epithelial cancers, malignant lymphomas, myeloid and lymphoblastic leukemias, and/or panmyeloses. The latter are usually preceded by a pre-leukemic phase of variable duration, often associated with cytopenia(s) and functional abnormalities of the blood cells (i.e. myelodysplastic syndromes). In most cases there are chromosomal alterations. Many features are similar to *de novo* AML: the patients suffer fatigue, weakness, fever, anemia, pallor, exertional dyspnea, infections and hemorrhage.

Bone marrow histology

The bone marrow in these syndromes reflects the stage in their development at which the biopsy was taken. Moreover, the bone marrow may be hypo-, normo- or hypercellular with morphological alterations in all three cell lines and marked stromal changes. Two main types of tMDS have been recognised: (1) tMDS after alkylating agents with chemotherapy in which there is a panmyelosis (plus abnormalities of chromosomes 3 and 7), and (2) after therapy with epipodophyllotoxin in which there is development of AML with a monocytic component. However, it should be remembered that transient depletion of all hematopoietic elements is seen after aggressive chemotherapy, together with extensive stromal reactions. Nevertheless, most of these post-chemotherapy bone marrows revert to near-normal on cessation of the treatment and after the regenerative phase. Thus, a detailed history is required for the correct interpretation of the biopsy sections, as some of them may not be distinguishable from secondary MDS in its preleukemic phase. The bone marrows in secondary MDS are not usually classifiable according to FAB criteria for the primary MDS as these criteria are based on bone marrow aspirate smears. Both an interstitial form in a hypo- or normocellular marrow, and a hypercellular form, with almost complete occupation of the marrow cavities, have been found in therapy-induced secondary MDS and leukemias. Myelofibrosis has also been observed, as well as atypical and clustered megakaryocytes, and marker techniques may be required for blast cell characterisation. However, by the application of immunohistology, secondary MDS can be classified according to biologic and clinical aggressiveness (see above).

Evolution of disease

tMDS usually progresses more quickly than primary MDS, and the subsequent acute leukemia, often a panmyelosis, is frequently not, or poorly, responsive to therapy.

Check list: Myelodysplastic Syndrome (MDS)

- Adequate biopsy: at least 30 mm after exclusion of cortex and subcortical areas.

- Cellularity of the bone marrow: hypo-, normo- or hypercellular?

- Disorganisation of marrow architecture?

- Topography of cell lines, altered?

- Presence of ALIPs? Confirmed by immunohistology (I.H.).

- Proportions of the three cell lines? I.H.: myeloid antigen, myeloperoxidase, CD34, CD68, Factor VIII will give some idea of the cell lines.

- Ratio of immature-to-mature precursors of each individual cell line?

- Dysplastic features: dyserythropoiesis, hypogranular leucocytes, coarse granulation, small and mononucleated megakaryocytes? I.H.: Factor VIII for small megakaryocytes.

- Macrophages with debris (ineffective hematopoiesis) plasma cells, mast cells, lymphocytic aggregates? I.H.: CD68, LCA, T cells, B cells.

- Evaluation of iron-stained section: normal, increased, sideroblasts increased? Storage iron reduced?

- Tentative diagnosis (often partly one of exclusion).

- Classification according to FAB based on peripheral blood and bone marrow aspirates, if available.

Clinical correlations

Primary MDS
- Mainly in adults >50 years, though MDS also occurs (rarely) in children.
- Presentation with uni-, bi- or tricytopenia and corresponding consequences.
- Primary MDS is a diagnosis of exclusion.
- Other conditions common to older age groups may be present.
- Characteristic cytogenetic changes present in many cases, >60% with the latest methods.
- Evolution to overt leukemia if fatal complications do not arise previously.
- Variable and limited response to chemotherapy.

Secondary MDS
- History of previous chemo- and radiotherapy, exposure to toxins.
- Variable time interval till overt MDS.
- Multiple chromosomal anomalies.
- Poor response to treatment.
- Rapid development of acute leukemia.
- Correlation with peripheral blood values, aspirate smears and FACS of peripheral blood and of nucleated cells in aspirate of bone marrow.
- Complex chromosomal aberrations: involvement of three or more chromosomes, occurs in approximately 50% of cases.

Clonal chromosomal characteristics

Primary MDS

−7	del(11)(q)	t(1;3)(p36;q21)	t(2;11) (p21;q23)
+8	del(12)(p)	t(6;9)(p23;q34)	t(11;21) (q24;q11)
del(5)(q12-q34)	del(13)(q)	t(5;12)(q33;p13)	i(17)(q)
translocations involving 5q	del(20)(q)		
del(7)(q)			
+7			

Continued

Therapy-related MDS			Other anomalies in MDS and also seen in AML and MPD		
del(5)(q)		del/t(3)(q)			
del(7)(q)		del/t(6)(p)	+4 +14		inv(16)(p13;q22)
−5	+8	del/t(17)(q)	+11 +15		t/ins(3)(q21;q26)
−7	−17	t/dup(X)(q13)	−Y		dup(1)(q)
del(12)(p)	+21	t(X)(p11)	t(3;5)(q21;q31)		t(9;22)(q34;q11)
t(1;7)(p11;p11)		del/t(17)(p)			

Therapy-related leukemia
Simple trisomies, e.g. of 8 or 21, as well as others
Monosomies 5, 7, 18

del(12)(p)	dup (1)(q)
del(1;7)(q10;p10)	t(3;21)(q26;q22)

Bibliography

Abeliovich D., Yehuda O., Ben Neriah S., Matzner Y. (1993) Therapy-related myelodysplastic syndrome: Two cytogenetically unrelated abnormal clones in a patient with multiple myeloma. *Cancer Genet. Cytogenet.*, **70 (2)**, 117–19.

Adachi M., Ryo R., Yoshida A. *et al.* (1989) Refractory anaemia terminating in acute megakaryoblastic leukaemia (M7). *Acta Haematol*, **81 (2)**, 104–8.

Anderson Jeanne E., Appelbaum F. (1997) Myelodysplasia and myeloproliferative disorders. *Curr. Opin. Hematol*, **4**, 261–7.

Auffermann W., Fohlmeister I., Bocking A. (1988) Diagnostic and prognostic value of DNA image cytometry in myelodysplasia. *J. Clin. Pathol.*, **41 (6)**, 604–8.

Bader-Meunier B., Mielot F., Tchernia G. *et al.* (1996) Myelsodysplastic syndromes in childhood: report of 49 patients from a French multicentre study. *Br J Haematol*, **92**, 344–50.

Barnard D.R., Kalousek D.K., Wiersma S.R. *et al.* (1996) Morphologic, immunologic, and cytogenetic classifiaction of acute myeloid leukemia and myelodysplastic syndrome in childhood: a report from the Childrens Cancer Group. *Leukemia*, **10 (1)**, 5–12.

Bastion Y., Thomas X., Felman P. *et al.* (1991) High risk myelodysplastic syndrome coexistent with chronic lymphocytic leukemia for more than 9 years: inhibtion of the myeloid clone by the lymphoid clone? *Leukemia*, **5 (11)**, 1006–9.

Beris P. (1989) Primary clonal myelodysplastic syndromes. *Semin. Hematol.*, **26 (3)**, 216–33.

Billstrom R., Thiede T., Hansen S. *et al.* (1988) Bone marrow karyotype and prognosis in primary myelodysplastic syndromes. *Eur. J. Hematol.*, **41 (4)**, 341–6.

Brusamolino E., Bernasconi C. (1992) Therapy-related myelodysplastic syndromes and acute leukemias. *Leukemia*, **6 (Suppl. 4)**, 23–5.

Buude R., Schaefer H.E. (1989) Smokers' dysmyelopoiesis – bone marrow alterations associated with cigarette smoking. *Pathol Res Pract.*, **185 (3)**, 347–50.

Chang J., Geary C.G., Testa N.G. (1990) Long-term bone marrow damage after chemotherapy for acute myeloid leukaemia does not improve with time. *Bt J Haematol*, **75 (1)**, 68–72.

Chessells J.M. (1991) Myelodysplasia. *Baillieres Clin. Hematol.*, **4 (2)**, 459–82.

Clatch R.J., Krigman H.R., Peters M.G., Zutter M.M. (1994) Dysplastic haemopoiesis following orthotopic liver transplantation: comparison with similar changes in HIV infection and primary myelodysplasia. *Br J Haematol*, **88 (4)**, 685–92.

Colon-Otero G., Malkasian G.D., Edmonson J.H. (1993) Secondary myelodysplasia and acute leukemia following carboplatin-containing combination chemotherapy for ovarian cancer. *J. Nat. Cancer Inst.*, **85 (22)**, 1858–60.

Creutzig U., Cantu-Rajnoldi A., Ritter J. *et al.* (1987) Myelodysplastic syndromes in childhood. Report of 21 patients from Italy and West Germany. *Am. J. Pediatr. Hematol. Oncol.*, **9 (4)**, 324–30.

Fenaux P., Morel P., Lai J.L. (1996) Cytogenetics of myelodysplastic syndromes. *Sem in Hematol.*, **33 (2)**, 127–38.

First MIC Cooperative Study Group (1986) Morphologic, immunologic, and cytogenetic (MIC) working classification of acute lymphoblastic leukemias. *Cancer Genet Cytogenet.*, **23**, 189–97.

Forman S.J. (1996) Myelodysplastic syndrome. *Current Opinion in Hematol*, **3 (4)**, 297–302.

Foti A., Cline M.J. (1994) Sequential relapses of blastic crisis may involve different clones of cells with different molecular abnormalities. *Br J Haematol*, **87**, 627–30.

Fox S.B., Lorenzen J., Herye A. *et al.* (1990) Megakaryocytes in myelodysplasia: an immunohistochemical study on bone marrow trephines. *Histopathology*, **17 (1)**, 69–74.

Frisch B., Bartl R. (1992) Minimal diagnostic criteria for the myelodysplastic syndrome (MDS) in clinical practice. *Leuk Res.*, **16 (1)**, 6–8.

Gadner H. (1991) Myelodysplasia in childhood. *Acta Pediatr. Hung.*, **31 (1)**, 3–12.

Gardner F.H.(1987) Refractory anemia in the elderly. *Adv Intern Med.*, **32**, 155–75.

Geary C.G. (1989) Myelodysplasia: clinical and morphological aspects and treatment. *Bone Marrow Transplant*, **4 (Suppl. 1)**, 138–40.

Geddes A.A., Bowen D.T., Jacobs A. (1990) Clonal karyotype abnormalities and clinical progress in the myelodysplastic syndrome. *Br. J. Hematol.*, **76 (2)**, 194–202.

Georgii A. (1997) Impact of histopathology on diagnosis, clinics and outcome of myelodysplastic syndromes. *Leuk Res*, **21 (1)**, S13.

Greenberg P., Cox C., LeBeau M.M. *et al.* (1997) International scoring system for evaluating prognosis in myelodysplastic syndromes. *Blood*, **89 (6)**, 2079–88.

Guinan E.C., Tarbell N.J., Tantravahi R., Weinstein H.J. (1989) Bone marrow transplantation for children with myelo-dysplastic syndromes. *Blood*, **73 (2)**, 619–22.

Haas O.A., Gadner H. (1996) Pathogenesis, biology, and management of myelo-dysplastic syndromes in children. *Seminars in Hematol*, **33 (3)**, 225–35.

Hilbr W., Eisterer W., Schmid C. *et al.* (1994) Bone marrow lymphocyte subsets in myelodysplastic syndromes. *J Clin Pathol*, **47 (6)**, 505–7.

Hoppe R.T. (1992) Secondary leukemia and myelodysplastic syndrome after treatment for Hodgkin's disease. *Leukemia*, **6 (Suppl. 4)**, 155–7.

Horny H.P., Wehrmann M., Schlicker H.U. *et al.* (1995) QBEND10 for the diagnosis of myelodysplastic syndromes in routinely processed bone marrow biopsy specimens. *J Clin Pathol*, **48 (4)**, 291–4.

Howard M.R., Kesteven P.J.L. (1993) Sea blue histiocytosis: a common abnormality of the bone marrow in myelodysplastic syndromes. *J. Clin. Pathol.*,**46 (11)**, 1030–32.

Jackson G.H., Carey P.J., Cant A.J. *et al.* (1993) Myelodysplastic syndromes in children. *Br. J. Hematol.*, **67 (5)**, 1156.

Kanter-Lewensohn L., Hellstrom-Lindberg E., Kock Y. *et al.* (1996) Analysis of CD34-positve cells in bone marrow from patients with myelodysplastic syndromes and acute myeloid leukemia and in normal individuals: a comparison between FACS analysis and immunochemistry. *Eur J Haematol*, **56 (3)**, 124–9.

Koeffler H.P. (1996) Myelodysplastic syndromes. *Semin Hematol.*, **33 (2)**, 87–94.

Lambertenghi-Deliliers G., Annaloro C., Oriani A. *et al.* (1993) Prognostic relevance of histological findings on bone marrow biopsy in myelodysplastic syndromes. *Ann Hematol*, **66 (2)**, 85–91.

Lambertenghi-Deliliers G., Orazi A., Luksch R. *et al.* (1991) Myelodysplastic syndrome with increased marrow fibrosis: a distinct clinico-pathological entity. *Br J Haematol*, **78 (2)**, 161–6.

Lesesve J.F., Troussard X., Bastard C. *et al.* (1996) p190[bcr/abl] rearrangement in myelodysplastic syndromes: two reports and review of the literature. *Br. J. Haematol*, **96**, 372–5.

Maschek H., Georgii A., Kaloutsi V. *et al.* (1992) Myelofibrosis in primary myelodysplastic syndromes: A retrospective study of 352 patients. *Eur J Haematol.*, **48**, 208–14.

Maschek H., Kaloutsi V., Werner M. *et al.* (1990) Myelosclerosis in myelodysplastic syndromes (MDS). Retrospective analysis of 232 patients with MDS. *Verh. Dtsch. Ges.Pathol.* **74**, 144–8.

Mazzone A., Ricevuti G., Pasotti D. *et al.* (1993) The CD11/CD18 granulocyte adhesion molecules in myelodysplastic syndromes. *Br. J. Hematol.*, **83 (2)**, 245–52.

McMullin M.J., Chisholm M., Hows J.M. (1991) Congenital myelodysplasia: a newly described disease entity? *Br. J. Hematol.*, **79 (2)**, 340–2.

Meckenstock G., Fonatsch C., Heyll A. *et al.* (1992) T-cell receptor gamma/delta expressing acute leukemia emerging from sideroblastic anemia: morphological, immunological, and cytogenetic features. *Leuk. Res.*, **16 (4)**, 379–84.

Miescher P.A., Jaffe E.R., Beris P. (eds) (1996) Myelodysplastic syndromes. *Seminars in Hematol*, **33 (2)**, 87–9.

Morra E., Lazzarino M., Castello A. *et al.* (1990) Risk assessment in myelodysplastic syndromes: value of clinical, hematological and bone marrow histologic findings at presentation. *Eur J Hematol*, **45 (2)**, 94–100.

Musilova J., Michalova K. (1988) Chromosome study of 85 patients with myelodysplastic syndrome. *Cancer Genet. Cytogenet.*, **33 (1)**, 39–50.

Navone R., Ranco V., Pich A. (1991) Evolution of acute leukemia in myelodysplastic syndromes: prognostic histopathological factors in a series of bone marrow biopsies. *Pathologica*, **83 (1083)**, 55–63.

Orazi A., Cattoretti G., Soligo D. *et al.* (1993) Therapy-related myelodysplastic syndromes: FAB classification, bone marrow histology, and immunohistology in the prognostic assessment. *Leukemia*, **7 (6)**, 838–47.

Oriani A., Annaloro C., Soligo D. *et al.* (1996) Bone marrow histology and CD34 immunostaining in the prognostic evaluation of primary myelodysplastic syndromes. *Br J Haematol*, **92 (2)**, 360–4.

Oscier D.G. (1997) ABC of clinical haematology: the myelodysplastic syndromes. *BMJ*, **314**, 883–8.

Passmore S.J., Hann I.M., Stiller C.A. *et al.* (1995) Pediatric myelodysplasia: a study of 68 children and a new prognostic scoring system. *Blood*, **85**, 1742–50.

Pedersen B. (1996) Anatomy of the 5q-deletion: different sex ratios and deleted 5q bands in MDS and AML. *Leukemia*, **10 (12)**, 1883–90.

Pointud P., Prudat M., Peron J.M. (1993) Acute leukemia after low dose methotrexate therapy in a patient with rheumatoid arthritis. *Nucleic Acids Research*, **21 (12)**, 2873–79.

Raynaud S.D., Baens M., Grosgeorge J. *et al.* (1996) Fluorescence in situ hybridization analysis of t(3;12)(q26;p13): a recurring chromosomal abnormality involving the TEL Gene (ETV6) in myelodysplastic syndromes. *Blood*, **88 (2)**, 682–9.

Raza A., Gezer S., Mundle S. *et al.* (1995) Apoptosis in bone marrow biopsy samples involving stromal and hematopoietic cells in 50 patients with myelodysplastic syndromes. *Blood*, **86 (1)**, 268–76.

Raza A., Mundle S., Iftikhar A. *et al.* (1995) Simultaneous assessment of cell kinetics and programmed cell death in bone marrow biopsies of myelodysplastics reveals extensive apoptosis as the probable basis for ineffective hematopoiesis. *Am J Hematol*, **48 (3)**, 143–54.

Rezuke W.N., Anderson C., Pastuszak W.T. *et al.* (1991) Arsenic intoxication presenting as a myelodysplastic syndrome: a case report. **36 (4)**, 291–3.

Rios A., Canizo M.C., Sanz M.A. *et al.* (1990) Bone marrow biopsy in myelodysplastic syndromes: morphological characteristics and contribution to the study of prognostic factors. *Br. J. Hematol.*, **75 (1)**, 26–33.

Rosati S., Anastasi J., Vardiman J. (1996) Recurring diagnostic problems in the pathology of the myelodysplastic syndromes. *Seminars in Hematol.*, **33 (2)**, 111–26.

Rosati S., Mick R., Xu F. *et al.* (1996) Refractory cytopenia with multilineage dysplasia: further characterization of an 'unclassifiable' myelodysplastic syndrome. *Leukemia*, **10 (1)**, 20–6.

Sanz M.A., Sempere A. (1996) Immuno-phenotyping of AML and MDS and detection of residual disease. *Baillieres Clin Haematol.*, **9 (1)**, 35–55.

Shi G., Weh H.J., Martensen S. *et al.* (1996) 3p21 is a recurrent treatment-related breakpoint in myelodysplastic syndrome and acute myeloid leukemia. *Cytogenet Cell Genet*, **74 (4)**, 295–9.

Shulze R., Schlimok G., Renner D. (1992) Coincidence of primary myelodysplastic syndrome and non-Hodgkin lymphoma. *Klinische Wochenschrift*, **70 (12)**, 1082–4.

Sole F., Espinet B., Woessner S. *et al.* (1997) Cytogenetic findings in 121 patients with refractory anemia: prognostic value. *Cytogenet Cell Genet.*, **77**, 138.

Thiele J., Quitmann H., Wagner S., Fischer R. (1991) Dysmegakaryopoiesis in myelodysplastic syndromes (MDS): an immunomorphometric study of bone marrow trephine biopsy specimens. *J Clin Pathol*, **44 (4)**, 300–5.

Third MIC Cooperative Study Group (1988) Recommendations for a morphologic, immunologic, and cytogenetic (MIC) working classification of the primary and therapy-related myelodysplastic disorders. *Cancer Genet Cytogenet.*, **32 (1)**, 1–10.

Thirman M.J., Larson R.A. (1996) Therapy-related myeloid leukemia. *Hematol/Oncol Clin N. Am*, **10 (2)**, 293–320.

Tuncer M.A., Pagliuca A., Hicsonmez G. *et al.* (1992) Primary myelodysplastic syndrome in children: the clinical experience in 33 cases. *Br J Haematol.*, **82**, 347–53.

Tuzuner N., Cox C., Rowe J.M. *et al.* (1995) Hypocellular myelodysplastic syndromes (MDS): new proposals. *Br J Haematol.*, **91 (3)**, 612–7.

Vallespi T., del Caar myelodysplastic syndrome *et al.* (1997) Laboratory presentation and morphological characteristics on myelodysplastic syndromes. *Fourth International Symposium on Myelodysplastic Syndromes*. Barcelona.

Van den Berghe H., Mecucci C. (Chairpersons) (1997) *Workshop on Cytogenetics, Fourth International Symposium on Myelodysplastic Syndromes*. Barcelona.

van den Tweel J.G. (1997) Preleukaemic disorders in children: hereditary disorders and myelodysplastic syndrome. *Current Diagnost Pathol.*, **4**, 45–50.

Van Lom K., Hagemeijer A., Vandekerckhove F. *et al.* (1996) Cytogenetic clonality analysis: typical patterns in myelodysplastic syndrome and acure myeloid leukaemia. *Br J Haematol.*, **93**, 594–600.

Verhoef G., Meeus P., Stul M. *et al.* (1992) Cytogenetic and molecular studies of the Philadelphia translocation in myelodysplastic syndromes. Report of two cases and review of the literature, *Cancer Genet. Cytogenet.*, **59 (2)**, 161–6.

Werner M., Maschek H., Kaloutsi V. *et al.* (1992) Chromosome analyses in patients with myelodysplastic syndromes: correlation with bone marrow histopathology and prognostic significance. *Virchows Arch A Pathol Anat Histopathol.*, **421 (1)**, 47–52.

Woessner S. (1997) Combined morphological, immunological and cytogenetic techniques in the diagnosis of myelodysplastic syndromes. *Fourth International Symposium on Myelodysplastic Syndromes*. Barcelona.

Wong K.F., Chan J.K. (1991) Are 'dysplastic' and hypogranular megakaryocytes specific markers for myelodysplastic syndrome? *Br J Haematol*, **77(4)**, 509–14.

Yoshida Y., Oguma S., Uchino H., Maekawa T. (1988) Refractory myelodysplastic anaemias with hypocellular bone marrow. *J. Clin. Pathol.*, **41 (7)**, 763–7.

21 Acute leukemias

General aspects

Hematological malignancies are derived from precursors of the myeloid or lymphoid cell lines, or from a precursor common to both which may give biphenotypic leukemias. The hematological malignancies are characterised by alterations in the architecture, topography, relative proportions of the bone marrow constituents and in some cases the more or less striking cytological features of the cell lines directly concerned, as well as concomitant alterations in the others. In the evaluation of biopsies with hyperplasias or proliferations of hematopoietic elements, a number of specific questions should be systematically considered:

1. Is there a hyperplasia or proliferation outside normal limits?

2. What is the cytology of the cells comprising the hyperplasia?

3. Is it monomorphic, or does it contain more than one cytological type?

4. Is there a particular spatial arrangement, is the growth nodular or diffuse, does it form a pattern, how much of the marrow cavities does it occupy?

5. Note the presence or absence of fibers (sclerosis); is there edema or exudation between the cells?

6. Note the presence or absence of histiocytes, macrophages and other cells such as lymphocytes and mast cells.

7. Is there an effect on the residual hematopoietic and fat tissues?

8. Is there an effect on the trabecular bone and bone cells?

9. Are there changes in blood vessels, or stimulation of neo-angiogenesis?

Traditionally, the diagnosis of acute leukemia has been, and still is, based on peripheral blood counts and on routinely stained smears of blood and bone marrow aspirates (except in cases of a dry tap). Electron microscopy, cytogenetics, cytochemistry, presence of Auer rods, immunological (monoclonal antibodies) and enzyme markers are required for categorisation and phenotyping. In some cases, especially those with some degree of differentiation, the type of leukemia may be recognised in sections of the biopsies; for example, erythroblastic, megakaryoblastic and monoblastic cell lines. In addition, if a panel of antibodies is applied the lineage of most acute leukemias can be identified.

In cases of early acute leukemia, there is a diffuse interstitial infiltration of blasts while the marrow architecture and fat cells are to some extent preserved. Alternatively, the interstitial infiltration is accompanied by an exudative or serous atrophy with partial disappearance of marrow and fat. In these cases the differential diagnosis includes hairy cell leukemia, early myelofibrosis, aplastic anemia, chronic myelomonocytic leukemia and possibly small cell lymphoma, neuroblastoma, and Ewing's sarcoma; these conditions will have been indicated clinically and the phenotype is demonstrable by flow cytometry as well as immunohistology.

Diagnosis of acute leukemia

1. Peripheral blood findings – counts and morphology especially nuclear and cytoplasmic characteristics of blasts.

2. Aspirate of bone marrow and bone marrow biopsy: morphology and phenotypic characterisation by enzyme cytochemistry; fluorescent activated cell sorting (FACS) and counts, i.e. percentage of blasts and their phenotypic characterisation by antibodies, and to rule out non-hematologic malignancies.

3. Supplementary examinations, such as cytogenetics and molecular biology.

4. State of residual hematopoiesis once a diagnosis of acute leukemia has been established.

Cell lineage in acute leukemia

For determination of lineage in acute leukemias it is essential to employ a panel of antibodies that react specifically with each of the cell lines, for example early progenitors cells CD34 (QBENDIO), HLA-DR, TdT; B lymphoid cells CD10, CD19, CD20, CD21, CD22, CD23, CD24, CD74, CD75; T lymphoid cells CD2, CD3, CD4, CD5, CD7, CD8; myeloid MPO, CD13, CD15, CD16, CD33, CDw65; monocytoid CD14, CD15; erythroid; glycophorin A; megakaryocytic CD36, CD41, CD42, CD61 (immunohistology and flow cytometry).

For special situations, various combinations are used, for example in a bone marrow with partial or complete replacement by what appears to be a lymphoproliferative disorder with extensive fibrosis, a panel of antibodies including T and B lymphoid cells, EMA, CD15 and CD30 as well as glycophyrin, CD68, CD33, myeloperoxidase and CD41 for residual normal hematopoiesis – erythroid, monocytoid, myeloid and megakaryocytic cell lines respectively. Results of reactions with such a panel should provide diagnostic information, for example B and T cells positive, EMA negative, CD15 and CD30 positive in the morphologically appropriate cells, will indicate Hodgkin's disease. The rest of the panel will identify residual normal hematopoiesis.

In addition, it should be remembered that the results of immunohistology are influenced by many factors (not always immediately evident) and that cross-reactivity must be taken into account as well as, in the acute leukemias, biphenotypic antigen expression. It is particularly useful to characterise the cells of a bone marrow aspirate by flow cytometry (FACS) as well as by immunohistology on the biopsy sections. In cases with fibrosis the cell population obtained by aspiration may not be representative of the proportions present in the bone marrow which can, however, be accurately ascertained in the biopsy sections.

Cellularity

There are two main types of bone marrow infiltration in the acute leukemias: the hypercellular and hypocellular (Figures 21.1–21.5). A few early cases may show a diffuse interstitial infiltration of blasts, with partial disappearance of hematopoiesis and fat which are replaced by exudative or serous atrophy; in some cases an increase in reticular fibers may be present (Figure 21.2). Occasionally, there are alternating areas of replacement by sheets of blasts or by fat cells, with scattered hematopoietic precursors among them (Figures 21.4–21.7).

Hypercellular type

The bone marrow is hypercellular with sheets of immature cells (mainly blasts) occupying the intertrabecular spaces or occurring as large aggregates (Figure 21.2). Few normal precursors or fat cells remain. The residual hematopoiesis may show dysplastic features; disrupted sinusoids and some macrophages with cellular debris complete the picture. When the cells are very densely packed, attempts at aspiration may result in a dry tap. Other cases may have a looser infiltration so that connective tissue elements, reticulin fibers, macrophages, erythrocytes and other cells are dispersed among the blasts. When rapid multiplication outstrips the blood supply, areas of necrotic cells may be found. The degree of fibrosis that accompanies these

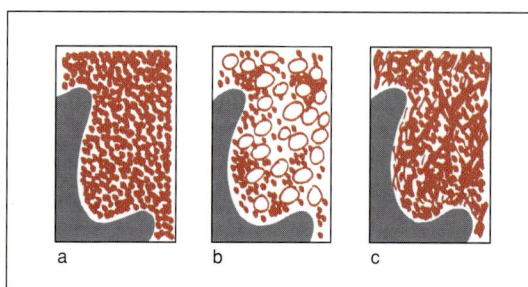

21.1 Representation of hyper- (a) and hypocellular (smoldering; b) acute leukemia, and acute myelosclerosis (or acute myelofibrosis) (c).

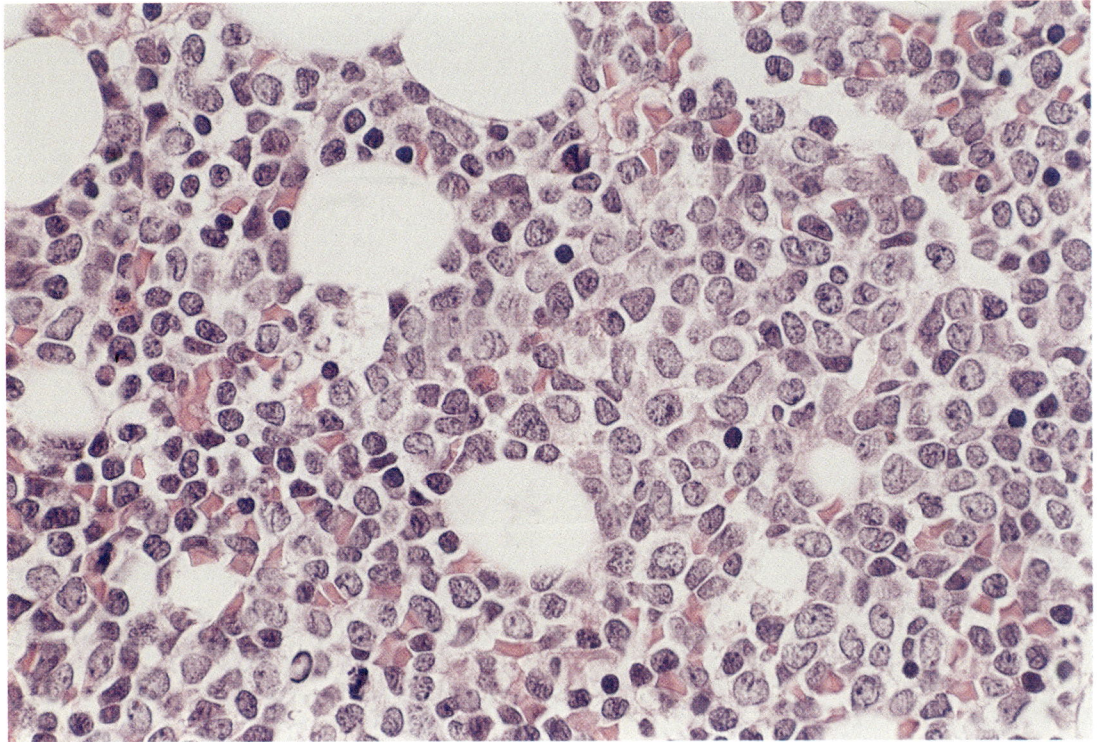

21.2 BMBS paraffin, H&E, hypercellular bone marrow; note fairly monomorphic picture of immature cells.

21.3 (left) BMBS plastic, Giemsa, hypercellular bone marrow, showing immature myeloid precursors and occasional erythroblasts.

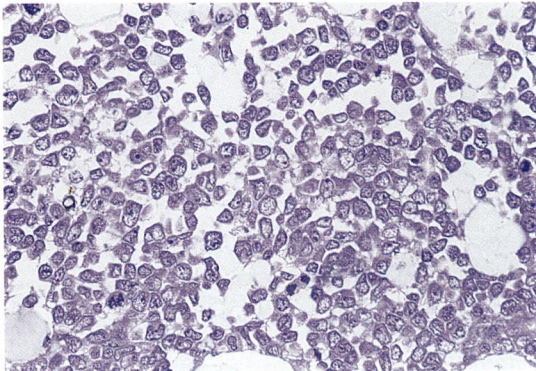

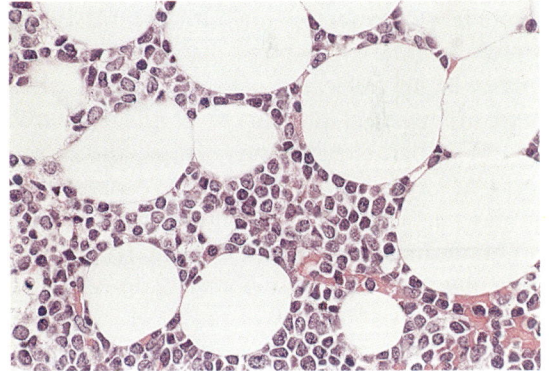

21.4 (right) BMBS paraffin, H&E, infiltration of myeloid precursors in hypocellular marrow.

21.5 (left) Same biopsy as for Figure 21.4, plastic, Giemsa, higher magnification, interstitial infiltration between the fat cells.

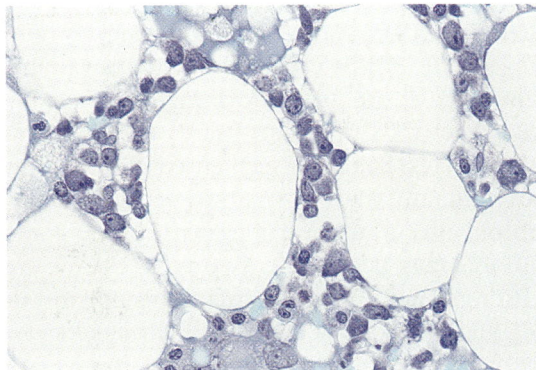

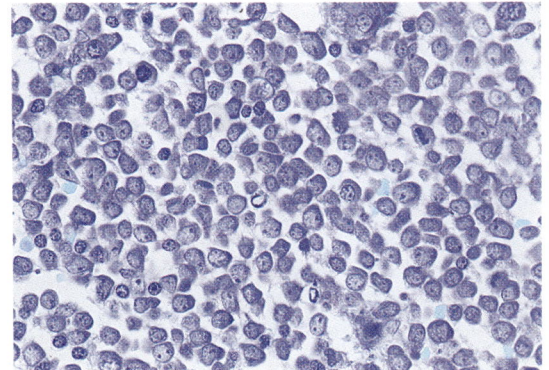

21.6 (right) Same biopsy as for Figure 21.5, Giemsa, mainly myeloblasts, from cellular area.

acute and subacute leukemias varies widely from mild to marked, as in acute myelofibrosis (AMF). Osteopenia, i.e. attenuation of the trabeculae with or without the presence of osteoclasts, is frequently seen. Occasionally increased osseous remodeling may be associated with hypercalcemia and osteolytic lesions; osteomalacia may develop during the course of therapy. Accelerated bone formation has also been reported. Dysplastic features may occur in cell lines other than the one directly involved in the acute leukemia, for example dysmegakaryopoiesis in acute myelomonocytic leukemia. Also proliferations affecting one myeloid cell line may predispose to acute leukemia in another; for example, myeloblastic leukemia in systemic mastocytosis.

Hypocellular type

There is a decrease in hematopoiesis and an increase in fat cells between which the blasts are dispersed (Figures 21.4 and 21.5). The residual hematopoiesis may show dysplastic features. Criteria for hypocellular acute leukemia include: (1) pancytopenia with few blasts, (2) <40% cellularity in bone marrow, (3) >30% blasts in all nucleated cells of bone marrow, and (4) myeloid phenotype of the leukemic blasts. When progression is slow, the hypocellular type corresponds to 'smoldering leukemia.' The degree of fibrosis varies widely in acute leukemias, from a slight increase in reticular fibers to coarse fibrosis as in AMF (see page 215).

Recently a comparative study was made of bone marrow aspirates and bone marrow biopsy findings at initial diagnosis in 51 patients with acute myeloid leukemia. Differences were observed in: (1) estimated overall marrow cellularity, (2) extent of blast cell infiltration, quantity and distribution of the different cell lines in the bone marrow and (3) bone marrow infiltration with inflammatory cells. These parameters were more reliably assessed in biopsies. The results suggest that bone marrow biopsies complement the findings of bone marrow aspiration in the acute leukemias and also provide additional information not otherwise obtained.

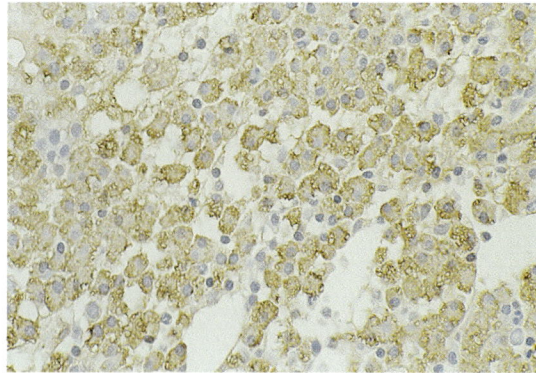

21.7 Same biopsy as for Figure 21.5, paraffin, I.H. with myeloperoxidase, most of the cells are positive.

Acute myeloid leukemias (AML)

The marrow is usually hypercellular, occasionally areas of replacement by fat cells may occur together with areas consisting of sheets of early myeloid precursors. The cytologic classification of the AML is given in Table 21.1.

Acute myeloblastic leukemia
(Figures 21.6–21.9)

M0
No cytologic maturation. CD13, CD33 and CD34-positive

M1
Minimal differentiation, Auer rods may be present. CD13, CD14, CD33-positive

M2
Significant maturation – granules are present; may be CD19-positive

Acute promyelocytic leukemia
(Figure 21.10)

M3
The bone marrow is hypercellular with broad paratrabecular seams of promyelocytes and myelocytes whose cytoplasm contains variable amounts of granules and bundles of needle-like Auer rods (faggots). Relatively few metamyelocytes, bands or segmented granulocytes are seen, and there is a marked decrease in erythroid precursors and megakaryocytes. Some fibrosis may be present. Two types of APL are distinguished: hypergranular and micro- or hypogranular. The blasts and promyelocytes express myeloid antigens.

TABLE 21.1 Classification of acute myeloid leukemia

Cell type	FAB
Acute myeloblastic leukemia, minimally differentiated	M0 (AML-M0)
Acute myeloblastic leukemia without maturation	M1 (AML-M1)
Acute myeloblastic leukemia with maturation	M2 (AML-M2)
Acute promyelocytic leukemia	M3 (AML-M3)
Hypergranular acute promyelocytic leukemia	APL
Microgranular (hypogranular) acute promyelocytic leukemia	M3V (APL-V)
Acute myelomonocytic leukemia	M4 (AML-M4)
Acute myelomonocytic leukemia with increased marrow eosinophils	(AML-M4EO)
Acute monocytic leukemia	M5 (AML-M5)
Acute monoblastic leukemia (acute monocytic leukemia, poorly differentiated)	M5A (AML-M5A)
Acute monocytic leukemia (acute monocytic leukemia. differentiated)	M5B (AML-M5B)
Erythroleukemia	M6 (AML-M6)
Acute megakaryoblastic leukemia	M7 (AML-M7)

21.8 (left) BMBS plastic, Gomori, acute myeloid leukemia, with fine reticular fibers between the rows of myeloid precursors.

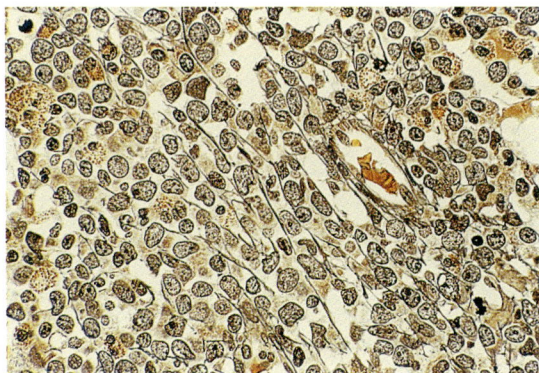

21.9 (right) Histogram of flow cytometry of nucleated cells of bone marrow aspirate of a patient with acute leukemia showing a single peak of CD33-positive cells. Same case as in Figures 21.4–21.8.

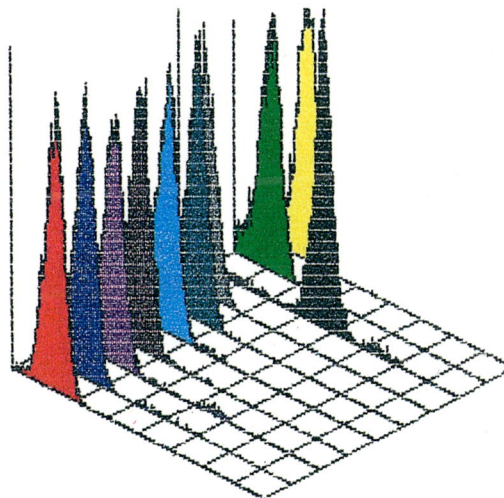

Acute myelomonocytic leukemia

M4

Hypercellular, hetero- – not monomorphic infiltration with decrease in erythroid and megakaryocytic cell lines and with increase in the proportions of granulocytic and monocytic precursors. Occasionally Auer rods are seen.

Varying proportions of cells express CD13, CD14, CD15, CD33 and CD36 and CD38 antigens.

M4 EO

Acute myelomonocytic with eosinophilia: M4 EO in which the eosinophils constitute about 5% of the non-erythroid blasts.

Acute monoblastic leukemia
(Figures 21.11 and 21.12)

M5A

The marrow is hypercellular with decrease in normal hematopoiesis. The infiltration consists of large cells with somewhat pleomorphic nuclei and abundant cytoplasm, no or few granules, no Auer rods.

M5B

Somewhat more differentiated type: the number of monocytes is usually higher in the peripheral blood than in the marrow. Varying proportions of cells express CD13, CD14, CD15, CD33, monocytic cells are CD36 positive and possibly CD38 on immunohistology (I.H.).

Acute erythroleukemia (Figure 21.13)

M6

A type of acute leukemia affecting the erythroid cell line to a greater extent than the myeloid (30%), so that erythroblasts >50% of the marrow cells. The histopathology depends on the proportions of erythroid and myeloid cells, and their degree of differentiation. Usually there is no difficulty in recognising the erythroid precursors because of their characteristic nuclei and cytoplasm: dysplastic multinucleated cells with abundant cytoplasm may be prominent. Megakaryocytes are often dysplastic and include micromegakaryocytes. Some degree of fibrosis is usually present. In rare cases, only the red cell series is apparently affected: erythremic myelosis. The erythroid cells express glycophorin A and may express CD36.

Acute megakaryoblastic leukemia
(Figure 21.14)

M7

The infiltration of blasts may show signs of differentiation so that the megakaryocytic cell line is recognised on morphology or special

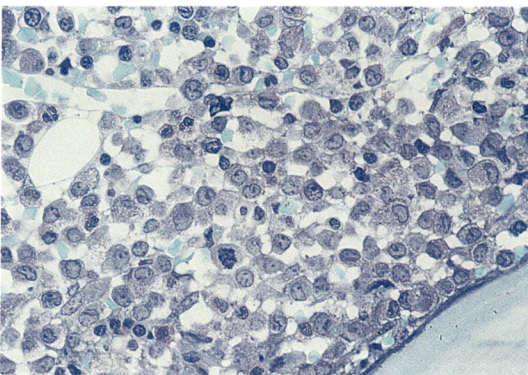

21.10 (left) BMBS plastic, from a case of promyelocytic leukemia, a broad seam of promyelocytes at the endosteal surface.

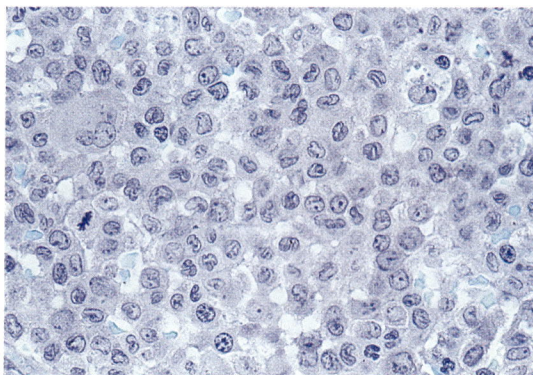

21.11 (right) BMBS plastic, Giemsa, case of moncytic leukemia.

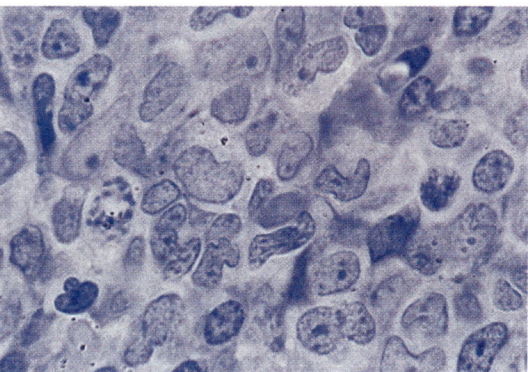

21.12 (left) BMBS plastic, Giemsa, high power, monocytic leukemia, illustrating the nuclear morphology.

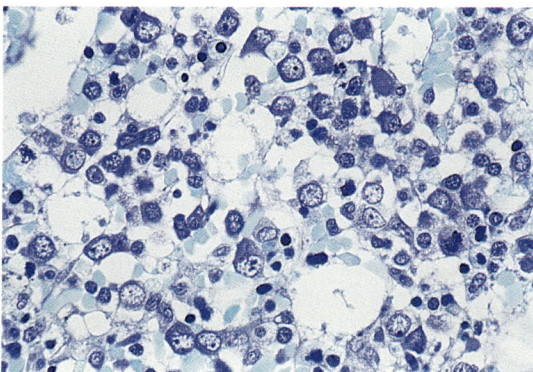

21.13 (right) BMBS plastic, Giemsa, erythroblastic leukemia, large erythroblasts with little maturation.

techniques may be required. Variable degrees of fibrosis occur, often in association with clusters of megakaryocytes which include micro, atypical and some typical ones. They react with Factor VIII-related antigen and CD41, and CD61; some are also positive with CD79a, which is a B cell marker.

Acute myelofibrosis (AMF)
(Figure 21.15)

Most cases of acute (or malignant) myelofibrosis/myelosclerosis have now been shown to be acute or subacute leukemias with a dominant fibrotic reaction. In many cases there is a panmyelosis, i.e. involvement of myelo-, erythro- and megakaryocytic cell lines, or a megakaryoblastic or myeloblastic myelosis; these can be distinguished on I.H.

Acute basophilic leukemia

Two types have been distinguished: (1) the typical granules are recognised in the light microscope and (2) electron microscopy is required for their identification.

Acute lymphoblastic leukemia
(Figures 21.16 and 21.17)

L1
Small uniformly sized blasts with scanty cytoplasm, round nucleus with small nucleolus.

L2
Larger irregularly shaped blasts with wider rims of cytoplasm, irregular nuclei with a single, prominent nucleolus.

L3
Large monomorphic blasts with abundant cytoplasm which has small vacuoles, round nuclei with prominent nucleoli.

The marrow is usually hypercellular, with almost complete absence of fat cells. There may also be foci of necrosis. Identification of the blasts is made by enzyme cytochemistry, flow cytometry and/or immunohistology in exceptional cases. Premature anaphase, as seen in the chromosomes of metaphase cells, has been interpreted as a sign of apoptosis (PCD) and proposed as a prognostic indicator in ALL.

Smoldering leukemia

1. A cell line similar to that in acute myeloblastic leukemia may be present in the bone marrow for months or years together with suppression, to a variable extent, of normal hematopoiesis. Clearly, there is a certain amount of overlap between these cases and hypoplastic acute leukemia and some forms of myelodysplastic syndrome, or even aplastic anemia.

2. Smoldering (or subacute or chronic) myelomonocytic leukemia. Though included in the classification of the myelodysplastic syndromes, which are considered to be preleukemic conditions by the FAB group, it would be more logical to classify this condition with the subacute leukemias as it is already an overt leukemia and can be recognised as such in peripheral blood, aspirate smears and in bone marrow histology. The marrow is hypo-, normo-, or hypercellular with preservation of the overall architecture and an interstitial

21.14 (left) BMBS plastic, Giemsa, mixed erythro- and megakaryoblastic leukemia.

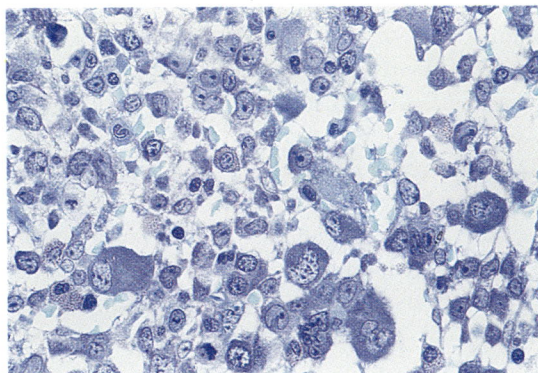

21.15 (right) BMBS plastic, Giemsa, viewed in polarised light, fibrosis in the bone marrow in case of AMF.

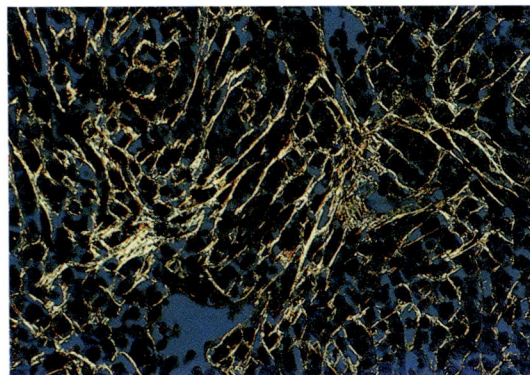

215

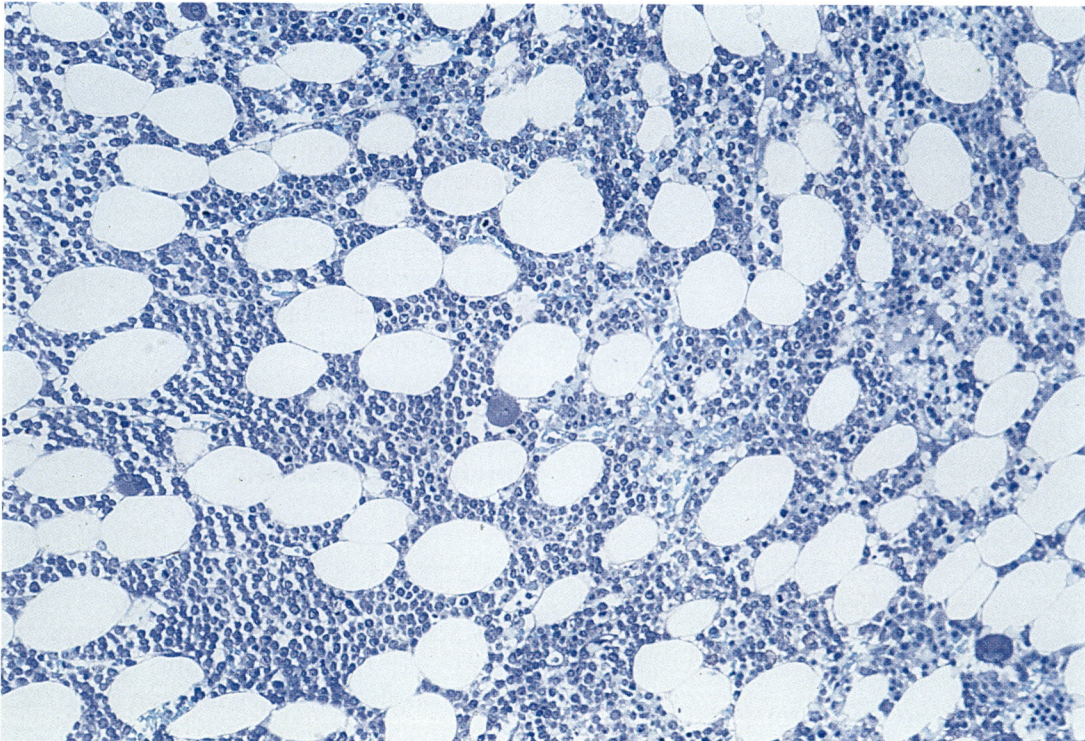

infiltration of monocytoid cells which may constitute 20–40% of the nucleated cell population present. These cells have round-to-oval or kidney-shaped nuclei, resembling those of hairy cells. A T cell lymphoma has been associated with myelomonocytic leukemia.

3. Chronic monocytic leukemia is presumed to be a separate entity as it affects primarily the monocytic cell line. The infiltration consists of a population of pleomorphic monocytic cells larger than hairy cells, without cytoplasmic extensions and more closely packed.

Subacute erythroid disorders

Subacute erythroid disorders, also called di Guglielmo syndrome or early erythroleukemias, are characterised by a hypercellular bone marrow consisting mainly of erythroid precursors, which are pleomorphic from small to gigantic and multinucleated with dyserythropoietic features. Myeloid elements are reduced while in some cases the megakaryocytic cell line is also involved. Erythroleu-

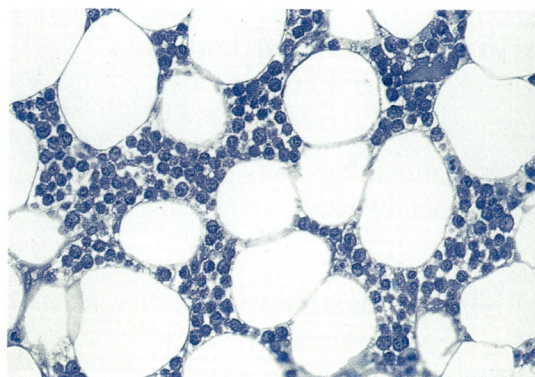

21.16 and 21.17 BMBS plastic, case of ALL low and high power hypo- to normocellular bone marrow extensively infiltrated by blasts.

kemia may also be accompanied by fibrosis. Erythremic myelosis has been observed in lymphoproliferative disorders.

Differential diagnosis of acute leukemia

Lymphadenopathy may be due to infections, to infectious mononucleosis, to a lymphoma. If there is splenomegaly – with or without enlargement of the liver, myelo- and lymphoproliferative disorders – storage or infectious disorders such as leishmaniasis should be considered. When pancytopenia is one of the presenting features aplastic anemia or bone marrow infiltration due to other malignancies may be the cause; in older patients, myelodysplasia.

Significance of bone biopsies in acute leukemia

It should be noted that the value of bone marrow biopsies in the acute, and especially the subacute, leukemias is gaining recognition both for diagnosis and monitoring of therapy. In cases with some degree of cellular differentiation the cells can be identified in the histological sections, and the amount of infiltration and the reactive fibrosis assessed; as well as recognition of areas of necrosis in fast-growing leukemias. Furthermore, in the erythroblastic and promegakaryocytic types a bone biopsy may be necessary for cell line recognition because of a subleukemic peripheral blood picture and a dry tap on aspiration. In treated patients bone marrow regeneration, as well as residual nests of blasts, are more easily recognised in sections than in smears of aspirates, which may not be representative of the proportions of cells left behind in the bone marrow.

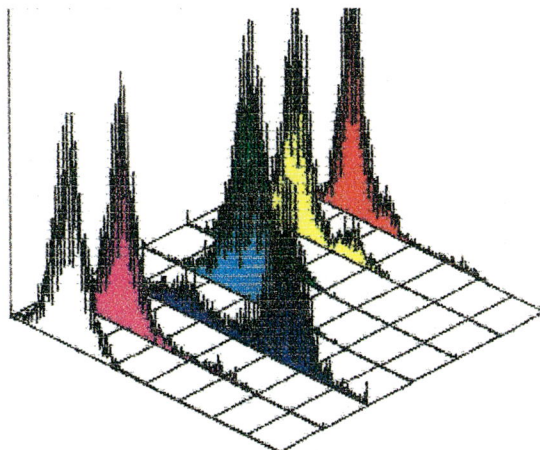

21.18 Histogram of flow cytometry. Left to right: white, control; pink, CD2 8%; dark blue, CD20 81%; light blue, CD19 50%; green, CALLA 6%; yellow, CD33 13%; red, CD14 11%; case of acute lymphoblastic leukemia.

Cell lines and phenotypic determination in the acute and subacute leukemias

As mentioned earlier, the diagnosis of these disorders has traditionally been based on peripheral blood counts and examination of peripheral blood and bone marrow smears which constitute the basis of the internationally recognised FAB classification of the acute leukemias. Blasts are recognised by their morphology, high nucleocytoplasmic ratio and the finer details of their nuclear structure and nucleoli. Leukemic blasts are assigned to a particular cell line by means of cytochemistry, electron microscopy, immunological and enzymatic studies. However, some of these investigations cannot be directly applied to bone marrow histology, though some may be performed on cryostat sections of fresh–frozen, unfixed bone biopsies. Studies for determination of phenotype are required, especially when the infiltration consists of very early undifferentiated precursors (Figure 21.18). In some cases malignant histiocytosis, malignant lymphomas and carcinomas must also be excluded. In children especially, osteosarcoma, Ewing's sarcoma, rhabdomyosarcoma, neuroblastoma, medulloblastoma and retinoblastoma have a tendency to involve the bone marrow. Moreover, leukemic blasts may sometimes show reactivity with non-hematopoietic antigens, but this does not exclude an acute leukemia. Conversely, increased hematogones (early lymphoid precursors) may be preferentially aspirated if bone marrow fibrosis is present, and possibly suggest an erroneous diagnosis of acute leukemia. In addition, such investigations have shown that more than one line may be involved, or that cells may possess characteristics of more than one cell-type: biphenotypic leukemias. This situation is readily clarified by the findings on bone marrow biopsy. When a dry tap occurs on attempts at aspiration in the acute leukemias the tests normally carried out on smears of aspirate can be made on imprints of the biopsy (enabling application of some of the FAB criteria for classification). Criteria for the acute leukemias of the individual cell lines as well as the mixed have been established.

Perspectives for the not-too-distant future

There has been accumulating criticism of the FAB classification of the acute leukemias, mainly because it was originally (and still is) based on morphologic criteria, which are subjective, depend on various technical factors and are open to different interpretations as well as practical difficulties. For example, there are differences in the way aspirates are taken that may influence the proportions of blasts and other cells in the cell counts and the aspirate smears. There are variations in cellularity (alternating cellular and fatty areas in the bone marrow) with different populations of cells, and this also influences the blast counts in the aspirates. Not only cellularity but also stromal factors – such as uneven increases in fibers, preventing egress of cells during aspiration – influences the blast counts in both peripheral blood and in smears of aspirates. Hence, an adequate biopsy is required to circumvent these obstacles and to present a more representative picture of the true state of the bone marrow. There are also some special situations in which mistakes are more likely to happen. For example, a blast count of up to 20% in a patient known to have myelofibrosis (MF) does not necessarily indicate transformation to an acute leukemia. In MF there is greatly disturbed bone marrow structure, as well as considerable stromal alterations which enable immature cells to leave the marrow; in addition, perhaps there is extramedullary hematopoiesis that is not subject to the intramedullary controlling mechanisms. A marrow aspirate taken from a site adjacent to an area of involvement by a nodular lymphoma within a network of fibers may show a preponderance of myeloid precursors, extracted from the areas between the nodules, so that again, erroneously, a diagnosis of a myeloid condition is suspected until the bone biopsy sections reveal the underlying pathology. Furthermore, FACS analysis of bone marrow aspirates in cases of involvement by lymphomas frequently does not reflect the lymphoma, and the values for B and T cells fall in the normal range simply because the lymphomatous infiltration is not aspirated into the syringe but remains in the marrow. Moreover, there are additional problems involved in attempting to correlate the expression of cell characteristics (immunophenotype) with the FAB classification since these were not considered (or were unknown) at the time this system was proposed, thus inevitably discrepancies may occur when the immunophenotype contradicts the morphologic diagnosis.

With the advent of the next millennium, there is no doubt that drastic revisions or new classifications will be introduced based on the new knowledge and insights acquired in immunology, cytogenetics and molecular biology, and thus on the pathogenesis of many of the clinical manifestations of the hematologic malignancies. Indeed, new classifications have already been proposed, see in particular Eikelboom et al. (1996). A case in point is CML in which the reciprocal translocation t(9;22)(q34;q11) results in the formation of two hybrid genes, one on each chromosome. The BCR-ABL fusion gene on chromosome 22 encodes a fusion protein with elevated tyrosine kinase and transforming activities, which in return are responsible for the phenotype of CML, and are central to the mechanism controlling the chronic phase of the disease. The breakpoint in the ABL gene can occur at different sites, and therefore there may be different amounts of BCR sequences in the BCR-ABL gene – and this has clinical consequences. The classical Ph+ CML phenotype derived from a p210 type of BCR-ABL fusion results in expansion of the granulocytic and megakaryocytic cell lines. Moreover, the data published so far suggest three (possibly more) entities depending on the fusion protein produced by the different BCR breakpoints: p210 CML; p190 CML and p230 CML, each with characteristic, but different hematologic manifestations. Quite possibly also new avenues of approach to therapy will involve antibodies targeted against the aberrant proteins produced by the fusion genes, when these are functional (which may not always turn out to be the case). In a

21.19 (left) Karyotype of a patient with AML, M2 showing 47, XY +4.

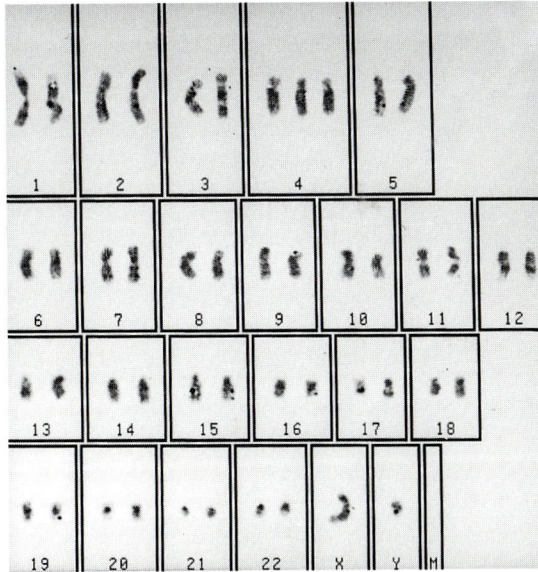

21.20 (right) Karyotype of a patient with AML, M4 showing t(3;5).

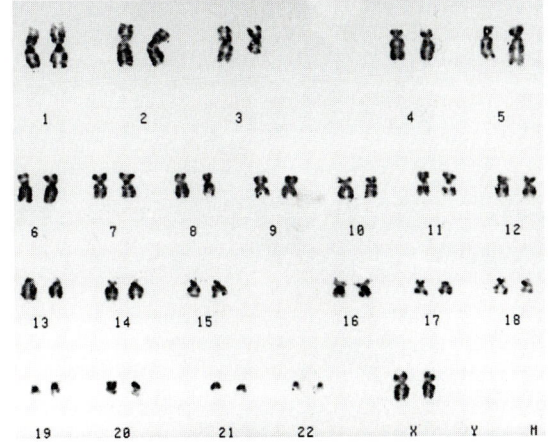

21.21 (left) Metaphase spread showing marker chromosome, bottom right, in case of acute leukemia. The origin of such chromosomes could be investigated by means of the FISH technique.

21.22 (right) Histogram of flow cytometry of patient with acute lymphoblastic leukemia, B cell. Left to right: red, control; gray, CD7; green, CD2; brown, CD19; blue, CD20; dark green, CD10; gray, CD34.

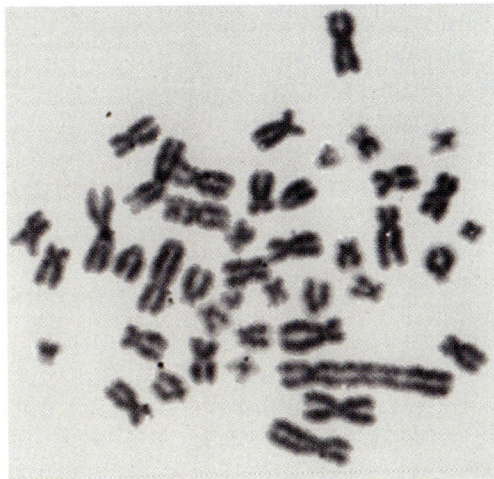

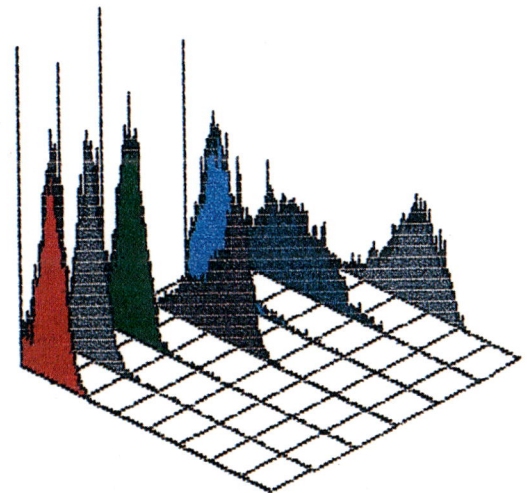

recent survey of 2500 patients, 130 breakpoints were involved in structural rearrangements in myeloid malignancies, of which only 16 were considered as primary as they were detected in more than five cases. Examples of representative karyotypes and histograms of flow cytometry are given in Figures 21.18–21.22.

Check list: Acute Leukemias

- Adequate biopsy?

- Cellularity – degree and uniformity?

- Infiltration – monomorphic, extent, topography?

- Precursors with or without indications of maturation and differentiation?

- Necrosis?

- Identification – if possible on morphology? I.H. appropriate antibodies according to suspected cell line.

- Residual normal hematopoiesis – which cell lines, how much, and where? I.H.: Factor VIII, myeloid and erythroid markers to identify normal cells within the infiltration.

- Stromal reactions: atrophy, fibrosis, osteoblastic or osteolytic reactions?

Clinical correlations

- May present as influenza-like disease.

- Anemia, fatigue, cardiac symptoms, pallor, dyspnea.

- Bleeding and infections.

- Bone pain – periosteal infiltration and/or expansion of marrow cavity.

- Meningeal infiltration: headache, nausea.

- Characteristic features in different types, for example: acute promyelocytic, disseminated intravascular coagulation (DIC); AMML, extramedullary involvement; T-ALL mediastinal masses; monocytic, swelling of gums.

- Correlation with peripheral blood values, FACS and cytochemistry of peripheral blood cells and bone marrow aspirates?

Clonal chromosomal characteristics

MO	M1	M2
−5	t(9;22)(q34;q11)	t(8;21)(q22;q22)
del(5)(q)	ins(3;3)(q26;q21q26)	t(6;9)(p23;q34)
−7	inv(3)(q21q26)	t(3;5)(q21–25;q31–34)
del(7)(q)	t(3;3)(q21;26)	t(7;11)(p14;p15)
+13	del(9)(q)	+4 (see Figure 21.19)
	+4	

M3	M4	M4 eos
M3(v)	+4	inv(16)(p13q22)
t(15;17)(q22;q11–21)	t(1;7)(p11;p11)	t(16;16)(p13;q22)
t(11;17)(q23;q11–21)	t(10;11)(p11;q23)	del(16)(q22)
	del/t(11)(q)	
	t(9;11)(p21–22;q23)	
	t(3;5)(q21–25;q31–34) (see Figure 21.20)	
	t(6;9)(p23;q34) with basophilia	

M5	M5a	M5b
del/t(11)(q23)	t(6;11)(q27;q23)	t(8;16)(p11;p13)
t(8;16)(p11;q13)	t(9;11)(p21–22;q23)	
t(11;17)(q23;q11–22)		
t(11;19)(q23;p13)		

Continued

M6
del(20)(q)
−5
−7
del(5)(q)
del(7)(q)
mar (see Figure 21.22)

M7
t(1;22)(p13;q13)
ins(3;3)(q26;q21q26)
t(3;3)(q21;q26)
t(16;21)(p11;q22)

Characteristics of AML (but also seen in other myeloid disorders)

+6	+19	del(5)(q)	del(11)(q)
+8	+21	del(7)(q)	del(20)(q)
+9	+22	del(9)(q)	i(17)(q)
+11	−X		
+13	−Y		

AML with/without atypical thrombocytes
t(3;3)(q21;q26)
inv(3;3)(q21/q26)
t(1;3)(p36;q21)
ins(5;3)(q14;q21q26)

Biphenotypic acute leukemia
t(4;11)(q21;q23)

Acute lymphoblastic leukemia

L1 or L2	Early B-precursor ALL	t(4;11)(q21;q23)	
		t(11;19)(q23;p13)	
		t(9;22)(q34;q11)	
L1 or L2	Common ALL	t(1;11)(q32;q23)	i(6)(p)
		t(9;22)(q34;q11)	i(7)(q)
		t(11;19)(q23;p13)	del(9)(p)
		t/del(12)(p11–p13)	i(9)(q)
		del(6)(q)	i(17)(q)
L1 or L2	Pre-B ALL	t(1;11)(p32;q23)	
		t(1;19)(q23;p13)	
		t(9;22)(q34;q11)	
		del(6)(q)	
		dic(7;9)(p11;p11)	
		also Burkitt's associated translocation	
L3	B ALL	t(2;8)(p12;q24)	
		t(8;14)(q24;q32)	
		t(8;22)(q24;q11)	
		dup(1)(q12–q31)	
		del(6)(q)	
L1 or L2	Early T ALL	t(1;14)(p32;q11)	
		t(7;9)(q35;q34)	
		t(7;19)(q35;p13)	
		t(8;14)(q24;q11)	
		del(9)(p13–22)	

Continued

L1 or L2	Common mature T ALL	t(11;14)(p13;q11)
		t(10;14)(q24;q11)
		t(9;17)(q34;q23)
		inv(14)(q11–q32)
		t/del(9)(q)
		t/del(14q11)
		inv/i(9)(q)
		t/del(12)(p11–p13)
		del(6)(q)

Bibliography

Abe R., Shiga Y., Uchida T., Kariyone S. (1989) Chromosome abnormalities in acute leukemia: its clinical implications and age of onset. *Indian J. Pediatr.,* **56 (6),** 719–31.

Akopian G.R., Sirenko A.G., Hulejuk N. *et al.* (1997) Premature anaphases as a possible cytogenetic indicator of apoptosis. *Cytogenet Cell Genet.,* **77,** 127.

Amadori S., Venditti A., Del Poeta G. *et al.* (1996) Minimally differentiated acute myeloid leukemia (AML-M0): a distinct clinico-biologic entity with poor prognosis. *Ann Hematol,* **72 (4),** 208–15.

Amberger D.M., Saleem A., Kemp B.L., Truong L.D. (1990) Acute myelofibrosis – a leukemia of pluripotent stem cell. A report of three cases and review of the literature. *Ann. Clin. Lab. Scie.,* **20 (6),** 409–14.

Arber D.A., Jenkins K.A. (1996) Paraffin section immunophenotyping of acute leukemias in bone marrow specimens. *Am J Surg.,* **106 (4),** 462–8.

Barnard D.R., Kalousek D.K., Wiersma S.R. *et al.* (1996) Morphologic, immunologic, and cytogenetic classification of acute myeloid leukemia and myelodysplastic syndrome in childhood: a report from the Childrens Cancer Group. *Leukemia,* **10 (1),** 5–12.

Baty J.M., Vogt E.C. (1935) Bone changes of leukemia in children. *Amer J Roentgenol.,* **34,** 310.

Beverloo H.B., Le Coniat M., Wijsman J. *et al.* (1995) Breakpoint heterogeneity in t(10;11) translocation in AML-M4/M5 resulting in fusion of AF10 and MLL is resolved by fluorescent in situ hybridization analysis. *Cancer Res.,* **55,** 4220–4.

Beverstock G.C., de Meijer P.H., ten Bokkel Huinink D. *et al.* A case of isodicentric 7p as sole abnormality in a patient with acute myeloid leukemia. *Cancer Genet Cytogenet.,* **89 (2),** 132–5.

Billstrom R., Heim S., Kristoffersson U. *et al.* (1990) Structural chromosomal abnormalities of 3q in myelodysplastic syndrome/acute myeloid leukemia with Sweet's syndrome. *Eur. J. Hematol.,* **45 (3),** 150–2.

Bloomfield C.D., de la Chapelle A. (1987) Chromosome abnormalities in acute nonlymphocytic leukemia: clinical and biologic significance. *Semin. Oncol.,* **14 (4),** 372–83.

Borowitz M.J., Guenther K.L., Shults K.E., Stelzer G.T. (1993) Immunophenotyping of acute leukemia by flow cytometric analysis: use of CD45 and right-angle light scatter to gate on leukemic blasts in three-color analysis. *Am. J. Clin. Pathol.,* **100 (5),** 534–40.

Braylan R.C. (1993) Acute Leukemias. In *Clinical Flow Cytometry.* Baltimore: Williams & Williams.

Brito-Babapulle V., Crawford A., Khokhar T. *et al.* (1991) Translocations T(14;18) with rearranged BCL-2 and C-MYC in a case presenting as B-ALL (L3). *Leukemia,* **5 (1),** 83–7.

Buccheri V., Matutes E., Dyer M.J. *et al.* (1993) Lineage commitment in biphenotypic acute leukemia. *Leukemia,* **7,** 919.

Bullorsky E.O., Shanley C.M., Stemmelin G. *et al.* (1990) Acute megakaryoblastic leukemia with massive myelofibrosis: complete remission and reversal of marrow fibrosis with allogeneic bone marrow transplantation as the only treatment. *Bone Marrow Transplant.*, 6 (6), 449–52.

Carbonell F., Swansbury J., Min T. *et al.* (1996) Cytogenetic findings in acute biphenotypic leukaemia. *Leukemia*, 10 (8), 1283–7.

Chessells J.M., Swansbury G.J., Reeves R. *et al.* (1997) Cytogenetics and prognosis in childhood lymphoblastic leukaemia: results of MRC UKALL X. *Br. J. Haematol.*, 99, 93–100.

Cohn S.L., Morgan E.R., Mallette L.E. (1987) The spectrum of metabolic bone disease in lymphoblastic leukemia. *Cancer*, 59, 346.

Cortes J.E., Kantarjian H., O'Brien S. *et al.* (1995) Clinical and prognostic significance of trisomy 21 in adult patients with acute myelogenous leukemia and myelodysplastic syndromes. *Leukemia*, 9 (1), 115–17.

Cuneo A., Ferrant A., Michaux J.L. *et al.* (1995) Cytogenetic profile of minimally differentiated (FAB M0) acute myeloid leukemia: correlation with clinicobiologic findings. *Blood*, 85 (12), 3688–94.

Cuneo A., Ferrant A., Michaux J.L. *et al.* (1996) Cytogenetic and clinicobiological features of acute leukemia with stem cell phenotype: study of nine cases. *Cancer Genet Cytogenet*, 92 (1), 31–6.

Cuneo A., Ferrant A., Michaux J.L. *et al.* (1996) Philadelphia chromosome-positive acute myeloid leukemia: cytoimmunologic and cytogenetic features. *Haematologica*, 81 (5), 423–7.

Cuneo A., Kerim S., Vandenberghe E. *et al.* (1989) Translocation t(6;9) occurring in acute myelofibrosis, myelodysplastic syndrome, and acute nonlymphocytic leukemia suggests multipotent stem cell involvement. *Cancer Genet. Cytogenet.*, 42 (2), 209–19.

Dokal I., Rule S., Chen F. *et al.* (1997) Adult onset of acute myeloid leukaemia (M6) in patients with Shwachman–Diamond syndrome. *Br. J. Haematol.*, 99, 171–3.

Dreyling M.H., Bohlander S.K., Le Beau M.M., Olopade O.I. (1995) Refined mapping of genomic rearrangements involving the short arm of chromosome 9 in acute lymphoblastic leukemias and other hematologic malignancies. *Blood*, 86 (50), 1931–8.

Eikelboom J., Cull G., Erber W. (1996) Time for a new acute myeloid leukaemia classification? *Br J Haematol.*, 92, 247–9

Fleischmann E.W., Volkova M.A., Frenkel M.A. *et al.* (1996) Translocation (2;3)(p13;q26) in two cases of myeloid malignancies. Acute myeloblastic leukemia (M2) and blastic phase of chronic myeloid leukemia. *Cancer Genet Cytogenet*, 87 (2), 182–4.

Gahn B., Haase D., Unterhalt M. *et al.* (1996) De novo AML with dysplastic hematopoiesis: cytogenetic and prognostic significance. *Leukemia*, 10 (6), 946–51.

Gallagher D., Heinrich S.D., Craver R. *et al.* (1991) Skeletal manifestations of acute leukemia in childhood. *Orthopedics*, 14, 485.

General Haematology Task Force of BCSH (1994) Immunophenotyping in the diagnosis of acute leukaemias. *J Clin Pathol*, 47, 777–81.

Grimwade D., Howe K., Langabeer S. *et al.* (1996) Establishing the presence of the t(15;17) in suspected acute promyelocytic leukaemia: cytogenetic, molecular and PML immunofluorescence assessment of patients entered into the M.R.C. ATRA trial. M.R.C. Adult Leukaemia Working Party. *Br J Haematol.*, 94 (3), 557–73.

Haase D., Feuring-Buske M., Schafer C. *et al.* (1997) Cytogenetic analysis of CD34+ subpopulations in AML and MDS characterized by the expression of CD38 and CD117. *Leukemia*, 11 (5), 674–9.

Haferlach T. (1996) More individual markers are necessary for patients with acute myeloid leukemia (AML). Does cytomorphology or cytogenetics define the biological entity? *Leukemia*, 10 (3), S5–9.

Harrington D.S., Peterson C., Ness M. *et al.* (1988) Acute myelogenous leukemia with eosinophilic differentiation and Trisomy 1. *Am. J. Clin. Pathol.*, 90 (4), 464–9.

Head D.R. (1996) Revised classification of acute myeloid leukemia. *Leukemia*, 10 (11), 1826–31.

Head D.R., Behm F.G. (1995) Acute lymphoblastic leukemia and the lymphoblastic lymphomas of childhood. *Semin Diagn Pathol.*, 12 (4), 325–34.

Helleberg C., Knudsen H., Hansen P.B. *et al.* (1997) CD34+ megakaryoblastic leukaemic cells are CD38−, but CD61+ and glycophorin-improved criteria for diagnosis of AML-M7? *Leukemia* 11 (6), 830–4.

Hiorns L.R., Swanbury G.J., Mehta J. *et al.* (1997) Additional chromosome abnormalities confer worse prognosis in acute promyelocytic leukaemia. *Br J Haematol.*, 96, 314–21.

Ingram L., Raimondi S.C., Mirro J. Jr. *et al.* (1989) Characteristics of Trisomy 11 in childhood acute leukemia with review of the literature. *Leukemia*, 3 (10), 695–8.

Islam A. (1993) Proposal for a classification of acute myeloid leukemia based on plastic-embedded bone marrow biopsy sections. *Leuk Res*, 17 (5), 421–7.

Islam A., Frisch B., Henderson E.S. (1989) Plastic embedded core biopsy: a complementary approach to bone marrow aspiration for diagnosing acute myeloid leukemia. *J Clin Pathol*, 42 (3), 300–6.

Janossy G., Campana D. (1991) Monoclonal antibodies in the diagnosis of acute leukemia. *The Leukemic Cell*, 2, 168–95.

Kanter-Lewensohn L., Hellstrom-Lindberg E., Kock Y. *et al.* (1996) Analysis of CD34-

positive cells in bone marrow from patients with myelodysplastic syndromes and acute myeloid leukemia and in normal individuals: a comparison between FACS analysis and immunohistochemistry. *Eur J Haematol.*, **56** (3), 124–9.

Katz F., Webb D., Gibbons B. *et al.* (1992) Possible evidence for genomic imprinting in childhood acute myeloblastic leukemia associated with monosomy for chromosome 7. *Br. J. Hematol.*, **80** (3), 332–6.

Knuutila S. (1997) Review: Lineage specificity in haematological neoplasms. *Br J Haematol.*, **96**, 2–11.

Kramer M.H., Raghoebier S., Beverstock G.O. *et al.* (1991) De Novo acute B-cell leukemia with translocation T(14;18): an entity with a poor prognosis. *Leukemia*, **5** (6), 473–8.

Lacombe F., Belloc F., Bernard P. *et al.* (1988) Cytogenetic study of cell sub-populations in human leukemias (AML, CML) sorted by flow cytometry. *Pathol. Biol. (Paris)*, **36** (1), 42–5.

Lampert F., Harbott J., Ritterbach J. (1992) Cytogenetic findings in acute leukaemias of infants. *Br J Cancer*, **18** (Suppl.), S20–2.

Lands R., Karnad A. (1991) Non T-cell lymphoblastic lymphoma with extensive osteolytic lesions and hypercalcemia. *South Med J.*, **84**, 1405.

Lee E.J., Schiffer C.A., Tomiyasu T., Testa J.R. (1990) Clinical and cytogenetic correlations of abnormal megakaryocytopoiesis in patients with acute leukemia and chronic myelogenous leukemia in blast crisis. *Leukemia*, **4** (5), 350–3.

Lewis S.M., Szur L. (1963) Malignant myelosclerosis. *Br. Med. J.*, **2**, 472–7.

Liesner R.J., Goldstone A.H. (1997) ABC of clinical haematology: The acute leukaemias. *BMJ*, **314**, 733–6.

Lim S.H., Culligan D., Couzens S. *et al.* (1996) Milecular evidence for a common leukaemic progenitor in acute mixed

lymphoid and myeloid leukaemia. *Br J Haematol.*, **92** (1), 131–3.

Machnicki J.L., Bloomfield C.D. (1990) Chromosomal abnormalities in myelodysplastic syndromes and acute myeloid leukemia. *Clin. Lab. Med.*, **10** (4), 755–67.

Marino G.G. (1989) Acute myelofibrosis: report of a case and review of current literature. *J A Osteopath Assoc.*, **89** (10), 1323–6.

Martin P.L., Look A.T., Schnell S. *et al.* (1996) Comparison of fluorescence in situ hybridization, cytogenetic analysis, and DNA index analysis to detect chromosomes 4 and 10 aneuploidy in pediatric acute lymphoblastic leukemia: a Pediatric Oncology Group Study. *J Pediatr Hematol Oncol*, **18** (2), 113–21.

Matutes E., Morilla R., Farahat N. *et al.* (1997) Definition of acute biphenotypic leukemia. *Haematologica* **82** (1), 64–6.

Mezger J., Permanetter W., Gerhartz H. *et al.* (1990) Philadelphia chromosome-negative acute haematopoietic malignancy: ultrastructural, cytochemical and immunocytochemical evidence of mast cell and basophil differentiation. *Leuk Res.*, **14** (2), 169–75.

Mijovic A., Rolovic Z., Novak A. *et al.* (1989) Chronic myeloid leukemia associated with pure red cells aplasia and terminating in promyelocytic transformation. *Am. J. Hematol.*, **31** (2), 128–30.

Minden M., Imrie K., Keating A. (1996) Acute leukemia in adults. *Current Opinion in Hematol*, **3** (4), 259–65.

Morgan D.L., Dunn D.M., Cobos E. *et al.* (1996) Translocation t(15;27) in acute myelogenous leukemia with atypical megakaryoblastic features: diagnostic, clinical, and therapeutic implications. *Cancer Genet Cytogenet.*, **92** (1), 50–3.

Nagai K., Kohno T., Chen Y.X. *et al.* (1996) Diagnostic criteria for hypocellular acute

leukemia: a clinical entity distinct from overt acute leukemia and myelodysplastic syndrome. *Leuk Res*, **20** (7), 563–74.

Nowak R., Oelschlaegel U., Schuler U. *et al.* (1997) Sensitivity of combined DNA/immunophenotype flow cytometry for the detection of low levels of aneuploid lymphoblastic leukemia cells in bone marrow. *Cytometry*, **30**(1), 47–53.

Ohyashiki K., Kodama A., Nakamura H. *et al.* (1996) Trisomy 10 in acute myeloid leukemia. *Cancer Genet Cytogenet.*, **89** (2), 114–17.

Olopade O.I., Thangavelu M., Larson R.A. *et al.* (1992) Clinical, morphologic, and cytogenetic characteristics of 26 patients with acute erythroblastic leukemia. *Blood*, **80** (11), 2873–82.

Partridge F., Richardson W., Kearns P. *et al.* (1996) Marked bone marrow eosinophilia at the time of relapse of acute myeloblastic leukaemia in association with the appearance of translocation t(12;20)(924;q11). *Leuk Lymphoma.*, **22** (1–2), 181–2.

Pui C.H. (1996) Acute leukemia in children. *Current Opinion in Hematol*, **3** (4), 249–58.

Pui C.H., Raimondi S.C., Head D.R. *et al.* (1991) Characterization of childhood acute leukemia with multiple myeloid and lymphoid markers at diagnosis and relapse. *Blood*, **78**, 1327.

Reading C.L., Estey E.H., Huh Y.O. *et al.* (1993) Expression of unusual immuno-phenotype combinations in acute myelogenous leukemia. *Blood*, **81**, 3083.

Richard G., Brody J., Sun T. (1993) A case of acute megakaryocytic leukemia with hematogones. *Leukemia*, **7** (11), 1900–3.

Roos R., Sol F., Montes C. *et al.* (1995) A new case of trisomy 5 as sole cytogenetic anomaly in acute myeloid leukemia. *Cancer Genet Cytogenet.*, **84** (2), 120–2.

Rothe G., Schmitz G. (1996) Consensus protocol for the flow cytometric immunophenotyping of hematopoietic malignancies. *Leukemia*, **10**, 877–95.

Rousselet M.C., Laniece A., Gardais J. *et al.* (1995) Immunohistochemical characterization of acute leukemia. *Ann Pathol*, **15 (2)**, 119–26.

Rubnitz J.E., Shuster J.J., Shuster L. *et al.* (1997) Case-control study suggests a favorable impact of *TEL* rearrangement in patients with B-lineage acute lymphoblastic leukemia treated with antimetabolite-based therapy: A Pediatric Oncology Group Study. *Blood*, **89 (4)**, 1143–6.

Ruck P., Horny H.P., Greschniok A. *et al.* (1995) Nonspecific immunostaining of blast cells of acute leukemia by antibodies against nonhemopoietic antigens. *Hematol Pathol*, **9 (1)**, 49–56.

Sanz M.A., Sempere A. (1996) Immuno-phenotyping of AML and MDS and detection of residual disease. *Baillière's Clin Haematol.*, **9 (1)**, 35–55.

Scott C.S., den Ottolander G.J., Swirsky D. *et al.* (1993) Recommended procedures for the classification of acute leukaemias. *Leuk and Lymph*, **2**, 37–50.

Secco C., Wiernik P.H., Bennett J.M., Paietta E. (1996) Acute leukemia with t(10;11)(p11–p15;q13–q23). *Cancer Genet Cytogenet*, **86 (1)**, 31–4.

Secker-Walker L.M., Mehta A., Bain B. (1995) Abnormalities of 3q21 and 3q26 in myeloid malignancy: a United Kingdom Cancer Cytogenetic Group study. *Br J Haematol*, **91 (2)**, 490–501.

Secker-Walker L.M. (1990) Prognostic and biological importance of chromosome findings in acute lymphoblastic leukemia. *Cancer Genet. Cytogenet.*, **49 (1)**, 1–13.

Shurtleff S.A., Buijs A., Behm F.G. *et al.* (1995) TEL/AML 1 fusion from a cryptic

t(12;21) is the most common genetic lesion in pediatric ALL and defines a subgroup of patients with an excellent prognosis. *Leukemia*, **9 (12)**, 1985–9.

Silverman F.N. (1948) Skeletal lesions in leukemia: clinical and roentgenographic observations in 103 infants and children with review of the literature. *Amer J Radiol.*, **59**, 819.

Sun G., Wormsley S., Sparkes R.S. *et al.* (1991) Hybrid leukemia and the 5q-abnormality. *Leuk. Res.*, **15 (5)**, 351–6.

Taguchi H., Morishita N., Murakami K. *et al.* (1996) Biphenotypic leukemia with a new translocation, t(2;6)(q31;q23). *Cancer Genet Cytogenet.*, **91 (2)**, 104–5.

Takeshita A., Shinjo K., Ohnishi K., Ohno R. (1996) Expression of multidrug resistance P-glycoprotein in myeloid progenitor cells of different phenotype: comparison between normal bone marrow cells and leukemia cells. *Br J Haematol*, **93 (1)**, 18–21.

Taubenberger J.K., Cole D.E., Raffeld M. *et al.* (1991) Immunophenotypic analysis of acute lymphoblastic leukemia using routinely processed bone marrow specimens. *Arch. Pathol. Lab. Med.*, **115 (4)**, 338–42.

Taylor C.G., Stasi R., Bastianelli C. *et al.* (1996) Diagnosis and classification of the acute leukemias: recent advances and controversial issues. *Hematopathol Mol Hematol*, **10 (1–2)**, 1–38.

Terstappen L.W., Loken M.R. (1990) Myeloid cell differentiation in normal bone marrow and acute myeloid leukemia assessed by multi-dimensional flow cytometry. *Anal. Cell Pathol.*, **2 (4)**, 229–40.

Terstappen L.W., Konemann S., Safford M. *et al.* (1991) Flow cytometric characterization of acute myeloid leukemia. Part 1 – Significance of light scattering properties. *Leukemia*, **5 (4)**, 315–21.

Thomas L.B., Forkner C.E., Frei E. *et al.* (1961) Skeletal lesions of acute leukaemia. *Cancer*, **14**, 608.

Traweek S.T. (1993) Immunophenotypic analysis of acute leukemia. *Am J Clin Pathol.*, **99**, 504.

Trueworthy R., Shuster J., Look T. *et al.* (1992) Ploidy of lymphoblasts is the strongest predictor of treatment outcome in B-progenitor cell acute lymphoblastic leukemia of childhood: a Pediatric Oncology Study Group study. *J Clin Oncol.*, **10**, 606.

Truong L.D., Saleem A., Schwartz M.R. (1984) Acute myelofibrosis. A report of four cases and review of the literature. *Medicine*, **63**, 182–7.

Van Lom K., Hagemeijer A., Vandekerckhove F. *et al.* (1996) Cytogenetic clonality analysis: typical patterns in myelodysplastic syndrome and acute myeloid leukaemia. *Br J Haematol.*, **93**, 594–600.

Vassilopoulou-Sellin R., Ramirez I. (1992) Severe osteopenia and vertebral compression fractures after complete remission in an adolescent with acute leukemia. *Amer J. Hematol.*, **39**, 142.

Velloso E.R.P., Michaux L., Ferrant A. *et al.* (1996) Deletions of the long arm of chromosome 7 in myeloid disorders: loss of band 7q32 implies worst prognosis. *Br J Haematol.*, **92**, 574–81.

Venditti A., Del Poeta G., Buccisano F. *et al.* (1997) Minimally differentiated acute myeloid leukemia (AML-M0): comparison of 25 cases with other French-American-British subtypes. *Blood*, **89 (2)**, 621–9.

Zhang Y., Poetsch M., Weber-Matthiesen K. *et al.* (1996) Secondary acute leukaemias with 11q23 rearrangement: clinical, cytogenetic, FISH and FICTION studies. *Br J Haematol*, **92 (3)**, 673–80.

22 Chronic myeloproliferative disorders

General aspects and pathogenesis

Myeloproliferative disorders (MPD) include the disorders listed in Table 22.1 as well as the variant, transitional and intermediate forms. The MPD are hematological neoplasias of clonal origin of pluripotent stem cells as shown by glucose 6-phosphate dehydrogenase determination and by molecular biology. As such they are primary disorders of the bone marrow. It is of interest that the erythrocytic, granulocytic, megakaryocytic and lymphocytic cell lines have all been identified as belonging to abnormal clones in the MPD, but no entity has yet been described with proliferation or involvement of the osteoclast, though it is thought also to be derived from the hematopoietic pluripotent stem cell, via the monocytic series. Though leukemic transformation represents clonal evolution from a neoplastic stem cell, it is capable in the MPD (for variable periods) of producing differentiated progeny with a consequent 'cytosis' in the peripheral blood – this over-production may be due to an increased sensitivity to interleukin 3 (IL-3) and defective feed-back mechanisms. In spite of this, the clone is inherently unstable and susceptible to maturation disturbances. Transformations to a blastic crisis or to myelofibrosis or osteomyelosclerosis (MF/OMS) have been documented in all the cMPD. Initially, at least, there are no unequivocal histological characteristics that distinguish the cMPD from their normal counterparts in the bone marrow; the megakaryocytes constitute an exception: the giant forms, nuclear configurations, and clustering characteristic of the cMPD are not typical features of the reactive conditions. The cMPD are characterised by anomalies in growth which result in a steadily increasing number of hematopoietic cells in the absence of an appropriate stimulus. In most cases the bone marrow is infiltrated diffusely and extensively so that a considerable tumor burden has accumulated before the disorder is diagnosed. Moreover, a 'normal' marrow cellularity may represent an increase in a previously hypocellular area, and does not exclude an MPD when other indications are present. Nevertheless, the overall histological pattern is almost invariably altered, and thereby permits reliable interpretation and diagnosis. Experience with a large number of biopsies in the MPD has shown that if the bone marrow histology does not appear to reflect a clinically evident cMPD in the first biopsy, it will do so subsequently. In the evaluation of the histological features of the bone marrow in patients with cMPD the values given in Table 4.1 (Chapter 4) serve as base lines for the estimation of increases or decreases in the parameters investigated. As the bone marrow is the source of myeloid cells, a bone marrow biopsy should be included in the investigation of all patients with MPD, and not only when a dry tap is obtained. Moreover, as far as polycythemia vera (PV) and its transformation is concerned, the criteria of the PV Study Group cannot always be met. Consequently, early, borderline, variant and transitional cases may be excluded from consideration in therapeutic protocols, comparative studies and clinical trials. The PV Study Group has recommended that a bone biopsy be taken at diagnosis and once annually thereafter.

Histologic criteria for cMPD

Histological recognition and classification is accomplished by means of three criteria: recognition of the predominant proliferative cell line(s), the degree of its (their) differentiation and the connective tissue reaction: reticulin and collagenous fibers, new bone formation with the accompanying vascular proliferation and frequently inflammatory infiltrations and lymphocytic nodules. Identification of a cell line as proliferative takes into consideration cytological, histological and histotopographical criteria. This classification by means of clearly defined characteristics enables categorisation of bone marrow biopsies of most patients who may therefore be assigned (in some cases tentatively or temporarily) to a clinical entity (Tables 22.1 and 22.2). This histological evaluation has yielded five main groups. It should be emphasised that these groups are not sharply divided; they overlap, and the position of any particular case within the groups will depend, at least to some extent, on the criteria of the investigator. The same holds true for the division of the major entities into subgroups. Moreover, a special requisite of a histological classification of the MPD is that it incorporates the possibility of indicating the subsequent course of the disease; these considerations underline the fact that a single biopsy represents only an instance in a constantly evolving process which may move in any one of several directions. Concurrent occurrence of myelo- and lymphoproliferative disorders also occurs: or a lymphoproliferative disorder may be superimposed on a pre-existing, usually chronic, myeloproliferative disorder.

Polycythemia vera (PV)

PV study group criteria
Major Criteria:
Increased red cell blood volume.
Normal arterial oxygen tension.
Splenomegaly.

TABLE 22.1 Histologic classification of MPD according to the proliferative cell line(s)

Proliferative cells lines	Clinical entities	Frequency (%)	Median survival (months)	Lymphoid nodules (%)	Metamorph.
ERY — —	PV	2	115	2	–
ERY GRA —	PV	3	99	3	–
ERY — MEG	PV	21	84	28	MF/OMS
ERY GRA MEG	PV	22	79	29	MF/OMS
— — MEG	IT	7	82	20	MF/OMS
— GRA MEG	CML	27	35	18	MF/OMS
— GRA —	CML	18	26	4	blast crisis

TABLE 22.2 Megakaryocytic hyper-plasia – Differential diagnosis

1. MPD – PV, CML, ET
2. LPD – HD
3. MDS – Sideroblastic, Refractory Anemia
4. Hemolysis
5. Tumors – metastases
6. Werlhof – Idiopathic Thrombocytopenia
7. Hemorrhage
8. Trauma – postoperative
9. Infections (e.g. AIDS)

Minor Criteria:
Platelet Count >400,000/mm^3 (>4 × $10^{11}/<$).
White blood cell count >12,000 mm^3.
Leucocyte alkaline phosphatase (LAP) >100.
Increased serum B$_{12}$, or B$_{12}$ binding capacity

Bone marrow histology in PV

The cell populations in the bone marrow show progressive development to mature elements. PV is not diagnosed from histology alone (particularly useful is the demonstration of erythropoietin-independent growth of erythroid colonies in culture), but this provides a valuable additional parameter. The bone marrow in PV shows an increase in the overall cellularity with a corresponding decrease in fat cells (Figures 22.1–22.5). The hyperplastic cell lines are found in their normal topographic loca-

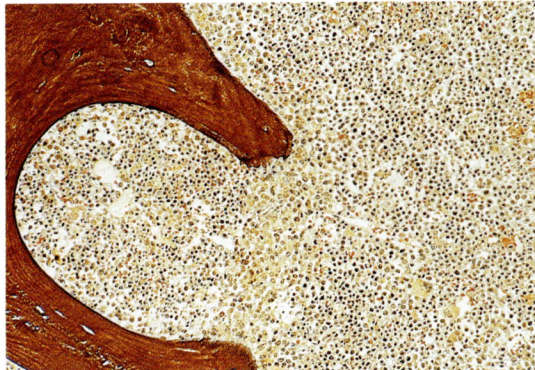

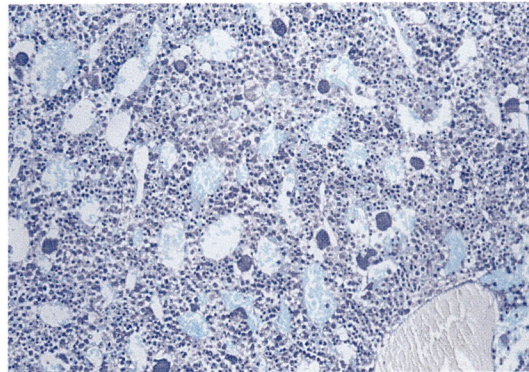

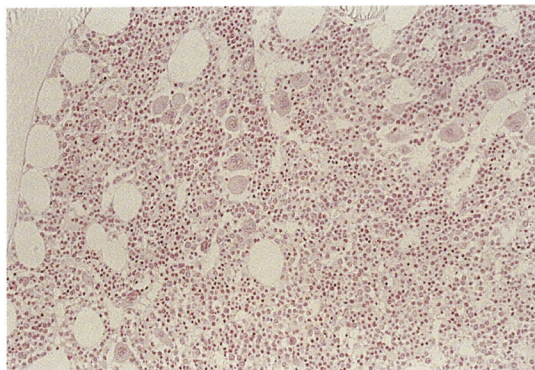

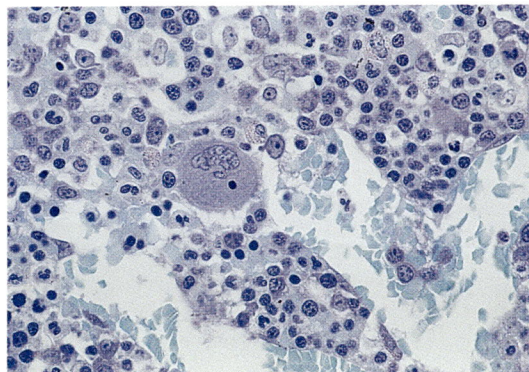

22.1–22.6 Aspects of bone marrow histology in PV.

22.1 (left) BMBS plastic, Gomori, classic PV hypercellular bone marrow with almost complete replacement by fat cells.

22.2 (right) BMBS plastic, Giemsa, trilinear PV; note engorged sinusoids.

22.3 (left) As for Figure 22.2, stain for iron, which is almost completely absent, as iron stores in PV are usually depleted.

22.4 (right) BMBS plastic, Giemsa, hyperplastic erythropoiesis and megakaryocyte in sinus.

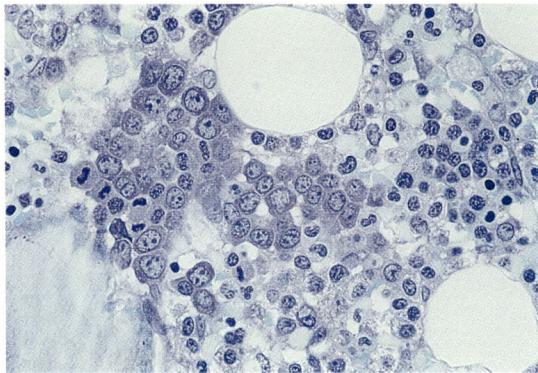

22.5 BMBS plastic, Giemsa, high magnification erythroblasts at trabecular surface, left; note mitotic figures and more mature erythroblasts, right.

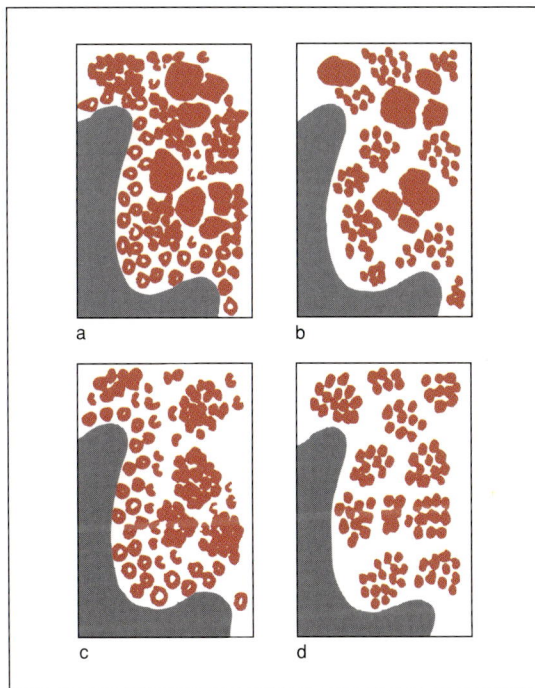

22.6 Four histological subtypes of PV: (a) trilinear, (b) bilinear, with erythrocytic and megakaryocytic lines, (c) bilinear, with erythrocytic and granulocytic lines, (d) unilinear.

round to highly convoluted – and variable cytoplasmic density; 'naked' megakaryocytic nuclei and emperipolesis are also common. There is an apparent increase in all the marrow blood vessels especially the sinusoids, occasionally with intravascular hematopoietic precursors; iron stores are depleted; a variable increase in reticular fibers, rarefaction of the trabecular bone without evidence of increased osseous remodeling, and infiltrations of lymphocytes, lymphoid nodules and plasma cells complete the picture. Extension of hematopoietic tissue into the lower extremities may occur. However, this full-blown picture may not yet be present in early PV and the picture may then resemble that seen in hemolysis or secondary erythrocytosis (see Chapter 17). The situation is usually clarified in follow-up biopsies.

Subtypes of PV in bone marrow histology (Figure 22.6)

The bone marrow histology in PV can be further divided into four subtypes as follows:

1. The classic trilinear type as described above, in which there is hyperplasia of the erythrocytic, megakaryocytic and granulocytic cell lines.

2. The bilinear type involving the erythrocytic and megakaryocytic lines.

3. The bilinear type involving the erythrocytic and granulocytic lines.

4. The unilinear type in which only the erythroid line exhibits hyperplasia in the bone marrow histology. The first – the classic trilinear – is the most frequent. The other types must also be distinguished from the other entities in the cMPD, by means of the appropriate investigations, and bearing in mind the overlap and transitions that may occur between the cMPD entities.

Evolution of disease

When 'spent' (or burned out) PV occurs, the peripheral blood levels begin to fall. The bone marrow then presents a mixed picture; with prominent stromal changes, serous atrophy, fibrosis with increased fibroblasts and fat cells, large erythroid islands consisting predominantly of immature cells, reduced granulopoiesis

tions: erythroid in the parasinusoidal zones, granulocytic in the paratrabecular and perivascular regions, and megakaryocytes in the intertrabecular areas, also adjacent to sinusoids, except when greatly increased in numbers, in which case they are also found along the endosteum, i.e. heterotopia. With increasing hyperplasia the megakaryocytes exhibit extreme polymorphism, ranging from 'giant' to 'micro' to pyknotic with variable nuclei – from single or multiple, small and

229

and dysplastic megakaryocytes (Figure 22.7). The marrow may even resemble that in some forms of aplastic anemia. Though an increase in reticulin is part of the disease picture, extensive myelofibrosis (MF/OMS) develops almost exclusively in cases with marked proliferation of megakaryocytes; osteolytic or, more rarely, osteosclerotic lesions may be found. Reorganisation of hematopoiesis into PV has been recorded following splenectomy for myelofibrosis. Further evolution to blast crisis, to another MPD or even development of a malignant lymphoma may occur, albeit rarely.

Differential diagnosis

In secondary erythrocytosis there is hyperplasia of the erythroid series only, and the other characteristic histological features of PV are absent. Megakaryocytes are not affected morphologically or quantitatively, fat cells are not markedly reduced, iron stores are not depleted (unless there is an identifiable cause of iron deficiency) and reticulin is not increased. In some hemolytic conditions, as well as autoimmune and hepatic diseases and refractory anemias, the marrow may also be hypercellular almost to the complete exclusion of fat cells, but other histological features should indicate the diagnosis.

Idiopathic thrombocythemia (IT)

Primary, idiopathic or essential thrombocythemia is a mature type of megakaryocytic myelosis, characterised by sustained increase in the platelet count at a level of $>10^{12}/1$iter. Recent evidence indicates that it is a clonal disorder with origin in a multipotent stem cell. Megakaryocytes (platelets), erythrocytes and granulocytes are involved; nevertheless, there are normal values for hemoglobin and leucocytes in the peripheral blood, and a normal leucocyte alkaline phosphatase level – LAP.

Criteria of IT recently published by the PV Study Group are as follows: platelet counts $>10^{12}/1$iter; megakaryocytic hyperplasia in the bone marrow, but a trilinear hyperplasia may also be present; Ph chromosome-negative (but

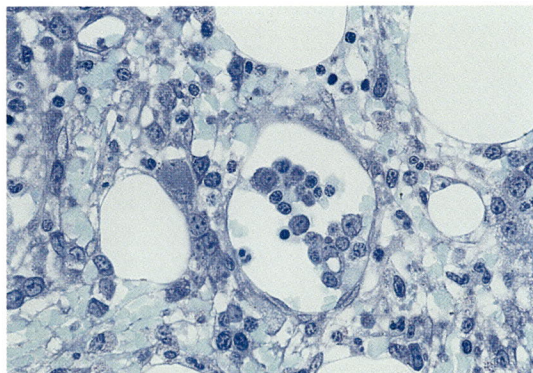

22.7 BMBS plastic, Giemsa, from case of PV with developing myelofibrosis; note intraluminal precursors.

occasional cases may be Ph chromosome-positive, in which case they could also be considered a subtype of CML, see page 232); absence of prominent fibrosis, but reticulin may be increased; absence of myeloid metaplasia; no increase in red cell mass; no marked iron deficiency in the bone marrow (as in PV); no previous myelosuppressive therapy; moderate splenomegaly and hepatomegaly may be present. Thus, bone marrow biopsy is important for establishing the diagnosis.

Bone marrow histology in IT

There is progressive maturation of the megakaryocytes, with production of platelets and their shedding and release directly into the bloodstream; moreover, portions of the megakaryocyte cytoplasm may separate off into the vascular lumen, or even whole megakaryocytes may migrate into the sinusoids, to be arrested in the lungs, broken up in the heart, completely or partially, and, more rarely, enter the capillary network of other organs.

Subtypes in bone marrow histology

The bone marrow in IT may be hypo-, normo- or hypercellular with hyperplasia of the megakaryocytes (Figures 22.8–22.10). These frequently form clusters of polymorphic cells, ranging in size from micro to gigantic forms with marked nuclear hyperlobulation, and they also include naked nuclei and pyknotic cells. The nuclei range from small, round and single to convoluted masses (Figures 22.11 and

22.8 (left) Bone biopsy in IT: dispersed (a) and (b) clustered pleomorphic megakaryocytes.

22.9 (right) BMBS plastic, Giemsa, low power showing hypocellular bone marrow with megakaryocytic hyperplasia – case of IT.

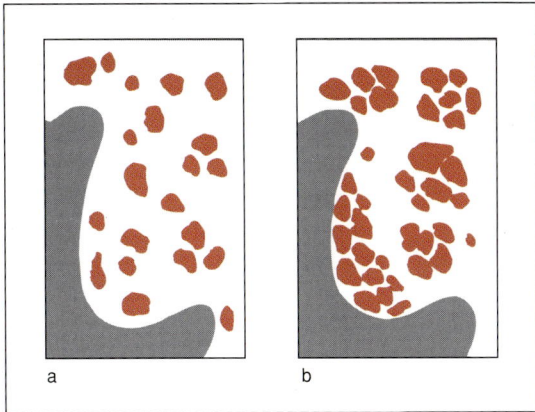

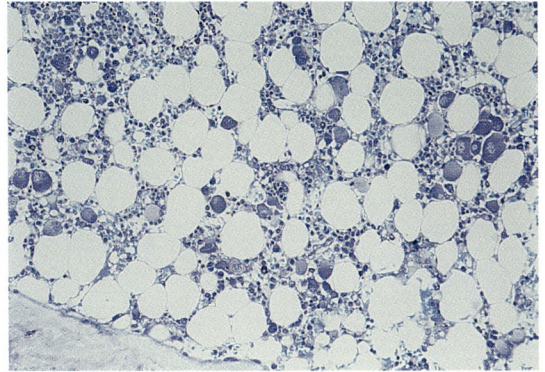

22.10 (left) BMBS plastic, Giemsa, cellular marrow with megakaryocytic hyperplasia.
22.11–22.13 Aspects of megakaryocytic hyperplasia and polymorphism in IT.
22.11 (right) BMBS, Giemsa, cluster of megakaryocytes ranging from small to large.

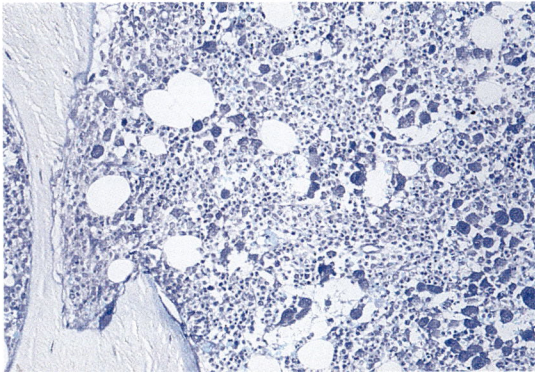

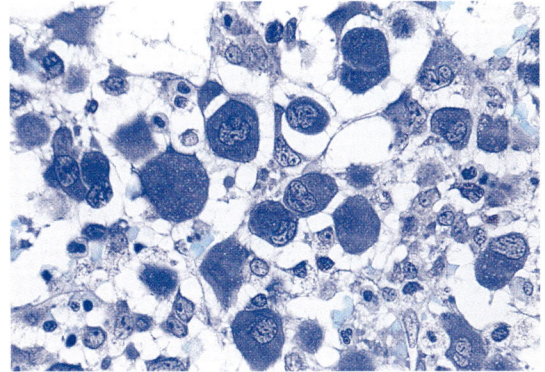

22.12 BMBS EM, showing disorganisation of bone marrow with interstitial platelets (arrows) and incipient fibrosis.

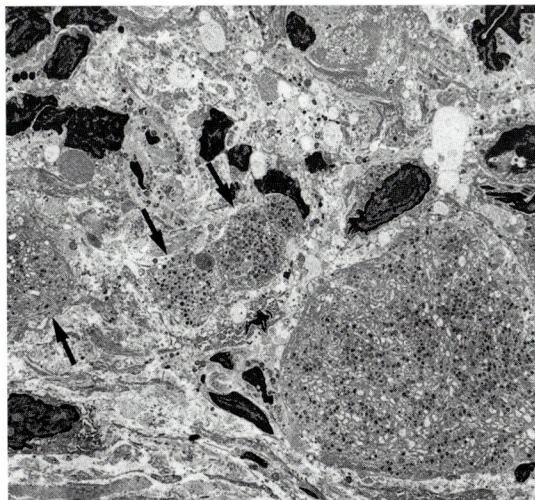

22.14). Emperipolesis (inclusion of other cells in megakaryocytic cytoplasm) is frequently observed. The normal architectural pattern of the bone marrow may be preserved or effaced. The erythroid and myeloid precursors may be reduced and at times show striking dysplastic features; more often, especially in the early stages, undergo normal maturation. Macrophages may be prominent, some with cellular debris and crystaline inclusions. Characteristic for IT is the localisation of the megakaryocytes at the walls of the sinusoids, or projecting into their lumina. The different bone marrow histological pictures which were found in a survey of patients, under the

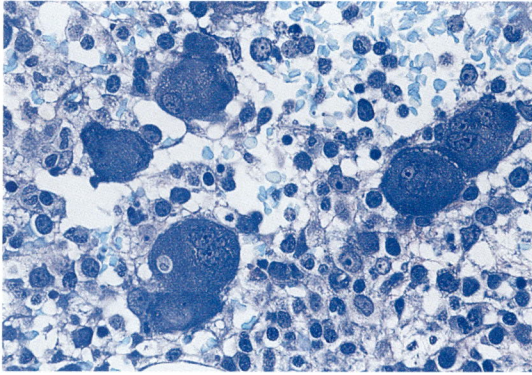

22.13 (left) BMBS Giemsa, large megakaryocytes in bone marrow interstitium.

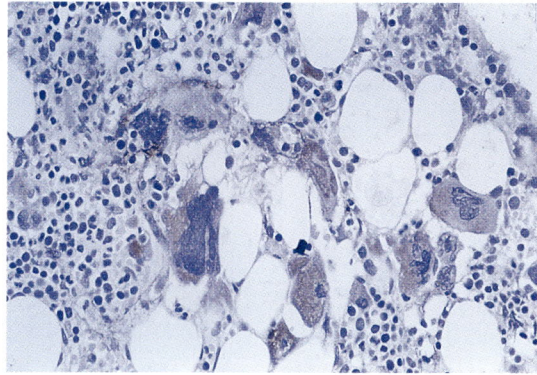

22.14 (right) BMBS paraffin, I.H., megakaryocytes positive for Factor VIII-related antigen – case of IT.

clinical syndrome of thrombocythemia are given in Table 22.2. This clearly demonstrates that IT is a syndrome with a variable underlying bone marrow histopathology and that it corresponds to a typical megakaryocytic myelosis, that is, a myeloproliferative disorder, in only 60% of cases.

Evolution of disease

Though IT generally has a slow and static course, the megakaryocytic hyperplasia may lead to fibroblastic stimulation and development of MF at any time, particularly when there is interstitial degeneration of megakaryocytes and/or release of platelets into the stroma instead of into the bloodstream. Moreover, a falling platelet count may not only indicate development of fibrosis but also transition to an immature type, with possibility of development of leukemia (myelosis).

Differential diagnosis

A raised platelet count may be due to many causes other than a myeloproliferative disorder (see Chapters 17 and 23).

Chronic myeloid leukemia (CML)

General aspects

CML is presumed to be a stem cell disorder. Chromosome studies have demonstrated that granulocytes, erythroid cells, megakaryocytes and lymphocytes all contain the characteristic Ph+ chromosome, t(9;22)(q34;q11). This char-

acteristic translocation produces the aberrant BCR-ABL gene which, in turn (1) induces cell proliferation, (2) induces transformation of hematopoietic precursors and (3) suppresses apoptosis *in vitro*. Depending on where exactly the breakpoint occurs, different Bcr Abl fusion genes are produced and multiparameter studies may be required to characterise them (cytogenetic, FISH, and molecular; see Chapter 21). In CML, there are abnormalities of stromal and progenitor cell interactions. A new line of approach for future treatment of CML (and other disorders with similar clonal anomalies, i.e. production of aberrant proteins responsible for the pathologic manifestations) is inactivation of the BCR-ABL gene and thereby reversal of the leukemic phenotype in CML. Studies of BMB of patients with clinically established CML have shown that it may be divided, broadly speaking, into two groups (Figure 22.15): the granulocytic and the mixed granulocytic and megakaryocytic, i.e. a uni- or bicellular proliferation. In both, the bone marrow is hypercellular with decrease in fat cells.

Bone marrow histology

In the former type there is hyperplasia of the white cells (the eosinophil precursors often appear prominent) with endosteal seams and perivascular cuffs of granulopoiesis which show increasing maturation towards the central parts of the marrow cavities. The proportion of immature to mature cells may be higher in the bone marrow than in the peripheral blood. Asynchronous maturation is evidenced by early cytoplasmic granulation and hyposegmentation of the nucleus. Eosinophils and basophils may be increased. There is a typical peripheral blood picture: leucocytosis of 50,000–200,000 may be found and though there is left shift, most are granulocytes with increased eosinophils and, typical for CML, a high basophil count. LAP is low. Hemoglobin is normal or decreased and platelets are normal or increased. In the mixed type of CML, hyperplasia of both myeloid and megakaryocytic elements is seen with a corresponding increase in both leukocytes and platelets in peripheral blood. The megakaryocytes exhibit polymorphism, heterotopia and clustering (small or large groups of megakaryocytes) in some cases and numerous small and micromegakary-

ocytes in others (Figures 22.16–22.19). The marrow in both types of CML is densely packed, with few residual fat cells. In addition, there may be macrophages with crystalloid inclusions, pseudo-Gaucher cells (Figures 22.20–22.29), and sea-blue histiocytes; plasma and mast cells, and lymphocytes in variable numbers are usually present. Decreased and ineffective erythropoiesis with maturation arrest is found in many patients with CML. There is some rarefaction of the cancellous bone (occasionally thick trabeculae especially in subcortical regions alternate with attenuated ones or with occasional areas of circumscribed osteolysis), a moderate (mainly perivascular) increase in reticulin, as well as in blood vessels are also fairly constant features. Histologic features of CML may be used for

22.15 (left) Granulocytic (a) and mixed granulocytic–megakaryocytic (b) types of CML.

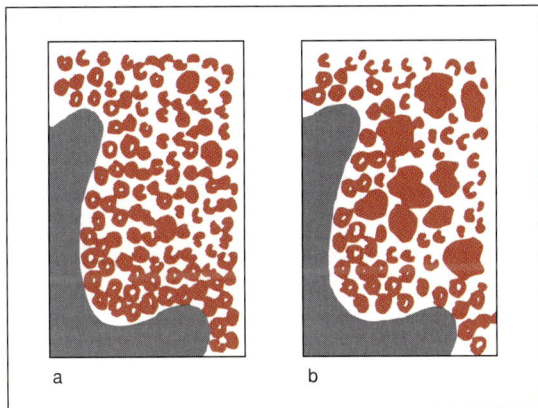

22.16 and 22.17 Two types of CML.
22.16 (right) BMBS plastic, Giemsa, low power, showing mainly myeloid hyperplasia with few megakaryocytes.

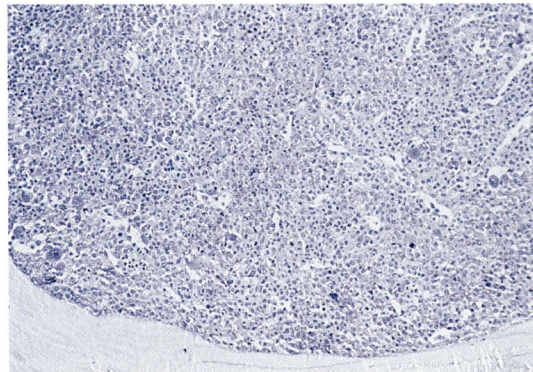

22.17 (left) BMBS plastic, Giemsa, illustrating mixed-type of CML with both myeloid and megakaryocytic hyperplasia.

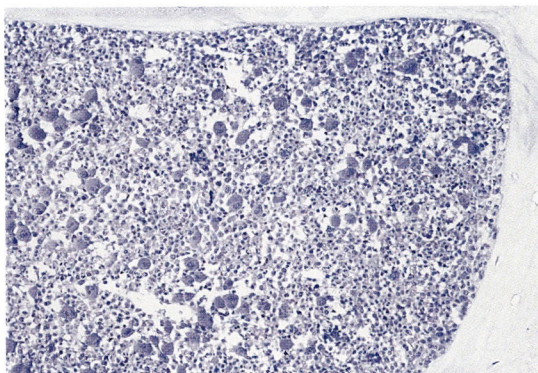

22.18 (right) BMBS plastic, Gomori, high magnification showing immature precursors adjacent to the bone and megakaryocytic hyperplasia.

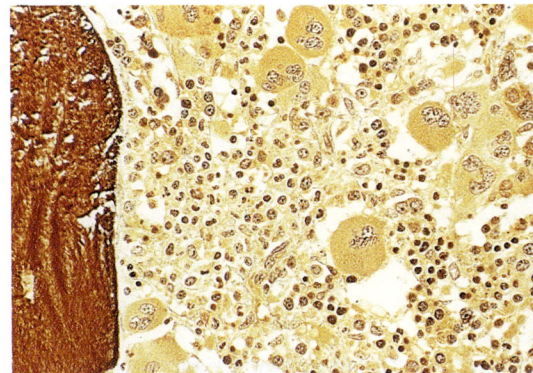

staging as well as diagnosis if done before therapy is given. Reversal of even severe bone marrow fibrosis has been achieved following bone marrow transplantation in CML. Cases have been described with predominant hyperplasia of one of the three series – neutrophilic, eosinophilic (Figure 22.22), basophilic (see below) – or involvement of one of the three to a greater extent that the others in individual patients with CML, and subgroups may be identified on this basis. Whether these have any clinical or prognostic significance has not yet been fully established. In addition, basophil production may be increased just before and during blastic transformation. Recent studies indicate that eosinophilia in the myeloproliferative disorders is an intrinsic part of the disease process.

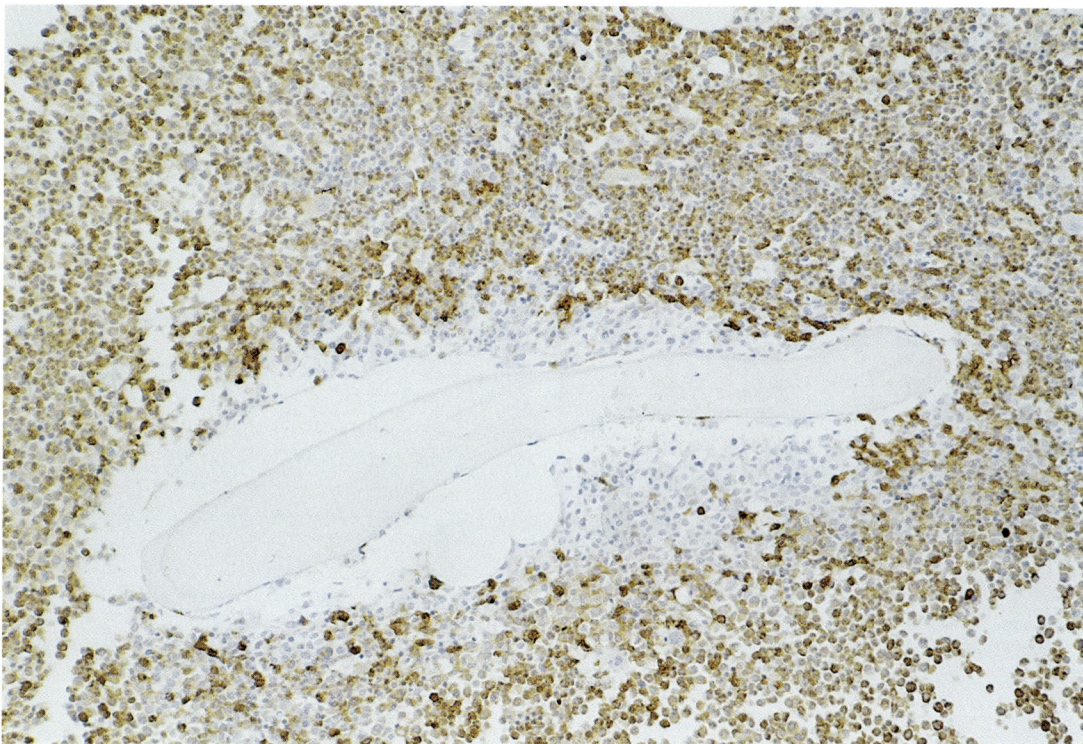

22.19 BMBS paraffin, I.H., myeloperoxidase, most of the myeloid cells are positive. Note negative myeloid precursors adjacent to the bone; these are probably CD34 positive myeloblasts though they did not react with QBENDIO (CD34) possibly for technical reasons.

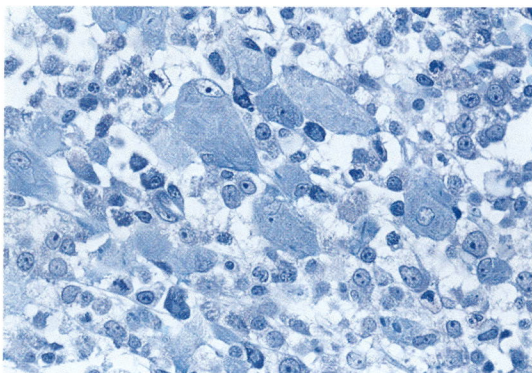

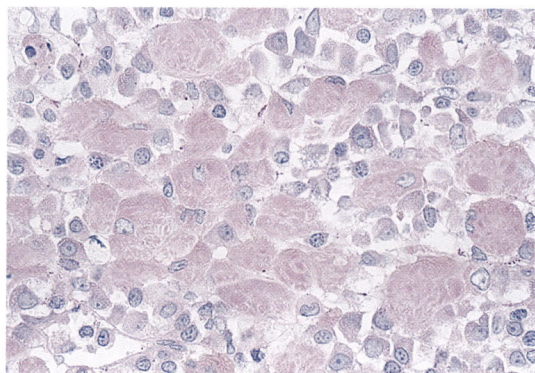

22.20 and 22.21 Pseudo-Gaucher cells in CML. 22.20 (left) BMBS plastic, Giemsa; pseudo-Gaucher cells are stained blue.

22.21 (right) BMBS paraffin; pseudo-Gaucher cells are stained pink. Such cells are formed when there is a high cell turnover.

22.22 (left) BMBS plastic, Giemsa, eosinophilic CML or hypereosinophilic syndrome.

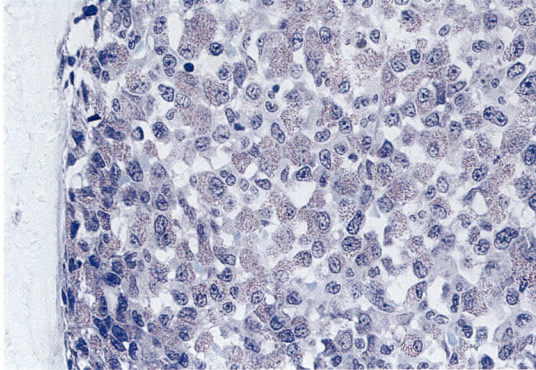

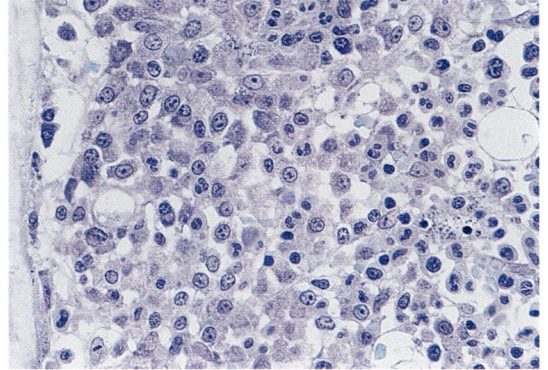

22.23 (right) BMBS plastic, Giemsa, broad seam of myeloid precursors in CML, accelerated phase.

22.24 and 22.25 Blast crisis in CML without and with participation of megakaryocytic cell line. **22.24** (left) BMBS plastic, Giemsa, showing sheet of blasts.

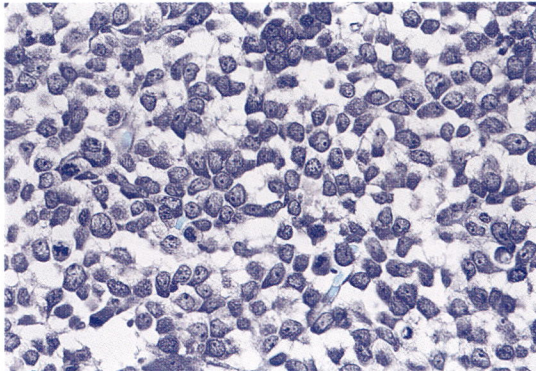

22.25 (right) BMBS plastic, aggregate of immature megakaryocytes and megakaryoblasts.

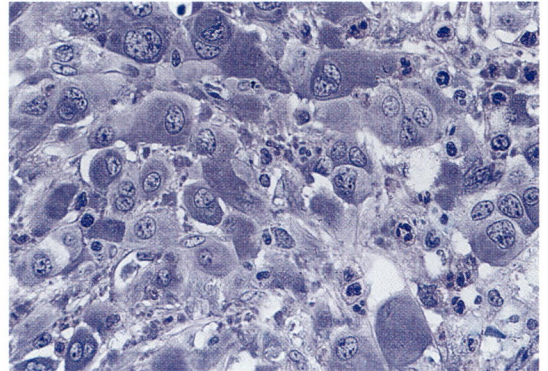

22.26 (left) Inter-relationships and evolution ('metamorphosis') of histologic subtypes in MPD, based on 1200 sequential biopsies taken in 550 patients. Frequency of transformation indicated by thickness of arrows. ERY, erythrocytic; GRA, granulocytic; MEG, megakaryocytic; PRO; promyelocytic, promegakaryocytic and/or proerythroblastic subtypes; SAL, subacute leukemias. **22.27** (right) Partial karyotype of patient with PV showing del(13)(q).

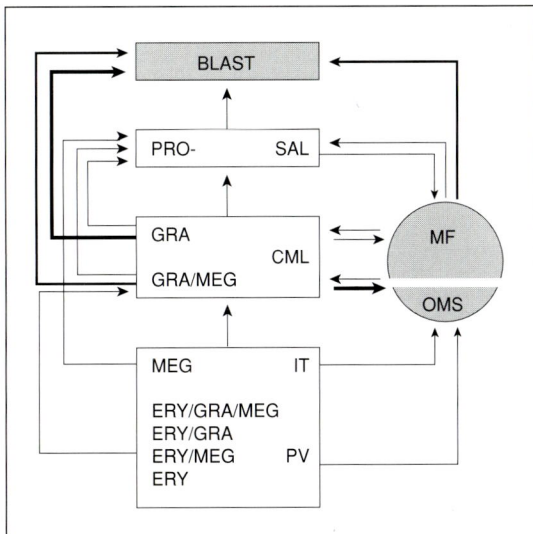

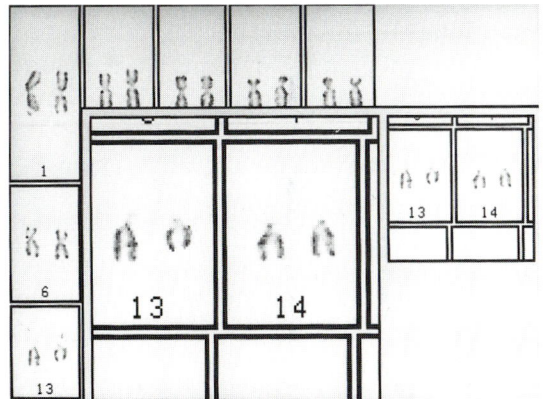

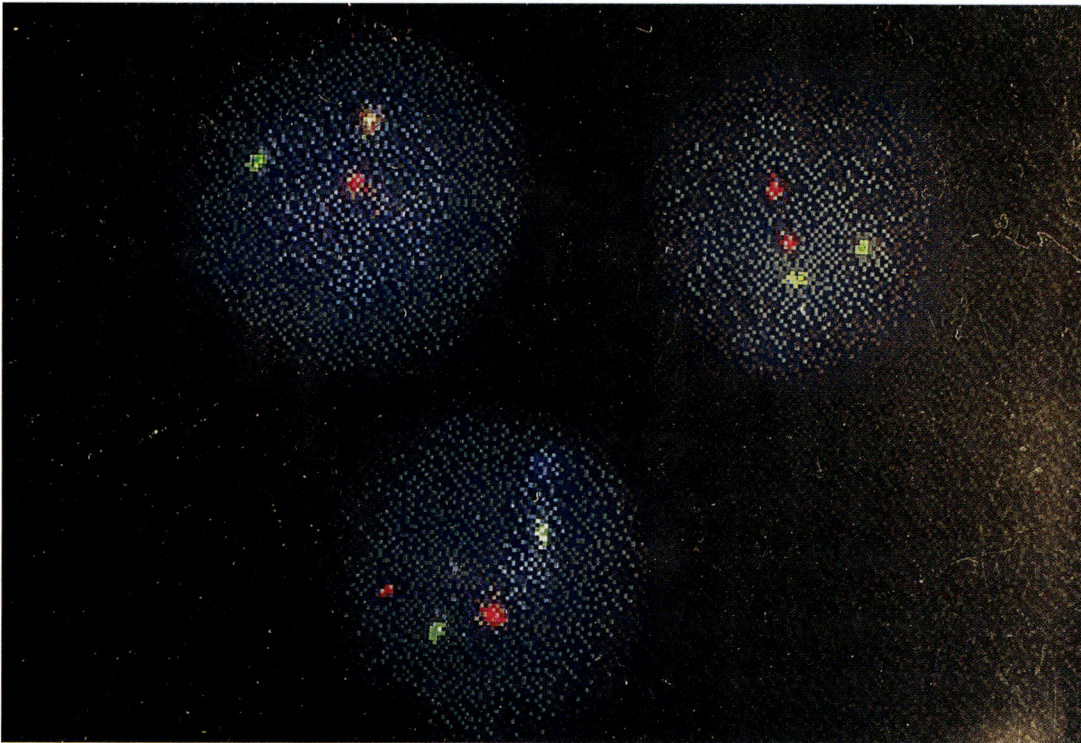

22.28 Interphase nuclei, FISH, one showing four signals corresponding to chromosomes 9 and 22, and the upper nucleus shows three signals, one green and one red corresponding to one each chromosome 9 and 22, and the yellow signal indicating the fused Bcr/Abl.

Evolution of disease

Roughly speaking, three phases of CML may be distinguished: (1) chronic, stable phase, (2) accelerated phase (Figure 22.23) and (3) blastic crisis (Figures 22.24 and 22.25).

As the disease progresses, it is thought that intraclonal mutation leads to changes in tempo, character and uncoupling of growth from differentiation. When this occurs, progressively wider osteoid seams of immature precursors herald the onset of blastic crisis. Immunohistology can be reliably used to demonstrate the increase of blasts in biopsies, which may not be readily aspirated when some degree of fibrosis is present. Classification of transformation in CML has so far only been made on smears of aspirates and increasingly, on flow cytometric analysis of the phenotypes of the blast cells in the aspirates. However, more information may be obtained from bone biopsies especially on the likelihood of imminent transformation as this is more frequently observed in the granulocytic type of CML,

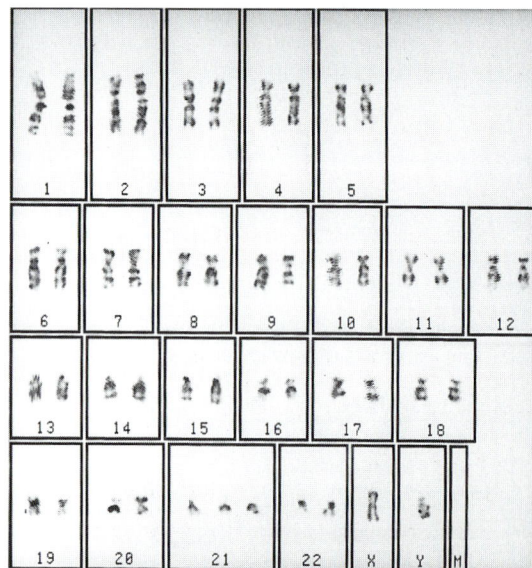

22.29 Karyotype of patient with CML showing t(9;22) (q34;q11), +21.

while the mixed type has a greater tendency to develop into MF/OMS (Figure 22.26). Blastic transformation to cells of both the myeloid, myeloblastic and erythroblastic, and lymphoid cell lines has been demonstrated in CML. Moreover, it has been shown that histologic features retain their prognostic significance under therapy with interferon.

In summary, assessment of sequential biopsies has shown that: (1) there are transitions between the two types of CML, (2) transformation to MF/OMS occurs only in the mixed type and (3) a terminal blast crisis usually occurs in the unilinear type.

Important for therapy is the observation that normal hematopoietic precursors are present in the bone marrow in patients with Ph+ positive CML, though special techniques may be required to detect them. However, it should be remembered that the agents used to treat CML may themselves be leukemogenic and contribute to the transformation to an acute phase.

Histological studies in CML in blast transformation, after ablative therapy, and after bone marrow autografting, have shown that bone biopsies are required for differential diagnosis, for detection of residual blasts, for assessment of overall cellularity and to monitor regeneration of hematopoiesis.

Variants of CML

Atypical CML
This is a chronic myeloproliferative disorder with features of both CML and CMML:
- PH and/or BCR-ABL-negative.
- There is some granulocytic dysplasia.
- Basophils are not increased.
- Leucocyte count is generally not very high.
- Monocytes in peripheral blood >3%.
- Platelets around 50,000.
- Hemoglobin variable.
- Hypercellular bone marrow with more erythropoiesis than in CML.

Chronic neutrophilic leukemia (CNL)
Usually there is neutrophilic leukocytosis with hepatosplenomegaly, without any evidence of infection. The bone marrow shows myeloid hyperplasia, and the leucocyte alkaline phosphatase (LAP), is high; B_{12} is also high. Reactive conditions and other MPDs must be excluded. CNL may be accompanied by bone marrow fibrosis, which decreases under therapy. However, there is still some uncertainty as to whether CNL is really a distinct disease entity, and probably the question will only be decided when many more cases have been observed and published.

Chronic myelomonocytic leukemia (CMML)
This overlaps with other MPDs; the patients may have hepatosplenomegaly and infiltrations in other organs. There is no baso- or eosinophilia, or Philadelphia chromosome; there is monocytosis in the peripheral blood. The bone marrow is hypercellular with myeloid and monocytic hyperplasia, the megakaryocytes are also increased.

Juvenile CML
This may occur in young children, more often in boys. LAP is decreased, fetal hemoglobin is increased, hemoglobin A_2 is decreased. The marrow is hypercellular, with an increase in blasts; there is dysplasia, an increase in monocytes and atypical megakaryocytes are present. Usually bone biopsies are not taken. Partial deletion of chromosome 7 has been found in some cases.

Chronic eosinophilic leukemia and hypereosinophilic syndrome
In both the bone marrow is hypercellular, with decrease in fat cells, increase in eosinophils, and in myeloblasts, megakaryocytes mostly within normal limits, or may even be decreased. Variable, mild fibrosis may be present. The difference between these two conditions is minimal (if at all) and their distinction on bone biopsy sections may not be possible, though a case of chronic eosinophilic leukemia (CEL) has recently been described as a distinct myeloproliferative disease terminat-

ing in AML, characterised by trisomy 15 and loss of the Y chromosome. Reactive conditions must be excluded. However, some structural chromosome abnormalities are associated with the myeloproliferative eosinophilia and their demonstration may help in the diagnosis. Moreover, eosinophilia may precede a myeloproliferative disorder for a number of years, as in a recently reported case of eosinophilia terminating in AML after 24 years.

Bone in the cMPD

Changes in cortical and trabecular bone occur in most patients. In PV there is osteopenia with attenuated trabecule, but preservation of the cancellous network. In CML and CMML osteolytic lesions have been reported in about 30% of the patients; but such lesions are more frequently seen in the accelerated and blastic phases. Mixed lesions (lytic and sclerotic) in the cMPD usually indicate transformation to MF/OMS (see chapter 23).

Check list: Chronic Myeloproliferative Disorders

- Adequate biopsy, at least 30 mm after exclusion of cortex and subcortical area.

- Cellularity: proportion of fat cells?

- Predominant proliferative cell line(s)? Confirm by immunohistology (I.H.).

- Pattern of proliferation?

- Compartmentalisation of cell lines?

- Degree of its (their) differentiation?

- Megakaryocytes: hyperplasia, morphology, topography, distribution? I.H.: Factor VIII for small and atypical ones.

- Stromal reactions: fibrosis, inflammatory infiltrations, new bone formation? Reticulin and collagen stains, vimentin, CD34 and stain for osteoid, i.e. toluidine blue.

- Blasts – topography and quantity? I.H.: myeloid and CD34.

- Bone structure and remodeling?
- Peripheral blood values.

In individual cases, according to the suspected diagnosis, and in addition to the above, other histologic features are considered:

Polycythemia vera (PV)

- Fe stain – stores depleted

- Sinusoids – increased and engorged. I.H.: Factor VIII, CD34

- In classical PV triple cell line involvement. Hypercellular bone marrow: few fat cells.

- Bone: thin trabeculae, little remodeling.

Idiopathic thrombocythemia (IT)

- Cellularity may be hypo (low) – normo (normal) – or hyper (increased).

- In all the above there is hyperplasia, polymorphism and clustering of megakaryocytes; I.H.: Factor VIII, CD41, CD61.

- Possibly fibrosis in vicinity of megakaryocyte clusters: stain for reticulin. I.H.: vimentin.

- Rule out pathologic infiltrations.

Chronic myeloid leukemia (CML)

- Cellularity increased.

- Fat cells decreased or absent?

- Myeloid hyperplasia – neutrophilic, eosinophilic and/or basophilic? I.H.: myeloperoxidase.

- Endosteal and perivascular seams of immature myeloid precursors, then abrupt transition to mature granulocytes, pseudo-Gaucher macrophages. I.H.: CD68.

- Erythropoiesis decreased and islands disrupted.

- Megakaryocytes (1) increased, mainly small and (2) not increased. I.H.: Factor VIII.

- Bone: some stout and some thin trabeculae with little remodeling and wide marrow spaces.

Clinical correlations

PV

- Typical facial appearance, headache, hypertension.
- Exclusion of secondary erythropoiesis.
- Intolerance to heat, pruritis.
- With high platelet count, frequent peripheral vascular complications – fingers and toes.
- Splenomegaly, abdominal fullness.
- Clonal +8
  Chromosomal +9
  Characteristics del(13)(q) (Figure 22.27)
  del(20)(q)
  structural abnormalities
  of chromosome 1.

IT

- Asymptomatic, incidental discovery.
- Young adults and older patients.
- Peripheral vascular effects, thrombosis and bleeding; digital microvascular ischemia, especially toes.
- Splenic vein thrombosis – Budd–Chiari syndrome.
- Clonal rearrangements of dup(1)(q)
  chromosome 3
  Chromosomal +8 del(13)(q)
  Characteristics +9 del(20)(q).

CML

- Early fortuitous discovery – asymptomatic.
- Splenomegaly: fullness upper left quadrant.
- Fatigue, weight loss, malaise, headaches.
- Bleeding or thromboses.
- Gout and arthritis.
- Gastrointestinal symptoms.
- Bone pains.
- Peripheral blood values and typical smear – basophilia and eosinophilia, LAP is low.
- Clonal chromosomal characteristics. The Philadelphia chromosome (Ph) results from a reciprocal translocation between the long arm (q) of chromosome 9 and 22, t(9;22)(q34;q11). The molecular consequences include disruption of the Bcr gene on chromosome 22 and transfer of the Abl gene from chromosome 9 to 22.

Philadelphia positive
Chronic phase
t(9;22)(q34;q11) (Figures 22.28 and 22.29)
Some CML patients have *complex translocations* in which three, four, or five chromosomes are involved (including chromosome 9 and 22) or *variant translocations* in which cytogenetic analysis demonstrates involvement of chromosome 22 and a chromosome other than 9, or vice versa.

Evolution to blast crisis
+8
second Philadelphia chromosome
i(17)(q)
+19
−7
−Y
t(3;21)(q26;q22).

Philadelphia negative
By karyotype, with Bcr or Abl rearrangements detected by molecular techniques.
normal diploid karyotype
+8
+11
−5
−7
−Y
i(17)(q).

Chronic neutrophilic leukemia
Ph-negative in the majority of cases.
Bcr/Abl rearrangement (molecular techniques).

Chronic myelomonocytic leukemia
Ph-negative/Bcr-negative.

Juvenile CML
Ph-negative.
Clonal chromosome abnormalities.
Over half the patients have normal karyotypes.

Chronic eosinophilic leukemia and hypereosinophilic syndrome
−7.

Bibliography

Ariad S., Dajee D., Willem P., Bezwoda W.R. (1993) Lack of involvement of T-lymphocytes in the leukemic population during prolonged chronic phase of Philadelphia chromosome positive chronic myeloid leukemia. *Leukemia and Lymphoma*, **10** (3), 217–21.

Asimakopoulos F.A., Holloway T.L., Nacheva E.P. *et al.* (1996) Detection of chromosome 20q deletions in bone marrow metaphases but not peripheral blood granulocytes in patients with myeloproliferative disorders or myelodysplastic syndromes. *Blood*, **87** (4), 1561–70.

Berlin N.I. (1997) Prologue: Polycythemia Vera: The Closing of the Wasserman–Polycythemia Vera Study Group Era. *Sem Hematol.*, **34** (1), 1–5.

Bitter M.A., Le Beau M.M., Rowley J.D. *et al.* (1987) Associations between morphology, karyotype, and clinical features in myeloid leukemias. *Hum. Pathol.*, **18** (3), 211–25.

Boavida M.G., Jorge G., Alves C. *et al.* (1997) Chromosomal and molecular heterogeneity of leukemia patients with *Bcr-Abl* fusion genes. *Cytogenet Cell Genet.*, **77**, 128.

Busche G., Buhr T., Georgii A. (1995) Histopathology of chronic myeloid keukemia in diagnostic biopsies of bone marrow. *Pathologe*, **16** (1), 70–4.

Campbell E., Maldonado W., Suhrland G. (1975) Painful lytic bone lesion in an adult with chronic myelogenous leukemia. *Cancer*, **33**, 1354.

Carulli G., Marini A., Baicchi U. *et al.* (1987) Chronic lymphocytic leukemia (B-cell) in the course of polycythemia vera. Description of a case with an unusual chromosomic anomaly. *Tumori*, **73** (6), 639–43.

Cervantes F., Rozman C., Feliu E. (1989) Prognostic evaluation of initial bone marrow histopathological features in chronic granulocytic leukemia. *Acta. Hematol.*, **82** (1), 12–15.

Chen Z., Morgan R., Berger C.S. *et al.* (1993) Identification of masked and variant Ph (complex type) translocations in CML and classic Ph in AML and ALL by fluorescence in situ hybridization with the use of *bcr/abl* cosmid probes. *Cancer Genet. Cytogenet.*, **70** (2), 103–7.

Chissoe S.L., Bodenteich A., Wang Y-F. *et al.* (1995) Sequence and analysis of the human ABL gene, the BCR gene and regions involved in the Philadelphia chromosomal translocation. *Genomics*, **27**, 67–82.

Chott A., Gisslinger H., Thiele J. *et al.* (1990) Interferon-alpha-induced morpholigcal changes of megakaryocytes: a histomorpho-metrical study on bone marrow biopsies in chronic myeloproliferative disorders with excessive thrombocytosis. *Br J Haematol*, **74** (1), 10–16.

Cuneo A., Mecucci C., Kerim S. *et al.* (1989) Multipotent stem cell involvement in megakaryoblastic leukemia: cytologic and cytogenetic evidence in 15 patients. *Blood*, **74** (5), 1781–90.

De Fabritiis P., Dowding C., Bungey J. *et al.* (1993) Phenotypic characterization of normal and CML CD34-positive cells: Only the most primitive CML progenitors include Ph-neg cells. *Leukemia and Lymphoma*, **11** (1–2), 51.

De Mascarel A. (1994) Contribution of bone marrow biopsy in the diagnosis and prognosis of polycythemia vera. *Nouv Rev Fr Hematol*, **36** (2), 165–6.

Diez-Martin J.L., Dewald G.W., Pierre R.V. (1988) Possible cytogenetic distinction between lymphoid and myeloid blast crisis in chronic granulocytic leukemia. *Am. J. Hematol.*, **27** (3), 194–203.

Dini D., Artusi T., di Prisco U. (1991) Idiopathic myelofibrosis associated with an IgM-secreting immunocytoma. *Recenti Prog. Med.*, **82** (2), 77–9.

Djulbegovic B., Hadley T., Yen F. (1991) Occurence of high-grade T-cell lymphoma in a patient with Philadelphia chromosome-negative chronic myelogenous leukemia with breakpoint cluster region rearrangement: case report and review of the literature. *Am. J. Hematol.*, **36** (1), 63–4.

Dokal I., Pagliuca A., Deenmamode M. *et al.* (1989) Development of polycythemia vera in a patient with myelofibrosis. *Eur. J. Hematol.*, **42** (1), 96–8.

Doorduijn J.K., van Lom K., Löwenberg. (1996) Eosinophilia and granulocytic dysplasia terminating in acute myeloid leukaemia after 24 years. *Br J Haematol*, **95**, 531–4.

Eberle F., Toiron Y., Camerlo J. *et al.* (1995) Persistence of BCR/ABL mRNA-expressing bone marrow cells in patients with chronic myelogenous leukemia in complete cytogenetic remission induced by interferon-alpha therapy. *Leuk Lymphoma*, **18** (1–2), 153–7.

Elmaagacli A.H., Wandl U.B., Berthel M. *et al.* (1993) Interferon alpha and gamma alter the binding of progenitor cells to fibronectin of patients with CML. *Leukemia*, **7** (8), 1300–1.

Enright H., McGlave P.B. (1996) Chronic myelogenous leukemia. *Current Opinion in Hematol*, **3** (4), 303–9.

Fioretos T., Nilsson P.G., Åman P. *et al.* (1993) Clinical impact of breakpoint position within M-bcr in chronic myeloid leukemia. *Leukemia*, **7** (8), 1225–31.

Frisch B., Bartl R., Jaeger K. (1989) Histologic diagnosis of chronic myeloproliferative disorders (CMPD). *Hematol Reviews*, **3**, 131–47.

Furukawa T., Narita M., Sakaue M. *et al.* (1997) Primary familial polycythaemia associated with a novel point mutation in the erythropoietin receptor. *Brit. J. Haematol*, **99**, 222–7.

Gaidano G., Guerrasio A., Serra A. *et al.* (1993) Mutations in the P53 and RAS family genes are associated with tumor progression of BCR/ABL negative chronic myeloproliferative disorders. *Leukemia*, **7**, 946–53.

Georgii A., Busche G., Kreft A. *et al.* (1996) Classification and staging of Ph1-negative myeloproliferative disorders by histopathology from bone marrow biopsies. *Leuk Lymphoma*, **22 (1)**, 15–29.

Georgii A., Vykoupil K.F., Buhr T. *et al.* (1990) Chronic myeloproliferative disorders in bone marrow biopsies. *Pathol Res Pract.*, **186 (1)**, 3–27.

Goldman J. (1997) ABC of Clinical Haematology – chronic myeloid leukaemia. *BMJ*, **314**, 657–60.

Goldman J.M. (1993) Chronic myeloid leukemia – the XXI century. *Leukemia and Lymphoma*, **11 (Suppl. 1)**, 7–9.

Gulati S.C., Lemoli R., van Poznak C. (1993) Newer approaches in treating chronic myelogenous leukemia. *Leukemia and Lymphoma*, **11 (Suppl. 1)**, 293–6.

Hehlmann R., Heimpel H. (1996) Current aspects of drug therapy in Philadelphia-positive CML: correlation of tumor burden with survival. *Leuk and Lymph*, **22 (Suppl. 1)**, 161–7.

Hirayama Y., Koda K., Matsumoto *et al.* (1994) A case of chronic neutrophilic leukemia accompanied with severe bone marrow fibrosis which was effectively treated by hydroxyurea. *Rinsho Ketsueki*, **35 (11)**, 1329–34.

Hochhaus A., Reiter A., Skladny H. *et al.* (1996) A novel BCR-ABL fusion gene (e6a2) in a patient with Philadelphia chromosome-negative chronic myelogenous leukemia. *Blood*, **6**, 2236–40.

Huret J.L. (1990) Complex translocations, simple variant translocations and Ph-negative cases in chronic myelogenous leukemia. *Hum. Genet.*, **85 (6)**, 565–8.

Kraus J., Henschke F., Decker M., Alliger K. (1989) Coincidence of chronic myeloid leukemia and Waldenstrom's disease. *Pathologe*, **10 (6)**, 349–53.

Kurtin P.J., Dewald G.W., Shields D.J., Hanson C.A. (1996) Hematologic disorders associated with deletions of chromosome 20q: a clinicopathologic study of 197 patients. *Am J Clin Pathol*, **106**, 680–8.

Kutti J., Wadenvik H. (1996) Diagnostic and differential criteria of esential thrombocythemia and reactive thrombocytosis. *Leuk and Lymph*, **22 (Suppl. 1)**, 41–5.

Lewis, J.P., Jenks, H., Walling, P. (1988) Ring chromosomes in chronic myelogenous leukemia: an ominous finding. *Leuk. Res.*, **12 (5)**, 379–83.

Li L., Ritterbach J., Harbott J. *et al.* (1993) Blastic phase chronic myeloid leukemia with a four-break rearrangement: t(11;9) (9;22) (q23;p22q34;q11). *Cancer Genet. Cytogenet.*, **68 (2)**, 131–4.

Liesner R.J., Machin S.J. (1997) ABC of clinical haematology: platelet disorders. *BMJ*, **314**, 809–11.

Macavei I., Galatar N. (1989) Bone marrow biopsy (BMB). II. Bone marrow biopsy in myeloproliferative disorders. *Morphol Embryol.*, **35 (2)**, 117–27.

Mancini M., Diverio D., Alimena G., Mandelli F. (1994) Recent advances in biological and therapeutic aspects of myeloproliferative disorders. *Current Opinion in Hematol*, **1**, 261–7.

Martell R.W., Myers H.S., Jacobs P. (1986) Bone lesions in chronic granulocytic leukaemia. *Br J. Haematol.*, **62**, 31.

Matano S., Nakamura S., Kobayashi K. *et al.* (1997) Deletion of the long arm of chromosome 20 in a patient with chronic neutrophilic leukemia: cytogenetic findings in chronic neutrophilic leukemia. *Am J Hematol*, **54 (1)**, 72–5.

Melo J.V. (1996) Overview: The molecular biology of chronic myeloid leukaemia. *Leukemia*, **10**, 751–6.

Melo J.V. (1996) The diversity of BCR-ABL fusion proteins and their relationship to leukemia phenotype. *Blood*, **88 (7)**, 2375–84.

Mijovic A., Rolovic Z., Novak A. *et al.* (1989) Chronic myeloid leukemia associated with pure red cells aplasia and terminating in promyelocytic transformation. *Am. J. Hematol.*, **31 (2)**, 128–30.

Mitelman F. (1993) The cytogenetic scenario of chronic myeloid leukemia. *Leukemia and Lymphoma*, **11 (Suppl. 1)**, 11–15.

Mittre H., Leymarie P., Macro M., Leporrier M. (1997) A new case of chronic myeloid leukemia with c3/a2 BCR/ABL junction. Is it really a distinct disease? *Blood*, **89 (11)**, 4239.

Najean Y., Rain J-D., Dresch C. *et al.* (1996) Risk of leukaemia, carcinoma, and myelofibrosis in ^{32}P- or chemotherapy-treated patients with Polycythaemia Vera: a prospective analysis of 682 cases. *Leuk and Lymph*, **22 (Suppl. 1)**, 111–19.

Najfeld V. (1997) FISHing among myeloproliferative disorders. *Sem Hematol.*, **34 (1)**, 55–63.

Najfeld V., Vlachos A., Parker R. *et al.* (1997) Evidence for the embryonic origin of partial chromosome 7 deletion in monozygotic twins with juvenile chronic myelogenous leukemia. *Leukemia*, **11 (2)**, 306–10.

Neri A., Fracchiolla N.S., Radaelli F. *et al.* (1996) P53 tumour suppressor gene and RAS oncogenes: molecular analysis in the chronic and leukaemic phases of essential thrombocythaemia. *Br J Haematol.*, **93**, 670–3.

Nolte M., Werner M., Ewig M. *et al.* (1996) Megakaryocytes carry the fused bcr-abl gene in chronic myeloid leukaemia: a fluorescence in situ hybridization analysis from bone marrow biopsies. *Virchows Arch*, **427 (6)**, 561–5.

Ohri S.K., Sharp D.J., Coutts G.B. (1990) Osteolytic lesions in chronic myelomonocytic leukaemia. *Br J Clin Pract.*, **44**, 672.

241

Ohyashiki K., Nagasu M., Hojo H. *et al.* (1989) Myelodysplastic syndrome with trisomy 11 associated with polycythemia vera. *Am. J. Hematol.*, **31** (2), 122–5.

Okamoto K., Karasawa M., Sakai H. *et al.* (1997) A novel acute lymphoid leukaemia type BCR/ABL transcript in chronic myelogenous leukaemia, **96**, 611–13.

Orazi A., Neiman R.S., Cualing H. *et al.* (1994) CD34 immunostaining of bone marrow biopsy specimens is a reliable way to classify the phases of chronic myeloid leukemia. *Am J Clin Pathol*, **101** (4), 426–8.

Orazi A., Cattoretti G., Sozzi G. (1989) A case of chronic neutrophilic leukemia with trisomy 8. *Acta. Hematol.*, **81** (3), 148–51.

Pane F., Frigeri F., Sindona M. *et al.* (1996) Neutrophilic-chronic myeloid leukemia: a distinct disease with a specific molecular marker (BCR/ABL with C3/A2 junction). *Blood*, **88** (7), 2410–14.

Pearson T.C., Messinezy M. (1996) The diagnostic criteria of Polycythaemia Rubra Vera. *Leuk and Lymph*, **22** (**Suppl. 1**), 89–93.

Peschel C., Aulitzky W.E., Huber C. (1996) Influence of Interferon-α on cytokine expression by the bone marrow microenvironment – impact on treatment of myeloproliferative disorders. *Leukemia and Lymphoma*, **22** (**Suppl. 1**), 129–34.

Rojas-Atencio A., Pineda-Del Villar L., Avila-Leon E. *et al.* (1996) Chronic myeloid leukemia. Karyotype changes. *Invest Clin*, **37** (3), 167–75.

Rozman C., Cervantes F., Rozman M., Urbano-Ispizua A. (1993) Prognosis of chronic myeloid keukemia: Studies from the Barcelona group. *Leukemia and Lymphoma*, **11** (**Suppl. 1**), 63–6.

Santucci M.A., Soligo D., Pileri S. *et al.* (1993) Interferon-alpha effects on stromal compartment of normal and chronic myeloid leukemia hematopoiesis. *Leukemia and Lymphoma*, **11** (**Suppl. 1**), 113–18.

Seong D.C., Kantarjian H.M., Ro J.Y. *et al.* (1995) Hypermetaphase fluorescence in situ hybridization for quantitative monitoring of Philadelphia chromosome-positive cells in patients with chronic myelogenous leukemia during treatment. *Blood*, **86** (6), 2343–9.

Seymour J.F., Grill V., Martin T.J. *et al.* (1993) Hypercalcemia in the blastic phase of chromic myeloid leukemia associated with elevated parathyroid hormon-related protein. *Leukemia*, **7** (10), 1672–5.

Shannon K.M., Watterson J., Johnson P. *et al.* (1992) Monosomy 7 myeloproliferative disease in children with neurofibromatosis, type 1: epidemiology and molecular analysis. *Blood*, **79** (5), 1311–18.

Shanske A.L., Kalman A., Grunwald H. (1996) A myeloproliferative disorder with eosinophilia associated with a unique translocation (3;5). *Br J Haematol*, **95**, 524–6.

Sullivan B.A., Schiffer C.A., Patil S.R. *et al.* (1995) Application of FISH to complex chromosomal rearrangements associated with chronic myelogenous leukemia. *Cancer Genet. Cytogenet.*, **82** (2), 93–9.

Takahira H., Shibata K., Hirata J. *et al.* (1989) Lymphoid blast crisis in a patient with Philadelphia-chromosome-negative chronic myelocytic leukemia. *Acta. Hematol.*, **81** (3), 155–9.

Tarachandani A., Advani S.H., Bhisey A.N. (1993) Chronic myeloid leukemia granulocytes have lower amounts of cytoplasmic actin. *Leuk. Res.*, **17** (10), 833–8.

Terpstra W.E., Meuwissen O.J., Hagemeijer A., Michiels J.J. (1990) Multiple myeloma and acute megakaryoblast leukemia in spent phase polycythemia vera. *Am. J. Clin. Pathol.*, **94** (6), 786–90.

Testoni N., Martinelli G., Farabegoli P. *et al.* (1996) A new method of 'in-cell reverse transcriptase-polymerase chain reaction for the detection of BCR/ABL ttranscript in chronic myeloid leukemia patients. *Blood*, **87** (9), 3822–7.

Thiele J., Hoeppner B., Wienhold S. *et al.* (1989) Osteoclasts and bone remodeling in chronic myeloproliferative disorders. A histochemical and morphometric study on trephine biopsies in 165 patients. *Pathol Res Pract.*, **184**, 591.

Thiele J., Kvasnicka H.M., Niederle N. *et al.* (1995) Clinical and histological features retain their prognostic impact under interferon therapy of CML: a pilot study. *Am J Hematol*, **50** (1), 30–9.

Thiele J., Zirbes T., Kvasnicka H.M. *et al.* (1996) Interferon therapy, but not busulfan restores normal-sized megakaryopoiesis in CML – a comparative histo- and immunomorphometric study. *Anal Cell Pathol*, **11** (1), 31–42.

Thiele J., Rompcik V., Wagner S., Fischer R. (1992) Vascular architecture and collagen type IV in primary myelofibrosis and polycythaemia vera: an immunomorphometric study on trephine biopsies of the bone marrow. *Br. J. Hematol.*, **80** (2), 227–34.

Thiele J., von Ammers E., Wagner S. *et al.* (1991) Megakaryocytopoiesis in idiopathic thrombocytopenic purpura: a morphometric and immunohistochemical study on bone marrow biopsies with special emphasis on precursor cells. *Hematol. Pathol.*, **5** (2), 75–82.

Thiele J., Kvasnicka H.M., Titius B.R. *et al.* (1993) Histological features of a prognostic significance in CML – an immuno-histochemical and morphometric study (multivariate regression analysis) on tephine biopsies of the bone marrow. *Annals of Hematology*, **66** (6), 291–302.

Urbano-Ispizua A., Cervantes F., Matutes E. *et al.* (1993) Immunophenotypic characteristics of blast crisis of chronic myeloid leukemia: Correlations with clinico-biological features and survival. *Leukemia*, **7** (9), 1349–54.

Van der Plas D.C., Grosveld G., Hagemeijer A. (1991) Review of clinical, cytogenetic, and molecular aspects of ph-negative CML. *Cancer Genet. Cytogenet.*, **52 (2)**, 143–56.

van Lom K., Hagemeijer A., Vandekerckhove F. *et al.* (1997) Clonality analysis of hematopoietic cell lineages in acute myeloid leukemia and translocation (8; 21): only myeloid cells are part of the malignant clone. *Leukemia*, **11 (2)**, 202–5.

Velloso E.R.P., Michaux L., Ferrant A. *et al.* (1996) Deletions of the long arm of chromosome 7 in myeloid disorders loss of band 7q32 implies worst prognosis. *Br J Haematol.*, **92**, 574–81.

Viniou N., Yataganas X., Abazis D. *et al.* (1995) Hypereosinophilia associated with monosomy 7. *Cancer Genet Cytogenet*, **80**, 68–71.

Weide R., Rieder H., Mehraein Y. *et al.* (1997) Chronic eosinophilic leukaemia (CEL): a distinct myeloproliferative disease. *Br J Haematol.*, **96**, 117–23.

Weinberg R.S. (1997) In vitro erythropoiesis in polycythemia vera and other myeloproliferative disorders. *Sem in Hematol.*, **34 (1)**, 64–9.

Westwood N.B., Pearson T.C. (1996) Diagnostic applications of haemopoietic progenitor culture techniques in Poycythaemias and Thrombocythaemias. *Leuk and Lymph*, **22 (Suppl. 1)**, 95–103.

Wetzler M., Talpaz M., Estrov Z., Kurzrock R. (1993) CML: Mechanisms of disease initiation and progression. *Leukemia and Lymphoma*, **11 (Suppl. 1)**, 47–50.

Widding A., Smolorz J., Franke M. *et al.* (1989) Bone marrow investigation with technetium-99m microcolloid and magnetic resonance imaging in patients with malignant myelolymphoproliferative diseases. *Eur. J. Nucl. Med.*, **15 (5)**, 230–8.

Yan L., Elkassar C., Gardin C., Briere J. (1996) Clonality assays and megakaryocyte culture techniques in essential thrombocythemia. *Leuk and Lymph*, **22 (Suppl. 1)**, 31–40.

Zeleznik-Le N.J., Nucifora G., Rowley J.D. (1995) The molecular biology of myeloproliferative disorders as revealed by chromosomal abnormalities. *Sem in Haematol.*, **32 (3)**, 201–19.

23 Myelofibrosis and osteomyelosclerosis and other fibroses in the bone marrow

Terminology

The normal bone marrow at all ages has few reticular or collagen fibers and these are found mainly in association with the trabecular bone surface and blood vessels. Myelofibrosis (MF) and/or myelosclerosis are terms applied to an increase in reticular and collagenous fibers in the bone marrow respectively. Osteomyelosclerosis (OMS) is used when increased new bone formation – appositional, woven or both – is also present.

Underlying conditions

MF and OMS as well as agnogenic myeloid metaplasia and their many synonyms are usually associated with the myeloproliferative disorders. Nevertheless, numerous other conditions may also be responsible for fibrosis in the bone marrow and they can be roughly divided into six major groups (Tables 23.1 and 23.2, Figures 23.1–23.4). In most cases, the patient's clinical condition, radiologic investigation, biochemical and hematologic profile will indicate the diagnostic possibilities and narrow the differential diagnosis to one or at most two of these major groups.

Stimuli that evoke fibrosis

Fibrosis in the bone marrow occurs as a response to many different stimuli – toxic, inflammatory, osteolytic and osteoblastic malignancies – and is mainly of collagen type III; various matrix proteins are also produced. These fibrotic reactions are always secondary; the basic disorders underlying or associated with fibrosis in the bone marrow are listed in Tables 23.1 and 23.2. Combinations of different cytokines and growth factors are responsible for the fibrosis in different disorders; for example, those produced by megakaryocytes and platelets in the myeloproliferative disorders (MPD), by lymphocytes in the lymphoproliferative disorders (LPD), by plasma, and mast cells and monocytes in conditions with inflammatory components and by the tumor cells in metastatic involvement of the bone marrow. In some disorders more precise mechanisms have been identified, as in hairy cell leukemia (HCL), in which it has been shown

244

23.1 Sketch of bone biopsy picture in full-blown MF (a) and OMS (b). In MF there is myelofibrosis, while in OMS the marrow cavities are also decreased by the additional bone. There are polymorphous megakaryocytes, ectatic sinusoids and intravascular hematopoietic precursors in both MF and OMS.

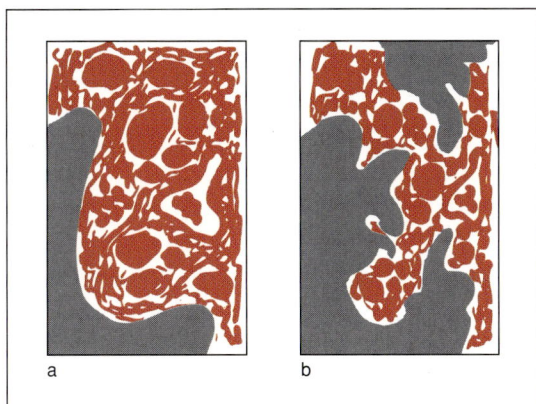

23.2 Three grades of bone marrow fibrosis: from a few interstitial fibers to obliterative fibrosis.

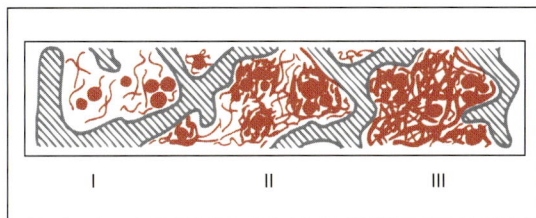

23.3 Three grades of bone increase from unobtrusive appositional bone formation and focus of woven bone to replacement of the trabecular network by the osteosclerosis.

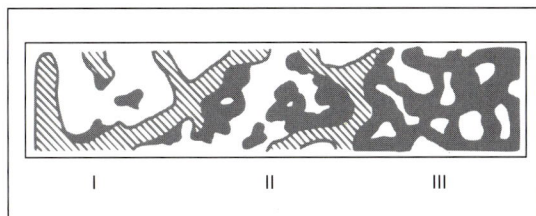

23.4 Underlying disorders and bone marrow fibrosis: (a) myeloproliferative disorder; (b) lymphoproliferative disorder; (c) Hodgkin's disease; (d) carcinoma; (f) inflammatory; (g) hyperparathyroidism.

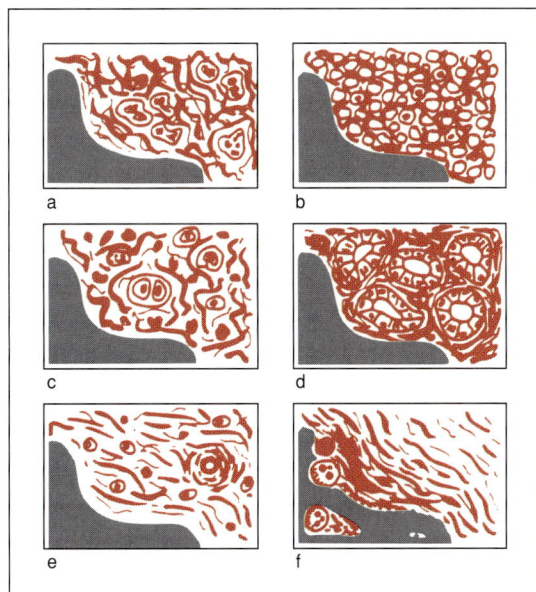

TABLE 23.1 Bone marrow fibrosis (grades II/III) and its basic disorders

Basic disorders	Patients
Hematological neoplasias	
Myeloproliferative disorders	1255
Acute/subacute leukemias	80
Multiple myeloma	250
Non-Hodgkin's lymphomas	797
Hodgkin's disease	69
Metastatic cancer	
Breast	156
Prostate	51
Lung	32
Others	27
Unknown primaries	90
Inflammatory reactions	
Toxic	38
Infectious	8
Unknown	42
Osteopathies	
Paget's disease	102
Primary hyperparathyroidism and Renal osteodystrophy	112
Myelodysplastic syndrome	43
Total	*3152*

that the bone marrow fibrosis is caused by the synthesis and assembly of a fibronectin matrix by the hairy cells. An increase in fibers is frequently observed in the myelodysplastic syndromes, and always in systemic mastocytosis. An increase in reticulin (myelofibrosis) is relatively easy to demonstrate, as with the commonly used stains for reticular fibers, the bone marrow shows very few when viewed in polarised light, apart from some near bone and blood vessels.

Effect of fibrosis on the marrow

The increase in fibers and in new bone leads to disorganisation of the bone marrow architec-

245

TABLE 23.2 Fibrotic Patterns and Basic Disorders

Basic Disorders in the Bone Marrow[a]	Number of Patients	Normal Fibers (%)	Fibrosis Grade I (%)	Fibrosis Grade II (%)	Fibrosis Grade III (%)	Woven Bone (%)
MPD	3393	28	35	11	14	12
AL	320	51	30	13	6	0
MM	813	32	37	20	9	2
NHL	1351	1	40	36	10	3
HD	95	0	27	30	39	4
Carcinoma	691	9	9	21	33	28
Sarcoma	60	2	20	28	30	20
HPT	280	15	45	20	16	9
Paget's disease	142	5	23	31	35	4

ture and trabecular bone network, dysplasia of the hematopoietic cell lines, fibrosis of vessel walls, especially sinusoids, and thereby impeded egress of mature cells from the bone marrow resulting in ineffective hematopoiesis, peripheral cytopenia (often the indication for the biopsy) and possibly myeloid metaplasia, which has been found in many organs, e.g. spleen, liver, lymph node, kidney and central nervous system. The diagnosis of myelofibrosis is often made by examination of the peripheral blood smear, which shows the typical appearances of the red blood cells, i.e. nucleated and teardrop erythrocytes, and leukoerythroblastic peripheral blood film, and a biopsy is required to establish the underlying cause.

Degree and extent of fibrosis and sclerosis

Both occur in varying degrees of severity and the extent of marrow and bone affected in each individual case is variable. Moreover, all degrees of severity may be present at the same time in a single biopsy, especially large ones, which makes not only morphologic classification very difficult, but also histomorphometric assessment of the different bone marrow compartments: fat cells, hematopoiesis, serous atrophy, blood vessels, fibrosis and newly formed bone. In spite of this, three grades have been distinguished (Figures 23.1–23.3).

Basic disorders causing fibrosis and sclerosis (Figure 23.4, Table 23.3)

Myeloproliferative disorders
(Figures 23.5–23.13)
Patients with pronounced involvement of megakaryocytes in any MPD are particularly prone to develop MF/OMS, and this is sometimes observed in the bone biopsy even at a very early stage, for example when hematopoietic hyperplasia includes polymorphism and clustering of megakaryocytes. In MF/OMS there are also changes in the blood vessels, with sclerosis of the walls and an increase in size and numbers of sinusoids, and a particular spatial relationship has been demonstrated

between megakaryocytes and the bone marrow sinus walls. However, megakaryocytic hyperplasia may also occur in many other conditions not only in the MPD, but the polymorphism and interstitial release of platelets and clustering typical of the MPD are rarely seen in most of these reactive states.

In essential thrombocythemia (ET) the bone marrow may be hyper-, normo- or hypocellular but there is always hyperplasia, polymorphism and a clustering of megakaryocytes with variable fibrosis ranging from a very mild increase in reticular fibers in proximity to clusters of megakaryocytes to an extensive fibrosis leading eventually to MF (or MF/OMS). Immunohistology has been particularly useful in identifying atypical and small megakaryocytes which would otherwise have remained unrecognised, in acute and subacute leukemias, in the MDS, and in all the chronic MPD. In acute myelofibrosis (AMF) as in some leukemias, fibrosis is present from the start. In chronic myeloid leukemia (CML) the bone marrow is hypercellular with well-nigh complete disappearance of fat cells, and two broad histologic categories are recognised: (1) granulocytic type (mainly neutrophilic, though eosinophilic and basophilic types are also

23.5–23.12 Aspects of MF/OMS in the MPD.

23.5 BMBS plastic, Giemsa, development of MF on basis of megakaryocytic myelosis, IT. Note megakaryocytic hyperplasia, intravascular hematopoiesis and fibrosis in the bone marrow surrounding the sinus.

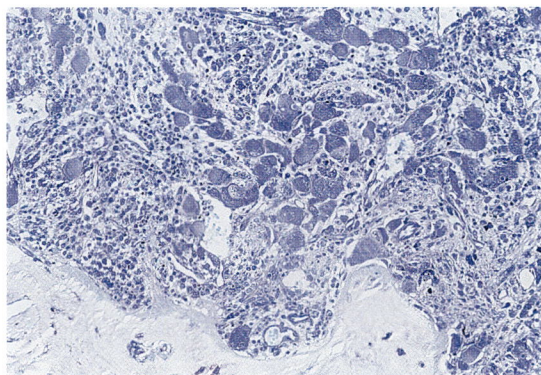

23.6 (left) BMBS plastic, Giemsa, showing MF after megakaryocytic myelosis, note fibrosis, disorganisation of marrow structure, megakaryocytes and interstitial platelets.

23.7 (right) BMBS plastic, Giemsa, large cluster of megakaryocytes in and around a dilated sinus.

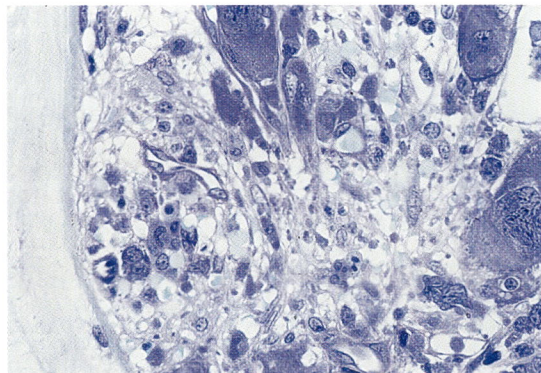
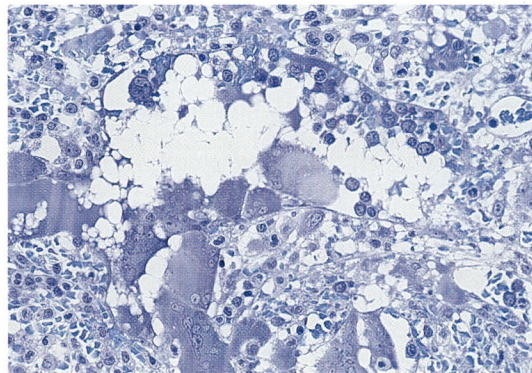

23.8 (left) BMBS plastic, Gomori, development of osteomyelosclerosis in case of PV with megakaryocytic hyperplasia; note presence of hematopoiesis.

23.9 (right) BMBS plastic, Gomori, viewed in polarised light, more advanced stage of OMS with increase in bone and decrease in hematopoiesis.

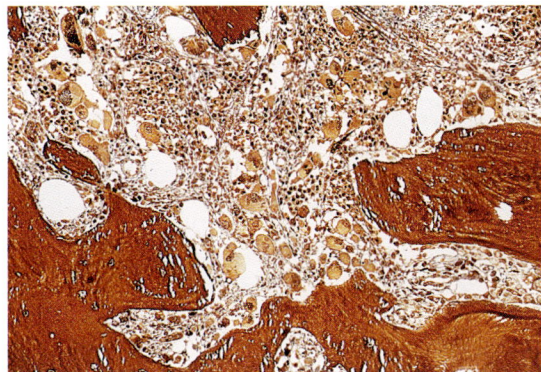
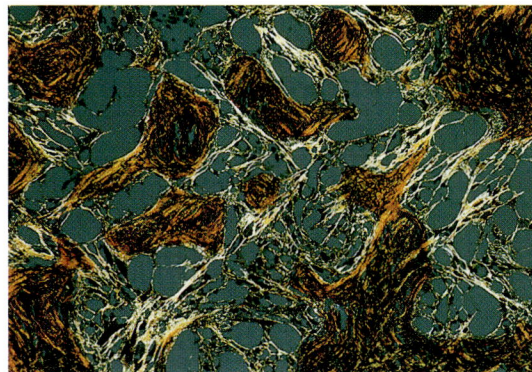

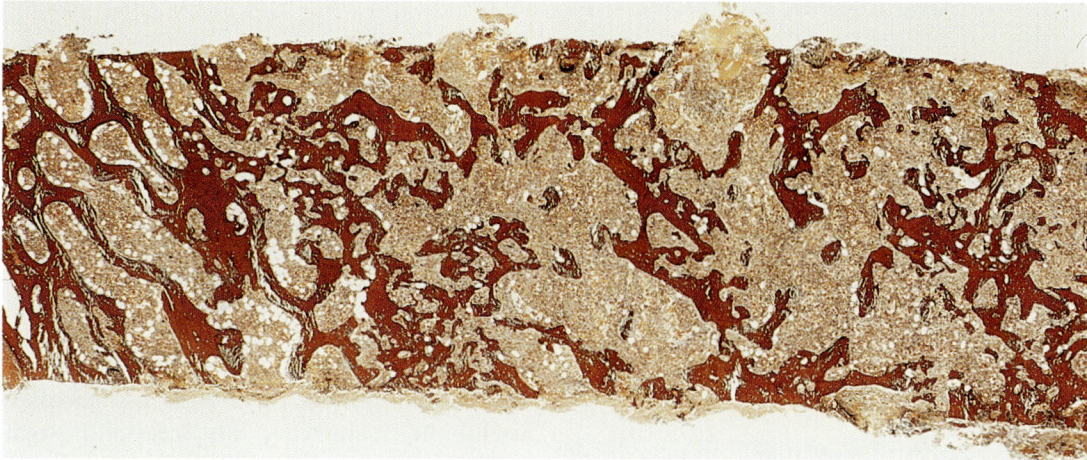

23.10 BMBS plastic, Gomori, low power, to illustrate uneven involvement of marrow and bone by MF/OMS.

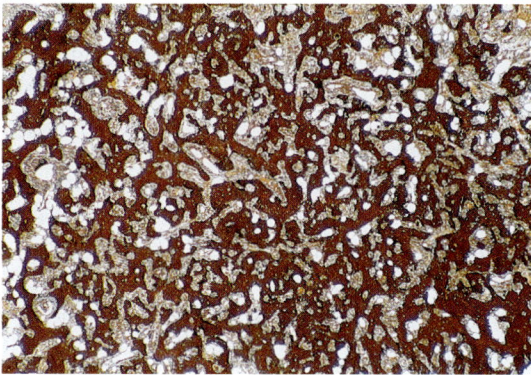

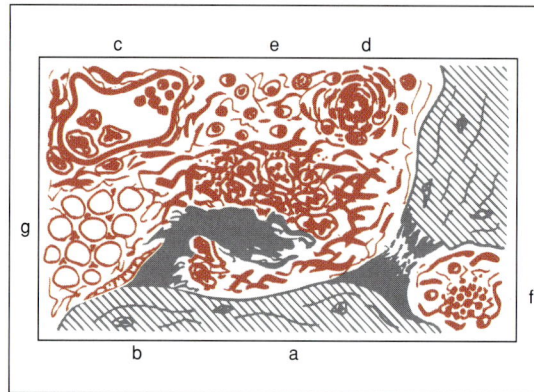

23.11 (left) BMBS plastic, Gomori, to show complete effacement of trabecular structure by osteosclerosis.

23.12 (right) Histological criteria in OMS. (a) and (b) Appositional and woven bone formation; periosseous clusters of megakaryocytes and interstitial platelets, center; (c) ectatic sinusoids with sclerotic walls and intravascular hematopoiesis; (d) perivascular inflammatory infiltration and fibrosis; (e) inflammatory infiltrates of plasma cells, mast cells and lymphoid cells; (f) benign lymphoid nodules; and (g) variable increase in fat cells.

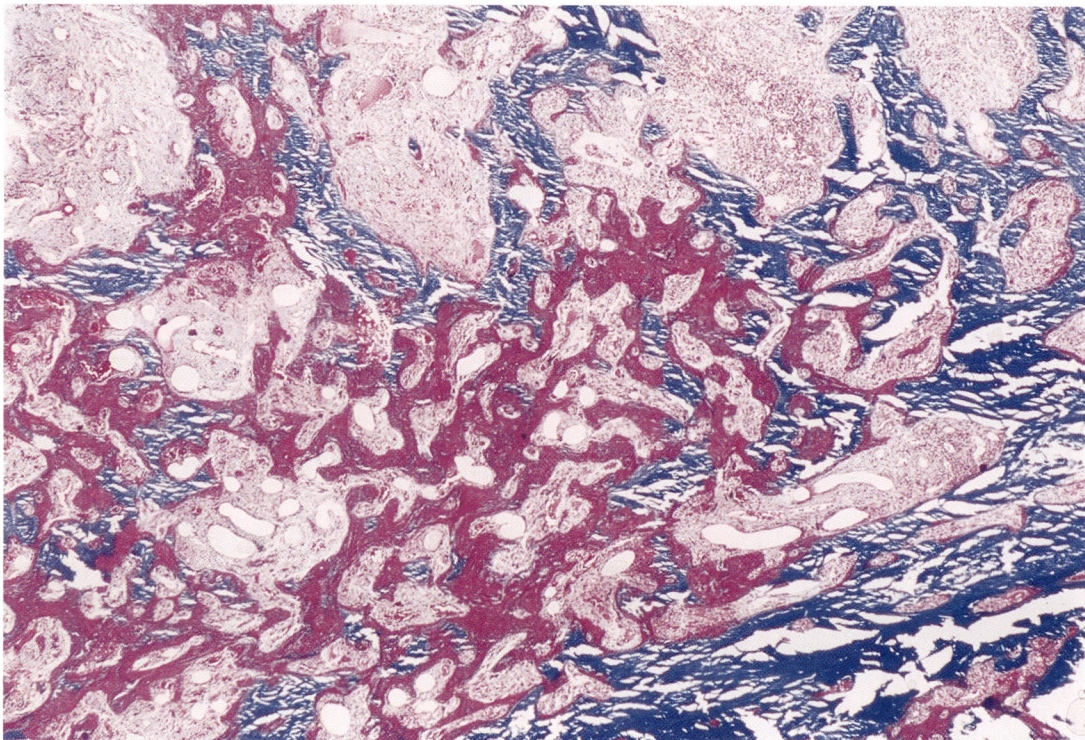

23.13 BMBS plastic Ladewig, highlighting component of osteoid (red) in the osteosclerotic bone.

248

TABLE 23.3 MPD megakaryocytes

Proliferative cell line(s)			Clinical entities	Biopsies (n)	Megakaryocytes (n) (SD) per mm² bone marrow area	1*	2	3	4	5	6
ERY	GRA	MEG	PV	135	6820 (8210)			+	+++	+++	++
——	——	MEG	IT	77	19810 (20139)	+	++	++	+++	+++	
——	GRA	MEG	CML	97	8987 (6737)	+	++	+	+	+	
——	GRA	——	CML	100	786 (520)		+	+			

* 1, Megakaryoblast; 2, promeagakaryocyte; 3, micro; 4, normal; 5, giant; 6, pyknotic.

occasionally seen) and (2) the mixed type of CML with concomitant hyperplasia of megakaryocytes, most of which are relatively small with small nuclei, accompanied by variable degrees of fibrosis, which is often patchy. Overlapping between the two histologic types of CML may occur, as in fact between all the clinical and histologic entities of the MPD. In some cases, two distinct cell lines may be affected, for example megakaryocytes and mast cells, as seen in coexistence of ET and systemic mastocytosis, in which there is often a striking fibrotic reaction, induced by both the affected cell lines. Moreover, progression of fibrosis over time has been recorded in some patients, though at varying rates.

Histology of bone marrow

The bone marrow to some extent reflects the development of the disease and three main phases (corresponding to three main types of histology) have been described: the hypercellular phase in which peripheral blood count values may be relatively high, the patchy phase with alternating areas of fibrosis and hematopoiesis, and low or normal peripheral blood count values, and the phase of obliterative sclerosis, which is reflected in pancytope-

nia usually with increasing transfusion requirements. However, these phases are not sharply separated, clinically or histologically, and overlap occurs between them. They need not be sequential and therefore may be found simultaneously in different parts of the skeleton, or even of the same section. This indicates spatial discordance in the evolution of the disease process. From the point of view of hematopoiesis they could be described as: (1) hematopoietic hyperplasia and (2) hematopoietic hypoplasia; both phases show a reduction in fat cells, increase in blood vessels and in fibroblasts, but even when few hematopoietic cells remain in the obliterative phase there are clusters of polymorphic megakaryocytes (in the MPD) with interstitially deposited platelets near them, areas of edema, gelatinous degeneration and infiltration with lymphocytes, plasma and mast cells, as well as macrophages containing hemosiderin or crystalloids and prominent islands of immature hematopoietic cells. Characteristic for MF in the MPD are the megakaryocytes, which may still be discerned within the dense fibrous tissue even when the other hematopoietic elements have disappeared. Frequently, naked nuclear masses are found, presumably remnants of megakaryocytes; little is known about how long they survive, or how they are eventually disposed of, in contrast with red cell nuclei which vanish rapidly into the voracious mononuclear phagocyte system. Naked nuclei may be seen in the sinusoids and possibly they are washed away and disintegrate in the bloodstream. It should be remembered that not all multinucleated or multilobulated cells in the bone marrow in various conditions are megakaryocytes; others are osteoclasts, monocytes and histiocytes, Langerhans' giant cells, metastatic neoplastic cells, anaplastic large cell lymphoma cells, Reed–Sternberg and mononuclear Hodgkin cells, and anaplastic plasmablasts. With progression of the disease process in MF/OMS, networks of reticulin merge with bundles of collagen and divide the marrow into compartments, causing sclerosis of the sinus walls, which no doubt is one reason for the appearance of intravascular islands of hematopoietic precursors, frequently observed in bone biopsies in both MF and OMS.

Histology of bone

In MF the overall trend is trabecular rarefaction, though occasional foci of osteoclastic activity may be found, while in OMS appositional new bone as well as irregular spicules of woven bone contribute to the progressive diminution of the marrow cavities, the contents of which, however, are often not so densely fibrotic as in obliterative MF; and some residual hematopoietic function is retained. Agnogenic myeloid metaplasia is the term applied to MF/OMS when the cause or the preceding disease is unknown, and there is extramedullary hematopoiesis in liver and spleen. It is now thought that most (if not all) cases are a consequence of a preceding MPD.

Lymphoproliferative disorders

(Figures 23.14–23.16)

Classic examples of fibrosis accompanying an LPD may be seen in hairy cell leukemia, centrocytic lymphoma, osteosclerotic multiple myeloma (MM) and Hodgkin's disease (HD). However, any lymphoproliferation – from benign lymphocytic aggregates to replacement of the marrow in chronic lymphocytic leukemia (CLL) – is accompanied by varying degrees of increase in reticular fibers, particularly in nodules if they are present; or around them as in some cases of nodular lymphomas and multiple myeloma. This is also the reason why an aspirate may not yield a high number of lymphocytes, even with considerable marrow involvement. Likewise for prolifera-

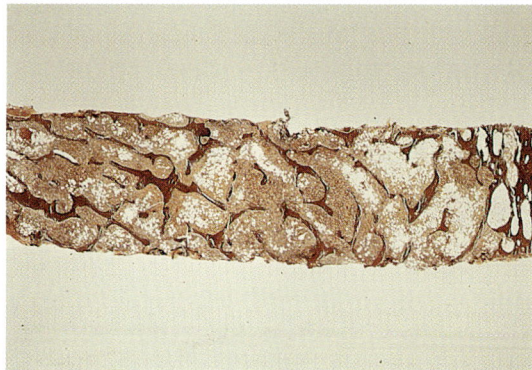

23.14 BMBS plastic, Gomori, low power, paratrabecular involvement by centrocytic lymphoma with fibrosis.

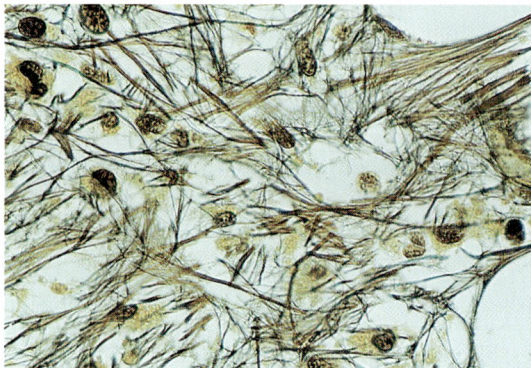

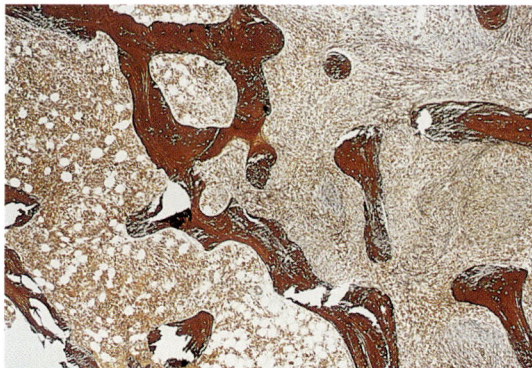

23.15 (left) BMBS plastic, Gomori, high power interstitial fibrosis in HCL.

23.16 (right) BMBS plastic, Gomori, HD involvement of bone marrow, left with fibrosis; hematopoiesis, right.

tions of the monocytic histiocytic cell lines, in which an almost obliterative fibrosis may develop.

Metastases in the bone marrow
(Figures 23.17–23.20)
In many cases of metastases in the bone marrow, a desmoplastic and osteoblastic reaction may occur as soon as the metastases attach to the endothelium and pass from the vascular lumen to the interstitial tissue of the bone marrow. Classic examples are metastases of breast and prostatic cancers and in some cases of paraneoplastic syndrome (Figure 23.20). This connective tissue and its blood vessels, especially the endothelium, react with Factor VIII-related antigen and CD34; as well as with actin and vimentin, which normal bone marrow connective tissue usually does not, though actin is present in blood vessels. However, these reactions are not confined to the connective tissue evoked by cancer cells;

they also occur in other reactive fibroses.

Osseous disorders (Figure 23.21)
The osseous conditions listed in Table 23.1 may all be focal, so that, for example, one of two bilateral biopsies may not be involved; or even one of two biopsies taken from the same iliac crest. In these cases prior radiologic guidance may be decisive. The paratrabecular areas are initially involved and the lesions then spread out into the marrow spaces, which may be obliterated in the involved regions. The degree of fibrosis varies in density but even in mildly fibrotic areas hematopoiesis is reduced though inflammatory infiltrating cells are present.

Deficiencies
1. Gaucher's disease is due to a deficiency of the enzyme glucose-cerebrosidase, as a consequence of which macrophages are unable to metabolise completely the breakdown prod-

23.17 (left) BMBS plastic, Gomori, polarised light, small focus of metastatic tumor cells in bone marrow with reactive fibrosis.

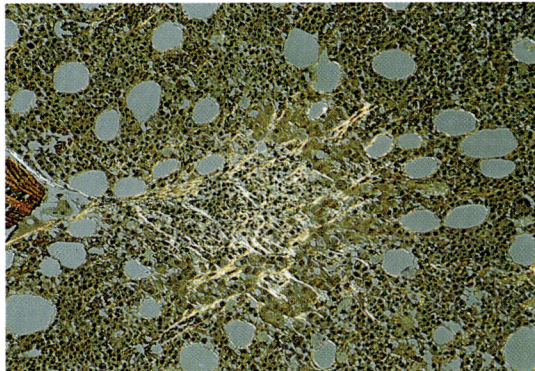

23.18 (right) BMBS paraffin H&E, metastases of prostatic carcinoma in dense fibrosis.

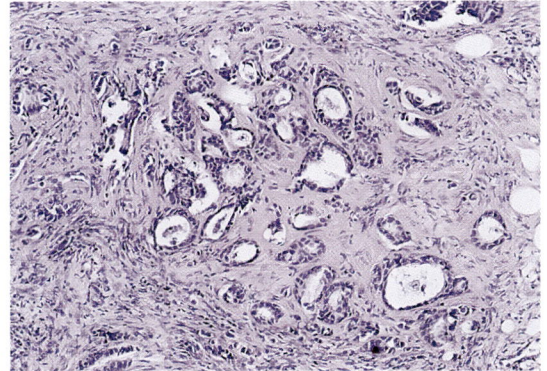

23.19 (left) BMBS plastic, Gomori, dense network of fibers surrounding metastatic tumor cells, case of breast cancer.

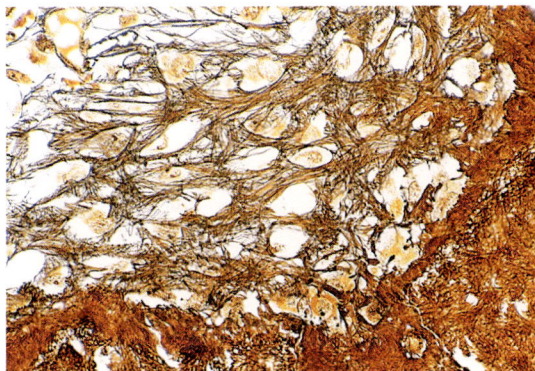

23.20 (right) BMBS plastic, Gomori, HPT in paraneoplastic syndrome, with paratrabecular fibrosis.

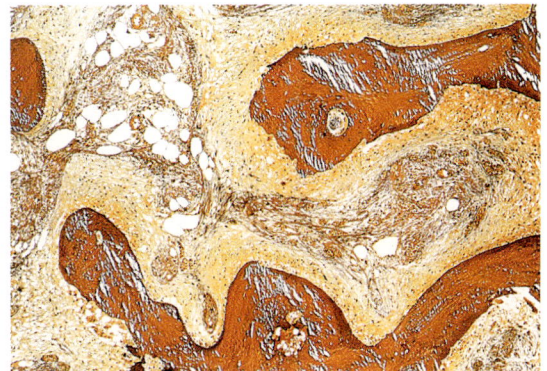

ucts of phagocytosed material, so that more and more phagocytic cells accumulate. As the typical Gaucher cells (macrophages, reticular cells, histiocytes, monocytes) accumulate in the bone marrow they replace both fat cells and hematopoiesis, are accompanied by a fibrotic reaction and frequently osteolytic bone lesions which cause intractable orthopedic problems as they develop (Figure 23.22). These late effects will be less frequently seen in the future as more patients are treated early on in the disease by the enzyme substitution therapy now available.

2. Vitamin D deficiency is still occasionally seen in young children and is associated with myelofibrosis and splenomegaly. The condition resolves completely after administration of appropriate therapy.

Inflammatory reactions

Some of the causes are listed in Table 23.1. Taken together, they form a fairly large group. The biopsies of these patients have in common the cellular components of an inflammatory reaction, though numerically the participating cells vary according to the provocative agent. Of particular clinical interest are the cytotoxic agents (therapy), infections such as tuberculosis (which is on the increase, especially in high-risk patients such as older age groups and those with decreased immunity), and AIDS in which, in addition to other findings, megakaryocytes are often increased and resemble those seen in myelodysplastic syndromes.

Five main morphologic types of inflammatory reactions have been described in the bone marrow (see Chapter 12): (1) exudative: this represents an acute inflammation with dilatation and disruption of the sinusoidal walls and subsequent hemorrhage and edema, and alterations in the stromal compartment; (2) atrophic type: chronic inflammatory reaction with replacement of hematopoiesis by fat cells, edema, gelatinous material, changes in the vessel walls, and inflammatory cell infiltrate. Such reactions may also terminate in fibrosis; (3) proliferative type: there is reduction in fat cells, hyperplasia of the cellular compartment, mainly of granulopoiesis, increased megakaryocytes, plasma and mast cells and lymphocytes. This type may be associated with neoplastic disease, bacterial infections, and drug abuse; (4) fibrotic type: also called sclerosing myelitis or cirrhosis of the bone marrow (Figure 23.23), in which development of coarse fibrosis is an early component, not, as it were, a late consequence. The fibrosis is accompanied by an exudative and inflammatory reaction, replacing most of the hematopoietic and fatty tissue; and (5) granulomatous type: characterised by the presence of nodules composed of macrophages, epithelioid cells, lymphocytes, multinucleated giant cells, fibroblasts, fibers and blood vessels. These nodules (granulomas) may be surrounded by a cuff of lymphocytes together with some plasma cells and eosinophils.

Pathogenesis and evolution of MF and OMS in the MPD (Figure 23.24)

Inflammation plays a central role in defense and healing processes and thus also contributes to their consequences: production of granulation tissue and fibrosis.

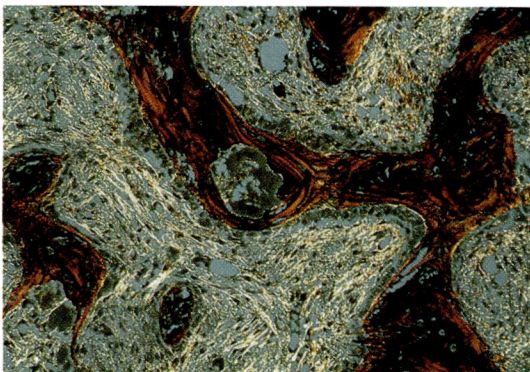

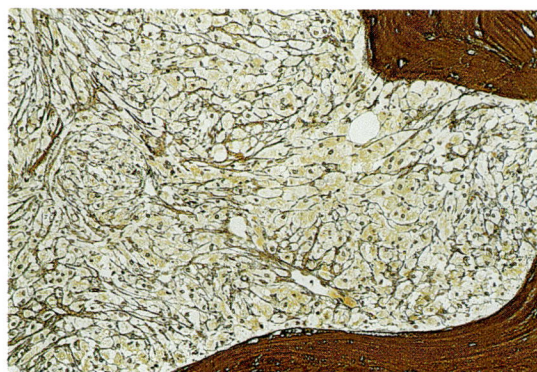

23.21 (left) BMBS plastic, Gomori, showing marked paratrabecular and intertrabecular fibrosis in PHPT.

23.22 (right) BMBS plastic, from case of Gaucher's disease, showing fibrosis in the foci of histiocytes.

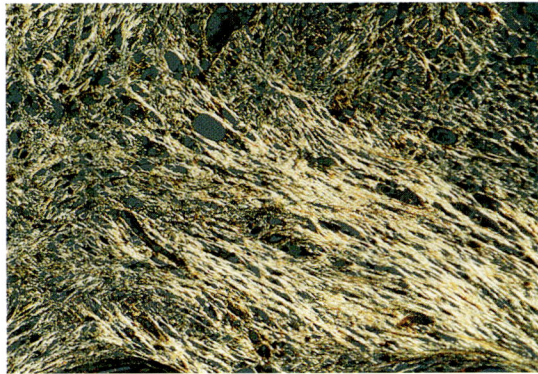

23.23 BMBS plastic, Gomori, showing atrophy and fibrosis in sclerosing myelitis.

23.24 Pathogenic mechanisms in MF/OMS; interactions between heterotopic megakaryocytes, interstitially deposited platelets, monocytes and lymphoid nodules induce the production of various growth factors, e.g. platelet-derived growth factor (PDGF), epidermal growth factor (EGF), transforming growth factor (TGF) β, endothelial cell growth factor (ECGF) and platelet factor IV (PLF IV). All induce fibroblast proliferation and fibrillogenesis: production of collagen types I (woven bone), III (coarse fibers in the marrow spaces) and IV (basement membrane material, sclerotic wall of the sinusoids).

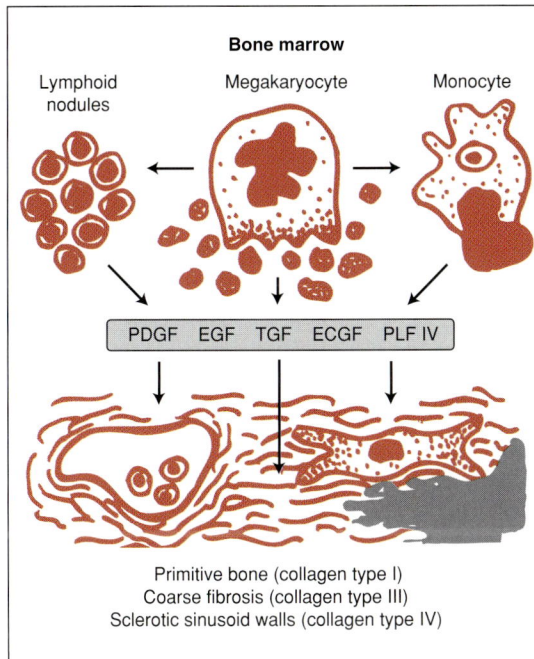

Bone marrow

Lymphoid nodules   Megakaryocyte   Monocyte

PDGF EGF TGF ECGF PLF IV

Primitive bone (collagen type I)
Coarse fibrosis (collagen type III)
Sclerotic sinusoid walls (collagen type IV)

fibrosis and the new bone formation. These effects are mediated by an increase in fibroblasts and increased secretion of fibers in MF, together with stimulation of osteoblasts and secretion of osteoid, resulting in appositional and primitive woven bone formation in OMS. In addition, the fibrosis also affects the blood vessels and though there is stimulation of capillaries and endothelial cell proliferation these are accompanied by development of continuous sheets of basement membrane without the fenestrations present in the normal marrow, so that egress of cells is impeded.

Myelofibrosis and osteomyelosclerosis occur together with additional stromal reactions, such as increased vascularisation and blood flow, usually also an increase in interstitial reticular cells, plasma and mast cells, lymphocytes and, in 15–30% of the cases, one or several lymphocytic aggregates. Hence, even in the myeloproliferative disorders, as in most of the other conditions, the pathogenic mechanisms are multiple, complex and interrelated. This probably explains the variability of the histologic findings, the uneven progression of the fibrosis and the ever present possibility of transformation to a different MPD; because the required regulatory factors are unevenly distributed in these heterogeneous environments.

Depending on the amount of fibrosis and of bone formation present three grades have been described, ranging from a moderate increase to an extensive replacement of the marrow and/or the normal trabecular bone. However, especially in large and long biopsies, different areas may show all the three grades so that morphologic classification is difficult, and the biopsy results must be interpreted within the framework of the peripheral blood values and other clinical data.

Evolution to MF/OMS has been observed in approximately 50% of patients with chronic MPD. On the basis of sequential biopsies it has been shown that OMS is not necessarily a more advanced stage of MF. These two types are qualitatively different modes of stromal reaction to the underlying myeloproliferation.

Though there may be relatively long periods between changes in bone marrow histology and their reflection in the peripheral blood

In the MPD, the fibrosis is thought to be due to a combination of mechanisms including: (1) a chronic inflammatory reaction mediated by immune complexes, (2) production of megakaryocyte and platelet-derived growth factors (PDGF) and collagenase inhibiting factor (platelet factor 4), and (3) production, release and activation of transforming growth factors β (TGFβ). Other growth factors are also involved, as well as matrix proteins.

Thus, the cytokines and growth factors released by plasma and mast cells, lymphocytes and monocytes as well as by megakaryocytes and platelets, are responsible for the picture, the myeloproliferations are non-static, constantly evolving disorders as evidenced also by cytogenetic analysis during their evolution. Likewise, though the rate of evolution may to some extent be influenced by therapy, this has little influence on the type of evolution the MPD may undergo, which is determined by the intrinsic characteristics of the cell lines involved and the stromal reactions evoked by them. A blast crisis could also ensue in any individual case after the transformation to MF/OMS. However, due to the disruption of the microenvironment and anomalies of maturation and egress of cells from the bone marrow (or sites of extramedullary hemato-poiesis) patients with an increased number of blasts in the peripheral blood do not necessar-ily have acute leukemia (Figure 23.25). Stages in the replacement of hematopoiesis have also been described, ranging from minimal to com-plete obliteration of the intertrabecular cavi-ties. Once the latter has occurred, difficulties in histologic diagnosis may arise if the under-lying myeloproliferative or other disorder can no longer be recognised. A biopsy from another site may then be required. Occasionally patients with longstanding MPD develop ML (Figure 23.26).

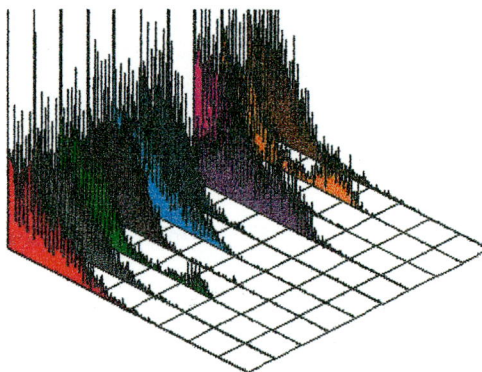

23.25 (left) Histogram of flow cytometry of bone marrow aspirate of patient with OMS and splenomegaly. Left to right: red, control; gray, CD7 8%; green, CD2 6%; dark purple, CD20 6%; blue, CD19 9%; dark blue, CD10 3%; red, CD33 5%; light brown, CD34 20%; dark brown, CD14 5%.

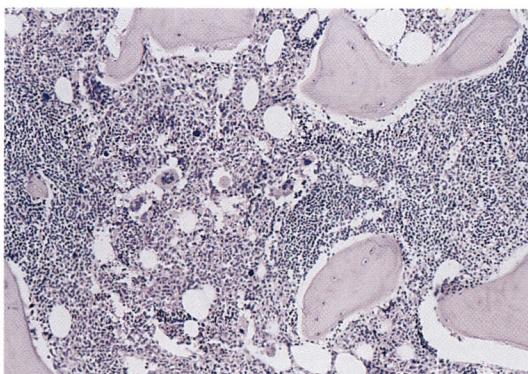

23.26 (right) BMBS paraffin, H&E, lymphoma developing in patient with longstanding MF.

Check list: Myelofibrosis and Osteomyelosclerosis and other Fibroses in the Bone Marrow

In cMPD
- Large biopsy required 3 × 40 mm.
- Microarchitecture of bone altered?
- Sclerosis or porosis?
- Mineralisation decreased? Toluidine blue, Ladewig or Goldner stain.
- Fibrosis: extent and topography? Reticulin and Masson's trichrome.
- Vascularity: sclerosis of vessels walls?
- Areas of hypocellularity, of atrophy?
- Hematopoiesis: quantity, topography, dysplastic features, maturation, intrasinusoidal?

- Clusters of abnormal megakaryocytes, sometimes also within the lumina of the sinusoids; I.H.: Factor VIII for megakaryocytes.
- Inflammatory infiltrations and lymphocytic aggregates? I.H.: LCA, T and B cells.

In other conditions
As well as points listed above:

- Osteoclasts and osteoblasts, woven bone?
- Osseous remodeling – primary disorder?
- Extent, type and density of fibrosis? Appropriate connective tissue stains. Vimentin and actin on I.H.
- Residual hematopoiesis? Myeloperoxidase, Factor VIII on I.H.

Continued

- Malignant infiltrations? Cytokeratin, S100, and EMA on I.H, other antibodies if required.
- Histiocytic infiltrations? CD68, lysozyme on I.H.
- Inflammatory reactions? LCA, T cells, kappa, lambda.
- Obliterative fibrosis? Consider another biopsy from other side?

Clinical correlations

- Clinical history – previous cMPD.
- Variable cytopenia(s) and corresponding complications.
- Splenomegaly, often massive.
- Leukoerythroblastic blood picture: even myeloblasts in peripheral blood.
- Extramedullary hematopoiesis in liver and spleen.
- High LAP in MF/OMS
- Peripheral blood values and leucoerythroblastic blood picture.
- Clonal   −5   del(5)(q)
  Chromosomal −7   del(13)(q)
  Characteristics +8   del(20)(q)
        +9   1q rearrangements.

Bibliography

Bartl R., Frisch B., Baumgart R. (1992) Morphologic classification of the myelodysplastic syndromes (MDS): combined utilisation of bone marrow aspirates and trephine biopsies. *Leukaemia Res.*, **16 (1)**, 15.

Bartl R., Frisch B., Burkhardt R. (1991) Bone marrow histology. In Catovsky, (ed) *Methods in Hematology: The Leukemic Cells.* Edinburgh: Churchill Livingstone, vol. 2, p. 47.

Bentley S.A., Herman C.J. (1979) Bone marrow fiber production in myelofibrosis: a quantitative study. *Br J Haematol.*, **42**, 51.

Bernabel P.A., Arcangeli A., Casini M. *et al.* (1986) Platelet-derived growth factor(s) mitogenic activity in patients with myeloproliferative disease. *Br J Haematol.*, **63**, 483.

Buhr T., Choritz H., Georgii A. (1992) The impact of megakaryocyte proliferation of the evolution of myelofibrosis. Histological

follow-up study in 186 patients with chronic myeloid leukemia. *Virchows Arch. A. Pathol. Anat. Histopathol.*, **420 (6)**, 473–8.

Burkhardt R., Bartl R., Jäger K. *et al.* (1984) Chronic myeloproliferative disorders (CMPD). *Pathol Res Pract.*, **179**, 131.

Burkhardt R., Bartl R., Beil E. *et al.* (1975) Myelofibrosis-osteosclerosis syndrome. Review of literature and histomorphometry. In *Advances in the Biosciences.* Oxford/ Braunschweig: Pergamon/Vieweg, vol. 16, pp. 9–56.

Caligaris Cappio F., Vigliani R., Novariono A. *et al.* (1981) Idiopathic myelofibrosis: a possible role for immune-complexes in the pathogenesis of bone marrow fibrosis. *Br. J. Haematol.*, **49**, 17–21.

Castro-Malaspina H. (1984) Pathogenesis of myelofibrosis: role of ineffective megakaryopoiesis and megakaryocyte components. In Berk, H. Castro-Malaspina and Wasserman (eds), *Myelofibrosis and the*

Biology of the Connective Tissue. New York: Alan R Liss, pp. 427.

Cervantes F., Lopez-Guillermo A., Piera C. *et al.* (1993) Initial iron deposits in idiopathic myelofibrosis. Analysis of 20 patients. *Sangre (Barc)*, **38 (4)**, 279–82.

Dini D., Artusi T., di Prisco U. (1991) Idiopathic myelofibrosis associated with an IgM-secreting immunocytoma. *Recenti Prog. Med.*, **82 (2)**, 77–9.

Fava R.A., Casey T.T., Wicox J. *et al.* (1990) Synthesis of transforming growth factor-β1 by megakaryocytes and its localization to megakaryocyte and platelet alpha-granules. *Blood*, **76**, 1946.

Frisch B., Bartl R., Burkhardt R. *et al.* (1984) Classification of myeloproliferative disorders by bone marrow histology. In B. Frisch and R. Bartl (eds), *Bone Marrow Biopsies Updated. New Prospects for Clinical Diagnostics.* Basel: Karger.

Frisch B., Bartl R. (1985) Histology of myelofibrosis and osteo-myelofibrosis. In: S.M. Lewis (ed), *Myelofibrosis*. New York: Marcel Dekker, pp. 51–86.

Frisch B., Bartl R. (1990) *Atlas of Bone Marrow Pathology*. Dordrecht: Kluwer Academic.

Frisch B., Bartl R. (1992) Bone marrow histology in myelodysplastic syndromes: an update. *Myelo-dysplastic Syndromes*, 103–6.

Frisch B., Bartl R., Jäger K. (1989) Histologic diagnosis of chronic myeloproliferative disorders. *Hematol. Rev.*, **3**, 131–47.

Frisch B., Lewis S.M., Burkhardt R., Bartl R. (1985) *Biopsy Pathology of Bone and Bone Marrow*. London, Chapman & Hall.

Georgii A., Vykoupil K.F., Thiele J. (1984) Classification of chronic myeloproliferative diseases by bone marrow biopsies. Hematological and cytogenic findings and clinical course. In B. Frisch and R. Bartl (eds), *Bone Marrow Biopsies Updated. New Prospects for Clinical Diagnostics*. Basel: Karger, pp. 41–56.

Hasselbalch H. (1990) Idiopathic myelofibrosis: a review. *Eur. J. Hematol.*, **45** (2), 65–72.

Hasselbalch H., Lisse I. (1991) A sequential histological study of bone marrow fibrosis in idiopathic myelofibrosis. *Eur. J. Hematol.*, **46** (5), 285–9.

Hasselbalch H., Jans H., Nielsen P.L. (1987) A distinct subtype of idiopathic myelofibrosis with bone marrow features mimicking hairy cell leukemia: evidence of an autoimmune pathogenesis. *Am J. Hematol.*, **25** (2), 225–9.

Hirata J., Takahira H., Kaneko S. *et al.* (1989) Bone marrow stromal cells in myeloproliferative disorders. *Acta. Hematol.*, **82** (1), 35–9.

Katoh O., Kimura A., Itoh T., Kuramoto A. (1990) Platelet derived growth factor messenger RNA is increased in bone marrow megakaryocytes in patients with myeloproliferative disorders. *Am J. Hematol.*, **35** (3), 145–50.

Kerim S., Rege-Cambrin G., Scaravaglio P. *et al.* (1991) Trisomy 8 and an unbalanced T(5; 17) (Q11; P11) characterize two karyotypically independent clones in a case of idiopathic myelofibrosis evolving to acute nonlymphoid leukemia. *Cancer Gent. Cytogenet.*, **52(1)**, 63–9.

Kimura A., Katoh O., Kuramoto A. (1988) Effects of platelet derived growth factor, epidermal growth factor and transforming growth factor-β on the growth of human marrow fibroblasts. *Br J Haematol.*, **69**, 1.

Kvasnicka H.M., Thiele J., Amend T., Fischer R. (1994) Three-dimensional reconstruction of histologic structures in human bone marrow from serial sections of trephine biopsies. Spatial appearance of sinusoidal vessels in primary (idiopathic) osteomyelofibrosis. *Anal Quant Cytol Histol*, **16** (3), 159–66.

Lisse I., Hasselbalch H., Junker P. (1991) Bone marrow stroma in idiopathic myelofibrosis and other hematological diseases. An immunohistochemical study. *APMIS*, **99** (2), 171–8.

Mccarthy D.M. (1985) Fibrosis of the bone marrow: content and causes (Annotation). *Br J Haematol.*, **59**, 1.

McCarthy D.M., Hibbin J.A., Goldman J.M. (1984) A role for 1,25-dihydroxyvitamin D3 in control of bone-marrow collagen deposition? *Lancet*, **i**, 78.

Murate T., Yamashita K., Isogai C. *et al.* (1997) The production of tissue inhibitors of metalloproteinases (TIMPs) in megakaryopoiesis: possible role of platelet- and megakaryocyte-derived TIMPs in bone marrow fibrosis. *Br. J. Haematol.*, **99**, 181–9.

Patton W.N., Bunce C.M., Larkins S., Brown G. (1991) Defective erythropoiesis in primary myelofibrosis associated with a chromosome 11 abnormality. *Br. J. Cancer*, **64** (1), 128–31.

Pereira A., Cervantes F., Brugues R., Rozman J.F. (1990) Bone marrow histopathology in primary myelofibrosis: clinical and hematologic correlations and prognostic evaluation. *Eur J Hematol*, **44** (2), 95–9.

Reilly, J.T. (1992) Pathogenesis of idiopathic myelofibrosis: role of growth factors. *J. Clin. Pathol.*, **45** (6), 461–4.

Roberts A.B., Sporn M.B., Assoian R.K. (1986) Transforming growth factor-β: rapid induction of fibrosis and angiogenesis in vivo and stimulation of collagen formation in vitro. *Proc Natl Acad Sci., USA*, **83**, 4167.

Smith R.E., Chelmowski M.K., Szabo E.J. (1988) Myelofibrosis: a concise review of clinical and pathologic features and treatment. *Am. J. Hematol.*, **29**, 174–80.

Spitzer T.R., Harris N.L. (1993) A 49-year-old man with myelofibrosis, myeloid metaplasia, and osteolytic lesions of the left femur. *New England Journal of Medicine*, **329** (6), 417–24.

Takahashi T., Akihama T., Yamaguchi A. *et al.* (1987) Lysozyme secreting tumor: a case of gastric cancer associated with myelofibrosis due to disseminated bone marrow metastasis. *Jpn. J. Med.*, **26** (1), 58–64.

Tasaka T., Nagai M., Murao S. *et al.* (1993) CD7, CD34-positive stem cell leukemia arising in agnogenic myeloid metaplasia. *Am. J. Hematol.*, **44** (1), 53–7.

Thiele J., Chen Y.S., Kvasnicka H.M. *et al.* (1994) Evolution of fibro-osteosclerotic bone marrow lesions in primary (idiopathic) osteomyelofibrosis – a histomorphometric study on sequential trephine biopsies. *Leuk Lymphoma*, **14** (1–2), 163–9.

Thiele J., Hoeppner B., Zankovich R., Fischer R. (1989) Histomorphometry of bone marrow biopsies in primary osteomyelofibrosis/-sclerosis (agnogenic myeloid metaplasia) correlations between clinical and morphological features. *Virchows Arch. A. Pathol. Anat. Histopathol.*, **415** (3), 191–202.

Truong L.D., Saleem A., Schwartz M.R. (1984) Acute myelofibrosis. A report of four cases and review of the literature. *Medicine*, **63**, 182.

Yetgin S., Ozsoylu S., Ruacan S. *et al.* (1989) Vitamin D-deficiency rickets and myelofibrosis. *J. Pediatr.*, **114** (2), 213–17

256

24 Systemic mastocytosis

Definition, classification and variants

Mast cells are a storehouse for many chemical mediators including histamine, serotonin, heparin, prostaglandins and proteoglycans (Table 24.1). It is the increased secretion of many of these substances that leads to the clinical manifestations of mastocytosis, such as pruritis, increased vasopermeability, gastric hypersecretion and bronchoconstriction (Table 24.2). Increases in mast cells in the bone marrow occur in many conditions (Figure 24.1), and have been dealt with in Chapters 17 and 19. Systemic mastocytosis is characterised by proliferation of mast cells in various organs and tissues. It is not yet clear whether the mast cell hyperplasia of systemic mastocytosis is clonal and neoplastic, or whether it represents a reactive hyperplasia. Several classifications have been published and a recent consensus classification describes four variants.

1. An indolent type that includes the majority of patients and which does not have a major influence on life expectancy.

2. A hematological type associated with a myeloproliferative or myelodysplastic disorder.

3. An aggressive type whose outcome is determined by the extent of mast cell proliferation in the parenchyme of various organs.

4. Mast cell leukemia, a rare and fatal disease.

Bone marrow histology

In the bone marrow, the characteristic histological lesion is the mast cell granuloma, which is located in endosteal, perivascular and intertrabecular regions, and is generally accompanied by variable increases in interstitial, perivascular and paratrabecular mastulla (Figures 24.2–24.6). These lesions are frequently found in the vertebrae and pelvic bones. The mast cell granulomas consist of variably granulated, mainly spindle-shaped mast cells, together with lymphocytes, plasma cells, eosinophils, sea-blue crystal-containing histiocytes and fibroblasts (Figure 24.7), all in a framework of fibers and blood vessels. Some cases may show a considerable increase in eosinophils, accompanied by peripheral blood eosinophilia. In advanced cases, the granulomas coalesce and occupy large areas of the marrow. Three stages can be distinguished: (1) small solitary granulomas, (2) multiple granulomas and (3) extensive granulomatous infiltration with marked fibrosis, replacement of hematopoiesis and increased osseous remodeling. Skeletal changes range from osteoporosis to osteolysis, or osteosclerosis, either focal or diffuse.

Paratrabecular granulomas always induce a local osseous reaction: osteoblastic, osteosclerotic or mixed; and on X-ray 70% of patients have skeletal lesions: osteopenia in 44%, multiple osteolysis in 27% and osteosclerotic lesions in 17%. Though malignant variants are rare, there is an increased risk of hematological malignancies in systemic mastocytosis

TABLE 24.1 Factors produced by mast cells

Lipid mediators	Granule mediators	Cytokines
LTB4	histamine	IL-1, 3, 4, 5, 6
LTC4	heparin proteoglycans	GM-CSF
PAF	serine proteases	TNF-alpha
PGD2	tryptase carboxypeptidase A	TGF-beta

TABLE 24.2 Responses to mast cell factors

Leukocyte responses	Fibroblast responses	Microvascular responses
Adherance	Proliferation	Augmented vascular permeability
Chemotaxis	Collagen production	Leukocyte adherence
Phagocytosis	Substrate responses	Constriction
IgE production	Protein degradation	Dilatation
Mast cell proliferation	Coagulation activation	
Eosinophil activation		

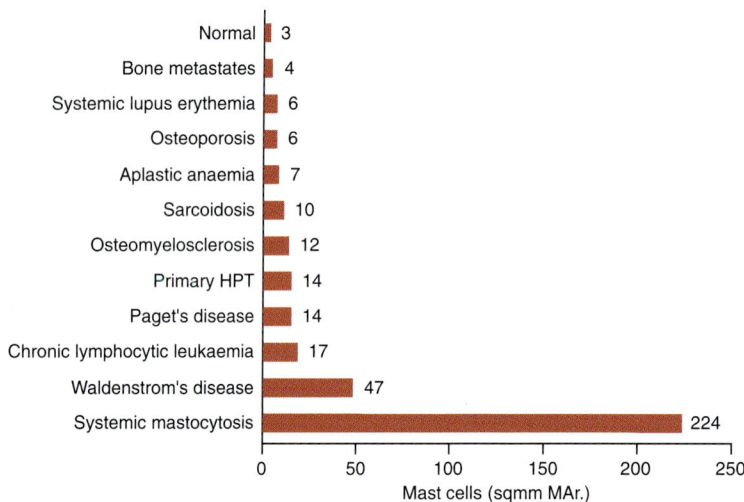

24.1 Conditions with increases in mast cells in the bone marrow.

24.2 (left) Systemic mastocytosis in the bone marrow. There is a patchy involvement: paratrabecular, intertrabecular and perivascular granulomas consisting of a heterogeneous cell population, though the majority are mast and lymphoid cells.

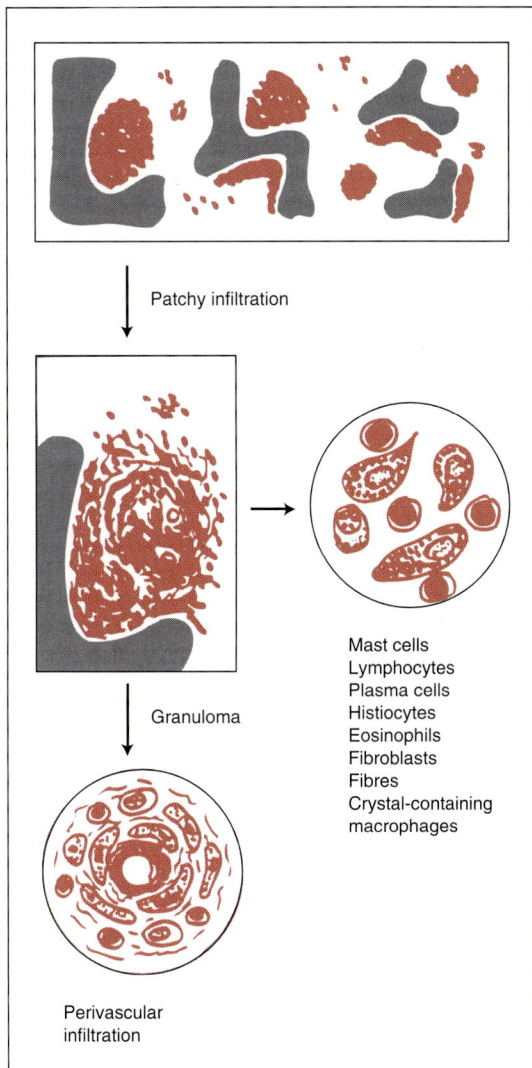

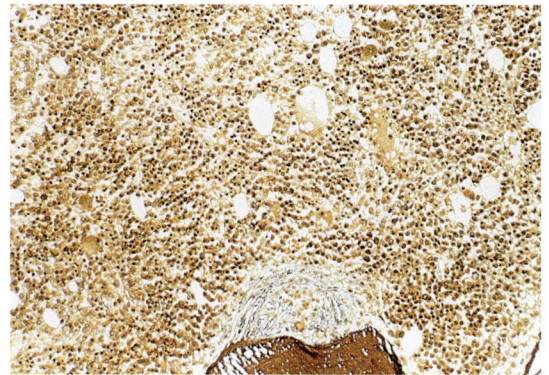

24.3 (right top) BMBS plastic, Gomori, small paratrabecular mast cell granuloma.

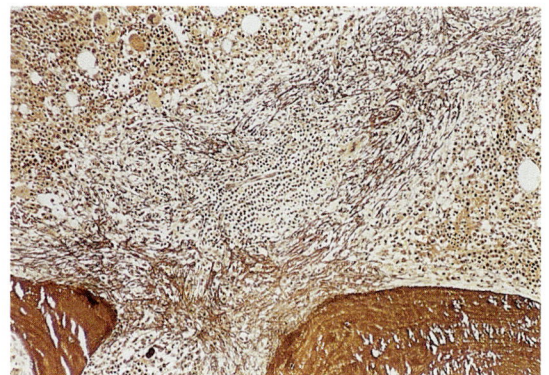

24.4 (right middle) BMBS plastic, Gomori, showing larger intertrabecular nodule, partly lymphocytic, surrounded by dense fibrosis.

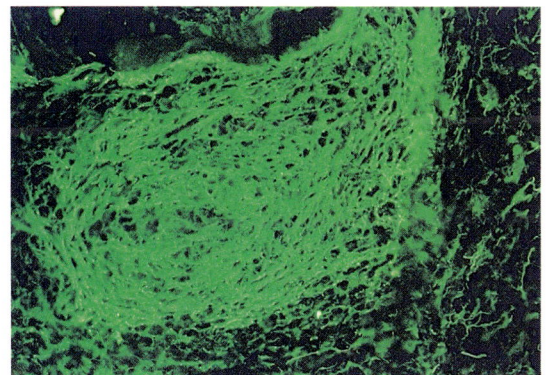

24.5 (right bottom) BMBS frozen section incubated with fluorescein-conjugated antibody to collagen type III in mast cell granuloma.

24.6 (left) BMBS plastic, Giemsa, moderate perivascular mastocytosis.

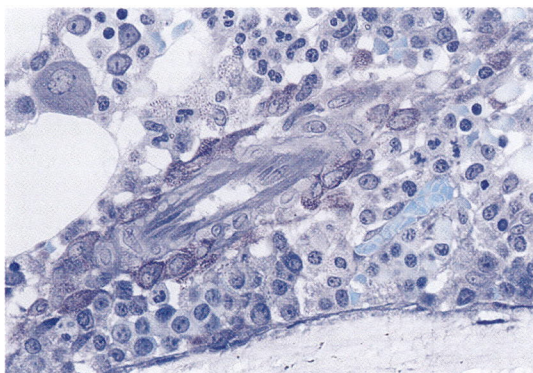

24.7 (right) BMBS plastic, Giemsa, part of mast cell granuloma, with elongated mast cells and numerous crystal-containing macrophages.

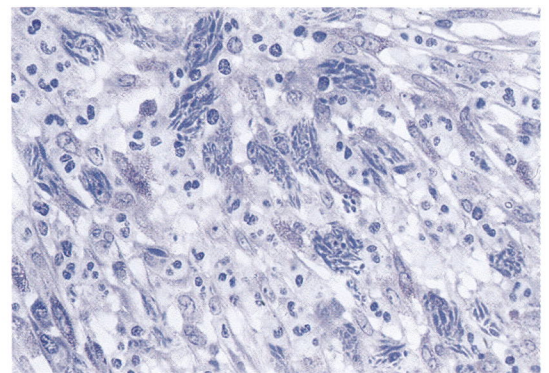

Patchy infiltration

Granuloma

Perivascular infiltration

Mast cells
Lymphocytes
Plasma cells
Histiocytes
Eosinophils
Fibroblasts
Fibres
Crystal-containing macrophages

259

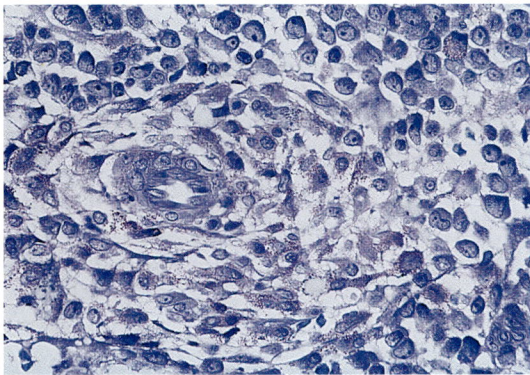

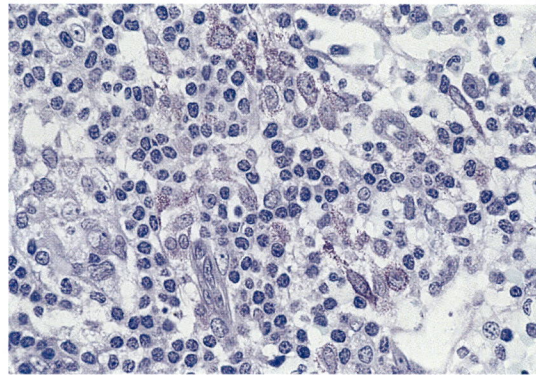

24.8 (left) BMBS plastic, Giemsa, showing myeloblasts surrounding perivascular mast cell granuloma, case of acute leukemia in patient with systemic mastocytosis.

24.9 (right) As for Figure 24.10, showing lymphocytic mast cell aggregate.

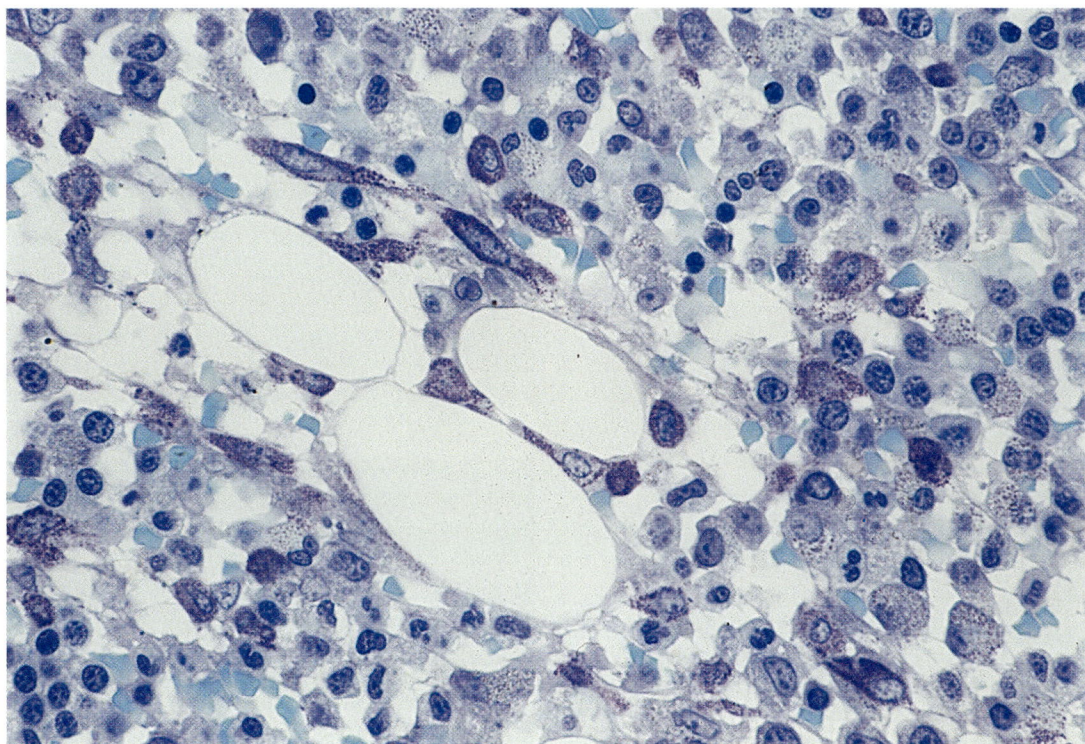

24.10 BMBS plastic, Giemsa, illustrating increased interstitial mast cells in biopsy of patient who later developed typical mast cell granulomas.

(Figure 24.8). The lymphocytic component of mast cell granulomas together with lymphocytic aggregates and nodules may occasionally be so extensive as to mimic a lymphoproliferative disorder.

In incipient or early cases, only increased interstitial, perivascular and paratrabecular or endosteal mast cells may be found, with or without a small lymphocytic and mast cell aggregate (Figures 24.9 and 24.10). These cases require close follow-up and sequential biopsies.

Check list: Systemic Mastocytosis

- Adequate biopsy with both cortex and cancellous bone.
- Undecalcified, as mast cell granules leach out during decalcification.
- In paraffin sections, IgE will stain mast cells on immunohistology (I.H.).
- Increased perivascular, paratrabecular and interstitial mast cells? Range in shape from round and oval to long and spindle-shaped.

Continued

- Aggregates – may be small in early cases – of mast cells, lymphocytes and plasma cells.
- Increased interstitial lymphocytes, plasma cells, eosinophils, crystal-containing macrophages?
- Presence of mast cell granulomas – perivascular, paratrabecular, interstitial, few or many, large or small, separate or confluent. Mast cells may be packed or have few granules, i.e. resemble fibroblasts. I.H.: T and B cells, vimentin, CD68, reticulin stain, kappa and lambda.

Example

Bone biopsy 3 × 40 mm. Undecalcified, Giemsa and toluidine blue stained sections. At low power fibrous nodules are seen. At high magnification typical mast cell granulomas with marked fibrosis are found – interstitial, perivascular and paratrabecular. There are increased interstitial and paratrabecular plasma cells, mast cells, lymphocytes, macrophages with crystals. The trabecular bone is osteopenic, with increased remodeling adjacent to the nodules. Overall decrease in hematopoiesis, present only between the mast cell granulomas. Summary: bone biopsy showing osteopenic trabecular bone, presence of paratrabecular, interstitial and perivascular typical mast cell granulomas. Hematopoiesis decreased. Diagnosis: systemic mastocytosis.

Clinical correlations

- Dermatologic manifestations: urticaria pigmentosa.
- Fluctuations of blood pressure, hypertension, flushing.
- Attacks of dyspnea due to bronchospasms.
- Osteoporotic, osteolytic and/or osteosclerotic skeletal lesions on scan and X-ray.
- Increased levels of histamine, and histamine metabolites in urine.
- Gastrointestinal symptoms: ulcers, malabsorption.
- Variable associated peripheral blood changes, e.g. neutropenia.
- Increased incidence of myeloproliferative and lymphoproliferative disorders.
- Possibly hepatosplenomegaly, lymphadenopathy.
- Generally indolent course; rare progression to rapidly fatal mast cell leukemia.
- Peripheral blood values, especially neutropenia.
- Clonal Chromosomal Characteristics: +8 t(X;8)(q2?6q21.3)

Bibliography

Austen K.F. (1992) Systemic mastocytosis. *N Engl J Med.*, **326**, 639.

Chessells J.M., Swansbury G.J., Reeves B. *et al.* (1997) Cytogenetics and prognosis in childhood and lymphoblastic leukaemia: results of MRC UKALL X. *Br. J. Haematol.*, **99**, 93–100.

Czarnetzki B.M., Kolde G., Schoemann A. *et al.* (1988) Bone marrow findings in adult patients with urtucaria pigmentosa. *J. Am. Acad. Dermatol.*, **18 (1)**, 45–51.

Dash S., Rao N.R., Deodhar S.D., Varma N. (1991) Malignant mastocytosis and myelodysplastic syndrome (letter). *Br. J. Hematol.*, **79 (3)**, 530–1.

Duschet P., Hanak H., Gschnait F. (1988) Systemic mastocytosis. *Z Hautkr*, **63 (11)**, 945–8.

Frisch B., Bartl R. (1990) *Atlas of Bone Marrow Pathology.* Dordrecht: Kluwer Academic.

Galli S.J. (1990) Biology of disease. New insights into 'The riddle of the mast cells': microenvironmental regulation of mast cell development and phenotypic heterogeneity. *Lab Invest.*, **62**, 5.

Gordon J.R., Burd P.R., Galli S.J. (1990) Mast cells as a source of multifunctional cytokines. *Immunol Today.*, **11**, 458.

Hills E., Dunstan C.R., Evans R.A. (1981) Bone metabolism in systemic mastocytosis. *J Bone Jt Surg.*, **63A**, 665.

Horny H.P., Ruck M., Wehrmann M., Kaiserling A. (1990) Blood findings in generalized mastocytosis: evidence of frequent simultaneous occurrence of myeloproliferative disorders. *Br J Haematol.*, **76**, 186.

Katsuda S., Okada Y., Oda Y. *et al.* (1987) Systemic mastocytosis without cutaneous involvement. *Acta Pathol. Jpn.*, **37**, 167.

Kettelhut B.V., Metcalfe D.D. (1991) Pediatric mastocytosis. *J Invest Dermatol.*, **96**, 15S.

Kluin-Nelemans H.C., Jansen J.H., Breukelman H. *et al.* (1992) Response to interferon alpha-2b in a patient with systemic mastocytosis. *N Engl J Med.*, **326**, 619.

Lawrence J.B., Friedman B.S., Travis W.D. *et al.* (1991) Hematologic manifestations of systemic mast cell disease: a prospective study of laboratory and morphologic features and their relation to prognosis. *Amer J Med.*, **91**, 612.

Lishner M., Confino-Cohen R., Mekori Y.A. *et al.* (1996) Trisomies 9 and 8 detected by fluorescence in situ hybridization in patients with systemic mastocytosis. *J Allergy Clin Immunol*, **98 (1)**, 199–204.

Lortholary O., Audouin J., Le Tourneau A., Diebold J. (1991) Le mastocyte et sa pathologie (2me partie). Histopathologie des mastocytoses. *Ann Pathol.*, **11**, 92–100.

Metcalfe D.D. (1991) Classification and diagnosis of mastocytosis: current status. *J Invest Dermatol.*, **96**, 2S.

Mezger J., Permanetter W., Gerhartz H. *et al.* (1990) Philadelphia chromosome-negative acute hematopoietic malignancy: ultrastructural, cytochemical and immunocytochemical evidence of mast cell and basophil differentiation. *Leukemia Res.*, **14**, 169.

Miranda R.N., Esparza A.R., Sambandam S., Medeiros L.J. (1994) Systemic mast cell disease presenting with peripheral blood eosinophilia. *Hum Pathol*, **25 (7)**, 727–30.

Orfao A., Escribano L., Villarrubia J. *et al.* (1996) Flow cytometric analysis of mast cells from normal and pathological human bone marrow samples: identification and enumeration. *Am J Pathol.*, **149 (5)**, 1493–9.

Parker R.I. (1991) Hematologic aspects of mastocytosis: II: Management of hematologic disorders in association with systemic mast cell disease. *J Invest Dermatol.*, **96**, 52S.

Raffi M., Firooznia H., Golimbu C., Balthaza E. (1983) Pathologic fracture in systemic mastocytosis. Radiographic spectrum and review of the literature. *Clin Orthop.*, **180**, 260.

Ridell B., Olafsson J.H., Roupe G. *et al.* (1986) The bone marrow in urticaria pigmentosa and systemic mastocytosis. *Arch Dermatol.*, **122**, 422.

Roberts L.J., Oates J.A. (1991) Biochemical diagnosis of systemic mast cell disorders. *J Invest Dermatol.*, **96**, 19S.

Tharp M.D. (1985) The spectrum of mastocytosis. *Amer J Med Sci.*, **289**, 119.

Travis W.D., Li C.Y., Bergsralh E.J. (1989) Solid and hematologic malignancies in 60 patients with systemic mast cell disease. *Arch Pathol Lab Med.*, **113**, 365.

Travis W.D., Li C.Y., Yam L.T. *et al.* (1988) Significance of systemic mast cell disease with associated hematologic disorders. *Cancer*, **62**, 965.

Travis W.D., Li C.Y., Yam L.T. *et al.* (1988) Systemic mast cell disease: analysis of 58 cases and literature review. *Medicine*, **67**, 345.

Yoo D., Lessin L.S. (1982) Bone marrow mast cell content in preleukemic syndrome. *Amer J Med.*, **73**, 539.

Yoo D., Lessin L.S., Jensen W.N. (1978) Bone marrow mast cells in lymphoproliferative disorders. *Ann Intern Med.*, **88**, 753.

Zhang Y., Schlegelberger B., Weber-Matthiesen K. *et al.* (1994) Translocation (X;8)(q2?6;q21.3) in a case of systemic mastocytosis. *Cancer Genet Cytogenet*, **78 (2)**, 236–8.

25 Lympho-proliferations in the bone marrow

General aspects

The bone marrow is an organ of lymphopoiesis, of passage in the migration of lymphoid cells and in the maturation of plasma cells. With the increasing investigation of bone biopsies in recent years it has become evident that lymphoid cells, nodules and follicles may frequently be encountered in bone marrow biopsies in a wide variety of reactive conditions as well as when involvement by malignant lymphomas is present. When dealing with possible bone marrow involvement by malignant processes of the lymphoid system, there are three main areas in which early or minimal involvement may be difficult to distinguish from reactive proliferations: (1) reactive lymphocytosis, (2) plasmacytosis and (3) granulomas. Their differential diagnosis is briefly considered below. In addition, it should be stressed that knowledge of the clinical setting is essential for the correct interpretation of the biopsy findings. As with lymphadenopathy, there is a long list of non-malignant conditions, as well as malignancies other than lymphomas, which can cause the bone marrow manifestations.

Benign and reactive lymphoproliferations and malignant lymphomas

Even under normal circumstances, lymphoid cells may constitute up to 20% of the population of nucleated cells in the bone marrow. However, there may be an absolute or a relative increase, the latter due to a reduction in hematopoietic tissue, as in some skeletal areas in advancing age, or in hypoplastic conditions.

Both B and T (LCA CD45-positive) cells are found in the normal bone marrow; range 0–8 for B cells CD20, but more for T cells CD2 (Figure 25.1). Though CD4 and CD8 T cells are generally regarded as distinct subsets, a small proportion of T cells (4%) coexpress these two antigens, in normal as well as in some malignant populations. There is a functional interaction between B and T cells and in the regulation of hematopoiesis. Moreover, T cells may not only determine the type of B cell immune response, but also provide stimulation for B cell lymphoma initiation and progression. This highlights the significance of T cells among the B cells in areas of bone marrow involvement in ML.

It is now clear that B lymphocytes, analogous to T lymphocytes can be subdivided into different subsets according to various cellular, phenotypic and functional characteristics; however, these aspects are not yet routinely taken into account.

Lymphoid cells are found in any of three forms in the bone marrow: (1) dispersed among the hematopoietic and fat cells, (2) in aggregates or nodules which may be intertrabecular or parasinusoidal (rarely paratrabecular), small or large, single or multiple, and (3) nodules with germinal centers – lymphoid follicles, but these are the least frequent (Figure 25.2). In most cases, a trabecular localisation indicates involvement by lymphoma, rather than benign hyperplasia. The malignant nodules are frequently irregular with lymphocytes extending outwards into the surrounding marrow, and consist of a more homogeneous or monomorphic cell population. As well as the pattern, size of the lymphocytes, amount of cytoplasm, and nuclear size and shape must be taken into account. Benign nodules range in size from 0.1 to 2 mm (average 0.4 mm), are usually round, discrete and well circumscribed (Figure 25.3). They consist of small, round lymphocytes with typical condensed chromatin and a narrow cytoplasmic rim, situated in a fine network of reticulin fibers, and accompanied by some capillaries, histiocytes, plasma cells, possibly immunoblasts, mast cells and occasionally eosinophils. They may be surrounded by a layer of fat cells. Though lymphoid nodules may be found in any marrow, they are more often encountered in the older age groups, and more in females. Their occurrences in hematological and other conditions are dealt with in the appropriate sections. It should be remembered that the incidence of both malignant lymphomas and benign lymphoid nodules in the bone marrow is higher in the older age groups, and it may be difficult to distinguish early involvement by malignant lymphoma from such nodules. This applies particularly to bone marrow lymphocytosis and early lymphocytic lymphomas with interstitial spread, and to multiple benign nodules (benign nodular hyperplasia) and a nodular lymphocytic lymphoma. Particularly useful in the differentiation of bone marrow lymphocytosis is the demonstration of B and T cells, together with the leucocyte common antigen LCA CD45, and separately with the appropriate antigens for B and T cell subsets. Demonstration of monoclonality may be required – but even that does not necessarily prove malignancy, as a clonal but nonneoplastic expansion to an antigenic stimulus may also occur. Multiclonal lymphomas have also been described, for example in immunosuppressed patients. Moreover, evolution from polyclonal proliferation to a malignant mono-

clonal process has also been documented. On immunohistology it has been shown that strong reactivity with the antigen to BCL2, together with other indications, can be used to distinguish benign from malignant nodules (Figure 25.4); though there is disagreement in the literature on this point. Such investigations may be particularly useful in cases of isolated lymphomas in the bone marrow. Other antibodies restricted to B cells are also useful in this respect. The accumulation of BCL2-positive cells may be due, in part at least, to its action in blocking apoptosis, i.e. programed cell death (PCD) in some cells without affecting proliferation, and it has been postulated that

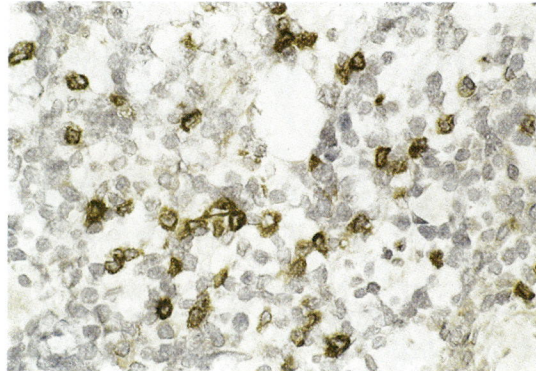

25.1 BMBS paraffin, I.H., T cells in bone marrow.

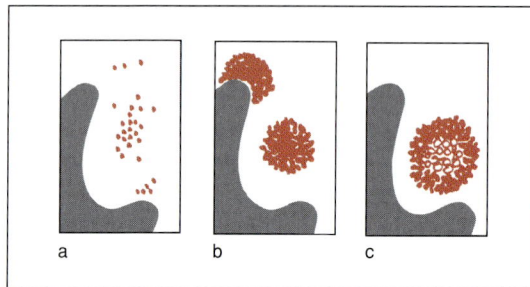

25.2 Lymphocytes in normal bone marrow: may be found dispersed among the hematopoietic and fat cells (a), in aggregates, in nodules (b), and in follicles with germinal centers (c).

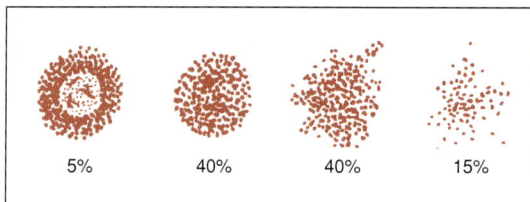

25.3 Frequency of types of lymphocytic accumulations in the bone marrow.

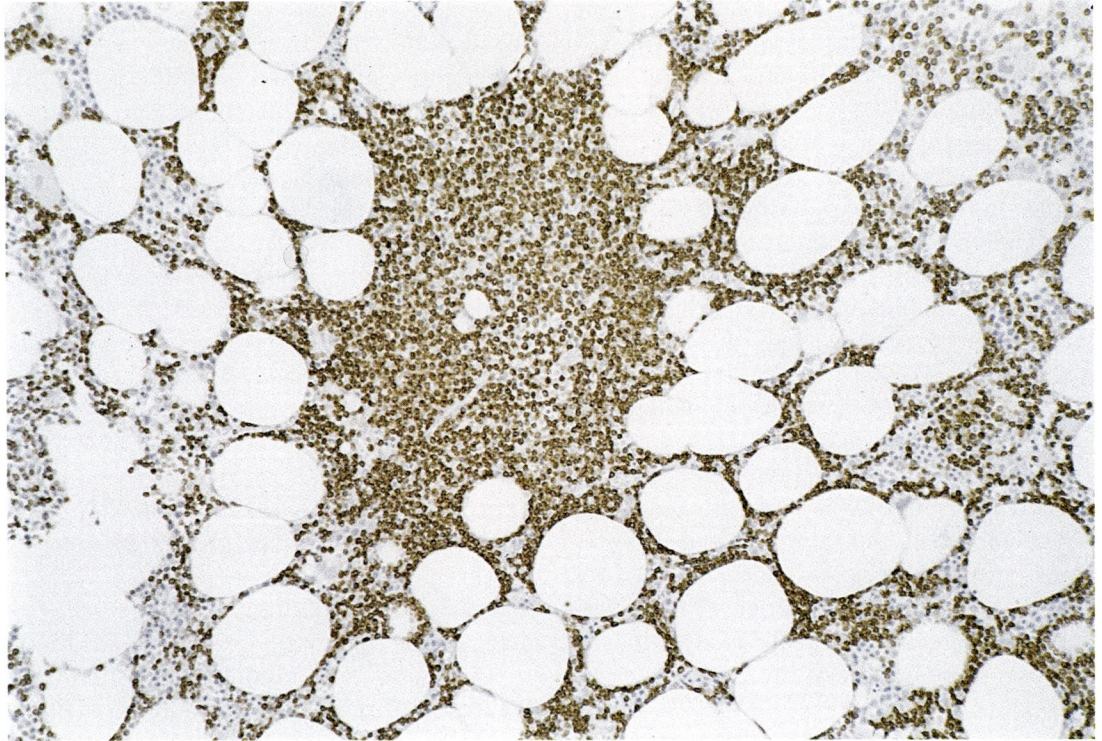

25.4 BMBS paraffin, strong reaction with BCL2 in the nodule and the lymphocytes.

the deregulation of PCD may be involved in the malignant transformation of lymphoid tissues.

Increased bone marrow lymphocytes and lymphoid nodules are found in rheumatoid and autoimmune disorders, in viral infections (e.g. infectious mononucleosis and cytomegalovirus; and mumps, measles, chicken pox); protozoan infections, such as toxoplasmosis; and in other conditions. Consequently, the clinical setting must always be considered in the evaluation and interpretation of such biopsies. This is of particular importance with respect to patients with disorders of the immune system, in view of their association with lymphoproliferative disorders. Lymphohistiocytic proliferations or aggregates have also been found in the bone marrow of patients with various infections, especially viral, as well as in patients with rheumatic and autoimmune diseases and immune deficiency syndromes; after transplantation or as a reaction to drugs, and to non-hematologic malignancies. In autoimmune disorders there is a different mechanism than in immunodeficient or suppressed patients, as the former have hyperactivity of the immune system. Sjogren's syndrome is a good example. It occurs both as a primary and a secondary disorder, the latter associated with well-defined entities such as rheumatoid arthritis, systemic lupus erythematosus, systemic sclerosis and polymyositis. The primary form is an autoimmune disorder with a multifactorial etiology, including various genes and possibly viral infection. The disease is characterised by lymphocytic infiltration, predominantly of CD4-positive T cells. Many other organs may be involved, including the lymphoreticular system: splenomegaly, lymphadenopathy and development of pseudolymphoma. Various cytopenias have been described, which may be due to the alterations in the lymphoreticular system as well as direct effects on the hematopoiesis in the bone marrow. Exclusion criteria for establishing the diagnosis include pre-existing lymphomas, AIDS, sarcoidosis and graft-versus-host disease. Consequently great care is required in the interpretation of lymphocytic aggregates, nodules and granuloma-like lesions in a patient with established Sjogren's syndrome. Bone marrow findings range from hypo to aplasia with or without lymphocytic nodules and granuloma-like lesions. In immuno-deficient patients, lymphomas are often advanced, aggressive and extranodal – in the central nervous system, gastrointestinal tract and bone marrow – when first diagnosed.

Some neoplastic conditions have more prominent peripheral blood than bone marrow involvement; these include T cell malignancies, large granular lymphocytosis and splenic lymphoma with villous lympho-cytes. In contrast, hairy cell leukemia may show extensive replacement in the bone marrow with relatively few lymphocytes in the peripheral blood. Adhesion molecules, partic-ularly of the integrin family, have been implicated in the dissemination of some lym-phomas. There has been a 50% increase in lym-phomas in the USA since the 1970s.

Reactive bone marrow plasmacytosis and multiple myeloma (MM)

It may not be possible to make a histological distinction between (1) the plasmacytosis of chronic inflammatory or other disease, (2) that of benign monoclonal gammopathy and (3) that of early or smoldering multiple myeloma. However, a monoclonal population may be identified by immunological investigation on smears of aspirates, on imprints of biopsies and on cryostat or paraffin sections (Figure 25.5). Though no single morphological feature of plasma cells is characteristic of a neoplastic

clone, a high incidence of any of the follow-ing features within a population suggests malignancy: large nuclei, prominent nucleoli, cellular and nuclear pleomorphism, multinu-clearity, crystaline or other inclusions and nucleocytoplasmic asynchronism. The bone marrow histology is similar in the three con-ditions listed above. Small groups of plasma cells are found near blood vessels and among the hematopoietic and fat cells. In early MM there are also small paratrabecular and periar-terial clusters of plasma cells. The incidence of multiple myeloma has also increased consider-ably in the last two decades.

Granulomatous bone marrow infiltrations and Hodgkin's disease

Granulomatous infiltrates – small or large, single or multiple – may be found in rheumatic and autoimmune conditions (Figures 25.6 and 25.7), infections, allergies

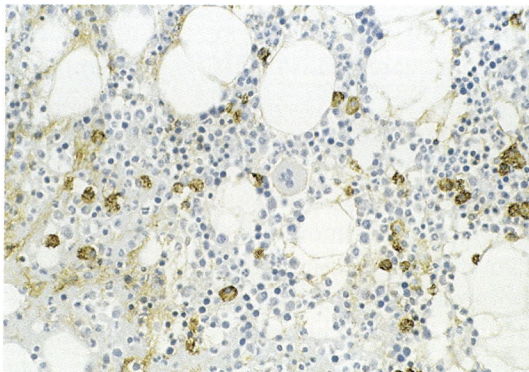

25.5 BMBS, paraffin, lambda, reactive plasma-cytosis in a patient with rheumatoid arthritis. Both lambda and kappa were positive indicating absence of light chain restriction.

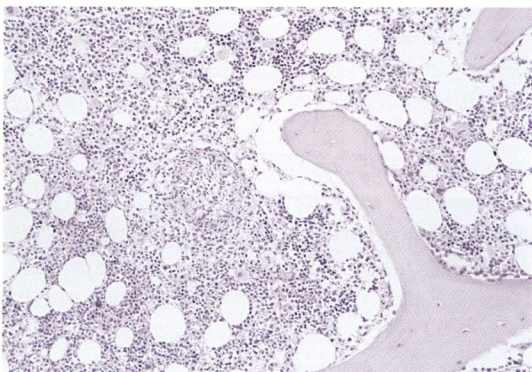

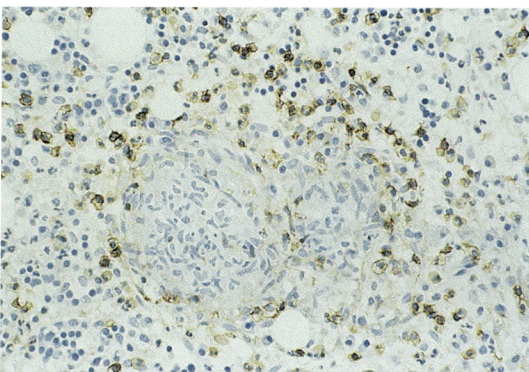

25.6 (left) BMBS paraffin, H&E, showing small gran-uloma near trabecula, left of center.

25.7 (right) As for Figure 25.4, I.H., showing T cells around small granuloma.

and immune deficiency syndromes, especially AIDS; in angioimmunoblastic lymphadenopathy (AILD) (Figure 25.8), in malignant histiocytosis (MH), and in systemic mastocytosis (SM). Lymphomatoid granulomatosis-like lesions have been described in 15% of 85 cases with malignant lymphomas.

The granulomas in some of these conditions may exhibit certain characteristic histological features: multinucleated giant cells in reactive or infectious bone marrow infiltrates, Reed–Sternberg cells and/or whorl-like vascular patterns in AILD, together with deposition of PAS-positive interstitial material; concentric layers of mast cells, fibroblasts and lymphocytes in SM, and clusters and diffuse spread of histiocytes in malignant histiocytosis (MH). The distinction between involvement by HD or by anaplastic large cell lymphoma may be particularly difficult. Should the biopsies be small, or the infiltrates single and small, or the characteristic features be absent, then purely histological distinction between these various entities is not possible. In such patients, if an adequate bone marrow biopsy (BMB) is not obtained at the first attempt, a second biopsy should immediately be taken, to ensure sufficient material for diagnostic evaluation.

Histology of bone marrow involvement in the malignant lymphomas

Bone marrow biopsy has now been firmly established as an integral part of the investigation of patients with known or suspected malignant lymphomas. Biopsies are routinely taken to estimate stage of disease at initial diagnosis. Moreover, a bone marrow biopsy may be diagnostic in patients without peripheral lymphadenopathy, it may aid classification when inconclusive or divergent histologies are found at other sites. Recently magnetic resonance imaging has been used to detect and estimate the extent of bone marrow involvement, and thus to complement bone marrow biopsy findings. The main histological parameters and their clinical correlations are given in Tables 25.1–25.3 and Figure 25.9. Malignant lymphomas may also sometimes develop in patients with myeloproliferative disorders (Figure 25.10).

Classification of the malignant lymphomas

Morphological and immunological criteria, as well as enzymic reactions, have been utilised to classify the malignant lymphomas. In recent years these have been supplemented by increasingly refined immunological markers, cytogenetics, serological studies and the newer techniques of molecular biology. However, as pointed out in the introduction to the updated Kiel classification, morphology remains the basis for lymphoma classification, at least in the foreseeable future. This refers mainly to lymph node histology, but applies equally well to the bone marrow, especially in view of the fact that there is a good correspondence between the two. In a study of the comparative histology of malignant lymphomas in lymph node and bone marrow of 120 patients with classifiable infiltrations in both organs, congruence was found in 91/120 (76%) of the patients. Moreover, as is true for morphology, there is also overlap between the immunophenotypes of the lymphoid neoplasias, which must be remembered when classifying or subclassifying the lymphoproliferative disorders.

In most cases, malignant lymphomas involving the bone marrow are classifiable by histology. In many patients the original diagnosis has already been established by lymph node biopsy, and the question is one of involvement for staging, or investigation of

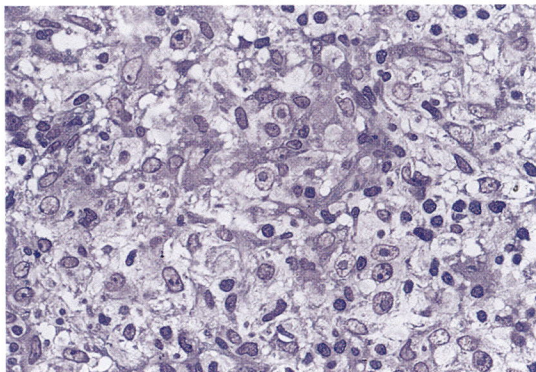

25.8 BMBS plastic, Giemsa, heterogeneous cell population in AILD. Note immunoblasts with large central nucleoli and numerous capillaries.

TABLE 25.1 Frequency and bone involvement in iliac crest biopsies in ML

Malignant lymphomas	Frequency (percentage of all cases)	Bone involvement (percentage in each group)
Lymphocytic (LC)	16	99
Lymphoblastic (LB)	2	45
Hairy cell leukemia (HCL)	8	95
Centrocytic (CC)	4	71
Centroblastic/cytic (CB/CC)	3	20
Centroblastic (CB)	1	25
Immunocytic (IC)	15	85
Immunoblastic (IB)	1	29
Plasmacytic (PC)	30	94
Plasmablastic (PB)	12	79
Hodgkin's disease (HD)	5	8
Angioimmunoblastic (AILD)	2	70
Unclassifiable (UCL)	2	–

TABLE 25.2 Frequency of patterns of bone involvement and their prognostic relevance in different types of ML (percentage in each histological class; median survival time, months, in parentheses)

ML	Nodular	Nodular/Interstitial	Interstitial	Paratrabecular	Focal	Packed
LC	–	32 (107)	42 (36)	–	–	26 (25)
IC	41 (74)	33 (56)	6 (34)	–	–	20 (17)
PC	4 (20)	9 (22)	58 (46)	13 (31)	–	15 (16)
CC	–	–	–	60 (29)	–	40 (19)
CB/CC	80 (50)	–	–	–	–	20 (12)
Blastic	–	–	–	–	–	100 (6)
HCL	–	–	–	–	75 (28)	25 (18)
HD	–	–	–	–	65 (35)	35 (29)
AILD	–	–	–	–	76 (34)	24 (12)

25.9 (left) Growth patterns and frequencies of lymphoproliferative disease in the bone marrow: NOD, nodular (9%); INT, interstitial (22%); NOD/INT, nodular/interstitial (29%); PAR, paratrabecular (2%); FOC, focal (10%); patchy, PAC, packed marrow (28%).
25.10 (right) BMBS plastic, Giemsa, biopsy of a patient with PV who developed a lymphoma.

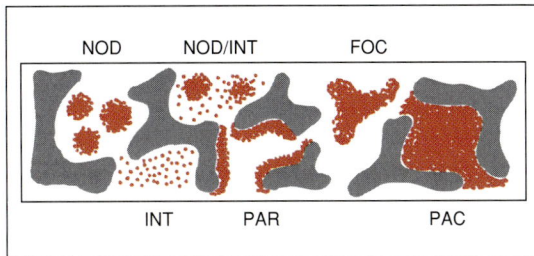

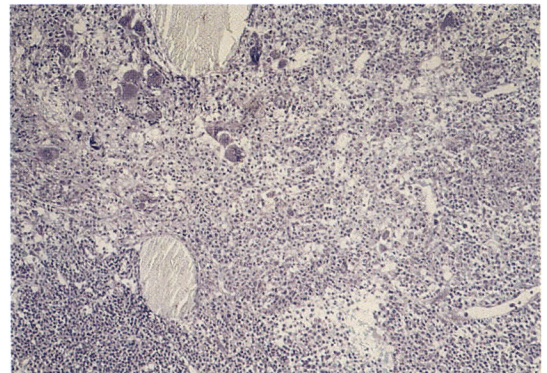

TABLE 25.3 Bone marrow biopsies in malignant lymphomas

Parameters	Correlation
Involvement	initial diagnosis
	clinical staging
Predominant cell type	classification
Proliferation pattern	subgrouping
Quantity	histological staging
Hematopoiesis	peripheral blood values
Bone structure	hypercalcemia, alkaline phosphatase levels
Cytological transformation	accelerated clinical course
Sequential BMB	effects of therapy, concurrent diseases

the other parameters listed in Table 25.3. In other cases a lymphoma is suspected on the basis of peripheral blood findings or results of imaging techniques. When the first histological diagnosis is by BMB, then immunological studies (FACS) are usually also made on an aspirate taken with the biopsy, on biopsy imprints or on cryostat sections of part of the bone biopsy; or on sections of paraffin-embedded biopsies (most widely used, though methods for plastic are also available).

Bone marrow involvement in the malignant lymphomas, mainly of B cell origin, showed six major types of spread, called growth patterns, which all merged into one pattern – the 'packed marrow' type with progression of disease and complete replacement of the marrow. It should be remembered that each B cell neoplasm includes cells in the different stages of the lymphocyte developmental pathway (lymphocytes, follicle center cells, immunoblasts and plasma cells) but their relative proportions differ in the various entities. It follows therefore, that any one of these may at any time be stimulated more than the others, so that in the course of its progression, a lymphoma may assume different guises, as suggested by Robb-Smith and Taylor many years ago, and as illustrated recently by a patient who developed four clinically, morphologically and immunophenotypically distinct low grade B cell lymphomas over 18 years

269

TABLE 25.4 Kiel classification

B-lineage

Low grade
    Lymphocytic
        Chronic lymphocytic leukemia
        Prolymphocytic leukemia
        Hairy cell leukemia
    Lymphoplasmacytic/lymphoplasmacytoid
        (immunocytoma)
        Lymphoplasmacytoid
        Lymphoplasmacytic
    Plasmacytic
    Centroblastic/centrocytic
        Follicular ± diffuse
        Diffuse
    Centrocytic

High grade
    Centroblastic
    Immunoblastic
    Large cell anaplastic
    Burkitt lymphoma
    Lymphoblastic

T-lineage

Low grade
    Lymphocytic
        Chronic lymphocytic leukemia
        Prolymphocytic leukemia
    Small, cerebriform cell
        Mycosis fungoides
        Sézary's syndrome
    Lymphoepithelioid (Lennert's lymphoma)
    Angioimmunoblastic
        (angioimmunoblastic lymphadenopathy with dysproteinemia
        lymphogranulomatosis X)
    T-zone
    Pleomorphic, small cell

High grade
    Pleomorphic, medium and large cell
    Immunoblastic
    Large cell anaplastic
    Lymphoblastic

from a single B cell clone. The relatively infrequent T cell lymphomas in the bone marrow show a diffuse, perivascular and/or intravascular spread. Nodular involvement is rare, but does occur. As more markers are applied, more lymphomas may be identified as separate entities, for example, an aggressive, non-nasal lymphoma expressing the natural killer cell marker CD56 which, however, has so far only been identified in people of Chinese origin.

The manifestations of the malignant lymphomas in the bone marrow will be briefly described; the updated Kiel classification, the Working Formulation and the more recent

TABLE 25.5 International working formulation

Low grade
    Malignant lymphoma, small lymphocytic – CLL
        Consistent with CLL
            Plasmacytoid
    Malignant lymphoma, follicular, predominantly small cleaved cell
        Diffuse areas
        Sclerosis
    Malignant lymphoma, follicular, mixed small cleaved and large cell
        Diffuse areas
        Sclerosis
Intermediate grade
    Malignant lymphoma, follicular, predominantly large cell
        Diffuse areas
        Sclerosis
    Malignant lymphoma, diffuse, small cleaved cell
        Sclerosis
    Malignant lymphoma, diffuse, mixed small and large cell
        Sclerosis
        Epithelioid cell component
    Malignant lymphoma, diffuse, large cell
        Cleaved
        Non-cleaved
High grade
    Malignant lymphoma, large cell immunoblastic
        Plasmacytoid
        Clear cell
        Polymorphous
        Epithelioid cell
    Malignant lymphoma, lymphoblastic
        Convoluted cell
        Non-convoluted cell
    Malignant lymphoma, small non-cleaved
        Burkitt's
        Non-Burkitt's
    Miscellaneous
        Composite
        Mycosis fungoides
        Histiocytic
        Extramedullary plasmacytoma
        Unclassifiable

TABLE 25.6 Revised European–American lymphoma classification (REAL)

B-cell neoplasms	T/NK-cell neoplasms

Indolent/chronic (untreated survival measured in years)
Indolent disseminated lymphoma/leukemia

B-cell neoplasms	T/NK-cell neoplasms
• B cell CLL/SLL/PLL	• T cell CLL/PLL
• Lymphoplasmacytic lymphoma	• Large granular lymphocyte leukemia (LGL)
• Hairy cell leukemia	
• Plasmacytoma/myeloma	
• Splenic marginal zone lymphoma/SLVL*	

Indolent extranodal lymphomas

• Extranodal marginal zone/MALT lymphoma	• Mycosis fungoides

Indolent nodal lymphomas
• Nodal marginal zone lymphoma*
• Follicle centre lymphoma (follicular lymphoma) (grades 1, 2, 3*)
• Mantle cell lymphoma

Aggressive (untreated survival measured in months)

• Diffuse large B cell lymphoma	• Anaplastic large cell lymphoma
	• Peripheral T cell lymphomas (subtypes*)

Highly aggressive/acute (untreated survival measured in months)

• Precursor B lymphoblastic leukemia/lymphoma	Precursor T lymphoblastic leukemia/ lymphoma
• Burkitt's lymphoma	Adult T cell lymphoma/leukemia

Hodgkin's disease

Lymphocyte predominance, nodular ± diffuse	• Classical Hodgkin's disease Nodular sclerosis Mixed cellularity Lymphocyte depletion Lymphocyte-rich classical HD*

Anaplastic large-cell lymphoma, Hodgkin's-like/related*

* Provisional.

REAL classification as well as the International Lymphoma Study Group's Classification are given for comparison (Tables 25.4–25.7). The phenotypic identification as B or T cell-derived is made on the basis of antibody reactions, the importance and clinical relevance of which has been emphasised in follow-up studies.

Post-transplantation lymphoproliferative disorders

These have been separately classified because of their diverse clinical, histopathologic, immunophenotypic and genotypic nature. The latest working classification (Swerdlow

TABLE 25.7 International Lymphoma Study Group Classification (including provisional categories)

B cell lymphoma	T/NK-cell lymphoma	Others
Precursor B lymphoblastic	Precursor T lymphoblastic	Composite lymphoma (types specified)
Small lymphocytic (CLL)	T cell chronic lymphocytic leukemia	Malignant lymphoma, unclassifiable low grade
Lymphoplasmacytic	Large granular lymphocyte leukemia	Malignant lymphoma, unclassifiable high grade
Mantle cell	Mycosis fungoides	Malignant lymphoma, unclassifiable
Follicle center, follicular	Peripheral T cell, unspecified	
Grade 1	*Medium-sized*	Hodgkin's disease
Grade 2	*Mixed medium and large cell*	Diagnosis other than lymphoma
Grade 3	*Large cell*	Case unclassifiable
Follicle center diffuse, small cell	*Lymphoepithelioid*	
Marginal zone B cell, MALT type	*Hepatosplenic*	
Marginal zone B cell, nodal	*Subcutaneous panniculitic*	
Marginal zone B cell, splenic	Angioimmunoblastic	
Hairy cell leukemia	Angiocentric, nasal	
Plasmacytoma	Intestinal	
Diffuse large B cell	Adult T cell lymphoma/leukemia	
Diffuse mediastinal large B cell	Anaplastic large cell (including null phenotype)	
Burkitt's	*Anaplastic large cell, Hodgkin's-like*	
High grade B cell, Burkitt-like	Unclassifiable low grade	
Unclassifiable low grade	Unclassifiable high grade	
Unclassifiable high grade		

Provisional categories are indicated in italics.
Abbreviations: CLL, chronic lymphocytic leukemia; MALT, mucosal-associated lymphoid tissue.

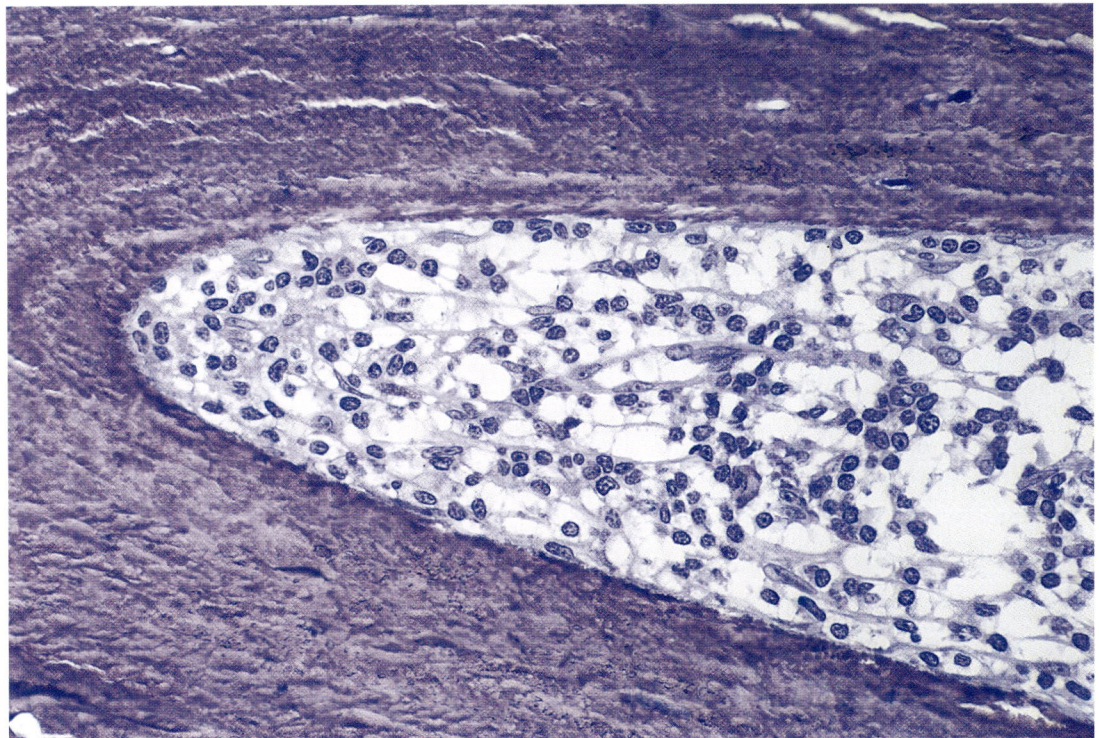

25.11 BMBS, plastic, toluidine blue, cortical bone with residual lymphoma after chemotherapy.

1997) is based on the preceding classifications of lymphoproliferative disorders in these patients.

Bone in the malignant lymphomas

Destruction of bone and hypercalcemia are seen in HD, CLL, Burkitt's lymphoma and some T cell lymphomas which produce osteoclast-activating factors, OAFs. The hypercalcemia may also be due, in part, to synthesis of calcitriol by lymphoma cells. The frequency of bone changes in the malignant lymphomas is given in Table 25.1. Local erosion of bone, mediated by osteoclastic activity, is frequently seen when there is paratrabecular involvement of the bone marrow. Cortical bone, especially a porous cortex should always be carefully examined for the presence of involvement, especially after therapy, as residual lymphoma may be present there (sanctuary site? See Figure 25.11).

Bibliography

Bartl R., Frisch B., Burkhardt R. *et al.* (1984) Lymphoproliferations in the bone marrow: identification and evolution, classification and staging. *J Clin Pathol.*, **37**, 233.

Ben-Ezra J.M., King B.E., Harris A.C. *et al.* (1994) Staining for Bcl-2 protein helps to distinguish benign from malignant lymphoid aggregates in bone marrow biopsies. *Mod Pathol*, **7 (5)**, 560–4.

Burger R., Wendler J., Antoni K. *et al.* (1994) Interleukin-6 production in B-cell neoplasias and Castleman's disease: evidence for an additional paracrine loop. *Ann Hematol.*, **69 (1)**, 25–31.

Chan J.K.C., Sin V.C., Wong K.F. *et al.* (1997) Non-nasal lymphoma expressing the natural killer cell marker CD56: a clinicopathologic study of 49 cases of an uncommon aggressive neoplasm. *Blood*, **89 (12)**, 4501–13.

Chetty R., Echezarreta G., Comley M., Gatter K. (1995) Immunohistochemistry in apparently normal bone marrow trephine specimens from patients with nodal follicular lymphoma. *J Clin Pathol*, **48 (11)**, 1035–8.

Crocker J. (1996) Lymphoid aggregates in bone marrow trephines: new approaches to a continuing problem. *J Pathol.*, **178**, 367–8.

Cuneo A., Castoldi G., van den Berghe H. (1991) Genomic alterations, origin and evolution of B-cell non-Hodgkin's lymphoma. *Hematologica*, **76 (1)**, 1–7.

Davis R.E., Longacre T.A., Cornbleet P.J. (1994) Hematogones in the bone marrow of adults. Immunophenotypic features, clinical settings, and differential diagnosis. *Am J Clin Pathol.*, **102 (2)**, 202–11.

DiGiuseppe J.A., LeBeau P., Augenbraun J., Borowitz M.J. (1996) Multiparameter flow-cytometric analysis of bcl-2 and Fas expression in normal and neoplastic hematopoiesis. *Am J Clin Pathol.*, **106 (3)**, 345–51.

Dohner H., Guckel F., Knauf W. *et al.* (1989) Magnetic resonance imagine of bone marrow in lymphoproliferative disorders: correlation with bone marrow biopsy. *Br J Haematol*, **73 (1)**, 12–17.

Drexler H.G., Gignac S.M. (1994) Characterization and expression of tartrate-resistant acid phosphatase (TRAP) in hematopoietic cells. *Leukemia*, **8 (3)**, 359–68.

Farahat N., Lens D., Zomas A. *et al.* (1995) Quantitative flow cytometry can distinguish between normal and leukaemic B-cell precursors. *Br J Haematol.*, **91 (3)**, 640–6.

Farhi D.C. (1989) Germinal centers in the bone marrow. *Hematol. Pathol.*, **3 (3)**, 133–6.

Ferme C., Brice P., Bourstyn E. *et al.* (1991) Surgical restaging of advanced Hodgkin's disease after first line chemotherapy. *Eur. J. Hematol.*, **46 (5)**, 306–11.

Ferrarini M., Caligaris-Cappio (eds) (1997) *Human B Cell Populations.* Basel: Karger.

Frisch B., Bartl R. (1990) *Atlas of Bone Marrow Pathology.* Dordrecht: Kluwer.

Frydecka I. (1994) Circulating cell differentiation antigens as markers of actvity in lymphoproliferative diseases. *Acta. Hematol. Pol.*, **25 (2 Suppl. 1)**, 50–5.

Gallo G. (1991) Renal complications of B-cell dyscrasias. *New Engl J Med.*, **324**, 1889.

General Haematology Task Force of BCSH (1994) Immunophenotyping in the diagnosis of chronic lymphoproliferative disorders. *J Clin Pathol*, **47**, 871–5.

Glass J., Hochberg F.H., Miller D.C. (1993) Intravascular lymphomatosis: a systemic disease with neurologic manifestations. *Cancer*, **71 (10)**, 3156–64.

Greiner A., Knorr C., Qin Y. *et al.* (1997) Low-grade B cell lymphomas of mucosa-associated lymphoid tissue (MALT-type) require CD40-mediated signaling and TH2-type cytokines for in vitro growth and differentiation. *Am J Pathol.*, **150**, 1583–93.

Guckel F., Brix G., Semmler W. *et al.* (1990) Systemic bone marrow disorders: characterization with proton chemical shift imaging. *J Comput Assit Tomogr.*, **14 (4)**, 633–42.

Guckel F., Dohner H., Knauf W. *et al.* (1989) MT tomography detection of bone marrow infiltration by malignant lymphomas. *Onkologie*, **12** (1), 34–7.

Guckel F., Semmler W., Dohner H. *et al.* (1989) NMR tomographic imaging of bone marrow infiltrates in malignant lymphoma. *ROFO Fortschr. Geb. Rontgenstr. Nuklearmed.*, **150** (1), 26–31.

Haddy T.B., Parker R.I., Magrath I.T. (1989) Bone marrow involvement in young patients with non-Hodgkin's lymphoma: the importance of multiple bone marrow samples for accurate staging. *Med Pediatr Oncol.*, **17** (5), 418–23.

Hiddeman W., Longo D.L., Coiffier B. *et al.* (1996) Lymphoma classification – the gap between biology and clinical management is closing. *Blood*, **88** (11), 4085–9.

Hiddemann W. (1996) Classification of malignant lymphomas – current status and clinical implications. *Ther Umsch.*, **53** (11), 816–19.

Hoane B.R., Shields A.F., Porter B.A., Shulman H.M. (1991) Detection of lymphomatous bone marrow involvement with magnetic resonance imaging. *Blood*, **78** (3), 728–38.

Horny H.P., Wehrmann M., Griesser H. *et al.* (1993) Investigation of bone marrow lymphocyte subsets in normal, reactive, and neoplastic states using paraffin-embedded biopsy specimens. *Am J Clin Pathol*, **99** (2), 142–9.

Horny H.P., Engst U., Walz R.S., Kaiserling E. (1989) In situ immunophenotyping of lymphocytes in human bone marrow: an immunohistochemical study. *Br. J. Hematol.* **73** (4), 576–7.

Huvos A.G. (1991) Skeletal manifestations of malignant lymphomas and leukemias. In A.G. Huvos (ed), *Bone Tumors: Diagnosis, Treatment, and Prognosis*. Philadelphia: W.B. Saunders, pp. 625.

Im T., Inoue T., Furukawa Y. *et al.* (1988) Evaluation of bone marrow involvement of malignant lymphoma by bone marrow aspiration and biopsy: necessity to evaluate both samples together. *Osaka City Med J.*, **34** (2), 147–58.

Jacobs J.C., Katz R.L., Shabb N. *et al.* (1992) Fine needle aspiration of lymphoblastic lymphoma: A multiparameter diagnostic approach. *Acta Cytologica*, **36** (6), 887–94.

Johansson B., Mertens F., Mitelman F. (1995) Cytogenetic evolution patterns in non-Hodgkin's lymphoma. *Blood*, **86** (10), 3905–14.

Juneja S.K., Wolf M.M., Cooper I.A. (1990) Value of bilateral bone marrow biopsy specimens in non-Hodgkin's lymphoma. *J Clin Pathol*, **44** (4), 350–1.

Kamel O.W., Van de Rijn M., Warnke R.A., Dorfman R.F. (1993) Reversible lymphomas. Reply. *New Eng. J. Med.*, **329** (22), 1658–58.

Kopper L., Ladanyi A., Mihalik R., Nagy P. (1994) Loss of transforming growth factor beta 1 regulatory activity in human non-Hodgkin lymphomas. *Anticancer Res.*, **14** (1A), 119–22.

Korsmeyer S. (1992) Bcl-2 initiates a new category of oncogenes: regulators of cell death. *Blood*, **80** (4), 879–86.

Krueger G.R., Manak M., Bourgeois N. *et al.* (1989) Persistent active herpes virus infection associated with atypical polyclonal lymphoproliferation (APL) and malignant lymphona. *Anticancer Res.*, **9** (6), 1457–76.

LeBien T.W. (1996) Lymphopoiesis. In E.S. Henderson, T.A. Lister, M.F. Greaves (eds), *Leukemia*. Philadelphia: W.B Saunders.

Leclercq G., Plum J. (1996) Thymic and extrathymic T-cell development. *Leukemia*, 10, 1853–9.

Leith C.P., Mangalik A., Fougar K. (1997) A B-cell 'Chameleon': striking clinical, morphological, and immunophenotypic diversity of a single low-grade B cell clone. *Human Pathol.*, **28** (1), 104–8.

Linden A., Zankovich R., Thiessen P. *et al.* (1989) Bone marrow scintigraphy and magnetic resonance tomography in malignant lymphomas: comparison with histologic results. *Nuklearmedizin*, **28** (5), 166–71.

Linden A., Zankovich R., Thiessen P. *et al.* (1989) Malignant lymphoma: bone marrow imaging versus biopsy. *Radiology*, **173** (2), 335–9.

Maio M., Pinto A., Carbone A. *et al.* (1990) Differential expression of CD54/intercellular adhesion molecule-1 in myeloid leukemias and in lymphoproliferative disorders. *Blood*, **76** (4), 783–90.

Malashenko O.S., Samoilova R.S., Bulycheva T.I. (1994) Evaluation of the proliferation and line of lymphoid cells in various lymphoproliferative diseases using a double immunocytochemical method. *Gematol Transfuziol.*, **39** (3), 3–7.

Melnyk A., Rodriguez A., Pugh W.C., Cabannillas F. (1997) Evaluation of the Revised European – American Lymphoma classification confirms the clinical relevance of immunophenotype in 560 cases of aggressive non-Hodgkin's lymphoma. *Blood*, **89** (12), 4514–20.

Meuge-Moraw C., Bernard M.C., Delacretaz F. (1993) Immunophenotyping of B lymphoma in bone marrow biopsies. Contribution of 4 monoclonal antibodies used on paraffin-embedded tissues: DDB.42, DNA.7, DNA.44 and DND.53. *Ann Pathol*, **13** (3), 151–6.

Michaux L., Mecucci C., Stul M. *et al.* (1996) BCL3 rearrangement and t(14;19)(q32;q13) in lymphoproliferative disorders. *Genes Chromosomes Cancer*, **15** (1), 38–47.

Molina T., Brouland J.P., Bigorgne C. *et al.* (1996) Pseudo-myelomatous plasmacytosis of the bone marrow in a multicentric Castleman's disease. *Ann Pathol*, **16** (2), 133–6.

Monni O., Joensuu H., Franssila K. *et al.* (1997) BCL2 Overexpression associated with chromosomal amplification in diffuse large B-cell lymphoma. *Blood*, **90** (3), 1168–74

Morse E.E., Yamase H.T., Greenberg B.R. *et al.* (1994) The role of flow cytometry in the diagnosis of lymphoma: a critical analysis. *Ann. Clin. Lab. Sci.*, **24** (1), 6–11.

Nah E.H., King D.E., Craig F.E. (1997) CD4 and CD8 antigen coexpression: a flow cytometric study of peripheral blood, bone marrow, body fluid, and solid lympho-reticular specimens. *Arch Pathol Lab Med.*, **121** (4), 381–4.

Negendank W., Soulen R.L. (1993) Magnetic resonance imaging in patients with bone marrow disorders. *Leuk-Lymphoma*, **10** (4–5), 287–98.

Nowotny H., Karlic H., Gruner H. *et al.* (1996) Cytogenetic findings in 175 patients indicate that items of the Kiel classification should not be disregarded in the REAL classification of lymphoid neoplasms. *Ann Hematol*, **72** (5), 291–301.

Nunez C., Nishimoto N., Gartland G.L. *et al.* (1996) B-cells are generated throughout life in humans. *J Immunol.*, **156**, 866–72.

O'Donnell L.R., Alder S.L., Balis U.J. *et al.* (1995) Immunohistochemical reference ranges for B lymphocytes in bone marrow biopsy paraffin sections. *Am J Clin Pathol*, **104** (5), 517–23.

Parker B.R., Marglin S., Castellino R.A. (1980) Skeletal manifestations of leukemia, Hodgkin disease, and non-Hodgkin lymphoma. *Semin Roentgenol.*, **15**, 302.

Perkins S.L., Kjeldsberg C.R. (1993) Immunophenotyping of lymphomas and leukemias in paraffin-embedded tissues. *Am. J. Clin. Pathol.*, **99** (4), 362–73.

Perreault C., Boileau J., Gyger M. *et al.* (1989) Chronic B-cell lymphocytosis. *Eur. J. Hematol.*, **42** (4), 361–7.

Petrasch S., Kosco M., Schmitz J. *et al.* (1992) Follicular dendritic cells in non-Hodgkin lymphoma express adhesion molecules complementary to ligands on neoplastic B-cells. *Br. J. Hematol.*, **82** (4), 695–700.

Pich A., Gastaldi M., Tragni G., Naývone R. (1991) Lymphocyte subsets in bone marrow lymphoid nodules and malignant lymphoma nodular involvement. *Eur. J. Basic. Appl. Histochem.*, **35** (1), 81–9.

Ponzoni M., Li C.Y. (1994) Isolated bone marrow non-Hodgkin's lymphoma: a clinicopathologic study. *Mayo Clin Proc*, **69** (1), 37–43.

Robb-Smith A.H.T., Taylor C.R. (1981) *Lymph Node Biopsy: A Diagnostic Atlas*. London: Miller, Heyden.

Said J.W., Barrera R., Shintaku I.P. *et al.* (1992) Immunohistochemical analysis of p53 expression in malignant lymphomas. *Am. J. Pathol.*, **141** (6), 1343–48.

Salisbury J.R., Deverell M.H., Cookson M.J. (1996) Three-dimensional reconstruction of benign lymphoid aggregates in bone marrow trephines. *J Pathol*, **178** (4), 447–50.

Shi G., Web H.J., Hossfield D.K. (1997) Reinterpretation of G-banded complex karyotypes by fluorescence in situ hybridization with chromosome-specific DNA painting probes and alpha-satellite centrome-specific DNA probes in malignant hematological disorders. *Am. J. Hematol.*, **55** (2), 69–76.

Shields A.F., Porter B.A., Churchley S. *et al.* (1987) The detection of bone marrow involvement by lymphoma using magnetic resonance imaging. *J. Clin. Oncol.*, **5** (2), 225–30.

Shiroky J.B., Mewkirk M.M. (1993) Reversible lymphomas. *New Engl J Med.*, **329** (22), 1657–58.

Simonian P.L., Grillor D.A.M., Nunez G. (1997) Bcl-2 and Bcl-XL can differentially block chemotherapy-induced cell death. *Blood*, **90** (3), 1208–16.

Singh T., Harjinder GM. (1989) Bone marrow biopsy in staging of malignant lymphomas. *J Assoc Physicians India*, **38** (8), 513–14.

Skalova A., Fakan F. (1997) Bcl-2 protein does not help to distinguish benign from malignant lymphoid nodules in bone marrow biopsy specimens. *J Clin Pathol.*, **50** (1), 87–8.

Smith S.R., Rowe D. (1996) Trisomy 15 in hematological malignancies: six cases and review of the literature. *Cancer Genet. Cytogen.*, **89**, 27–30.

Swerdlow S.H. (1997) Post-transplant lymphoproliferative disorders: a working classification. *Curr Diagnost Pathol.*, **14**, 28–35.

Tang D.G., Porter A.T. (1996) Apoptosis: a current molecular analysis. *Pathol Oncol Res.*, **2** (3).

Thaler J., Dietze O., Denz H. *et al.* (1991) Bone marrow diagnosis in lymphoproliferative disorders: comparison of results obtained from conventional histomorphology and immunohistology. *Histopathology*, **18** (6), 495–504.

The Non-Hodgkin's Lymphoma Classification Project (1997) A clinical evaluation of the International Study Group classification of non-Hodgkin's lymphoma. *Blood*, **89** (11), 3909–18.

Thiele J. (1995) Differential 'lymphoid cell infiltrates' diagnosis in bone marrow. *Pathologe*, **16** (2), 106–19.

van Erp P.E., Brons P.P., Boezeman J.B. *et al.* (1988) A rapid flow cytometric method for bivariate bromodeoxyuridine/DNA analysis using simultaneous proteolytic enzyme digestion and acid denaturation. *Cytometry*, **9** (6), 627–30.

Veldman T., Vignon C., Schröck E. *et al.* (1997) Hidden chromosome abnormalities in haematological malignancies detected by multicolour spectral karyotyping. *Nature Genetics*, **15**, 406–10.

Warzynski M.J., Otto R.N., Steingart R.H. *et al.* (1991) MY4 expression on B-lymphocyte malignancies may be associated with a more adverse prognosis. *Leuk. Res.*, **15** (5), 357–65.

Wass J., Motum P., Vincent P.C., Young G.A. (1987) Fine needle aspiration sampling of bone marrow for DNA flow cytometric analysis. *Exp. Hematol.*, **15** (8), 908–10.

Widding A., Smolorz J., Franke M. *et al.* (1989) Bone marrow investigation with technetium-99m microcolloid and magnetic resonance imaging in patients with malignant myelolymphoproliferative diseases. *Eur. J. Nucl. Med.*, **15** (5), 230–8.

Williams M.P., Olliff J.F. (1990) Magnetic resonance imaging in extranodal pelvic lymphoma. *Clin. Radiol.*, **42** (4), 264–8.

Yarkoni S., Lishner M., Tangi I. *et al.* (1996) B-cell non-Hodgkin's lymphoma: evidence for the t(14;18) translocation in all haematopoietic cell lineages. *J Natl Cancer Inst.*, **88** (14), 973–9.

26 Chronic lymphocytic leukemia (CLL), Hairy cell leukemia (HCL) and related disorders

B cell chronic lymphocytic leukemia (CLL)

General aspects and bone marrow histology

CLL is the commonest leukemia and malignant lymphoma; it involves the pathologic systemic accumulation of long-lived lymphocytes. The bone marrow is always involved and the infiltration consists mainly of small round lymphocytes with heavily clumped chromatin, which are generally closely packed and show few mitotic figures. There are also variable numbers of nucleolated cells, usually not more than 10%. These are larger, have less clumped chromatin and a somewhat wider rim of cytoplasm; a high proportion indicates prolymphocytic leukemia. Lymphoid nodules with structures resembling follicle centers are present in about 25% of the cases. Hematopoietic tissue and fat cells are reduced in proportion to the amount of infiltration, though in some cases there is selective depression of hematopoiesis with preservation of fat cells or selective inhibition of a particular cell line, e.g. erythroid or megakaryocytic. But erythroid hyperplasia is found when CLL is complicated by hemolysis. A network of reticulin fibers is present in the infiltrations and a few mast and plasma cells are also found. There is trabecular osteopenia without increased remodeling. Though rare cases of B-CLL with osteoblastic or osteolytic lesions have been reported, marked osteoclastic activation is more characteristic of T cell lymphoproliferations. B-CLL is a clonal proliferation of lymphoid cells which appear mature morphologically, but are maturationally immature, and do not necessarily represent the neoplastic counterpart of the circulating peripheral blood B lymphocyte. Occasionally, CLL B lymphoid cells may mature, leading to clinical multiple myeloma. In a small number of cases, transformation to a large cell lymphoma occurs (Richter's syndrome). The onset is often abrupt and extramedullary.

Patterns of spread

B-CLL demonstrates three main patterns of spread in the bone marrow (Figure 26.1): (1) nodular, (2) interstitial and (3) packed marrow. These three bone marrow patterns have prognostic significance at all clinical stages (median survivals of 90, 46 and 28 months respectively). The favorable prognosis of an initial nodular growth pattern in the bone marrow has been confirmed in several reports (Figures 26.2–26.10). Close study of the growth patterns in sequential biopsies, especially by

26.1 (left) Three main proliferation patterns of CLL in the bone marrow: (a) nodular, (b) interstitial, (c) packed.

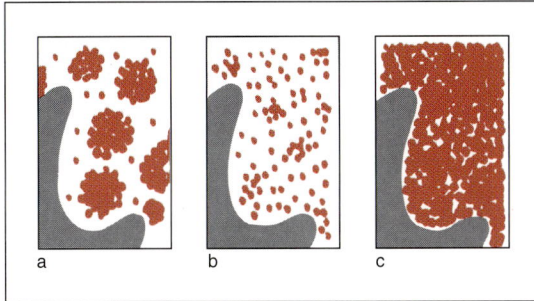

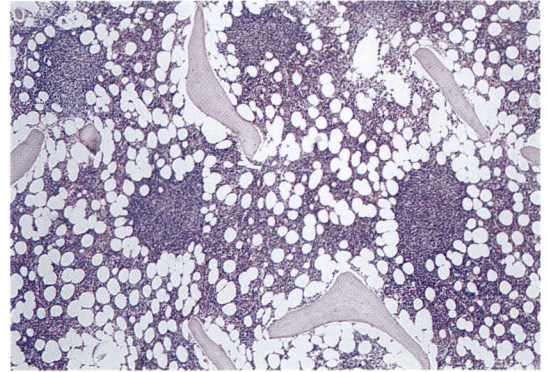

26.2 (right) BMBS paraffin, H&E, small lymphocytic nodules in hypocellular bone marrow.

26.3 (left) As for Figure 26.2, paraffin, I.H., nodules and interstitial cells positive with B cell antigen.

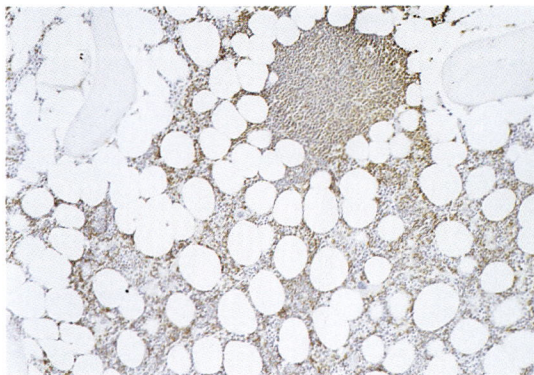

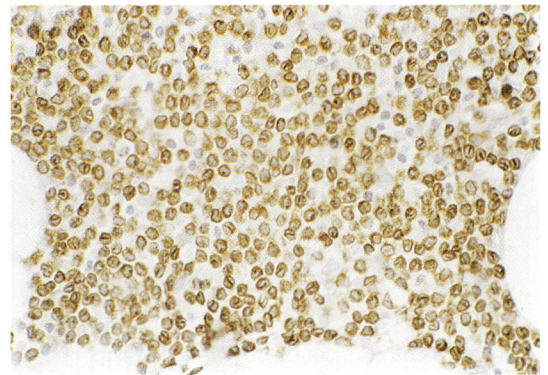

26.4 (right) As for Figure 26.2, I.H., higher magnification of nodule positive for BCL2.

26.5 (left) BMBS paraffin, H&E, large nodules occupying much of the bone marrow space.

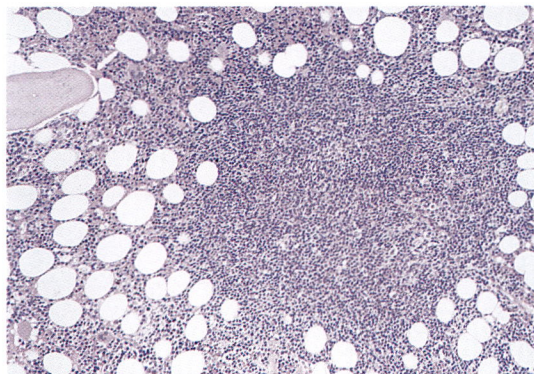

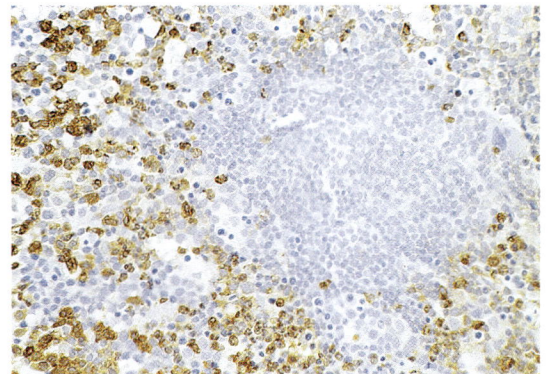

26.6 (right) BMBS paraffin, I.H., for myeloperoxidase which is strongly positive in many cells around the nodule.

26.7 (left) BMBS paraffin, I.H., for CD79a, an early B cell marker, many cells in the nodule are positive.

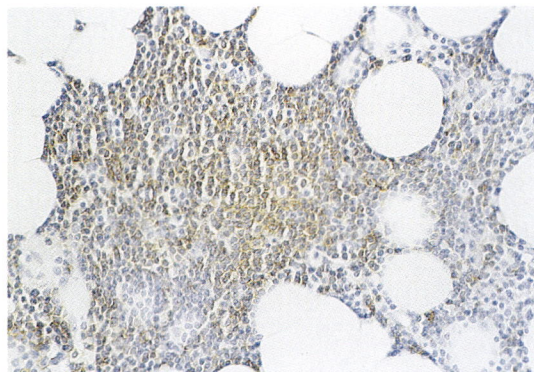

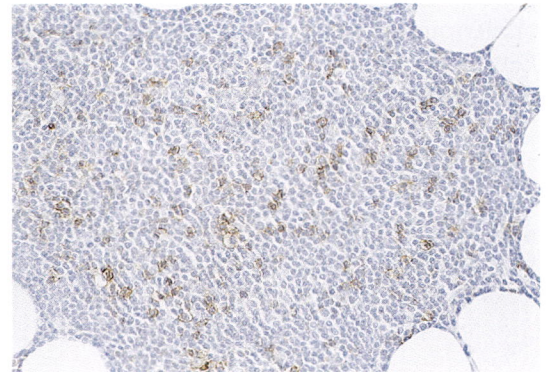

26.8 (right) BMBS paraffin, I.H., for T cells, also present in the nodule.

279

means of the Gomori stain for reticulin fibers, have shown that both nodular and interstitial patterns eventually progressed to the packed marrow type (Figure 26.10).

Cytologic classification

CLL could also be classified into three histological types on the basis of cellular characteristics: small round nuclei, notched nuclei, large round nuclei and presence of nucleoli (Figures 26.11–26.13): the three histologic types are small round, small notched and mixed with median survivals of 53, 26 and 28 months respectively. A long survival in B-CLL has also been correlated with a surface IgM phenotype. Conversely, expression of the adhesion molecule CD54 and low expression of CD18 have been associated with poor prognostic features. Recently, an association has been established between CLL and mantle cell lymphoma (MCL); the translocation t(11:14)(q13:q32) is considered a marker of MCL but has also been found in atypical CLL, and the term mantle cell leukemia has been proposed for this group.

Histologic staging and evolution of disease

Estimation of the quantity of infiltration in the biopsy could be used for histological staging and correlated with the clinical stages, according to the staging systems most widely used. In most cases histological progression, i.e. increase in tumor cell burden, reflects the clinically advanced stages, especially when clinical stages 3 and 4 are combined to form the group of 'bone marrow failure'. This is also indicated by the correlation between tumor cell burden in the BMB, peripheral lymphocytosis and platelet counts, i.e. increases in tumor cell burden are accompanied by increases in the lymphocyte count and decreases in platelet counts and hemoglobin. Both growth patterns and the proliferative cell system reflect the aggressiveness of the disease and have clinical and prognostic relevance. The type, degree and rate of change that occur over time in histologic pattern and amount of infiltration can be investigated in serial biopsies to supplement the clinical monitoring and follow-up. There is thought to be a continuous migration of lym-

phocytes to and from the bone marrow (Figures 26.14 and 26.15). Terminal transformations of CLL into acute forms are recognised in BMB in their initial stages. Moreover, the simultaneous presentation of CLL with multiple myeloma, polycythemia vera, and myeloblastic leukemia has been described. The association of CLL with erythremic myelosis and composite CLL and HD have also been reported. In some cases CLL may be superimposed on a myeloproliferative disorder, for example polycythemia vera.

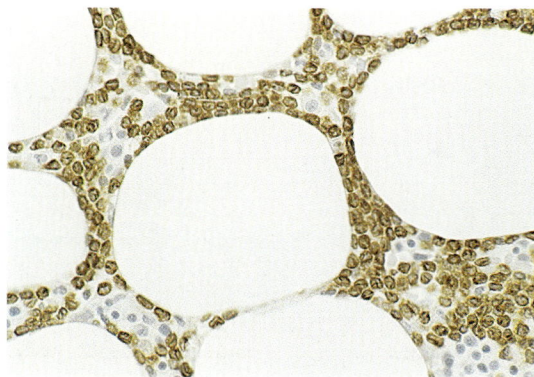

26.9 BMBS paraffin, I.H., showing a diffuse interstitial infiltration of lymphocytes, BCL2-positive.

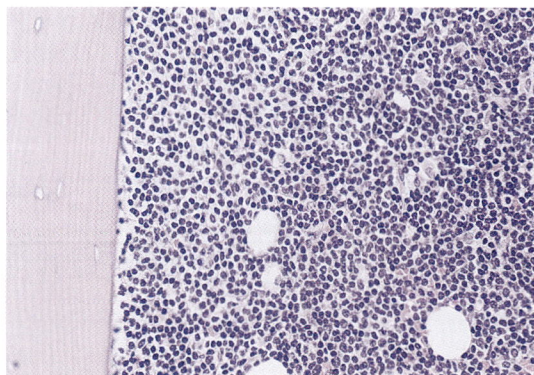

29.10 BMBS paraffin, H&E, packed marrow pattern, with no remaining hematopoiesis in this biopsy area.

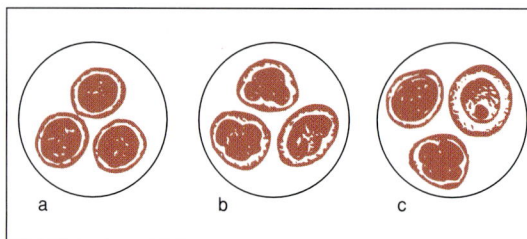

26.11 Main types of lymphocytes in CLL showing range in cell size and nuclear configuration: (a) small round, (b) notched, (c) mixed.

26.12a (left) BMBS plastic, nodular-to-packed marrow consisting mainly of small round lymphocytes.

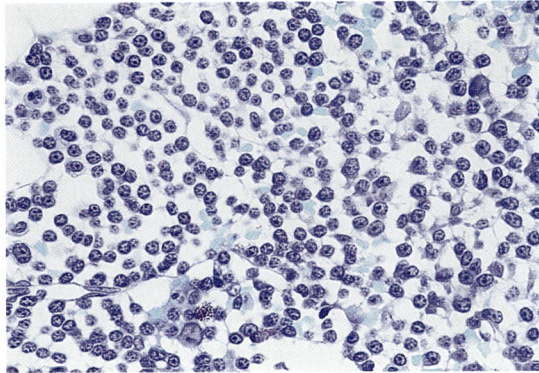

6.13a (right) BMBS plastic, diffuse-to-packed marrow consisting mainly of notched type.

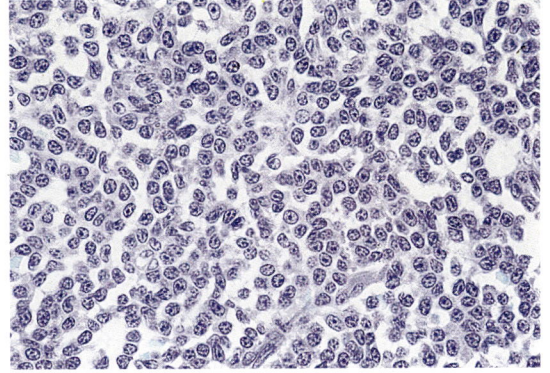

26.12b (left) BMBS, EM, mainly small round lymphocytes in CLL.

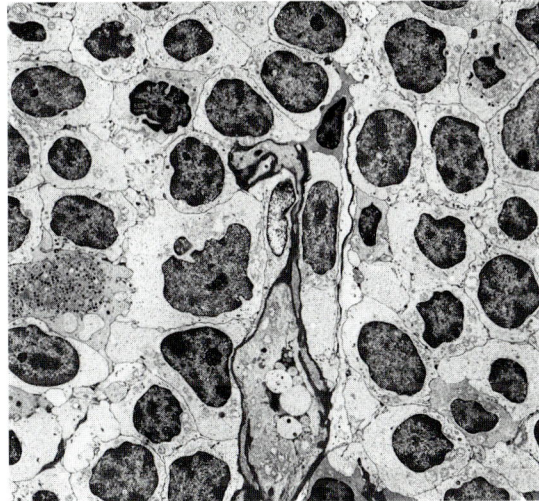

26.13b (right) BMBS, EM, mainly notched lymphocytes in CLL.

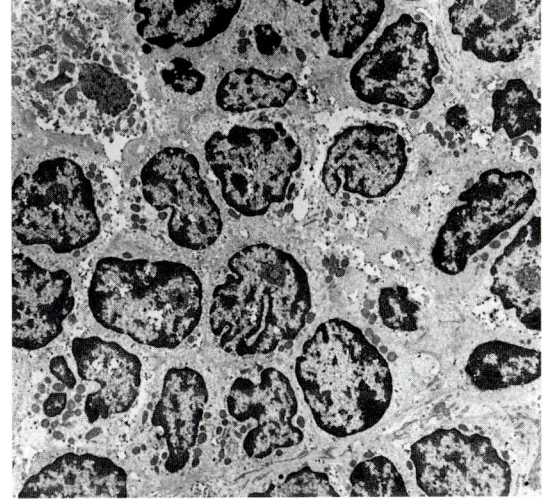

26.14 (left) Presumptive migration of lymphocytes to and from the bone marrow. S-sinusoid.

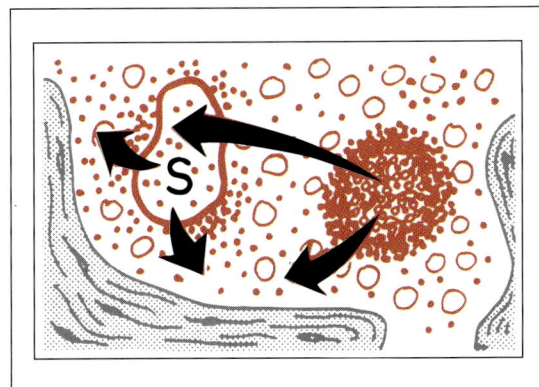

26.15 (right) BMBS, plastic, Giemsa, dilated sinusoid surrounded by lymphocytic infiltrate in CLL.

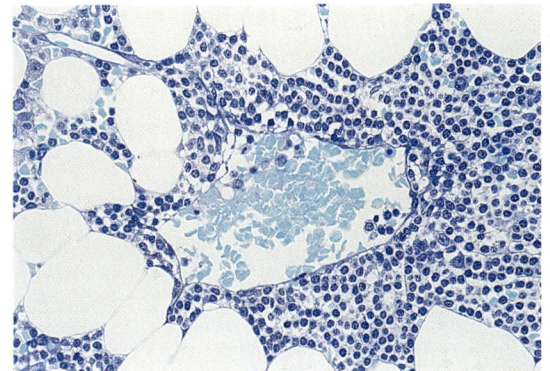

Differential diagnosis

Though usually there is little doubt, reactive lymphocytoses and other malignant lymphomas must be included in the differential diagnosis. These include lymphocytosis in infections such as toxoplasmosis and cytomegalovirus; PLL, HCL, SLVL, leukemic phase of other lymphomas and Waldenstrom's macroglobulinemia, each of which has characteristic features which distinguish it from CLL (Figure 26.16).

Early CLL, and smoldering CLL

(Figures 26.17–26.20)

Occasionally bone biopsies and peripheral blood counts are taken during the initial phases of CLL for other reasons, and the patients subsequently develop the full-blown clinical and histological pictures of CLL. In these retrospectively diagnosed early cases, which at the time did not fulfil the criteria for CLL, the lymphoid cells were dispersed between fat and hematopoietic elements and around the sinusoids in the interstitial pattern while a few aggregates were present in the nodular pattern. The quantity in both cases was low. In 'smoldering CLL' the initial tumor cell burden was also minimal, usually of the nodular type, and remained so for long periods, without disease progression. A benign variant of CLL, called benign monoclonal B cell lymphocytosis corresponding to stage 0 CLL, which remained static for long periods,

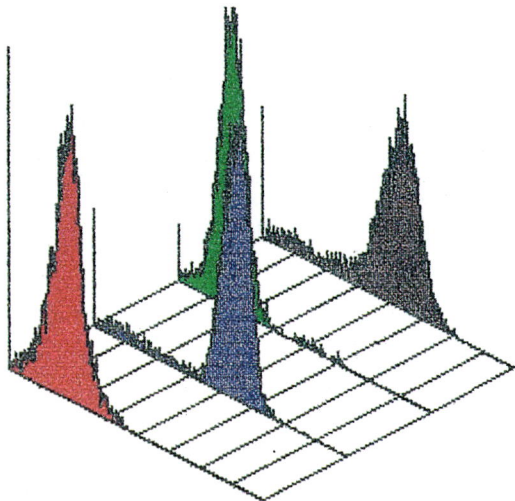

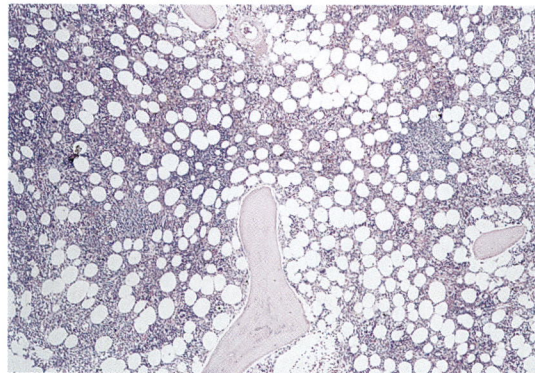

26.16 (left) Histogram of flow cytometry of bone marrow aspirate; red, control; purple, CD5 90%; green, CD2 3%; brown, CD20 82%.

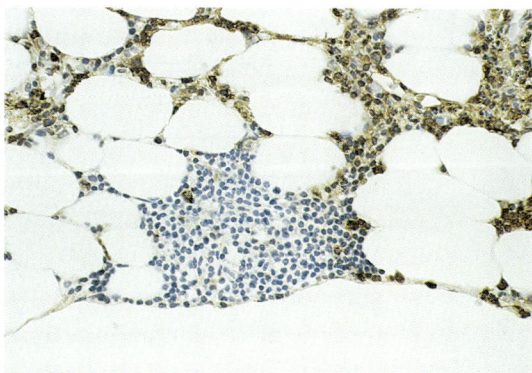

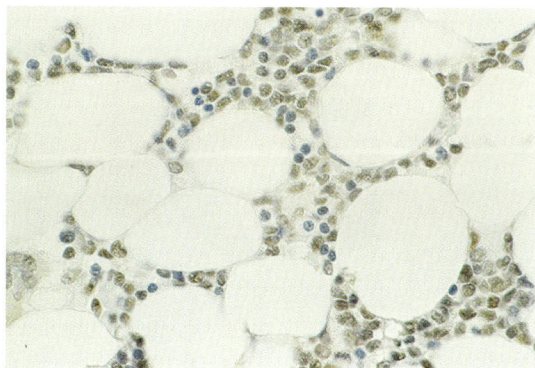

26.17–26.20 Early minimal or smoldering CLL.
26.17 (right) BMBS paraffin, H&E, intertrabecular nodules and incipient interstitial infiltration.
26.18 (left) BMBS paraffin, I.H., myeloperoxidase positive in the bone marrow cells near the paratrabecular aggregate.

26.19 (right) BMBS paraffin, I.H., showing interstitial infiltration in hypocellular bone marrow lymphocytes positive for P53.

26.20 (left) BMBS, plastic, Giemsa, overview of BMB with minimal nodular infiltration in lymphocellular marrow in early CLL.

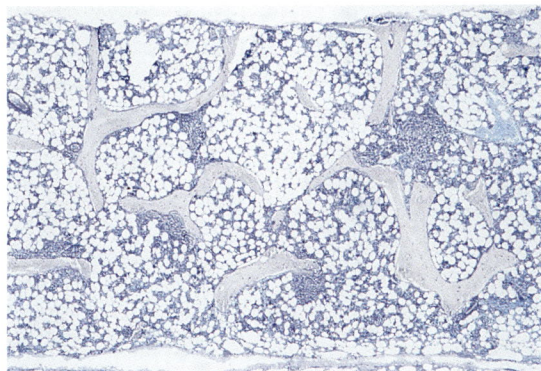

26.21 (right) BMBS plastic, Giemsa, patient with T cell lymphoma showing perivascular infiltration.

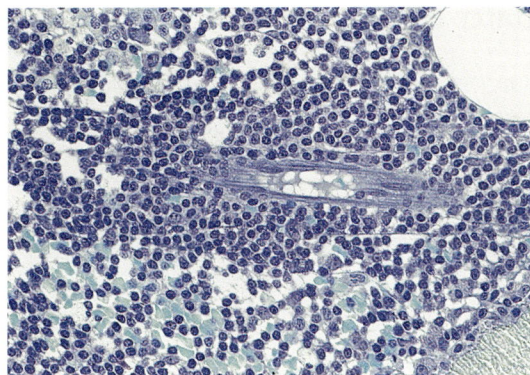

has also been described. It should be pointed out that the purely morphological distinction between benign lymphoid nodules and bone marrow lymphocytosis on the one hand, and early lymphomatous infiltrations on the other, may not be possible, and immunohistology may be required to demonstrate the increase in B lymphocytes. Even that may not be decisive, because both B and T cells are present in the benign as well as the neoplastic proliferations.

Prolymphocytic CLL

The lymphoid cells are small to medium with moderate amounts of cytoplasm and a high proportion of nucleolated cells; generally a packed marrow pattern is observed. There is a positive acid phosphatase reaction in the lymphoid cells when the test is performed on smears, imprints and cryostat sections.

T cell CLL (Figure 26.21)

T cell CLL with a nodular growth pattern in the bone marrow has rarely been described. Most cases reported so far have shown interstitial, diffuse, perivascular and packed marrow types; a few lymphoid cell aggregates may also be present. The nuclei are often convoluted and the cytoplasm more abundant than that of B CLL. The T cell origin must be established by means of immunological studies on peripheral blood, smears of aspirates, imprints of the biopsies, cryostat sections or on paraffin

sections of decalcified bone biopsies. Rare T cell lymphoproliferative disorders that are S100-positive, have also been described: bone marrow involvement is minimal or absent.

Large granular lymphocyte disorders

Large granular lymphocyte disorders refers to proliferations of T cells. These include disorders of both cytotoxic/suppressor T cells and NK (natural killer) cells.

Adult T cell leukemia/lymphoma usually involves the bone marrow and may range from focal lesions to complete replacement. The trabecular bone is generally affected and both osteoclastic and osteoblastic activity are seen. There is frequently hypercalcemia, presumably due to production of transforming growth factor β and interleukin 1 (IL-1).

Sezary syndrome and mycosis fungoides

Both are cutaneous T cell lymphomas of CD4 phenotypes. The number of Sezary cells in the peripheral blood is variable, though usually present. In spite of this, bone marrow involvement is relatively infrequent (10–20%) and often minimal and difficult to detect. However, when present the cells are readily identified by their cerebriform nuclei. In a small number of cases, transformation to a large cell, immunoblastic lymphoma may occur.

283

Hairy cell leukemia (HCL)

This is now classified as a malignant lymphoma of B cell lineage on the basis of immunologic, enzyme and electron microscopic studies. Nevertheless, recent studies have demonstrated reactivity of hairy cells with an antibody usually restricted to early thymocytes and Langerhans cells, thereby again introducing an element of ambiguity into the postulated derivation of hairy cells.

HCL is primarily manifest in spleen, bone marrow and peripheral blood. Both clinical course and therapeutic response are variable, which has led some observers to the conclusion that HCL represents a spectrum rather than a single disease entity

Bone marrow histology
(Figures 26.22–26.25)
Involvement of the bone marrow is nearly always present. Initially there is a patchy

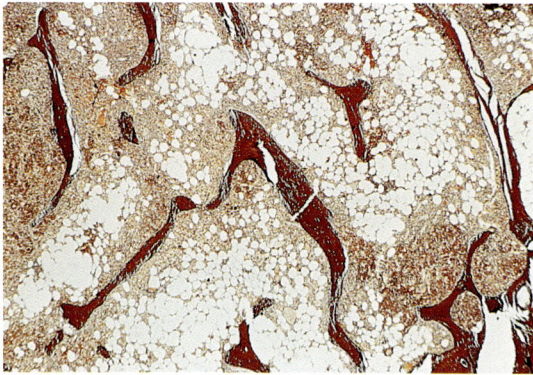

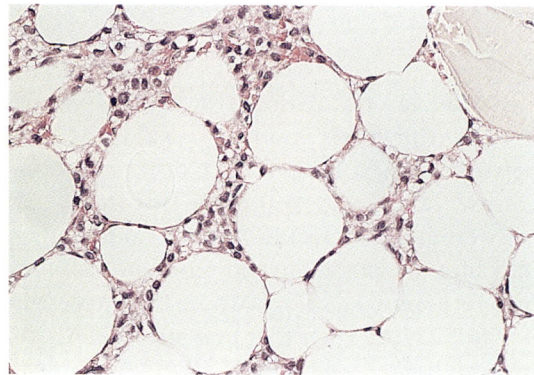

26.22–26.29 Aspects of hairy cell leukemia in the bone marrow.

26.22 (left) BMBS plastic, Gomori, low power showing paratrabecular infiltrates and hypocellular bone marrow.

26.23 (right) BMBS paraffin, H&E, interstitial infiltration of hairy cells.

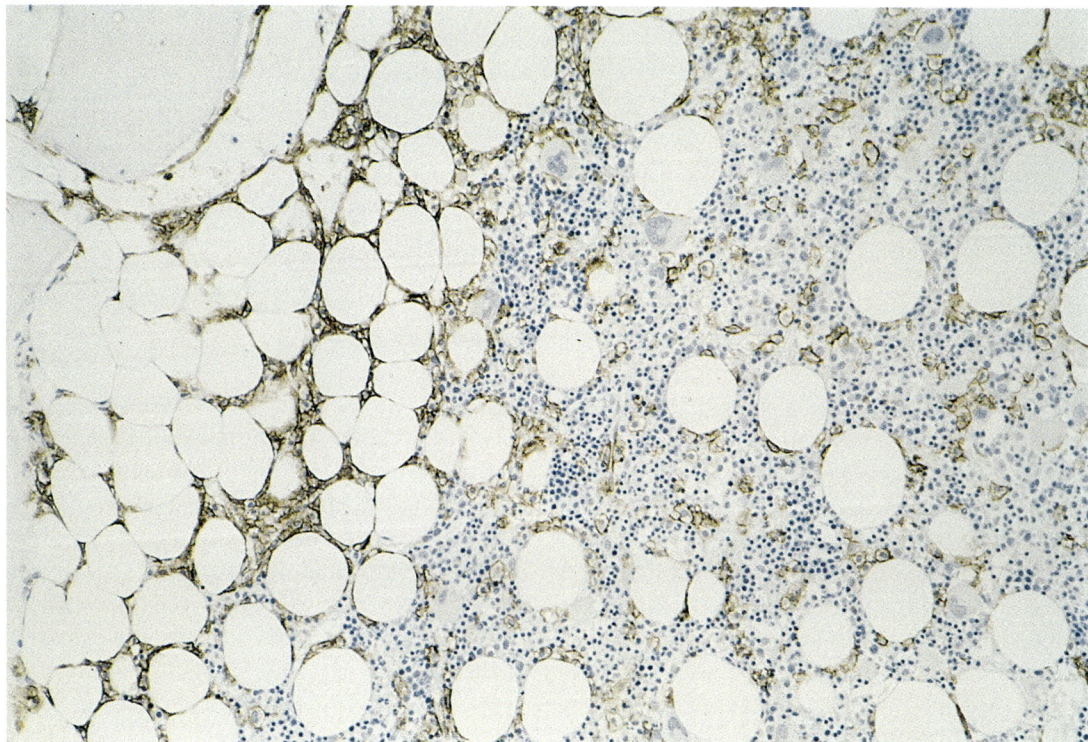

26.24 BMBS paraffin, I.H., hairy cells stained by HCL marker, left as well as cells dispersed in the marrow, right.

284

infiltration, interstitial and perivascular, of small-to-large clusters or aggregates of hairy cells. Subsequently large areas of the bone marrow may be completely replaced by hairy cells. There is variable preservation of fat cells and of islands of hematopoietic tissue. These lymphoid cells have round to oval, indented or convoluted nuclei; they usually have fairly abundant cytoplasm with lateral, long, interdigitating extensions – the processes which give them their name of 'hairy' cells. There are rod-like cytoplasmic inclusions in about half of the cases – visible as bars or circles under oil in the light microscope. On electron microscopy the typical ribosome lamellar complexes may be seen. However, these are not specific, as they have been found in a wide variety of diseases; and in benign plasma cells. The hairy cells are situated in a characteristic background, except in the early cases described above. This microenvironment consists of a reticular fiber network that also encloses lym-

phocytes, plasma and mast cells, extravasated erythrocytes and precursors of red and white cells and megakaryocytes. Erythropoietic islands showing maturation arrest and megaloblastoid features are often present within a hairy cell infiltrate. There are also numerous blood vessels, histiocytes or reticular cells, and fibroblasts. The loose network of widely separated lymphoid cells is typical of hairy cell infiltration in the bone marrow, in contrast with other lymphomatous infiltrations in which the cells are more densely packed together. In some cases, especially early ones with minimal infiltrations, the differential diagnosis includes other malignant lymphomas and monocytic infiltrates.

Subtypes of HCL (Figures 26.26–26.30)

When examined under high magnification, hairy cell nuclei display a wide range of size and configuration with three main types: ovoid, convoluted and indented. Usually one

26.25 (left) As for Figure 26.24, I.H., hairy cells stained with B cell antibody.

26.26 (right) Representation of the three main configurations of hairy cell nuclei: ovoid (a), convoluted (b) and indented (c).

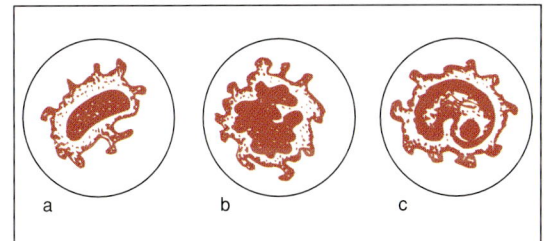

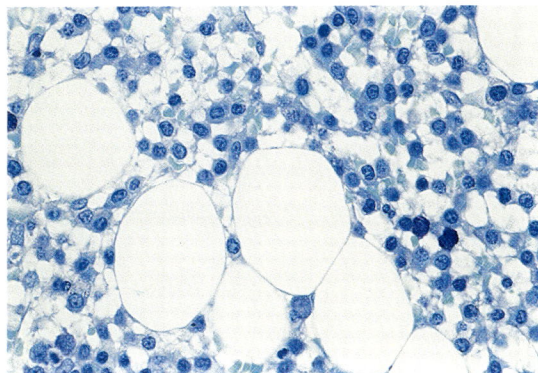

26.27 (left) BMBS plastic, Giemsa, showing morphology of hairy cells, mainly ovoid type.

26.28 (right) BMBS plastic, Gomori, illustrating mainly notched hairy cells; note the reticular fibers and erythrocytes (brown).

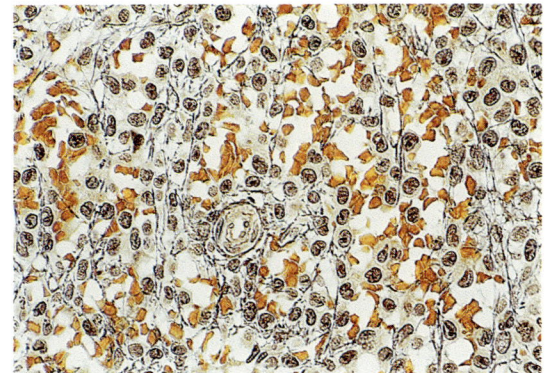

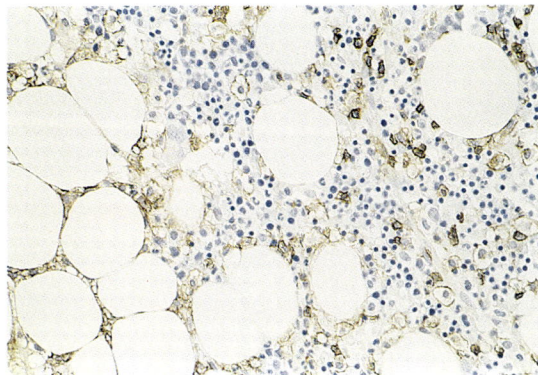

285

type predominates in each individual case. The ovoid type has the best, and the indented type has the least, favorable prognosis. These three cell types are more easily distinguished in sections of plastic-embedded BMB than in hematoxylin and eosin-stained sections of decalcified and paraffin-embedded BMB. The reaction for tartrate-resistant acid phosphatase can be performed on peripheral blood smears (not indicated if the lymphocyte count is low), on smears of aspirates or on imprints of the biopsy, especially in cases of 'dry tap' on attempts at aspiration. The karyotype of a patient with HCL is given in Figure 26.31.

Evolution of disease

Studies on the evolution of the disease have shown that the hairy cell burden in the bone marrow correlates with the clinical course, and a rapid increase of tumor mass indicated an unfavorable prognosis. Transformation of the mainly ovoid to the indented type also signaled a rapid progression. These findings have been supported by a recent report of a blastic variant of HCL. HCL must be differentiated from B cell CLL, cleaved type (centrocytic) lymphomas, myelomonocytic and monocytic infiltrations, monocytoid B cell lymphomas and splenic B cell lymphomas with 'villous' lymphocytes in the peripheral blood. Reduction in the amount of hairy cell mass, and repopulation by hematopoietic elements, has been demonstrated in some patients in response to therapy. The occurrence of HCL with myeloid metaplasia and myelofibrosis has also been described.

Hairy cell variants are characterised by morphology intermediate between HCL and B cell prolymphocytic leukemia. HCL together with another B cell clone producing a paraprotein has also been reported.

Splenic lymphoma with villous lymphocytes (SLVL)

The lymphocytes in this malignant lymphoma morphologically resemble hairy cells in the peripheral blood, though there is usually a leu-

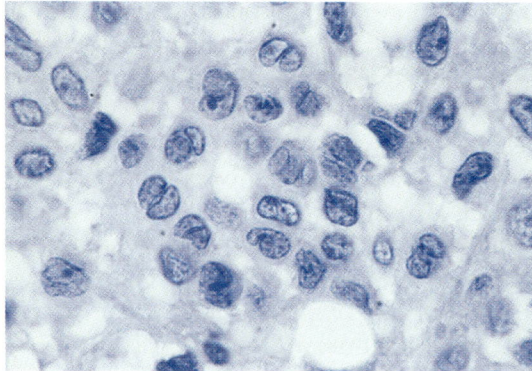

26.29 BMBS plastic, Giemsa, showing hairy cells with convoluted nuclei.

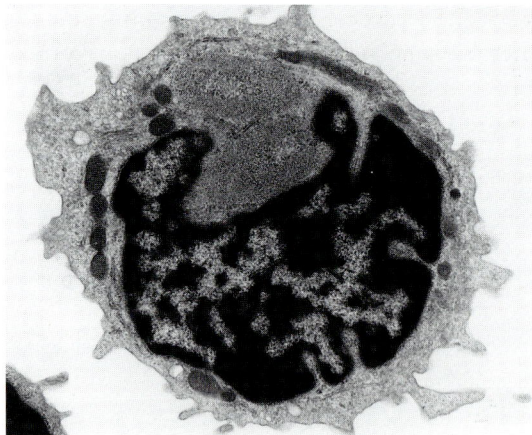

26.30 BMBS, EM, convoluted subtype with ribosome–lamellar complex.

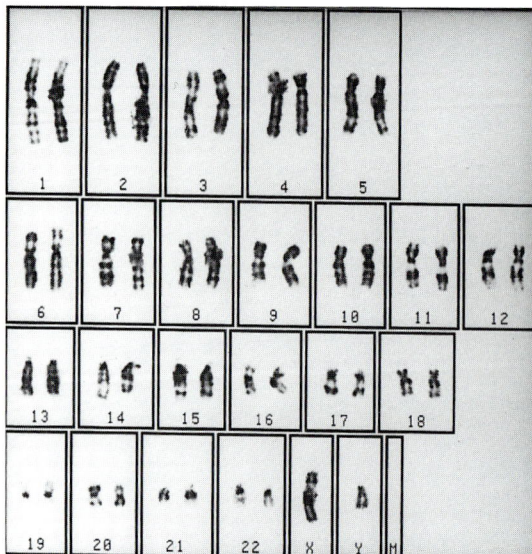

26.31 Karyotype of patient with HCL showing del(14)(q).

cocytosis and not a leucopenia as in HCL. The bone marrow is usually involved to a variable extent, in both a nodular and interstitial pattern. Unlike in HCL, the cells are closely packed, and there is little fibrosis. When there is minimal involvement, immunohistology may be helpful in establishing a B cell phenotype.

Malignant lymphoma lymphoplasmacytic/cytoid (immunocytoma, Waldenström's macroglobulinemia)

This is a B cell lymphoma of low-grade malignancy secreting monoclonal lgM or lgG. Bone marrow involvement is found in about 80% of patients. The predominant cell type is a small lymphocyte with variable plasmacytoid differentiation, but there is a wide spectrum of lymphoid cells, ranging from small lymphocyte with variable plasmacytoid differentiation, to immunoblasts and plasma cells (Figure 26.32). In a typical case there are nuclear inclusions, consisting of immunoglobulins, the so-called Dutcher bodies (PAS-positive) in a variable number of the infiltrating plasma cells. Initially, the infiltrations are present in a hypo- or normocellular bone marrow. Three proliferation patterns are recognised (Figures 26.32 and 26.33): (1) nodular with multiple nodules adjacent to sinusoids and trabeculae, (2) interstitial/nodular in which there is a loose interstitial infiltration in addition to the nodules, and (3) packed marrow in which there is complete replacement of hematopoietic and fat cells. EM and immunohistology often reveal the plasmacytoid nature of cells identified as lymphocytes in the light microscope.

Subtypes of immunocytoma

There are three histological subdivisions, comparable with the subtypes recognised in the lymph nodes: (1) lymphoplasmacytoid, (2) lymphoplasmacytic and (3) polymorphous (Figures 26.32–26.35). However, as in the lymph nodes, there is some overlap between them. The first generally has a nodular pattern, the second an interstitial/nodular pattern with numerous plasma and mast cells, and the third usually presents with a packed marrow pattern whose cell population consists of lymphocytes,

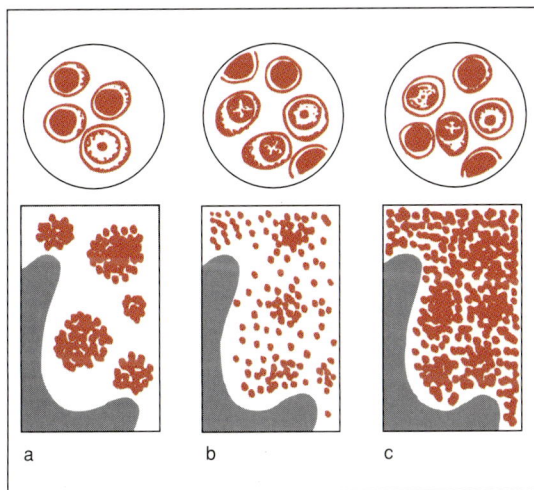

26.32 Bone marrow involvement in the three types of Waldenström's macroglobulinemia: (a) lymphoplasmacytoid, (b) lymphoplasmacytic, (c) polymorphous.

26.33 (left) BMBS plastic, Gomori, showing nodules in hypocellular bone marrow.

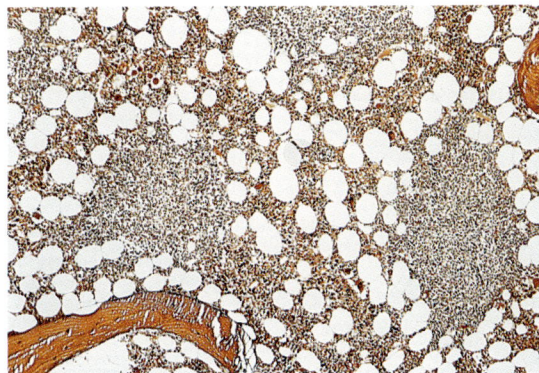

26.34 (right) BMBS plastic, Giemsa, showing marrow replaced by polymorphic type.

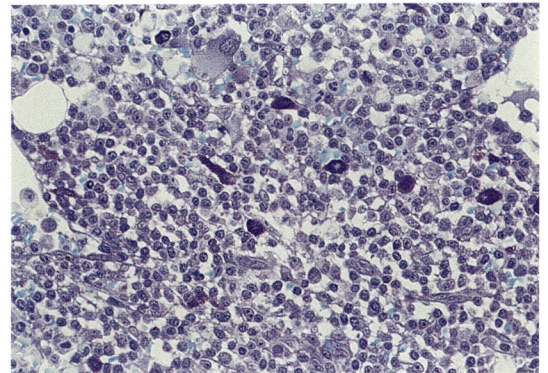

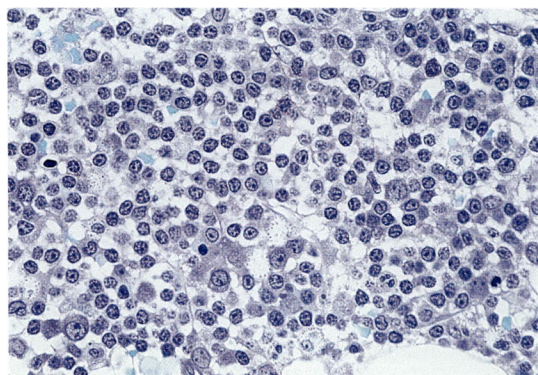

26.35 (left) BMBS plastic, Giemsa, showing mast cells in lymphoid nodule, lymphoplasmacytoid type.

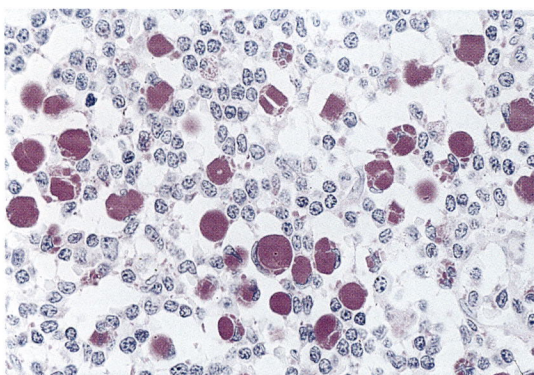

26.36 (right) BMBS plastic, PAS stain showing numerous plasma cells packed with PAS-positive material.

plasma cells, centrocytes, centroblasts and immunoblasts. These types are characterised by differences in growth patterns, clinical features, anatomic extent and median survivals. Bone marrow mast cells are increased in all types (Figure 26.35). Hematopoietic precursors are located in the infiltrates as well as between them. Hyperplastic and ectatic sinusoids with sclerosis of the endothelium, and prominent histiocyctes, are especially characteristic of the lymphoplasmacyctic type. The blood vessels in any case of immunocytoma may be filled with a homogeneously stained PAS-positive material, which may also be found in the interstitium, where it is secreted by plasma cells instead of into the vascular lumen. This material may also be partly responsible for the interstitial staining sometimes observed in immunohistology (Figures 26.36 and 26.37).

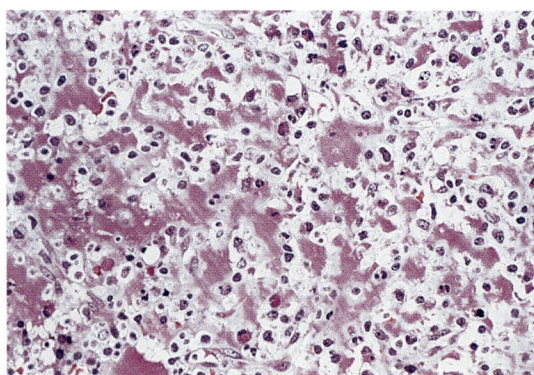

26.37 BMBS plastic, PAS stain, deposition of PAS-positive material in the bone marrow interstitium.

Evolution of disease

In the evolution of disease conversion of an immunocytoma to an immunoblastic lymphoma has also been described. Diagnostic difficulties may arise in the absence of PAS-positive inclusions, and when the infiltration is minimal. The picture may resemble nodular lymphoid hyperplasia, or CLL. However, mast cells are more numerous in immunocytoma. Immunohistology is required in borderline cases. Post-therapy sections of bone biopsies of patients with WM may show residual interstitial, perivascular and paratrabecular infiltrations.

Check list: Chronic Lymphocytic Leukemia and Related Disorders

CLL

- Cortical and trabecular structure?
- Cellularity?
- Growth patterns: interstitial, nodular or both?
- Extent of infiltration: mild, moderate, massive: packed marrow?
- Hematopoiesis: quantity and topography? I.H.: for identification of normal hematopoiesis within the infiltration.
- Amount of fat cells?
- Cytologic features of infiltrating cells: types and their relative proportions?
- Immunohistology: B and T cell markers, BCL2, LCA, and CD79[a].

Continued

HCL

- Adequate biopsy: frequently patchy distribution of the infiltration, or paratrabecular.
- Typical cytology and topography and accompanying features – widely spaced hairy cells.
- Fine fibrosis, especially in infiltrated areas.
- Megaloblastoid erythropoiesis.
- Plasma and mast cells in areas of hairy cell infiltration.
- On immunohistology, hairy cells positive with markers for B cells and hairy cells, DB4 44, TRAP.
- On cytochemistry, positive for tartrate resistant acid phosphatase (TRAP) on smears and imprints of the biopsy.
- Hairy cells nuclei on high magnification are coffee-bean-shaped, oval, round or indented, have abundant cytoplasm and projections visible in good sections.
- One of these three types usually predominates in any individual case.

ML lymphoplasmacytic (immunocytoma)

- Adequate biopsy: 30 mm excluding cortex.
- Histologic pattern at low magnification?
- Nodular, interstitial, packed?
- Fat cells: present, decreased, absent?
- Bone – trabecular network preserved, thin – remodeling?
- Hematopoiesis – quantity, topography – dysplasia.
- Infiltration-proliferation pattern

  topography

  composition

  cytologic features

  Dutcher bodies: PAS stain shows intranuclear inclusions.
- Fibrosis – extent, location, reticulin stain.
- Mast cells.
- Immunohistology: monoclonality with kappa or lambda antigens, LCA, B and T cells, CD79[a].

Clinical correlations

CLL

- Early detection – asymptomatic, only mild or moderate lymphocytosis in peripheral blood.
- Enlarged peripheral lymph nodes, painless.
- Fatigue, weight loss.
- Fever, night sweats, anemia and infections increase with progressive disease.
- Hepatosplenomegaly and other organ infiltration.
- Immune red cell aplasia, neutropenia, thrombocytopenia.
- Transformation of CLL, possibly in extranodular site.
- Peripheral blood values, lymphocytosis: increases with progression.
- Clonal chromosomal characteristics

Chronic lymphocytic leukemia

B cell chronic lymphocytic leukemia

+12

13q14 rearrangements

14q+ breakpoints at 14q32

t(11;14)(q13;q32)

t(14;19)(q32;q13)

6q anomaly.

T cell chronic lymphocytic leukemia

inv(14)(q11q32)

t/del(14)(q11)

+8q

structural abnormalities on chromosome 7.

Prolymphocytic leukemia

PLL

14q32 rearrangements, including
   t(11;14)(q13;q32)

t(6;12)(q15;p13)

del(3)(p13)

+12

6q−

1q−.

T-PLL

inv(14)(q11q32) and other rearrangements
   with 14q11 breakpoints

+8q

rearrangements with 8p12 breakpoints.

Continued

Sezary syndrome and mycosis fungoides

chromosome 1 rearrangements
t/del(6)(p).

HCL

- Male predominance 4:1. Median age 50 years.
- Fatigue, fever, weight loss, possibly vasculitis.
- Splenomegaly, abdominal discomfort; usually no lymphadenopathy.
- Anemia, granulocytopenia, monocytopenia with relative lymphocytosis.
- Propensity to recurrent infections.
- Lymphadenopathy and lytic bone lesions – unusual.
- Correlation with peripheral blood values leucopenia, pancytopenia.
- Clonal chromosomal characteristics

Hairy cell leukemia

14q+
rearrangements of 14q32
6q anomaly

changes on 5q13
       1q42
       2q11
trisomy 3,12,18,Y.

Splenic lymphoma with villous lymphocytes

t(11;14)(q13;q32)
t(2)(p)
i(17)(q10)
del/t (7)(q).

Waldenstroem's macroglobulinemia (immunocytoma)

- Older age groups affected, especially males.
- Suggestive profile in peripheral blood.
- Evidence of other organ disease.
- Evidence of bone marrow failure.
- Evidence of concomitant conditions.
- Clonal chromosomal characteristics

abnormalities of chromosome 1
+12
14q+
t(8;14)(q24;q32).

Bibliography

Agnarsson B.A., Loughran T.P. Jr., Starkebaum G., Kadin M.E. (1989) The pathology of large granular lymphocyte leukemia. *Hum. Pathol.*, **21 (4)**, 458–9.

Arber D.A., Lopategui J.R., Brynes R.K. (1993) Chronic lymphoproliferative disorders involving blood and bone marrow. *Am J Clin Pathol.*, **99**, 494–503.

Arkel Y.S., Lake-Lewin D., Savopoulos A.A., Berman E. (1984) Bone lesions in hairy cell leukemia. A case report and response of bone pains to steroids. *Cancer*, **53**, 2401.

Bardawil R.G., Ratain M.J., Golomb H.M. *et al.* (1987) Changes in peripheral blood and bone marrow specimens during and after alpha 2b-interferon therapy for hairy-cell leukemia. *Leukemia*, **1 (4)**, 340–3.

Bartl R., Frisch B., Hill W. *et al.* (1983) Bone marrow histology in hairy celly leukemia: identification of subtypes and their prognostic significance. *Amer J Clin Pathol.*, **79**, 531.

Bartl R., Frisch B., Mahl G. *et al.* (1983) Bone marrow histology in Waldenstroem's macroglobulinaemia. Clinical relevance of subtype recognition. *Scand J Haematol.*, **31**, 359.

Berthiot G. (1993) Hairy-cell leukemia and sarcoidosis (letter). *Eur. J. Med.*, **2 (1)**, 61.

Berthold, F., Krueger, G.R., Tesch, H., Hiddemann, W. (1989) Monoclonal B cell proliferation in lymphoproliferative disease associated with herpes virus type 6 infection. *Anticancer Res.*, **9 (6)**, 1511–18.

Bouroncle B.A. (1987) Unusual presentations and complications of hairy cell leukemia. *Leukemia*, **1 (4)**, 288–93.

Braylan R.C. (1993) Flow cytometric DNA analysis in the diagnosis and prognosis of lymphoma. *Am J Clin Pathol.*, **99**, 374–80.

Brito-Babapulle V., Maljaie S.H., Matutes E. *et al.* (1997) Relationship of T leukaemias with cerebriform nuclei to T-prolymphocytic leukaemia: a cytogenetic analysis with in situ hybridization. *Br J Haematol.*, **96**, 724–32.

Brito-Babapulle V., Matutes E., Oscier D. *et al.* (1994) Chromosome abnormalities in hairy cell leukemia variant. *Genes. Chromosom. Cancer.*, **10 (3)**, 197–202.

Brynes R.K., McCourty A., Sun N.C., Koo C.H. (1995) Trisomy 12 in Richter's transformation of chronic lymphocytic leukemia. *Am J Clin Pathol.*, **104 (2)**, 199–203.

Burthem J., Baker P.K., Hunt J.A., Cawley J.C. (1994) Hairy cell interactions with extracellular matrix: expression of specific integrin receptors and their role in the cell's response to specific adhesive proteins. *Blood*, **84** (3), 873–82.

Burthem J., Cawley J.C. (1994) The bone marrow fibrosis of *hairy cell leukemia* is caused by the synthesis and assembly of a fibronectin matrix by the hairy cells. *Blood*, **83** (2), 497–504.

Cavallero G.B., Bonferroni M., Gallamini A. *et al.* (1994) Scleroderma and hairy cell leukemia. (letter). *Eur. J. Hematol.*, **52** (3), 189–90.

Cha I., Herndier B.G., Glassberg A.B., Hamill T.R. (1996) A case of composite Hodgkin's disease and chronic lymphocytic leukemia in bone marrow. Lack of Epstein–Barr virus. *Arch Pathol Lab Med*, **120** (4), 386–9.

Cherepakhin V., Baird S.M., Meisenholder G.W., Kipps T.J. (1993) Common clonal origin of chronic lymphocytic leukemia and high-grade lymphoma of Richter's syndrome. *Blood*, **82 (10)**, 3141–7.

Copeland A.R., Bueso-Ramos C., Liu F.J. *et al.* (1997) Molecular study of hairy cell leukemia variant with biclonal paraproteinemia. *Arch Pathol Lab Med*, **121**, 150–4.

Criel A., Wlodarska I., Meeus P. *et al.* (1994) Trisomy 12 is uncommon in typical chronic lymphocytic leukaemias. *Br J. Haematol.*, **87**, 523–8.

Dascalescu C., Gressin R., Callanan M. *et al.* (1996) T(11;14)(q13;q32): Chronic lymphocytic leukaemia or mantle cell leukaemia? *Br J Haematol*, **95**, 570–6.

Demanes D.J., Lane N., Beckstead J.H. (1982) Bone involvement in hairy cell leukemia. *Cancer*, **49**, 1697.

Desablens B., Claisse J.F., Piprot-Choffat C., Gontier M.F. (1989) Prognostic value of bone marrow biopsy in chronic lymphoid leukemia. A study of 98 initial bone marrow biopsies. *Nouv Rev Fr Hematol.*, **31** (3), 179–82.

Domingo A., Gonzalez-Barca E., Castellsague X. *et al.* (1997) Expression of adhesion molecules in 113 patients with B-cell chronic lymphocytic leukemia: relationship with clinico-prognostic features. *Leuk Res.*, **21** (1), 67–73.

Dorfman D.M., Longtime J.A., Weinberg D.S., Pinkus G.S. (1993) Small lymphocytic non-Hodgkin's lymphoma of surpressor/cytotoxic T-cell phenotype [CD4(−), CD8(+)]. *Human Pathol.*, **24** (11), 1253–6.

Dyer M.J., Zani V.J., Lu W.Z. *et al.* (1994) BCL2 translocations in leukemias of mature B cells. *Blood*, **83** (12), 3682–8.

Fineberg S., Marsh E., Alfonso F. *et al.* (1993) Immunophenotypic evaluation of the bone marrow in non-Hodgkin's lymphoma. *Hum Pathol.*, **24** (6), 636–42.

Finn W.G., Thangavelu M., Yelevarthi K.Y. *et al.* (1996) Karyotype correlates with peripheral blood morphology and immunophenotype in chronic lymphocytic leukemia. *Am J Clin Pathol*, **105**, 458.

Frassoldati A., Lamparelli T., Federico M. *et al.* (1994) Hairy cell leukemia: a clinical review based on 725 cases of the Italian Cooperative Group (ICGHCL). *Leuk Lymphoma*, **13** (3–4), 307–16.

Frisch B., Bartl R. (1988) Histologic classification and staging of chronic lymphocytic leukemia. *Acta Haematol.*, **79**, 140–52.

Geisler C.H., Larsen J.K., Hansen N.E. *et al.* (1991) Prognostic importance of flow cytometric immunophenotyping of 540 consecutive patients with B-cell chronic lymphocytic leukemia. *Blood*, **78**, 1795.

Greil R., Fasching B., Huber H. (1991) Expression of the c-myc proto-oncogene in multiple myeloma and chronic lymphocytic leukemia: an in situ analysis. *Blood*, **78** (1), 180–91.

Haglund U., Juliusson G., Stellan B., Gahrton G. (1994) Hairy cell leukemia is characterized by clonal chromosome abnormalities clustered to specific regions. *Blood*, **83** (9), 2637–45.

Hanson C.A., Gribbin T.E., Schnitzer B. *et al.* (1990) CD11c (LEU-M5) expression characterizes a B-cell chronic lymphoproliferative disorder with features of both chronic lymphocytic leukemia and hairy cell leukemia. *Blood*. **76** (11), 2360–7.

Hassan I.B., Sunstrom C., Hagberg H. (1989) Bone marrow morphology during alpha-interferon treatment in hairy cell luekemia. *Eur. J. Hematol.* **43** (2), 120–6.

Jonveaux P., Daniel M.T., Martel V. *et al.* (1996) Isochromosome 7q and trisomy 8 are consistent primary, non-random chromosomal abnormalities associated with hepatosplenic T gamma/delta lymphoma. *Leukemia*, **10** (9), 1453–5.

Juliusson G., Gahrton G. (1990) Chromosome aberrations in B-cell chronic lymphocytic leukemia. Pathogenetic and clinical implications. *Cancer Genet. Cytogenet.*, **45** (2), 143–60.

Juliusson G., Gahrton G. (1993) Cytogenetics in CLL and related disorders. *Baillieres Clin. Hematol.*, **6** (4), 821–48.

Juliusson G., Lenkei R., Liliemark J. (1994) Flow cytometry of blood and bone marrow cells from patients with hairy cell leukemia: phenotype of hairy cells and lymphocyte subsets after treatment with 2-chlorodeoxyadenosine. *Blood*, **83** (12), 3672–81.

Koduru P.R.K., Lichtman S.M., Smilari T.F. *et al.* (1993) Serial phenotypic, cytogenetic and molecular genetic studies in Richter's syndrome: Demonstration of lymphoma development from the chronic lymphocytic leukemia cells. *Br. J. Hematol.*, **85** (3), 613–16.

Konwalinka G., Dchirmer M., Hilbe W. *et al.* (1995) Minimal residual disease in hairy-cell leukemia after treatment with

2-chlorodeoxyadenosine. *Blood Cells Mol Dis*, **21** (2), 142–51.

Loghran T.P. (1993) Clonal diseases of large granular lymphocytes. Review article. *Blood*, **82**, 1–14.

Lee J.S., Dixon D.O., Kantarjian H.M. *et al.* (1987) Prognosis of chronic lymphocytic leukemia: a multivariate regression analysis of 325 untreated patients. *Blood*, **69** (3), 929–36.

Littlewood T.J., Lydon A.P.M., Barton C.J. (1990) Hypercalcaemia and osteolytic lesions associated with chronic lymphatic leukaemia (CLL). *Br Med J.*, **43**, 877.

Macak J., Krc I., Cihal K., Scudla V. (1988) Morphological correlates between bone marrow findings in patients with lymphocytic ML (CCL and immunocytoma) and clinical staging. *Acta. Univ. Palacki. Olomuc. Fac. Med.*, **120**, 211–22.

Macon W.R., Kinney M.C., Glick A.D., Collins R.D. (1993) Marrow mast cell hyperplasia in hairy cell leukemia. *Mod. Pathol.*, **6** (6), 695–8.

Malik S.T., Amess J., D'Ardenne A.J., Lister T.A. (1989) Hairy cell leukemia – mediastinal involvement. A report of two cases and review of the literature. *Hematol Oncol.*, **7** (4), 303–6.

Marti R.M., Estrach T., Reverter J.C. *et al.* (1996) Utility of bone marrow and liver biopsies for staging cutaneous T-cell lymphoma. *Int J Dermatol*, **35** (6), 450–4.

Merup M., Spasokoukotskaja T., Einhorn S. *et al.* (1996) Bcl-2 rearrangements with breakpoints in both vcr and mbr in non-Hodgkin's lymphomas and chronic lymphocytic leukaemia. *Br J Haematol*, **92** (3), 647–52.

Monserrat E., Villamor N., Reverter J.C. *et al.* (1996) Bone marrow assessment in B-cell chronic lymphocytic leukaemia: aspirate or biopsy? A comparative study in 258 patients. *Br J Haematol*, **93** (1), 111–16.

Mossafa H., Troussard X., Valensi F. *et al.* (1996) Isochromosome i(3q) and premature chromosome condensation are recurrent findings in chronic B-cell lymphocytosis with binucleated lymohocytes. *Leuk Lymphoma*, **20** (3–4), 267–73.

Nathwani B.N., Hernandez A.M., Deol I., Taylor C.R. (1997) Marginal zone B-cell lymphomas: an appraisal. *Human Pathol.*, **28** (1), 42–6.

O'Brien S., del Giglio A., Keating M. (1995) Advances in the biology and treatment of B-cell chronic lymphocytic leukaemia. *Blood*, **85**, 307–18.

Oka K., Mori N., Yatabe Y. (1993) Immunohistochemical characteristics of monocytoid B cell lymphoma, mantle zone lymphoma, small lymphocytic lymphoma (or B chronic lymphocytic leukemia), and hairy cell leukemia. *Acta. Hematol.*, **90** (2), 84–9.

Oscier D.G., Gardiner A., Mould S. (1996) Structural abnormalities of chromosome 7q in chronic lymphoproliferative disorders. *Cancer Genet Cytogenet*, **92** (1), 24–7.

Pangalis G.A., Boussiotis V.A., Kittas C. (1993) Malignant disorders of small lymphocytes: Small lymphocytic lymphoma, lymphoplasmacytic lymphoma, and chronic lymphocytic leukemia: Their clinical and laboratory relationship. *Am. J. Clin. Pathol.*, **99** (4), 402–8.

Pangalis G.A., Kittas C., Viniou N. *et al.* (1987) Hairy cell leukemia: bone marrow changes following splenectomy and alpha-interferon therapy. *Leukemia*, **1** (4), 343–6.

Paulson J.A., Marti G.E., Fink J.K. *et al.* (1989) Richter's transformation of lymphoma complicating Gaucher's disease. *Hematol Pathol*, **3** (2), 91–6.

Polliack A., Dann E.J. (1994) Rapid massive splenic relapse of hairy cell leukemia (HCL) during bone marrow remission after 2-chlorodeoxyadenosine therapy: the spleen as a sanctuary site in HCL? (letter). *Blood*, **84** (6), 2057–8.

Rai K.R., Montserrat E. (1987) Prognostic factors in chronic lymphocytic leukemia. *Semin. Hematol.*, **24** (4), 252–6.

Rai K.R., Sawitsky A. (1987) A review of the prognostic role of cytogenetic, phenotypic, morphologic, and immune function characteristics in chronic lymphocytic leukemia. *Blood cells*, **12** (2), 327–8.

Robertson T.L., Byth K. (1993) Sequential changes in the bone marrow trephine biopsy in B-cell chronic lymphocytic leukaemia. *Aust NZ J Med*, **23** (5), 470–6.

Schwarzmeier J.D., Gasche C.G., Hilgarth M.F. *et al.* (1994) Myelosuppression in HCL: role of hairy cells, T cells and hematopietic growth factors. *Eur. J. hematol.*, **52** (5), 257–62.

Shamsi T.S., Hasmi K.Z. (1994) Hairy cell leukemia – diagnosis and current treatment. *J. Pak. Med. Assoc.*, **44** (6), 149–55.

Traweek S.T., Liu J., Johnson R.M. *et al.* (1993) High-grade transformation of chronic lymphocytic leukemia and low-grade non-Hodgkin's lymphoma: genotypic confirmation of clonal identity. *Am. J. Clin. Pathol.*, **100** (5), 519–26.

Valens F., Duran V., Bast B., Flýandrin G. (1990) Splenic B-cell lymphoma with villous lymphocytes (SLVL). A lymphocytic lymphoma simulating hairy cell leukemia. A study of 8 cases. *Nouv. Rev. Fr. Hematol.*, **32** (6), 409–14.

Vescio R., Rosen L., Schmulbach E., Berenson J. (1996) Multiple myeloma and chronic lymphocytic leukemia. *Current Opinion in Hematol*, **3** (4), 288–96.

Wasman J., Rosenthal N.S., Farhi D.C. (1996) Mantle cell lymphoma. Morphologic findings in bone marrow involvement. *Am J Clin Pathol*, **106** (2), 196–200.

Yam L.T., Janckila A.J., Li C.Y., Lam W.K. (1987) Cytochemistry of tartrate-resistant acid phosphatase: 15 years' experience. *Leukemia*, **1** (4), 285–8.

27 Malignant lymphomas

Mantle cell lymphoma (Malignant Lymphomas centrocytic, Kiel Classification)

These are also known as cleaved cell lymphomas, or follicle center cell lymphomas. More recently, 'mantle cell or zone lymphoma' has been suggested for this group of malignant lymphomas, based on their relationship to lymphocytes in the follicles of the lymph nodes. There is a characteristic bone marrow involvement in about 70% of cases, consisting of paratrabecular infiltrations of small-to-medium-sized lymphoid cells with somewhat angulated 'cleaved' nuclei containing fairly dense chromatin and narrow rims of cytoplasm (Figures 27.1–27.8). The lymphoma cells are closely packed. A few centroblasts or centroblast-like cells are often present. These infiltrations are generally enmeshed in a fairly dense network of coarse fibers radiating out from the trabeculae and which stops at the boundary between the infiltration and the central, residual hematopoietic tissue. According to size and nuclear morphology, three subtypes are distinguished: (1) small centrocytic, cleaved, (2) large centrocytic, cleaved, and (3) polymorphous. A follicular lymphoma may also undergo conversion to a blastic type.

'Mantle cell leukemia' is now also used for those cases of apparent but atypical CLL with the t(11:14)(q13:q32) translocation, as these cases are now envisioned as the leukemic expression of mantle cell lymphomas. However, rare cases of typical CLL may also have this chromosome abnormality. Mantle cell lymphomas may be distinguished from other small cell B lymphomas including marginal zone lymphoma, by means of cyclin D on immunohistology.

Monocytoid B cell lymphoma

This also has a relationship to the lymph node follicle; marrow involvement is rare. In BMB with a packed marrow the morphological distinction between centrocytes and CLL of the B2 notched or the T-CLL types, or immunocytoma, may not be possible. The same holds true for the distinction between large centrocytes and monocytic infiltrations. The diagnosis in these cases will depend on supplementary enzymic and immunological methods, as well as the clinical findings. Monocytoid B cell lymphomas is the term used for classifying the so-called marginal zone lymphomas, of which three types have been described, depending on the predominant cell type: (1) malignant monocytoid B cells and follicle center cells, (2) malignant monocytoid B cells, follicle center cells and plasma cells; and (3) malignant monocytoid B cells and malignant mantle cells. However, there appears to be some confusion in the distinction of lymphomas in these two groups (mantle cell and monocytoid), especially since 'monocytoid B cell lymphoma' is not generally used in the international classification.

Malignant lymphoma centroblastic/centrocytic

Bone marrow involvement in this lymphoma is relatively infrequent, in about 20% of the cases. The pattern is nodular (Figure 27.1):

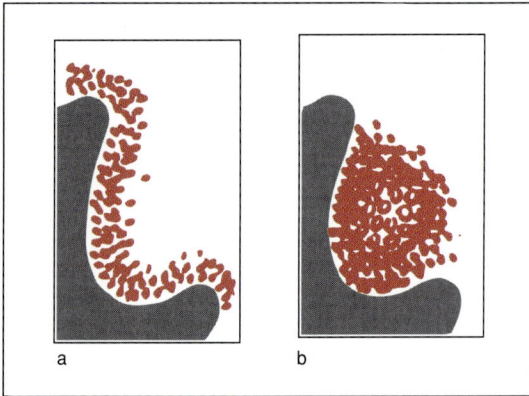

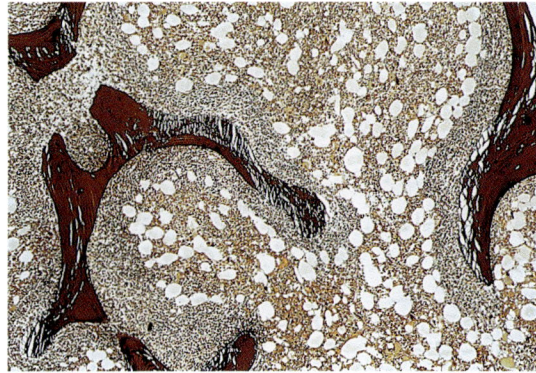

27.1 (left) Bone marrow involvement in centrocytic (a) and centroblastic/centrocytic (b) lymphomas, showing the characteristic paratrabecular and nodular patterns.

27.2 (right) BMBS plastic, Gomori, showing extensive paratrabecular localisation of the lymphoma – mantle cell or as previously called centrocytic (Kiel Classification).

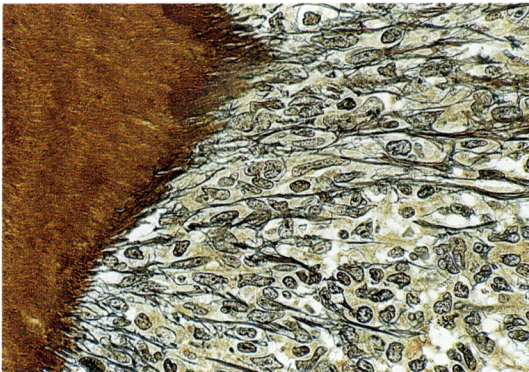

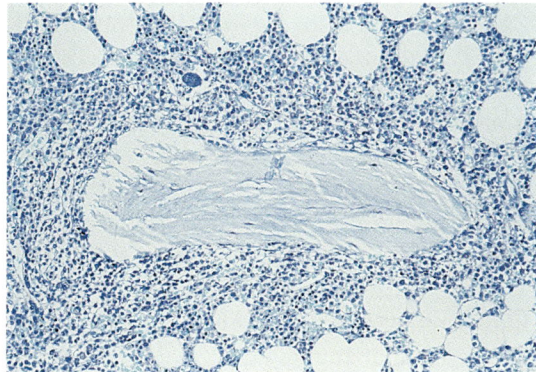

27.3 (left) BMBS plastic, Gomori, high power to illustrate the fibers; note their direct connection to the surface of the trabecular bone.

27.4 (right) BMBS plastic, Giemsa, showing centrocytes small, cleaved cells; note the fibers.

follicles with germinal centers consisting of centroblasts, centrocytes, lymphocytes, reticular cells, blood vessels and fibers (Figures 27.9 and 27.10). Some lymphoid nodules may not have germinal centers. At the periphery of the follicles eosinophils, plasma cells and mast cells may form a transition between them and the normal bone marrow. In some cases a packed marrow pattern is found, and then the nodularity is blurred. The distinction between minimal involvement and nodular immunocytoma or benign lymphoid nodules or follicles is not possible on histology alone. The nodules and follicles have a typical localisation at the endosteal surface of the trabecular bone where they stimulate osseous remodeling.

Malignant lymphoma centroblastic

Involvement is relatively rare (20%) and shows a packed marrow pattern. The characteristic

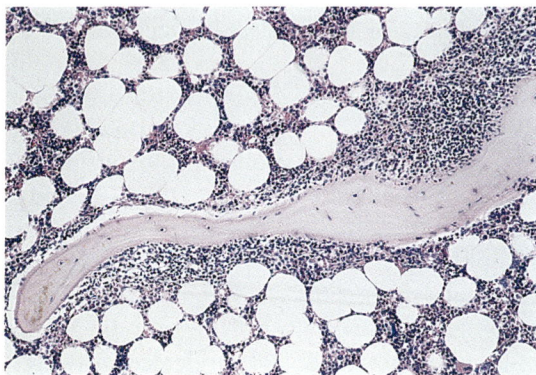

27.5 BMBS paraffin, H&E, paratrabecular involvement by mantle cell lymphoma, both left and right.

nuclear structure and the nucleoli indicate the cell type so that little difficulty is encountered (Figures 27.11–27.14). In some cases, the centroblasts have a signet-ring-like appearance.

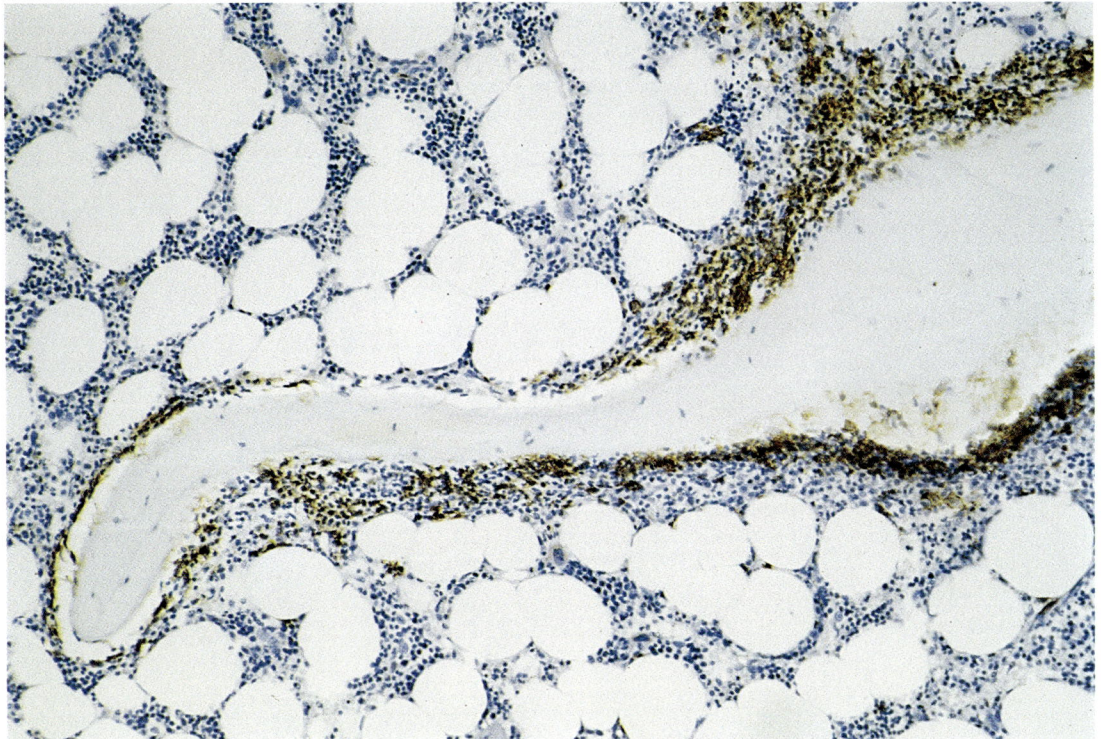

27.6 As for Figure 27.5, I.H., B cell antigen; note that only the infiltration is positive.

27.7 (left) As for Figure 27.5, I.H., T cell antigen; T cells also present in the infiltration.

27.8 (right) BMBS, paraffin, H&E, same biopsy as for Figure 27.5, showing considerably broader paratrabecular infiltration.

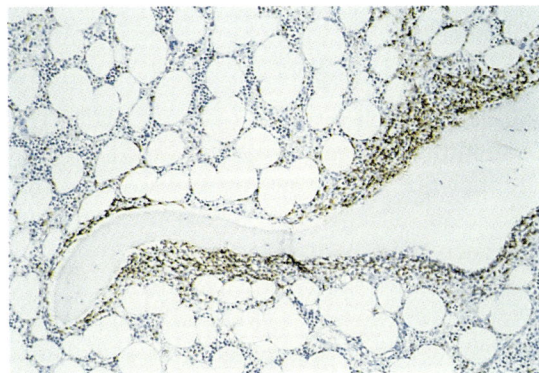

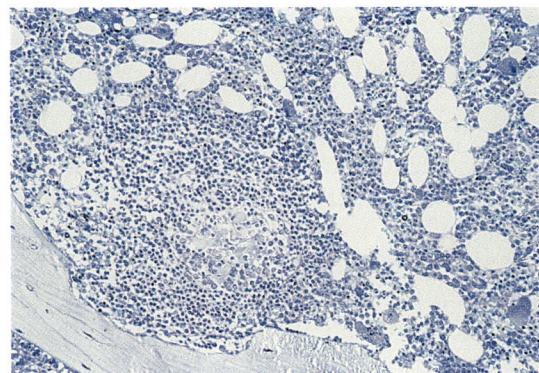

27.9 (left) BMBS plastic, Giemsa, involvement of the bone marrow by centroblastic-centrocytic lymphoma; note nodule adjacent to bone and eroding the trabecula, lower left.

27.10 (right) BMBS plastic, Giemsa, showing part of nodule with centroblasts, left, and centrocytes.

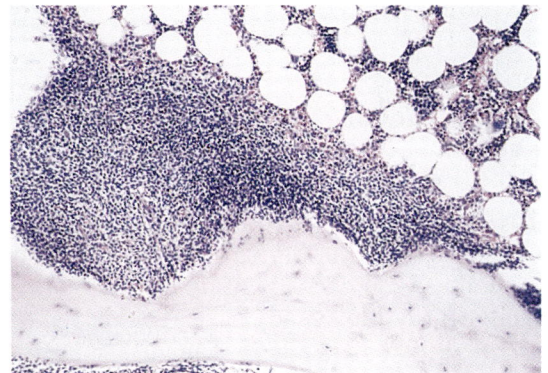

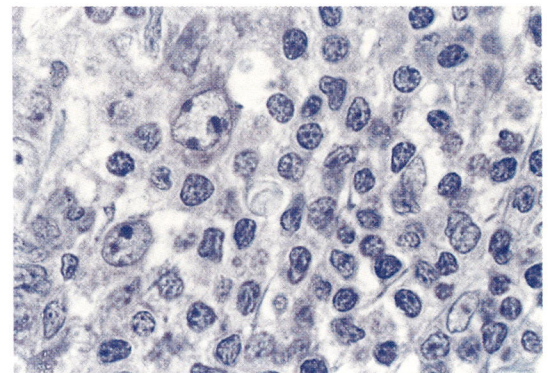

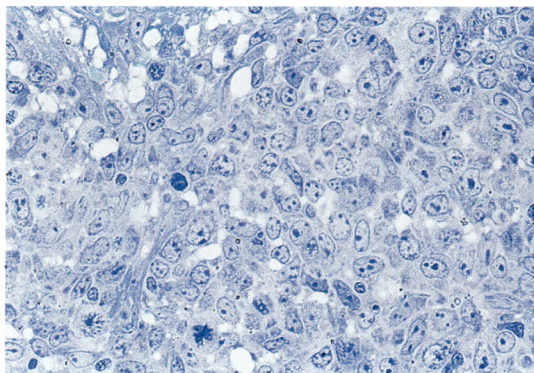

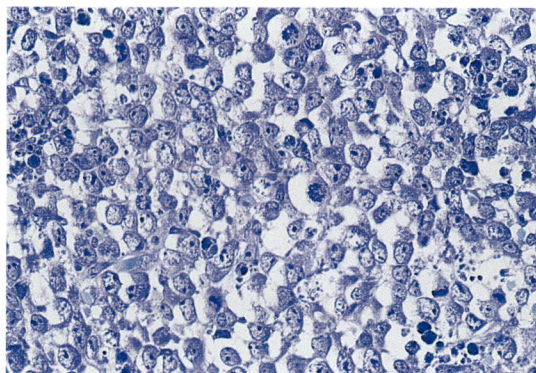

27.11 (left) BMBS plastic, Giemsa, showing packed marrow in case of involvement by centroblastic lymphoma.

27.12–27.14 Case of ML centroblastic.
27.12 (right) BMBS, plastic, Giemsa, showing the typical centroblasts.

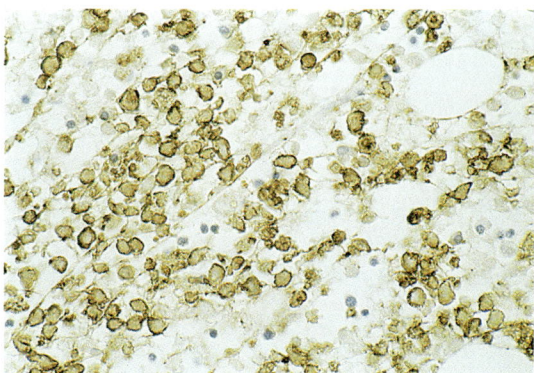

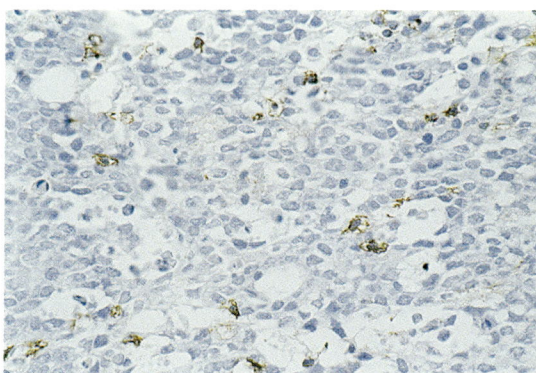

27.13 (left) BMBS, paraffin, I.H., with CD20-positive in all the centroblasts.

27.14 (right) BMBS, paraffin, I.H., reaction with the T cell antigen, only isolated cells are positive.

Anaplastic large cell lymphomas (ALCL)

These are high-grade usually T cell lymphomas characterised by a strongly positive reaction with the Ki antigen. Bone marrow involvement shows the typical large cells dispersed among the hematopoietic elements, in aggregates and in the sinusoids. Characteristically these cells often express the epithelial membrane antigen (EMA), while the leucocyte common antigen (LCA) may be negative, though the pan T cell antigen is positive in most cases.

A major difficulty in differential diagnosis may arise when cells resembling Reed–Sternberg cells are also present. However, in anaplastic large cell lymphomas these cells are negative for CD15 and CD30, while in HD they are positive for these markers. Moreover, in HD the RS cells and the mononuclear Hodgkin's cells will be present in the characteristic environment, which is not the case for ALCL. The possibilities of transformation of HD at one site, but not at another; or of discordant histologies, must also be considered if an ALCL has been diagnosed elsewhere and the bone marrow shows the typical picture of HD (see Chapter 28). Moreover, nodal ALCL may show the typical translocation t(2;5)(p23;q35) which is not present in HD.

Malignant lymphoma immunoblastic

In this lymphoma also, the bone marrow is infrequently involved. When it occurs the marrow is usually packed, to the exclusion of hematopoietic and fat cells. B immunoblasts have round nuclei with prominent central nucleoli and basophilic cytoplasm (Figure 27.15). In contrast, T immunoblasts are polymorphic, have pleomorphic nuclei but definitive identification requires immunological studies.

Burkitt lymphoma

Marrow involvement is rare; it is a subtype of the small non-cleaved follicle center cell lymphoma.

Malignant lymphoma lymphoblastic

The phenotype (e.g. common ALL, B ALL, T ALL) must be established by marker studies (adult patients – see also section on acute leukemia). A diffuse marrow pattern is characteristic, with little residual hematopoiesis or fat cells. In T cell variants there is a pronounced perivascular infiltration of lymphoid cells with oval, notched or convoluted nuclei, and variable amounts of cytoplasm (Figure 27.16).

Lennert's lymphoma (lymphoepithelioid) (Figure 27.17)

This is classified with the T cell lymphomas. Nevertheless, a few patients had a B cell phe-

notype, though these lymphomas were morphologically indistinguishable from their T cell counterparts. This lymphoma is thought to mark the border between Hodgkin's disease and the malignant lymphomas. Bone marrow involvement is characterised by aggregates of epithelioid cells together with macrophages, lymphocytes, plasma cells, immunoblasts and sometimes eosinophils. Occasional Hodgkin's or RS-like cells may be found.

Angioimmunoblastic lymphadenopathy with dysproteinemia (AILD) (Lymphogranulomatosis X)

This is now also classified with the T cell lymphomas (Figures 27.18 and 27.19). However, AILD is considered (by some investigators) to occupy a position, at least initially, somewhere between benign lymphoid proliferation and clonal lymphoid transformation. Studies with monoclonal antibodies have shown a variable

27.15 (left) BMBS plastic, Giemsa, illustrating packed marrow in case of immunoblastic lymphoma; note large central nucleoli in many of the cells.
27.16 (right) BMBS plastic, Giemsa, of patient with mediastinal T cell lymphoma, fairly monomorphic cells with high nucleo-cytoplasmic ratio replacing the bone marrow.

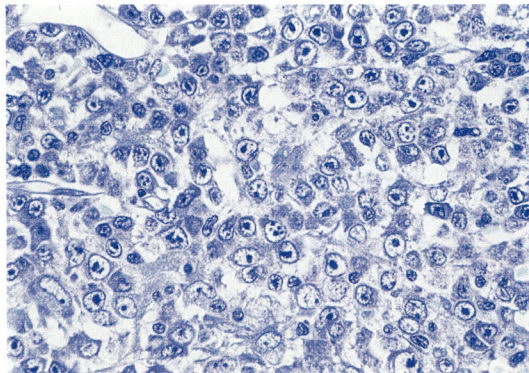

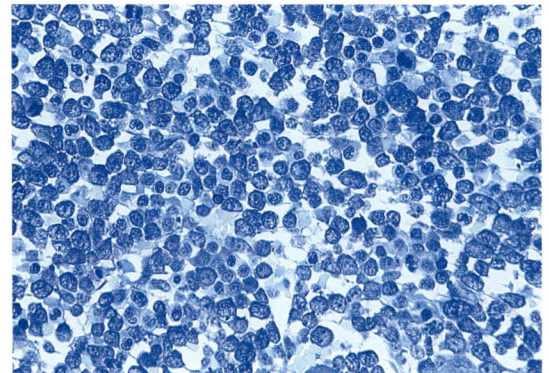

27.17 (left) BMBS plastic, Gomori, high power view of focus of involvement by Lennert's lymphoma (lymphoepithelioid); note lymphocytes and epithelioid cells in network of fibers.
27.18 (right) BMBS plastic, Giemsa, heterogeneous cell population of lymphoctyes and immunoblasts; note vascular proliferation.

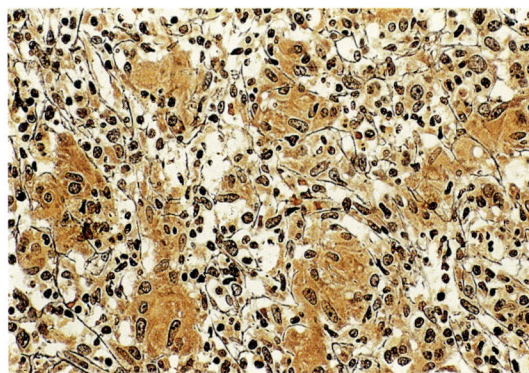

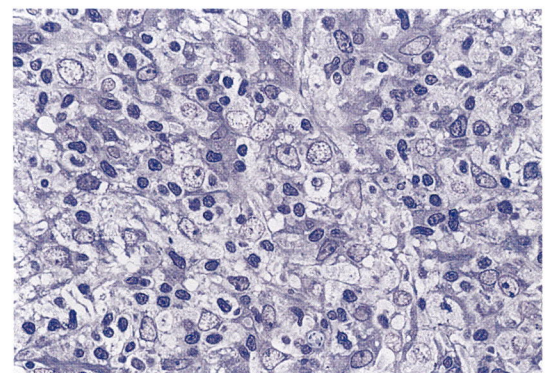

antigenic profile in frozen sections of lymph node biopsies in AILD; but expression of the proliferation-associated antigen recognised by the antibody Ki67 in >25% of lymphoid cells is thought to constitute an unfavorable prognostic marker in AILD. Bone marrow involvement occurs in about half of the cases. There are usually multiple infiltrates consisting of a heterogeneous cell population including immunoblasts, lymphocytes, centrocytes, plasma cells and eosinophils within a reticular framework. Interstitial deposits of PAS-positive material may be pronounced. Marked vascular proliferation may result in arborising capillaries, which form whorl-like arrangements together with reticulin fibers. These infiltrates may resemble those seen in involvement of the bone marrow by HD.

Other T cell lymphomas such as mycosis fungoids and Sezary syndrome, and peripheral T cell lymphomas rarely spread to the bone marrow except in advanced stages of disease. In general, peripheral blood involvement in the lymphomas usually indicates progressive disease. Identification with the appropriate antibodies are required for their recognition.

Mucosa-associated lymphoid tumors (MALT)

These are sometimes called maltomas and may arise in the stomach, thyroid, and parotid glands and lung. They may develop from pre-existing autoimmune (Sjorgen's syndrome) or inflammatory disorders (gastritis due to *Helicobacter pylori*). Such lymphomas usually do not involve the bone marrow, though involvement of peripheral blood and bone marrow has been reported. Moreover, they can progress to more aggressive forms and spread to other tissues. Some may be cured by antibiotic therapy, others by local resection and/or radiotherapy.

Angiotropic lymphoma

Also known as intravascular lymphomatosis. This is a lymphoproliferative disorder, of B or

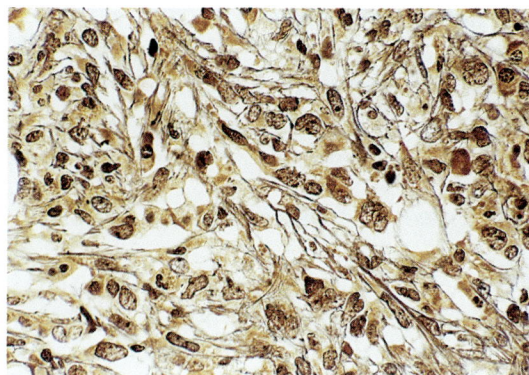

27.19 BMBS plastic, Gomori, showing appearance of an area of involvement by AILD; there is a large component of T cells and a network of reticular fibers and blood vessels.

T cells, characterised by widespread intravascular proliferation, without the presence of focal disease. A similar condition with histiocytic phenotype has also been reported. Intravascular lymphomatosis has been seen in bone marrow blood vessels.

Histologically unclassifiable malignant lymphomas in the bone marrow

In a small percentage of cases the lymphoid infiltrations in the bone marrow cannot be classified without multiparameter enzyme and marker studies, and even these are not always unequivocal.

Additional bone biopsy findings in LPD

Histological discordance, variability, conversion or transformation, concurrent neoplasias, development of other neoplasias have all been documented in the bone marrows of patients with lymphoproliferative disorders. For example, malignant lymphoma centroblastic/centrocytic in the lymph node biopsy and malignant lymphoma immunocytic in the bone marrow; development of Richter's syndrome in CLL, development of a myeloproliferative disorder together with a pre-existing malignant lymphoma, or vice versa.

Complications such as phagocytic histiocytosis may also be found by examination of the bone marrow. Effects of therapy on both the malignant lymphomas in BMB of patients with involvement, as well as on the hematopoietic tissue, may be monitored by bone biopsy. In many cases, though a considerable reduction in amount of lymphomatous infiltration is achieved, some residual foci remain even when the marrow has become severely hypoplastic. Such foci are usually not extracted on aspiration, but are found in BMB

sections. Deletions of p53 have been found in some cases of large cell lymphomas. Foci may also be found in the cortical bone. In the absence of fibrosis, flow cytometry or bone marrow aspirates may be helpful. Some examples are given in Figures 27.21–27.23. The frequency of bone marrow involvement in the malignant lymphomas is given in Table 25.1 (see Chapter 25).

27.20 (left) Partial karyotype of patient with ML showing −2 and +3.

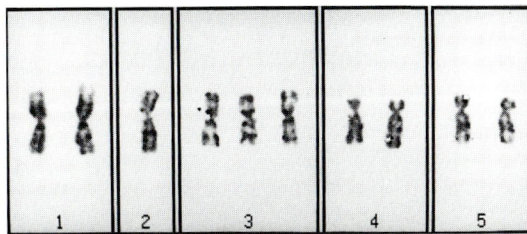

27.21 (right) Histogram of flow cytometry of nucleated cells of bone marrow aspirate, interstitial involvement of the bone marrow by B cell lymphoma. Left to right: red, control; gray, CD5 94%; green, CD2 10%; brown, CD19 91%; blue, CD20 31%; dark green, CD34 1%.

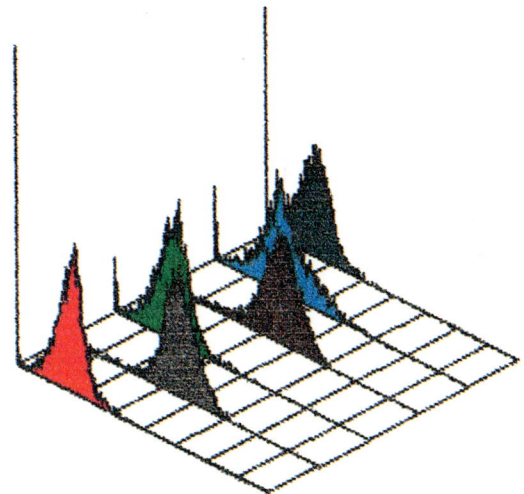

27.22 (left) Histogram of flow cytometry of nucleated cells of bone marrow aspirate. Left to right: red, control; gray, CD7 6%; green, CD3 10%; brown, CD19 56%; blue, CD20 72%; dark green, CD10 1%; gray, CD13 3%; red, CD4 13%; green, CD33 3%; yellow, CD34 0%; case of diffuse, mainly small, cleaved cell lymphoma.

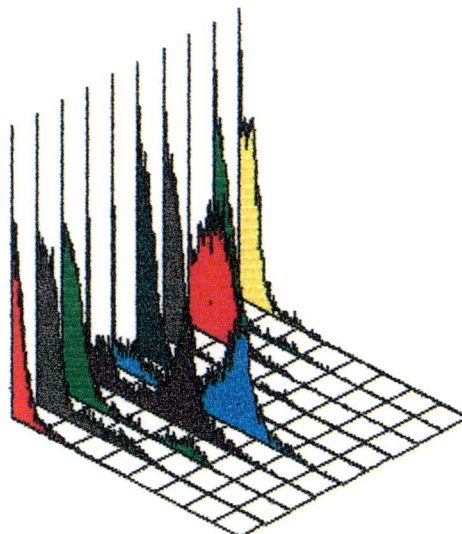

27.23 (right) Histogram of bone marrow aspirate of a 44-year-old patient with large cell lymphoblastic lymphoma. Left to right: red, control; purple, CD3 10%; green, CD19 77%; brown, CD20 53%; blue, CD10 80%; dark green, CD14 4%; gray, CD33 2%; dark blue, CD34 68%.

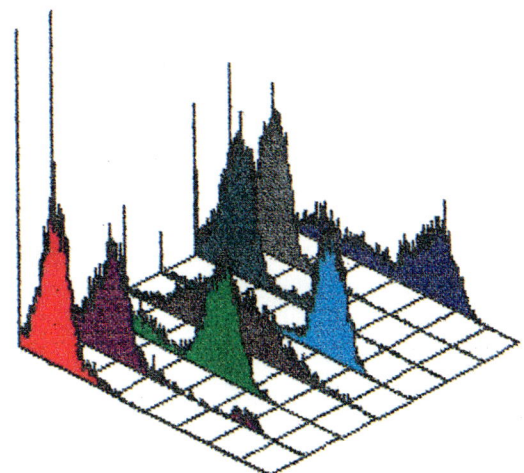

Check List: Malignant Lymphomas

ML Centrocytic – mantle cell lymphoma

- Adequate biopsy: 30 mm excluding cortex.
- State of trabecular bone.
- Paratrabecular infiltrations.
- Extent of infiltrations – trabeculae involved, width of infiltrations.
- Composition of infiltrating cells predominantly small or large cleaved lymphocytes.
- Degree of fibrosis and its location: reticulin stain.
- Quantity of residual hematopoiesis.
- Immunohistology especially in case of a packed marrow, LCA, T and B cells, BCL2, CD79[a], cyclin DI, CD68.

ML Centroblastic/centrocytic

- Adequate biopsy.
- Nodular pattern of involvement.
- Typical endosteal localisation.
- Osseous remodeling of adjacent bone.
- Nodules or follicles with germinal centers. I.H.: LCA, B and T cells, BCL2, cyclin DI, CD68.

- Cellular composition – heterogenous population.
- Quantity of residual hematopoiesis.
- In cases of packed marrow: nodularity effaced.
- Reticulin stain – highlights nodularity.
- Minimal involvement – differential diagnosis ML immunocytoma and benign lymphoid hyperplasia.

AILD (Lymphogranulomatosis)

- Adequate biopsy size.
- Multiple variably large infiltrates.
- Heterogenous cell population in infiltrates.
- Lymphocytes, plasma cells, immunoblasts.
- Vascularisation and fibrosis: reticulin stain.
- Whorl-like patterns of capillaries and fibers.
- PAS in interstitial material.
- Immunohistology – variable results with LCA, B and T cells, kappa and lambda, CD68, Factor VIII and CD34 for endothelium.

Clinical correlations

- History and clinical presentation: varies with type of ML, nodal or extranodal.
- Assessment of systemic symptoms: fever, night sweats, weight loss.
- Physical examination: lymphadenopathy, splenomegaly, pain in involved areas.
- Blood and biochemical profiles: immunoglobulin levels.
- Peripheral blood count – lymphocytosis?

- Staging: imagining of chest, abdomen, skeleton.
- Cytology of cerebrospinal fluid.
- Bone biopsy: for staging.
- Most lymphomas are not curable by presently available treatment modalities.
- Incidence of lymphomas is increasing overall as well as increasing incidence with age.
- Clonal chromosomal characteristics

Continued

Centroblastic/Centrocytic:
t(14;18)(q32;q21)

Mantle zone lymphoma:
t(11;14)(q13;q32)

Centroblastic:
t(14;18)(q32;q21)
t(3;14)(q27;q32)
t(3;22)(q27;q11)

Anaplastic large cell lymphoma:
t(2;5)(p23;q35)

Immunoblastic:
t(14;18)(q32;q21)
del(3)(p)

Burkitt's lymphoma:
t(8;14)(q24;q32)
t(2;8)(p11–p13;q24)
t(8;22)(q24;q11)

Lymphoblastic:
t(9;17)(q34;q23)
t(8;13)(p11;q11–12)

Lennert's lymphoma:
rearrangement of 3q22

Angioimmunoblastic
lymphadenopathy:
+3 (see Figure 27.20)
+5

Additional chromosomal abnormalities

+2	+22
+3	+X
+7	−14
+12	−17
+18	i(17)(q)
+20	−X
+21	−Y

Bibliography

Aisenberg A.C. (1995) Coherent view of non-Hodgkin's lymphoma. *J Clin Oncol.*, **13**, 307–18.

Arber D.A., Sun H.L., Weiss L.M. (1996) Detection of the t(2;5)(p23;q35) chromosomal translocation in large B-cell lymphomas other than anaplastic large cell lymphoma. *Hum Pathol*, **27 (6)**, 590–4.

Bartl R., Frisch B., Burkhardt R. (1985) *Bone Marrow Biopsies Revisited: A New Dimension for Haematologic Malignancies.* Basel: Karger.

Bierman P.J., Armitage J.O. (1996) Non-Hodgkin's lymphoma. *Current Opinion in Hematol*, **3 (4)**, 266–72.

Blayney D.W., Jaffe E.S., Fisher R.I. (1983) The human T-cell lymphoma virus, lymphoma, lytic bone lesions and hypercalcemia. *Ann Intern Med.*, **98**, 144.

Braunstein E.M. (1980) Hodgkin disease of bone: radiographic correlation with histological classification. *Radiology*, **137**, 643.

Braunstein E.M., White S.J. (1980) Non-Hodgkin lymphoma of bone. *Radiology*, **135**, 59.

Breslau N.A., McGuire J.L., Zerwekh J.E. *et al.* (1984) Hypercalcemia associated with increased serum calcitriol levels in three patients with lymphoma. *Ann Intern Med.*, **100**, 1.

Carbone A., Poetti A., Manconi R. *et al.* (1989) Intermediate lymphocytic lymphoma encompassing diffuse and mantle zone pattern variants. A distinct entity among low-grade lymphomas? *Eur J Cancer Clin Oncol*, **25 (1)**, 113–21.

Carbone A., Gloghini A., Volpe R. (1992) Immunohistochemistry of Hodgkin and non-Hodgkin lymphomas with emphasis on the diagnostic significance of the BNH9 antibody reactivity with anaplastic large cell (CD30 poitive) lymphomas. *Cancer*, **70 (11)**, 2691–8.

Carbone A., Gloghini A., Pinto A. *et al.* (1989) Monocytoid B-cell lymphoma with bone marrow and peripheral blood involvement at presentation. *Am. J. Clin. Pathol.*, **94 (1)**, 117–18.

Caulet S., Delmer A., Audouin J. *et al.* (1990) Histopathological study of bone marrow biopsies in 30 cases of T-cell lymphoma with clinical, biological and survival correlations. *Hematol Oncol.*, **8**, 155–68.

Cha I., Herndier B.G., Glassberg A.B., Hamill T.R. (1996) A case of composite Hodgkin's disease and chronic lymphocytic leukemia in bone marrow. Lack of Epstein-Barr virus. *Arch Pathol Lab Med*, **120 (4)**, 386–9.

Chott A., Kaserer K., Augustin I. *et al.* (1990) Ki-1 positive large cell lymphoma.

301

A clinicopathologic study of 41 cases. *Am. J. Surg. Pathol.*, **14 (5)**, 439–48.

Chubachi A., Miura I., Hashimoto K. *et al.* (1993) High incidence of leukemic phase in follicular lymphoma in Akita, Japan: Clinicopathologic, immunological and cytogenetic studies. *Eur. J. Hematol.*, **50 (2)**, 103–9.

Diebold J., Kanavaros P., Audouin J. *et al.* (1987) Centroblastic and centrocytic centroblastic malignant lymphomas, predominantly splenic (or primary of the spleen). Anatomo-clinical study of 17 cases. *Bull. Cancer*, **74 (4)**, 437–53.

Dierlamm J., Michaux L., Wlodarska I. *et al.* (1996) Trisomy 3 in marginal zone B-cell lymphoma: a study based on cytogenetic analysis and fluorescence in situ hybridization. *Br J Haematol*, **93 (1)**, 242–9.

Emile J-F., Boullard M-L., Haioun C. *et al.* (1996) CD5⁻ CD56⁺ T-cell receptor silent peripheral T-cell lymphomas are natural killer cell lymphomas. *Blood*, **87 (4)**, 1466–73.

Ferry J.A., Yang W.I., Zukerberg L.R. *et al.* (1996) CD5+ extranodal marginal zone B-cell (MALT) lymphoma. A low grade neoplasm with a propensity for bone marrow involvement and relapse. *Am J Clin Pathol.*, **105 (1)**, 31–7.

Fisher D.E., Jacobson J.O., Ault K.A., Harris N.L. (1990) Diffuse large cell lymphoma with discordant bone marrow histology. Clinical features and biological implications. *Cancer*, **64 (9)**, 321–35.

Frisch B., Bartl R. (1988) Histologic classification and staging of chronic lymphocytic leukaemia. A retrospective and prospective study of 503 cases. *Acta Haematol.*, **79**, 140.

Gaulard, P., Kanavaros, P., Farcet, J.P. *et al.* (1991) Bone marrow histologic and immunohistochemical findings in peripheral T-cell lymphoma: a study of 38 cases. *Hum. Pathol.*, **22 (4)**, 331–8.

Gautier M.S., Piérard G.E., Andrien F. *et al.* (1993) High-grade pleomorphic T cell lymphoma with restricted involvement of skin and bone marrow. *Dermatology*, **186 (4)**, 287–9.

Griesser H., Kaiser U., Au W. *et al.* (1990) B-cell lymphoma of the mucosa-associated lymphatic tissue (MALT) presenting with bone marrow and peripheral blood involvement. *Leuk Res.*, **14 (7)**, 617–22.

Head D.R., Behm F.G. (1995) Acute lymphoblastic leukemia and the lymphoblastic lymphomas of childhood. *Semin Diagn Pathol.*, **12 (4)**, 325–34.

Huvos A.G. (1991) Skeletal manifestations of malignant lymphomas and leukemias. In A.G. Huvos (ed.),: *Bone Tumors; Diagnosis Treatment and Prognosis*. Philadelphia: W.B. Saunders.

Imamura N., Kusunoki Y., Kawa Ha K. *et al.* (1990) Aggressive natural killer cell leukemia/lyphoma: report of four cases and review of the literature. *Br J Haematol.*, **76 (3)**, 444–8.

Jacobson J.O., Wilkes B.M., Kwiatkwoski D.J. *et al.* (1993) *Bcl*-2 Rearrangements in de novo diffuse large cell lymphoma. *Cancer*, 72, 231–6.

Jaffe E.S. (1996) Classification of natural killer (NK) cell and NK-like T-cell malignancies. *Blood*, **87 (4)**, 1207–10.

Joos S., OtaXo-Joos M.I., Ziegler S. *et al.* (1996) Primary mediastinal (thymic) B-cell lymphoma is characterized by gains of chromosomal material including 9p and amplification of the *REL* gene. *Blood*, **87 (4)**, 1571–8.

Kadin M.E. (1993) Lymphomatoid papulosis and associated lymphomas: how are they related? *Arch. Dermatol.*, **129 (3)**, 351–3.

Kalla J., Ott G., Katzenberger T. *et al.* (1997) Detection of the t(2;5)(p23;q35) in nodal and primary extranodal CD30+ anaplastic large cell lymphomas. *Cytogenet Cell Genet.*, 77, 133.

Kalmanti M., Kalmantis T. (1989) Committed erythroid progenitors and erythropoietin levels in anemic children with lymphomas and ctumors. *Pediatr. Hematol. Oncol.*, **6 (2)**, 85–93.

Kneba M., Eick S., Herbst H. *et al.* (1991) Frequency and structure of t(14; 18) major breakpoint regions in non-Hodgkin's lymphomas typed according to the Kiel classification: analysis by direct DNA sequencing, *Cancer Res.*, **51 (12)**, 3243–50.

Kornblau S.M., Goodacre A., Cabanillas F. (1991) Chromosomal abnormalities in adult non-endemic Burkitt's lymphoma and leukemia: 22 new reports and a review of 148 cases from the literature. *Hematol. Oncol.*, **9 (2)**, 63–78.

Krishnan J., Wallberg K., Frizzera G. (1994) T-cell rich large B-cell lymphoma. A study of 30 cases supporting its histologic heterogeneity and lack of clinical distinctiveness. *Am J Surg Pathol.*, **18**, 455–65.

Kwong Y.l., Wong K.F., Chan L.C. *et al.* (1994) The spectrum of chronic lymphoproliferative disorders in Chinese people. An analysis of 64 cases. *Cancer*, **74 (1)**, 174–81.

Lands R., Karnad A. (1991) Non T-cell lymphoblastic lymphoma with extensive osteolytic lesions and hypercalcemia. *South Med. J.*, **84**, 1405.

Levine E.G., Bloomfield C.D. (1990) Cytogenetics of non-Hodgkin's disease lymphoma. *Monogr. Natl. Cancer Inst.*, **10**, 7–12.

Littlewood T.J., Lydon A.P.M., Barton C.J. (1990) Hypercalcemia and osteolytic lesions associated with chronic lymphatic leukaemia. (CLL). *Br Med J.*, **43**, 877.

Macon W.R., Williams M.E., Greer J.P. *et al.* (1996) Natural killer-like T-cell lymphomas: aggressive lymphomas of T-large granular lymphocytes. *Blood*, **87 (4)**, 1474–83.

Magrini U., Castello A., Boveri E. *et al.* (1991) Histopathology of bone marrow involvement in T-cell lymphomas. *Leukemia*, **5 (1)**, 24–5.

Marti R.M., Estrach T., Reverter J.C. *et al.* (1996) Utility of bone marrow and liver biopsies for staging cutaneous T-cell lymphoma. *Int J Dermatol*, **35 (6)**, 450–4.

Matutes E., Morilla R., Owusu-Ankomah K. *et al.* (1994) The immunophenotype of splenic lymphoma with villous lymphocytes and its relevance to the differential diagnosis with other B-cell disorders. *Blood*, **83 (6)**, 1558–62.

McCluggage W.G., Bharucha H., El-Agnaf M., Toner P.G. (1995) B cell signet-ring lymphoma of bone marrow. *J Clin Pathol*, **48 (3)**, 275–8.

Mead G.M. (1997) ABC of clinical haematology: malignant lymphomas and chronic lymphocytic leukaemia. *BMJ*, **314**, 1103–6.

Merlio J.P., De Mascarel A., Goussot J.F. (1990) Bone marrow involvement in large granular lymphocyte leukemia. *Hum Pathol.*, **21 (4)**, 458–9.

Milla F., Junca J., Flores A. *et al.* (1989) Multilobulated non-Hodgkin lymphoma of B-cell type: leukemization and multiorganic involvement. *Am J Hematol.*, **32 (4)**, 311–13.

Montalbán C., Obeso G., Gallego A. *et al.* (1993) Peripheral T-cell lymphoma: A clinicopathological study of 41 cases and evaluation of the prognostic significance of the updated Kiel classification. *Histopathology*, **22 (4)**, 303–10.

Ohta Y., Shimamura K., Lertprasertsuke N. *et al.* (1989) An autopsy case of so-called midline malignant reticulosis followed by extensive dissemination with immuno-histochemical evidence for its T cell malignancy. *Acta Pathol Jpn*, **39 (7)**, 446–50.

Ortiz-Hidalgo C., Wright D.H. (1992) The morphological spectrum of monocytoid B-cell lymphoma and its relationship to lymphomas of mucosa-associated lymphoid tissue. *Histopathology*, **21 (6)**, 555–61.

Ott G., Kalla J., Ott M.M. *et al.* (1997) Blastoid variants of mantle cell lymphoma: frequent bcl-1 rearrangements at the major translocation cluster region and tetraploid chromosome clones. *Blood*, **89 (4)**, 1421–9.

Parker B.R., Marglin S., Castellino R.A. (1980) Skeletal manifestations of leukemia, Hodgkin disease, and non-Hodgkin lymphoma. *Semin Roentgenol.*, **15**, 302.

Pedrazzoli P., Cazzola M., Stella C.C. *et al.* (1987) Lymphoproliferative disorder of large granular lymphocytes: reversal of lymphocyte proliferation, anemia and meutropenia with chlorambucil. *Tumori*, **73 (2)**, 117–19.

Pistoia V., Roncella S., Di Celle P.F. *et al.* (1991) Emergence of a B-cell lymphoblastic lymphoma in a patient with B CLL: evidence for the single-cell origin of the two tumors. *Blood*, **78 (3)**, 797–804.

Raffeld M., Sander C.A., Yano T., Jaffe E.S. (1992) Mantle cell lymphoma: an update. *Leukemia and Lymphoma*, **8 (3)**, 161–6.

Ribeiro I., Costa M.M., Fernandes B.A. *et al.* (1992) Splenic lymphoma with villous lymphocytes in two sisters. *J. Clin. Pathol.*, **45 (12)**, 1111–13.

Rosenwald A., Ott G., Kalla J. *et al.* (1997) p53 deletion in non-Hodgkin's lymphomas (NHL): detection by fluorescence in situ hybridization (FISH). *Cytogenet Cell Genet.*, **77**, 137.

Rossi J.F., Chappard D., Marcelli C. *et al.* (1990) Micro-osteoclast resorption as a characteristic feature of B-cell malignancies other than multiple myeloma. *Br. J. Hematol.*, **76 (4)**, 469–75.

Salhany K.E., Greer J.P., Cousar J.B., Collins R.D. (1989) Marrow involvement in cutaneous T-cell lymphoma. A clinicopathologic study of 60 cases. *Am J Clin Pathol.*, **94 (1)**, 119–20.

Schlegelberger B., Zwingers T., Hohenadel K. *et al.* (1996) Significance of cytogenetic

findings for the clinical outcome in patients with T-cell lymphoma of angio-immunoblastic lymphadenopathy type. *J Clin Oncol*, **14 (2)**, 593–9.

Shin S.S., Sheibani K. (1993) Monocytoid B-cell lymphoma. *Am. J. Clin. Pathol.*, **99 (4)**, 421–5.

Shiroky J.B., Mewkirk M.M. (1993) Reversible, lymphomas. *New Eng. J. Med.*, **329 (22)**, 1657–8.

Singh N., Wright D.H. (1997) The value of immunohistochemistry on paraffin wax embedded tissue sections in the differentiation of small lymphocytic and mantle cell lymphomas. *J Clin Pathol.*, **50**, 16–21.

Snowden J.A., Angel C.A., Winfield D.A. *et al.* (1997) Angiotropic lymphoma: report of a case with histiocytic features. *J Clin Pathol.*, **50**, 67–70.

Stein R.S., Magee M.J., Lenox R.K. *et al.* (1987) Malignant lymphomas of follicular center cell origin in man. VI. Large cleaved cell lymphoma. *Cancer*, **60 (11)**, 2704–11.

Sun T., Susin M., Brody J. *et al.* (1994) Splenic lymphoma with circulating villous lymphocytes: report of seven cases and review of the literature. *Am. J. Hematol.*, **45 (1)**, 39–50.

Tanaka K., Hagari Y., Sano Y. *et al.* (1990) A case of T-cell lymphoma associated with panniculitis, progressive pancytopenia and hyperbilirubinemia. *Br. J. Dermatol.*, **123 (5)**, 649–52.

Tassies D., Cervantes F., Feliu E. *et al.* (1993) T-cell lymphoblastic lymphoma with blood eosinophilia and associated myeloid malignancy. *Am. J. Surg. Pathol.*, **17 (1)**, 92–3.

Tsujimoto Y., Jaffe E., Cossman J. *et al.* (1985) Clustering of breakpoints on chromosome 11 in human B-cell neoplasms with the t(11;14) chromosome translocation. *Science*, **15**, 340–3.

Wang J.H., Chang T.K., Hsieh Y.I., Hwang B.T. (1989) Non-Hodgkin's lymphoma in childhood: five years survey in VGH-Taipei. *Chung Hua I Hsueh Tsa Chih*, **44 (4)**, 249–55.

Wasman J., Rosenthal N.S., Farhi D.C. (1996) Mantle cell lymphoma. Morphologic findings in bone marrow involvement. *Am J Clin Pathol*, **106 (2)**, 196–200.

Weisenburger D.D., Armitage J.O. (1996) Mantle cell lymphoma – an entity comes of age. *Blood*, **11**, 4483–94.

Weisenburger D.D., Gordon B.G., Vose J.M. *et al*. (1996) Occurrence of the t(2;5)(p23;q35) in non-Hodgkin's lymphoma. *Blood*, **87 (9)**, 3860–8.

White D.M., Smith A.G., Whitehouse J.M., Smith J.L. (1989) Peripheral T-cell lymphoma: value of bone marrow trephine immunophenotyping. *J Clin Pathol*, **42 (4)**, 403–8.

Wong K.F., Chan J.K., Ng C.S. *et al*. (1991) Anaplastic large cell Ki-1 lymphoma involving bone marrow: marrow findings and association with reactive hemo-phagocytosis. *Am J. Hematol.*, **37 (2)**, 112–19.

Ye B.H., Lista F., Lo Coce F. *et al*. (1993) Alterations of a zinc finger-encoding gene, bcl-6, in diffuse large-cell lymphoma. *Science*, **262**, 747–50.

Yuan R., Dowling P., Zucca E. *et al*. (1993) Detection of bcl-2/JH rearrangement in follicular and diffuse lymphoma: Concordant results of peripheral blood and bone marrow analysis at diagnosis. *Br. J. Cancer*, **67 (5)**, 922–5.

28 Hodgkin's disease (HD)

General aspects

The origin or derivation of the typical Hodgkin (H) or Reed–Sternberg (RS) cell still remains controversial, though in some cases immunological phenotyping of H's cells revealed a B cell origin, not necessarily monoclonal. Recent studies have shown that involvement of the bone marrow is low at initial presentation (6%) in patients with stages I and II disease and in nodular sclerosis (1, 2 and 4% respectively). A higher incidence (22%) has been found in patients with lymphocytic depletion type in the lymph node biopsy. However, since one of the criteria for systemic spread (stage IV) is involvement of the bone marrow, a bone marrow biopsy is still an integral part of the initial investigation of patients with HD. Various factors may influence the rate of detection: (1) selection of the patients and therefore unequal proportions in the different lymph node histologies and clinical stages; (2) biopsy techniques, size and histological preparation; and (3) differences in the interpretation of the histological findings (Figure 28.1).

Criteria of involvement

To make the initial diagnosis of HD in the bone marrow, RS cells in an appropriate stromal setting are required. The involved foci (Figures 28.1 and 28.2) may replace part or all of the normal bone marrow in the section. Such foci consist of fibrous tissue with blood vessels (often with prominent endothelial cell nuclei) within which are eosinophils, plasma cells, macrophages, histiocytes and a variable degree of lymphocytic infiltration (Figures 28.3–28.6). Considerable plasmocytosis, and occasionally massive monocytosis (histiocytosis), may be found in the vicinity of and around the foci of HD in the bone marrow. Mononuclear HD, binuclear HD and lacunar cells may also be present. The marrow in the non-involved areas may be normal or hyperplastic with reduction in fat cells. In other cases the normal marrow between the foci may be replaced by a loose connective tissue stroma containing fibers, lymphoid cells, plasma and mast cells, and some hematopoietic precursors. Small, epithelioid cell clusters may also be found. The lesions in involved biopsies range from small paratrabecular foci to large, patchy areas of lymphogranulomatous tissue. However, RS cells are not pathognomonic for HD as RS-like cells may also be found in a variety of large cell lymphomas, or lymphoproliferations with a large cell component, and in plasmablastic myeloma.

When Hodgkin's disease has already been diagnosed elsewhere, mononuclear Hodgkin's cells (Figure 28.7) in an appropriate setting are considered evidence of bone marrow involvement. The differential diagnosis has been considered in Chapter 25.

Subtypes of HD in the bone marrow
(Figure 28.8)

Three criteria are utilised: (1) a high content of lymphocytes (Figure 28.4), (2) a low content of lymphocytes (Figures 28.9 and 29.11) and (3) a high content of epithelioid cells. Bone marrow involvement by definition indicates stage IV. The trabecular bone structure is usually affected when the involved areas are

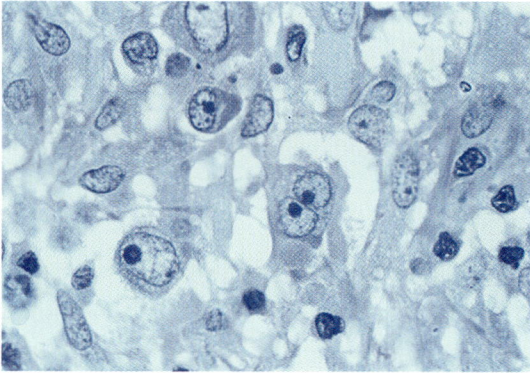

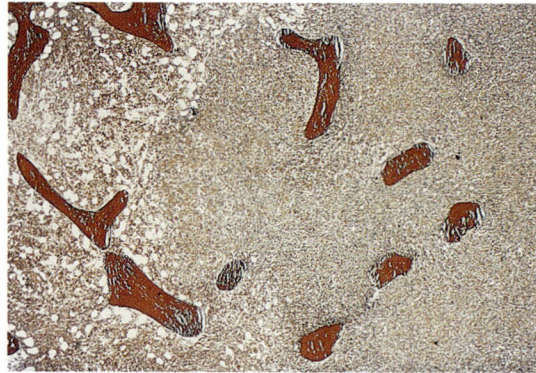

28.1 (left) BMBS plastic, Giemsa, of a patient with Hodgkin's disease; note RS cell, center, in the appropriate environment (partly shown).

28.2 (right) BMBS plastic, Gomori, low power showing area of involvement by HD, right.

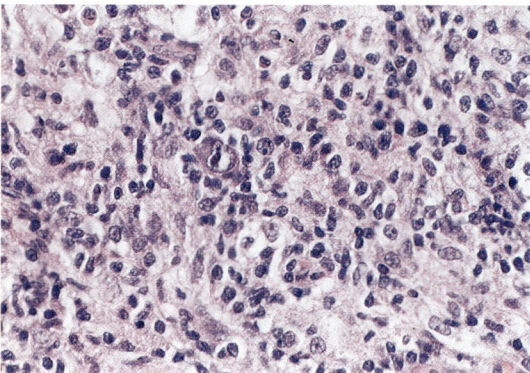

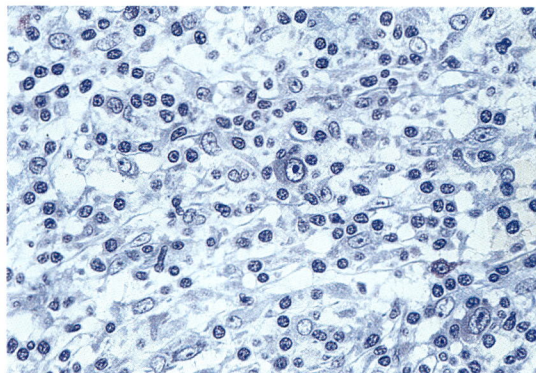

28.3 (left) BMBS paraffin, H&E, showing heterogeneous cell population in focus of HD in the bone marrow.

28.4 (right) BMBS plastic, Giemsa, showing lymphocytic infiltration.

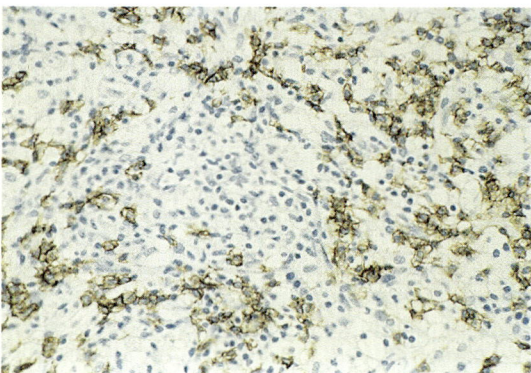

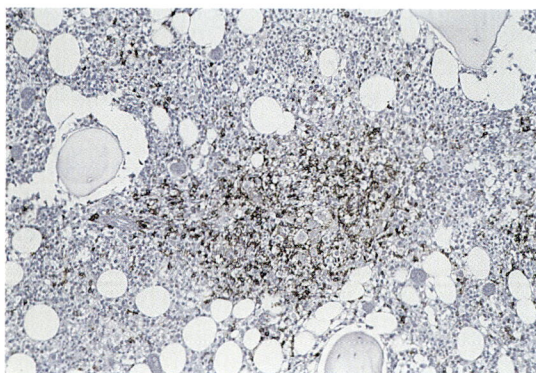

28.5 (left) BMBS paraffin, I.H., with CD68 demonstrating histiocytes and monocytes around the nodule.

28.6 (right) As for Figure 28.5, paraffin, I.H., with T cell antigen showing T cells in nodule.

large: osteosclerosis, osteolysis or osteoporosis, or a combination of these have all been described. Hypercalcemia and elevated 1,25-dihdroxy-vitamin D levels have been found, presumably due to metabolism of vitamin D by the granulomas as in sarcoidosis and tuberculosis.

Epithelioid cell granulomas are foci of fibrous tissue or lymphocytic nodules without the presence of RS or H cells. These may be found in bone marrow biopsy (BMB) patients with HD documented elsewhere, but are not by themselves considered as evidence of bone marrow involvement (Figure 28.10).

Nodular lymphocyte predominance HD of B cell origin (in lymph node histology) has recently been shown to have important phenotypic as well as clinical differences from

28.7 (left) BMBS plastic, Giemsa, showing large mononuclear HD cell in bone marrow in area of involvement.

28.8 (right) Histological types of bone marrow involvement in Hodgkin's disease: (a) high content of lymphocytes, (b) low content of lymphocytes, (c) high content of epithelioid cells.

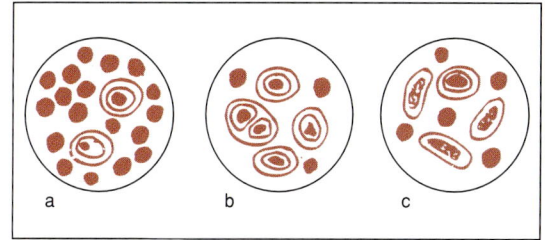

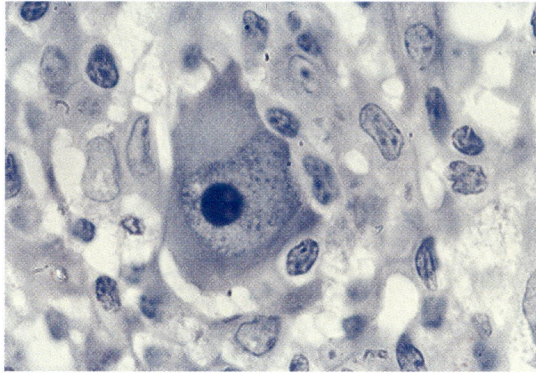

28.9 (left) BMBS plastic, Giemsa, showing bone marrow involvement with a low content of lymphocytes.

28.10 (right) BMBS plastic, Gomori, low power view showing small paratrabecular nodule with lymphocytes and epithelioid cells. Other large, typical foci were also present in this biopsy.

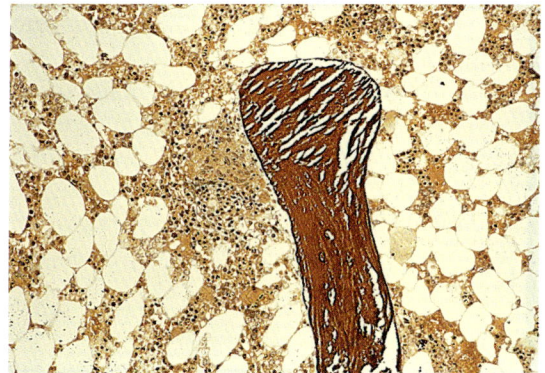

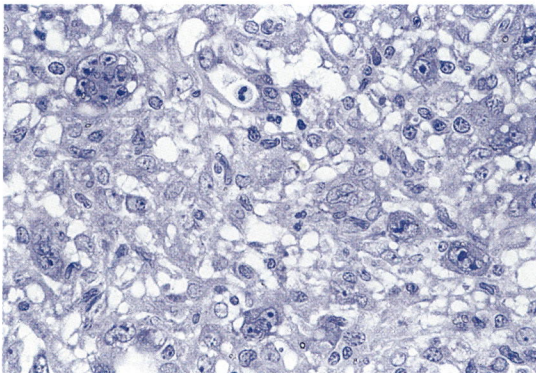

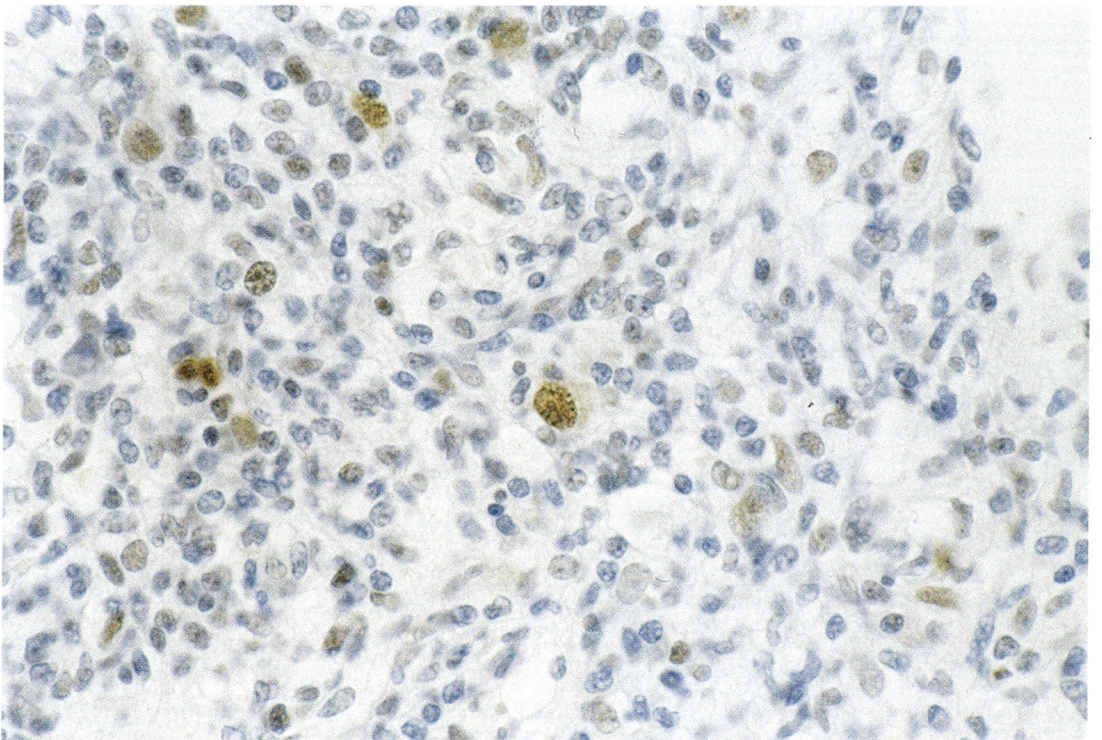

28.11 BMBS paraffin, I.H., p53, positive in HD cell, center, and in a few other cells.

other forms of HD, including the possibility of late relapse, as well as that of the development of a large B cell lymphoma.

Non-involved bone marrow in HD

Bone biopsies of many patients with histologically documented HD elsewhere but without marrow involvement exhibit a variety of reactions. These include lymphoid cell nodules, epithelioid cell granulomas, increased phagocytic macrophages, focal accumulations of fibrous tissue and leukemoid reactions. Alternatively, the biopsy may show infiltrations of lymphoid, plasma and mast cells and maturation inhibition of hematopoietic precursors. Areas of replacement of hematopoiesis by fat cells, or serous atrophy, may also be present and be quite extensive. If a long core is examined, different manifestations may be found in one biopsy. Macrophages packed with cellular debris may be pronounced, especially in hyperplastic bone marrows.

- Hypercellular marrow with megakaryocytic and granulocytic hyperplasia: reactive picture.
- In case of fibrosis: stepwise serial sections to detect specific cells, HD or RS cells, or both, which are CD15- and CD30-positive on I.H. as well as showing the characteristic morphologic features.

Check list: Hodgkin's Disease

- Adequate biopsy: 30 mm without periosteum and cortex.
- For initial Diagnosis: RS cells in appropriate environment.
- For involvement if diagnosed elsewhere – mononuclear HD (or RS, or both) in appropriate environment.
- Immunohistology (I.H.): CD15, CD30; CD68 as well as LCA, T and B cells to characterise environment. PAS and reticulin stains.
- In absence of RS or HD cells, definite involvement cannot be diagnosed.
- Differential diagnosis especially large cell anaplastic ML. EMA: positive in ALCL, negative in HD.
- Small granulomas alone are not indicative of involvement.

Clinical correlations

- Variable clinical manifestations: cervical, mediastinal, para-aortic, lymphadenopathy.
- Possibly fever, weight loss, sweats – B symptoms.
- CT for internal lymphadopathies.
- Bone scan and bone biopsy for staging.
- Nodular-sclerosis (NS) type of HD constitutes 70–80% of cases.
- NS mostly in young women with mediastinal and cervical disease.
- Mixed cellularity HD mainly in older men.
- Lymphocyte depletion HD is rare.
- HD has a good prognosis: 70–80% cure in young patients.
- Clonal chromosomal characteristics

  +3
  +7
  +18
  +21
  +22

  Structural changes:

1q	7q
1p	8q
3p	11q
3q	12p
4q	14q
6q	15q

Bibliography

Anastasi J., Bitter M.A., Vardiman J.W. (1989) The histopathologic diagnosis and subclassification of Hodgkin's disease. *Hematol. Oncol. Clin. North Am.*, **3** (2), 187–204.

Bartl R., Frisch B., Burkhardt R. *et al.* (1982) Assessment of bone marrow histology in Hodgkin's disease: correlation with clinical factors. *Br J Haematol*, **51**, 345–60.

Bergter W., Fetzer I-C., Sattler B., Ramadori G. (1996) Granulomatous hepatitis preceding Hodgkin's disease. *Pathol Oncol Res.*, **2** (3), 177–80.

Carbone A., Gloghini A., Volpe R. (1992) Immunohistochemistry of Hodgkin and non-Hodgkin lymphomas with emphasis on the diagnostic significance of the BNH9 antibody reactivity with anaplastic large cell (CD30 positive) lymphomas. *Cancer*, **70** (11), 2691–8.

Cowie F., Benghiat A., Holgate C. (1991) Primary Hodgkin's disease of bone. *Clin Oncol.*, **3**, 233.

Deerberg-Wittram J., Weber-Matthiesen K., Schlegelberger B. (1996) Cytogenetics and molecular cytogenetics in Hodgkin's disease. *Ann Oncol*, **7** (4), 49–53.

DeVita V.T., Hubbard S.M. (1993) Hodgkin's disease. *N Engl J Med.*, **328**, 560–5.

Di Benedetto G., Cataldi A., Verde A. *et al.* (1989) Gamma heavy chain disease associated with Hodgkin's disease. Clinical, pathologic, and immunologic features of one case. *Cancer*, **63** (9), 1804–9.

Ellis M.E., Diehl L.F., Granger E., Elson E. (1989) Trephine needle bone marrow biopsy in the initial staging of Hodgkin's disease: sensitivity and specificity of the Ann Arbor staging procedure criteria. *Am J Hematol.*, **30** (3), 115–20.

Guckel F., Semmler W., Brix G. *et al.* (1989) Bone marrow changes in Hodgkin's disease: MR tomo and chemical shift imaging. *ROFO Fortschr. Geb. Rontgenstr. Nuklearmed.*, **150** (6), 670–3.

Heitger A., Gadner H., Bucksy P. *et al.* (1989) Large cell anaplastic lymphoma in children – clinical experience with a newly defined histologic entity. *Klin Padiatr.*, **201** (4), 237–41.

Johnston P.G., Ruscetti F.W., Connaghan D.G. *et al.* (1991) Transient reversal of bone marrow aplasia associated with lymphocyte depleted Hodgkin's disease after combination chemotherapy. *Am. J. Hematol.*, **38** (1), 54–60.

Juliusson G., Hast R., Ljungman P. *et al.* (1991) Simultaneously presenting aplastic anemia and Hodgkin's disease successfully treated with allogeneic bone marrow transplantation. *Eur. J. Hematol.*, **46** (5), 314–6.

Macavei I., Galatar N. (1990) Bone marrow biopsy (BMB). III. Bone marrow biopsy in Hodgkin's disease (HD). *Morphol. Embryol.*, **36** (1), 25–32.

MacIntyre E.A., Vaughan-Hudson B., Linch D.C. *et al.* (1987) The value of staging bone marrow trephine biopsy in Hodgkin's disease. *Eur. J. Hematol.*, **39** (1), 66–70.

Meadows L.M., Rosse W.R., Moore J.O. *et al.* (1989) Hodgkin's disease presenting as myelofibrosis. *Cancer*, **64** (8), 1720–6.

Moormeier J.A., Williams S.F. Golomb H.M. (1989) The staging of Hodgkin's disease. *Hematol Oncol Clin North Am.*, **3** (2), 237–51.

Munker R., Hasenclever D., Brosteanu O. *et al.* for the German Hodgkin's lymphoma study group. (1995) Bone marrow involvement in Hodgkin's disease. An analysis of 135 consecutive cases. *J Clin Oncol.*, **13**, 403–9.

Nakamine H., Okamoto Y., Tsuda T. *et al.* (1987) Hodgkin's disease in hairy cell leukemia. Phenotypic characterization of neoplastic cells. *Cancer*, **60** (8), 1751–6.

Schicha H., Franke M., Smolorz J. *et al.* (1989) Diagnostic strategies and staging procedures for Hodgkin's lymphoma: bone marrow scintigraphy and magnetic resonance imaging. *Recent Results Cancer Res.*, **111**, 112–19.

Thangavelu M., Le Beau M.M. (1989) Chromosomal abnormalities in Hodgkin's disease. *Hematol. Oncol. Clin. North Am.*, **3** (2), 221–36.

Wolf J., Kapp U., Bohlen H. *et al.* (1996) Peripheral blood mononuclear cells of a patient with advanced Hodgkin's lymphoma give rise to permanently growing Hodgkin-Reed Sternberg cells. *Blood*, **87** (8), 3418–28.

Yuen A.R., Horning S.J. (1996) Recent advances in Hodgkin's disease. *Current Opinion in Hematol*, **3** (4), 273–8.

29 Multiple myeloma (MM) and related disorders

Pathogenesis

The pathogenesis of multiple myeloma (MM) is not known, though prolonged antigenic stimulation has been postulated. The malignant stem cell in MM has not been conclusively identified though early B lymphocytes, developing through a CD10- and CD11b-positive stage into CD138-positive myeloma cells, have been implicated. Identification of early stages, B lymphocytes, which belong to the malignant clone, is of practical significance, as these may not be eliminated before BMT or PBSCT and therefore may be reinfused into the patient, in contrast with plasma cells which are CD138+ and CD34−. A cascade of interactions between pre-myeloma cells and endothelial cells, stromal cells and extracellular matrix regulates their adhesion and maturation to plasma cells. MM is a monoclonal B cell neoplasm of terminally differentiated B cells – plasma cells, and is primarily a bone marrow disorder, and the bone marrow microenvironment, in turn controlled by and producing a battery of cytokines, including IL-6, determines the growth and manifestations of MM in the bone marrow. IL-6 in particular is important in myeloma cell growth and the accompanying skeletal disease.

Primary site and spread

Most bone marrow myelomas are systemic when first diagnosed; rarely, solitary plasmacytomas in the bone marrow may be cured by local excision, though a biopsy from another site is required to rule out an early stage of systemic MM. Extramedullary plasmacytomas are more likely to be solitary. At initial diagnosis,

only a few patients have no involvement in the iliac crest biopsy. The majority, >90%, show widespread dissemination from the start – myelomatosis. In this context, it has been shown that adhesion molecules, e.g. CD44, CD56, CD58, VLA4, VLA5, MPC1, RHAMM and syndecan 1, play a pathogenic role in MM: homing, growth and survival of the malignant cells in the bone marrow; development of hematogenous spread and seeding of extramedullary MM, are all regulated by adhesion molecules. Demonstration of these molecules will play an increasingly important part in diagnosis and in evaluation of prognosis, as well as in providing targets for new treatment strategies in MM.

Diagnostic criteria of MM

Clinical, laboratory and radiologic findings are always considered together with the bone marrow morphology. Traditionally, diagnosis of MM requires at least two of the following criteria: (1) >10% atypical plasma cells in smears and/or biopsies, (2) a serum and/or urinary monoclonal protein and (3) osteolytic bone lesions. The majority of cases may be diagnosed on morphology alone (Figures 29.1 and 29.2) – the few equivocal cases can be elucidated by checking for monoclonality utilising kappa and lambda light chains (Figures 29.3–29.8). This can be done on sections as well as on smears and imprints.

Clinically there are five aspects of MM:

1. Growth and expansion leading to destruction of bone.

2. Consequences of paraprotein in blood and/or urine.

29.1 (left) BMBS plastic, Giemsa, illustrating cytologic features of the malignant plasma cells, polymorphism of the cells, and nuclei, nucleoli and variability in cytoplasmic staining.

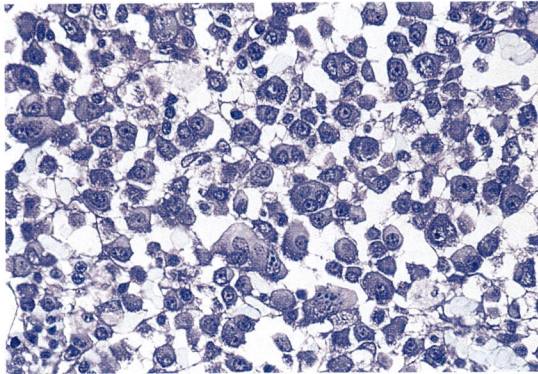

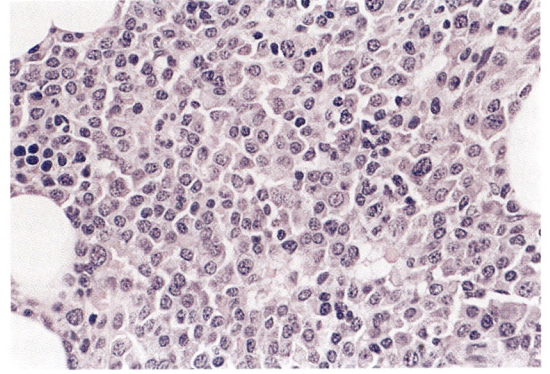

29.2 (right) BMBS paraffin, H&E, showing extensive infiltration of myeloma in the bone marrow.

29.3 (left) As for Figure 29.2, BMBS paraffin, I.H., for kappa light chains; most of the plasma cells are positive.

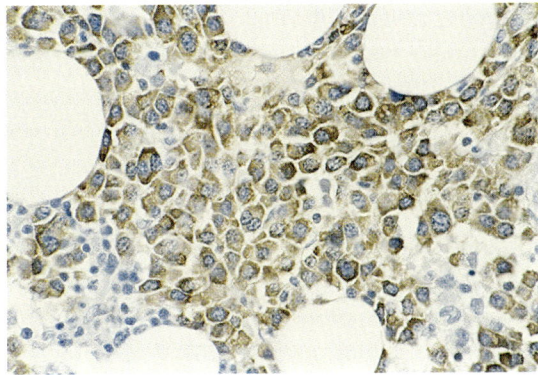

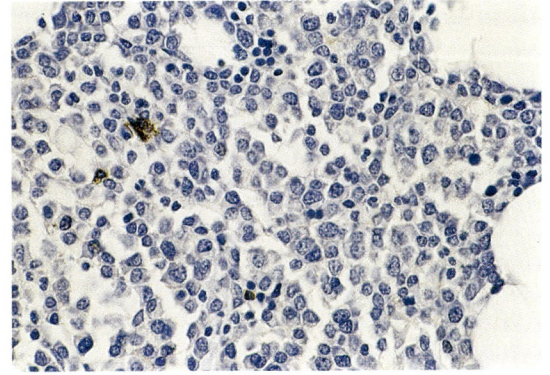

29.4 (right) As for Figure 29.2, I.H., reaction for lambda, most of the myeloma cells are negative.

29.5–29.8 Case of MM, aggressive type.

29.5 (left) BMBS, plastic, Giemsa, massive infiltration by polymorphic plasma cells.

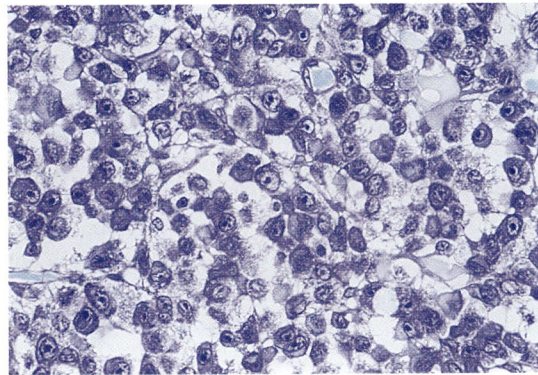

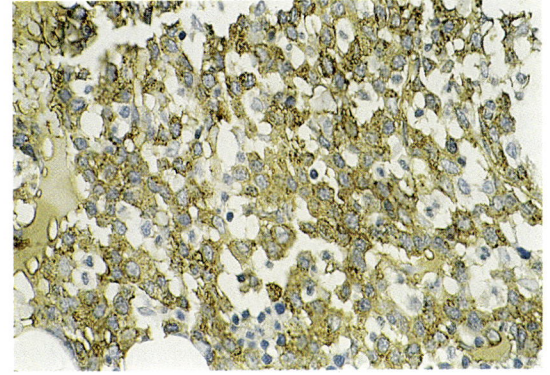

29.6 (right) BMBS, paraffin, I.H., lambda, all the plasma cells are stained, reaction for kappa was negative.

29.7 (left) BMBS, paraffin, I.H., BCL2, positive in almost all the plasma cells.

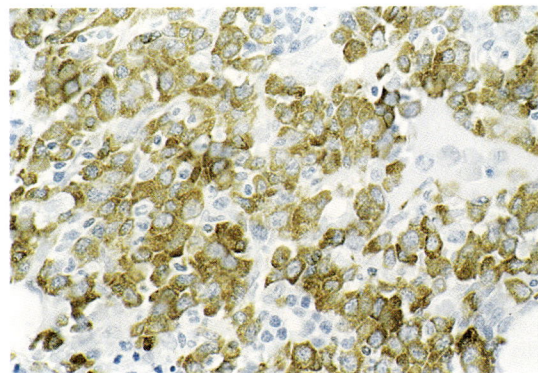

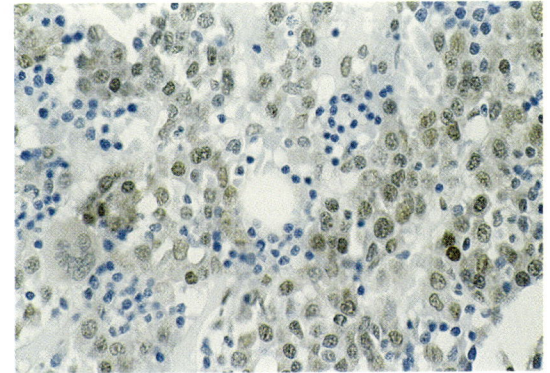

29.8 (right) BMBS, paraffin, I.H., p53, positive in the plasma cells.

3. Hypogammaglobulinemia leading to immune deficiency.

4. Marrow replacement leading to marrow failure.

5. Renal impairment, usually multifactorial.

A marked increase in plasma proteins may lead to a hyperviscosity syndrome, which may present insiduously or acutely, with symptoms and signs such as headache, neurological disturbance, visual disturbances, genitourinary and gastrointestinal bleeding.

Quantity of plasma cells

In most centers the diagnosis of MM is still based on percentages of plasma cells in an aspirated marrow sample, ranging from 5–10 to 30% of the nucleated cell population, though equal or higher numbers of plasma cells may be present in other non-neoplastic conditions: reactive plasmacytosis is common in association with chronic inflammatory and infectious conditions, hepatic cirrhosis, Hodgkin's disease, especially after therapy and diabetes mellitus. Moreover, patients with MGUS (monoclonal gammopathy of unspecified significance) may also have a bone marrow plasmacytosis in the 5–10% range.

Occasionally, discrepancies may occur between numbers of plasma cells in aspirate smears and biopsy sections. This is due to fibrosis or nodular bone marrow infiltrations preventing aspiration of the plasma cells and thereby giving low numbers in the smears. Conversely, aspirates of patients with reactive plasmacytosis and/or MGUS may contain >30% plasma cells, and in many of these cases the biopsy sections reveal a hypocellular bone marrow. In addition, because of the inhibition of hematopoiesis in some cases, the bone marrow may be hypocellular, containing mainly fat cells, which further invalidates percentages of plasma cells as a criterion of MM.

Plasma cell labeling index (PCLI)

As MM is a slowly growing tumor only about 1–2% of plasma cells are in the S phase of the cell cycle, as shown by the PCLI, which is useful for distinguishing MM from MGUS. Ki67, a nuclear antigen of proliferating cells, as well as other antibodies and flow cytometry, may also be applied for this purpose. Classical cytogenetic studies in MM have been limited because of this low proliferative activity. Nevertheless abnormalities involving chromosomes 11 or 13 have been considered as unfavorable prognostic factors. However, more recent data derived from flow cytometry and FISH analyses indicate the presence of chromosomal aberrations in 80–90% of patients, implying that the normal karyotypes of previous studies were those of hematopoietic and not myeloma cells.

Qualitative abnormalities of plasma cells

These may be as important as the quantity of plasma cells. Though there are no characteristics pathognomonic for MM, many are suggestive: variations in cell size and nuclear size and shape, multinuclearity and hypersegmentation, presence of Dutcher bodies in the nucleus, Russell and other inclusion bodies (Figure 29.9), grape cells, Mott cells, flaming cells, tadpole-like cells, thesaurocytes, and cytoplasmic heterogeneity in staining quality and enzyme reactions (Figure 29.10). Conversely plasmacytic satellitosis (histiocyte surrounded by plasma cells) and increased eosinophils, mast cells and megakaryocytes are typical of reactive plasmacytosis.

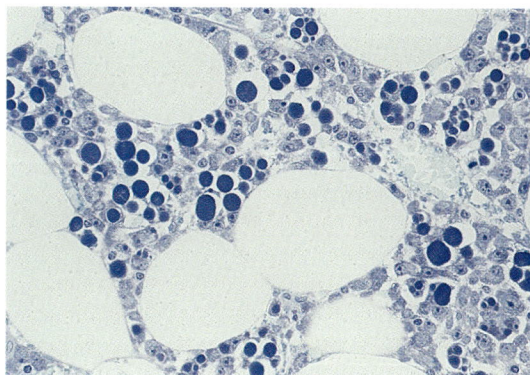

29.9 BMBS plastic, Giemsa, plasma cells with Russell bodies in MM.

Nuclear-cytoplasmic asynchrony

Instead of the typical spoke-wheel pattern seen in normal and reactive plasmacytoses, the nuclear chromatin in MM is often finely dispersed like that of a blast, and contains a large, sharply demarcated nucleolus. The shape of the nuclei in MM is often variable: notched, cleaved, multilobulated, convoluted or cerebriform, sometimes with multiple nucleoli or inclusion bodies (Figures 29.11 and 29.12). At the ultrastructural level, three types of nuclear inclusions have been described:

1. Cytoplasmic invagination into the nucleus.

2. Invagination of the inner nuclear membrane.

3. Nuclear blobs.

No differences were found in plasma cell morphology when the patients were grouped according to the type of M-component. Histochemically, there are considerable variations in reactivity between plasma cells and between MM, MGUS and reactive plasmacytosis. Therefore, these reactions cannot be used as discriminants.

In summary, the presence of three cytologic features enables a morphologic diagnosis of MM regardless of a low number of plasma cells (<5%) in aspirate smears: (1) nuclear-cytoplasmic asynchrony with large nucleoli, (2) irregularities of nuclear configuration and (3) variations in cell size and cytoplasmic staining.

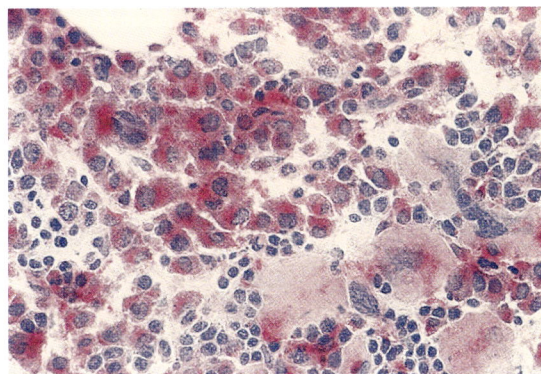

Histotopography of plasma cells

This is also useful in distinguishing reactive from neoplastic plasmacytosis (Figures 29.13–29.16). In the former, many typical reticular plasma cells are located around the small blood vessels. In the latter there is in addition a random interstitial infiltration among fat and hematopoietic cells initially and subsequently

29.10 BMBS cryostat section, reaction for acid phosphatase, the myeloma cells show a positive (red) reaction product.

29.11 (left) BMBS, EM, neoplastic plasma cell showing deep invagination of cytoplasm containing endoplasmic reticulum in the nucleus.

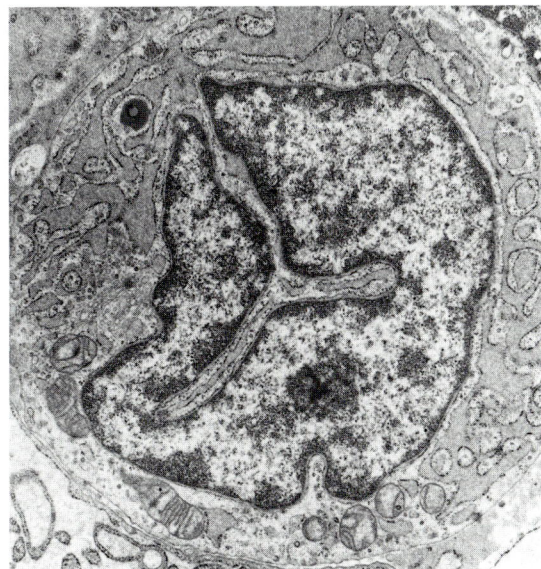

29.12 (right) BMBS, EM, myeloma cell showing loose chromatin pattern with prominent nucleolus. The cytoplasm contains numerous mitochondria as well as large amounts of endoplasmic reticulum.

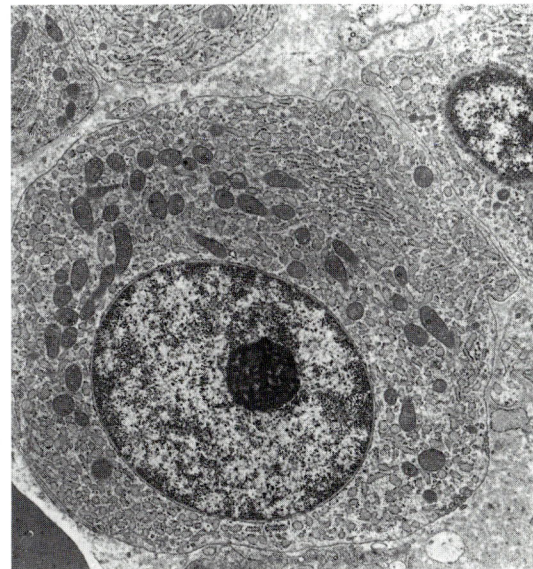

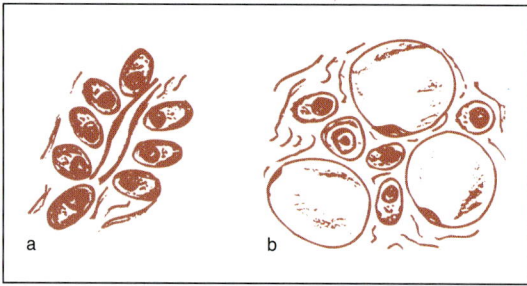

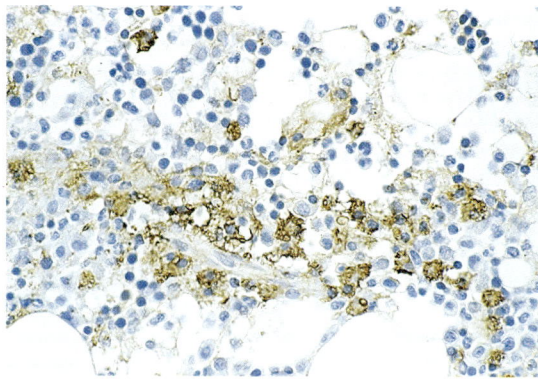

29.13 (left) Topographic significance of reactive (a) and neoplastic plasmacytosis (b) as well as the cytological differences between the two groups of plasma cells.

29.14 (right) BMBS paraffin, I.H., kappa, reactive especially perivascular plasmacytosis. Another section of same biopsy incubated for lambda also showed positive plasma cells.

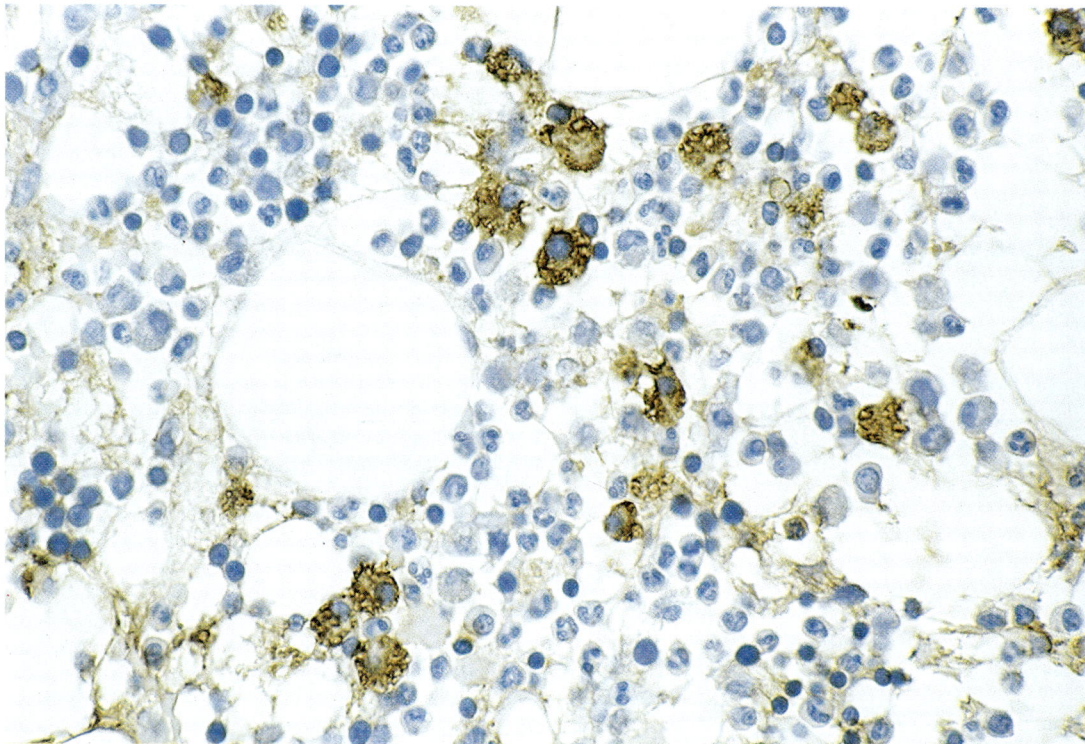

29.15 BMBS paraffin, I.H., lambda, interstitial plasma cells in case of smoldering MM with lambda light chain restriction.

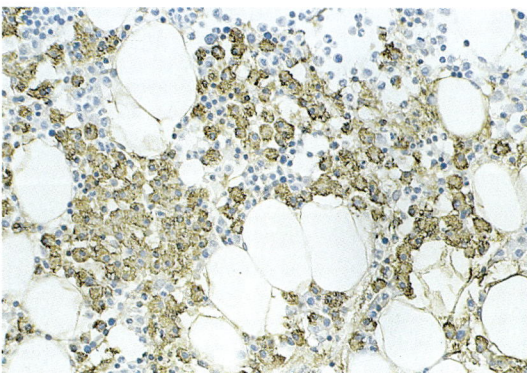

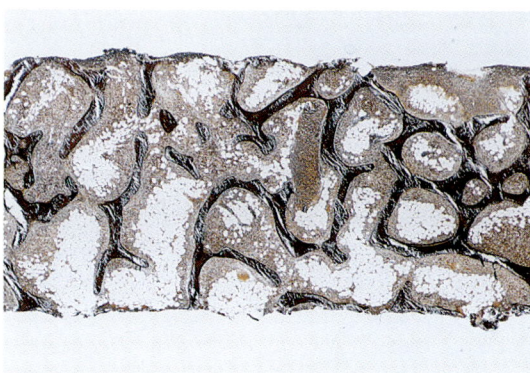

29.16 (left) BMBS paraffin, I.H., kappa, partial replacement of bone marrow by monoclonal plasma cells.

29.17 (right) BMBS plastic, Gomori, low power showing unusual case of paratrabecular MM with hypocellular fatty marrow.

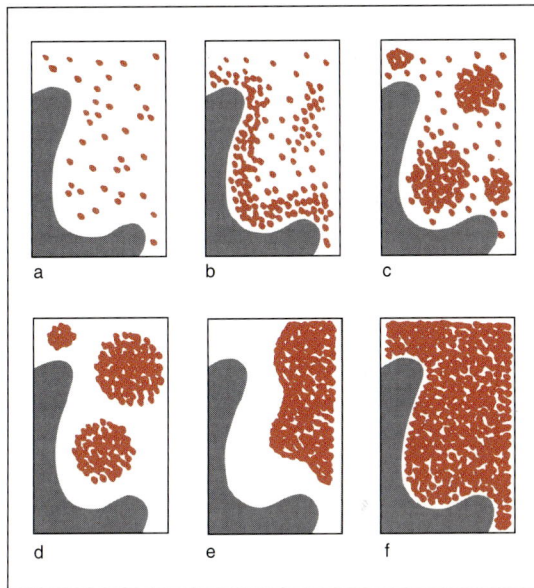

29.18 Growth patterns in MM: (a) interstitial, (b) interstitial/sheets, (c) interstitial/nodular, (d) nodular, (e) sarcomatous, (f) packed marrow.

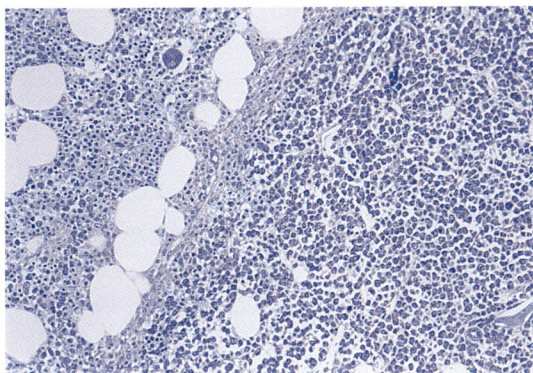

29.19 BMBS plastic, Giemsa, showing edge of myeloma nodule, in a case of mainly nodular MM, separated by layer of fat cells from hematopoietic tissue, left.

29.20 Expansion and interactions of MM in bone marrow: myeloma stem cells proliferate and circulate in the blood. On return to the bone marrow the premyeloma cells attach to the cytokine-rich stroma and differentiate to plasma cells. Complex interactions between myeloma and stromal cells induce a range of cytokines (e.g. IL-6), which determine tumor growth as well as osseous and hematopoietic reactions (OAF, osteoclast-activating factors; OIF, osteoblast-inhibiting factor; HDF, hematopoietic-depressing factor).

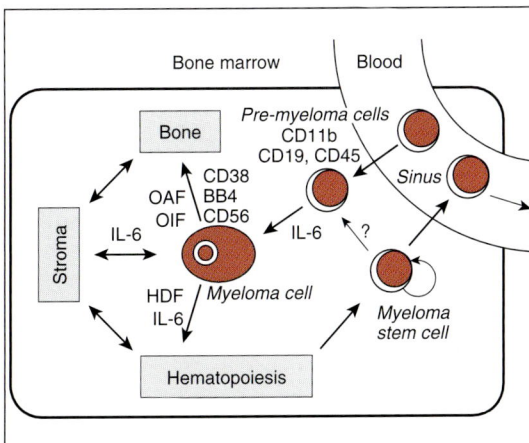

denser aggregates of myeloma cells accumulate along endosteal surfaces and around ectatic sinusoids and arteries, eventually forming nodules or sheets which replace the hematopoietic and fat tissues (Figure 29.17). Six architectural patterns have been observed in the biopsy sections (Figure 29.18). An exclusively nodular infiltration was rare (Figure 29.19): it characterises the multifocal variant of MM, which may be the cause for a negative aspirate/biopsy at initial presentation. Magnetic resonance imaging (MRI) can be used to show the type and extent of bone marrow infiltration in MM.

Hematopoiesis, stroma and bone in MM

Myeloma cells produce a variety of cytokines that influence hematopoiesis, stroma and bone (Figure 29.20).

Hematopoiesis

Failure of hematopoiesis in myeloma patients is due to replacement by the plasma cell infiltration as well as to severe marrow atrophy (Figure 29.17), hypothetically caused by hematopoiesis-inhibiting factors produced by the myeloma cells (HIF, IL-6). Myelodysplasia may lead to ineffective hematopoiesis and thus also contribute to the peripheral cytopenia. Reduction of the plasma cell mass under chemotherapy is usually also followed by a decrease in the amount of the fatty tissue and regeneration of hematopoiesis.

Bone marrow stroma

This is a complex system of cellular and extracellular (matrix) elements that regulate the growth and differentiation of hematopoietic cell lines in the bone marrow. Under the influence of myeloma cells the stromal cells produce large quantities of adhesion and extracellular matrix molecules which together with the cytokines influence the rate and type of tumor growth in MM, as well as the blood vessels, fibroblasts and fibbers. Development of coarse fibrosis (collagen type III) accompanied by an inflammatory reaction proved to be unfavorable prognostic signs (Figure 29.21).

Bone

Skeletal destruction is characteristic of MM (Figures 29.20 and 29.22) and causes many of its complications, such as bone pain, pathologic fractures, hypercalcemia and renal damage. Generalised osteoporosis with or without lytic lesions is seen in 60% of patients at diagnosis. Patients with interstitial and packed marrow patterns usually had generalised osteoporosis. The presence of nodules usually correlated with osteolytic lesions. Osteoclast-activating factors (OAFs) appear to act locally mainly in close proximity to accumulations of myeloma cells (Figure 29.22); hence the clinical efficacy of primarily antiosteoclastic agents such as the bisphosphonates. Moreover there is a direct relationship between skeletal destruction, plasma cell burden and amount of OAF produced (Figures 29.20 and 29.23). In addition, osteoblasts are inhibited, further upsetting the balance ('coupling') between bone resorption and bone formation; moreover therapy of MM with prednisone further decreases bone formation, stimulates resorption and so augments osteoporosis.

Bisphosphonate therapy reduces osteoclastic resorption and stimulates osteoblastic repair (Figures 29.24 and 29.25). Once monthly injections are effective, given indefinitely or as long as there is evidence of disease.

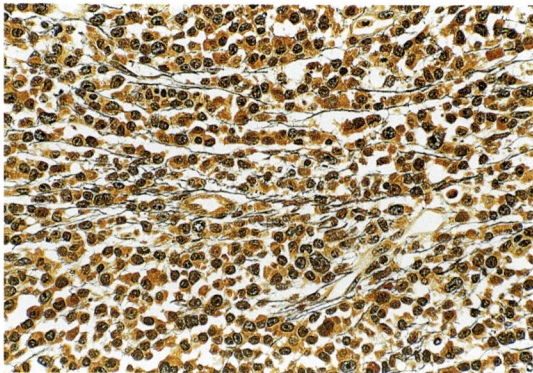

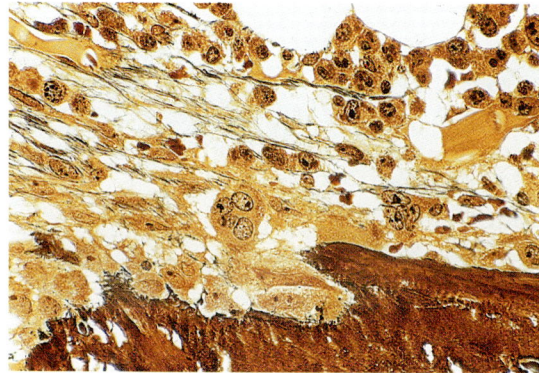

29.21 (left) BMBS plastic, Gomori, illustrating fibers in MM.

29.22 (right) BMBS plastic, Gomori, osteoclastic bone resorption near myeloma cells.

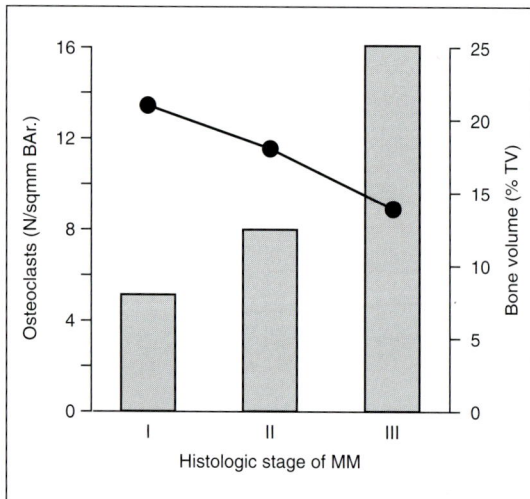

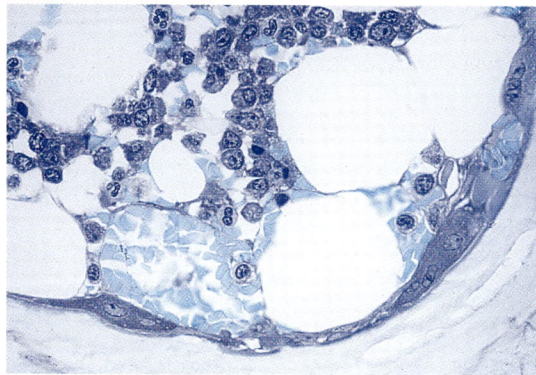

29.23 (left) Correlation of histological stage of MM with osteoclastic resorption. Stages I: <20 vol% plasma cells in the biopsy; II, 20–50 vol%; III, >50 vol%. Osteoclasts, ●.

29.24 (right) BMBS plastic, Giemsa, MM 14 days after therapy with bisphosphonates; note flat osteoclasts and only very shallow surface erosion.

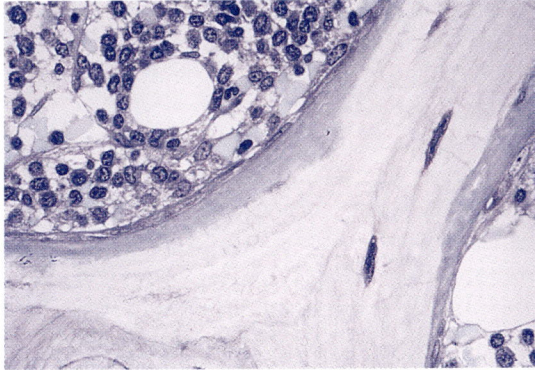

29.25 BMBS plastic, Giemsa, MM 2 months after therapy with bisphosphonates, note osteoid seam, repair of trabecula and no osteoclastic activity.

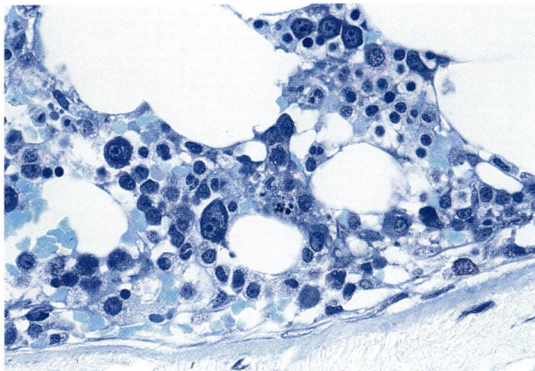

29.26 BMBS plastic, Giemsa, example of smoldering MM with minimal plasma cell infiltration but distinctly atypical plasma cells.

MM variants

Smoldering MM (SMM) (Indolent MM) (Figure 29.26)

The diagnosis of SMM depends on: presence of M protein of >3 g/dl in serum, >10% atypical plasma cells in the bone marrow and the absence of anemia, renal insufficiency and skeletal lesions. The bone marrow showed the following characteristics: (1) minimal plasma cell infiltration <5% in biopsy sections, (2) interstitial growth pattern, (3) mainly typical reticular plasma cells and (4) low <1.5 PCLI.

Plasma cell leukemia

This diagnosis requires that atypical plasma cells comprise 20% of the differential count of the peripheral blood. The patients frequently have hepatosplenomegaly, a progressive course and poor response to therapy. Biopsy sections show a packed marrow pattern with a marked infiltration of small and/or cleaved plasma

cells within the sinusoids. Sometimes these cells are lymphoplasmacytoid or even lymphoblastoid in appearance.

Non-secretory MM

These patients have no M-protein in the serum or the urine – their plasma cells either do not produce (non-producers) or do not secrete (non-secretory) monoclonal immunoglobulins or their light chains; although with the most sophisticated methodology minimal amounts of M protein may be detected in some cases. There are no characteristic cytologic features or histologic growth patterns and since most patients are in an advanced stage when first investigated, they are readily diagnosed by conventional morphology in bone biopsies, since there is usually extensive involvement.

Osteosclerotic MM

Of patients with MM, 1–2% have osteosclerotic bone lesions, possibly associated with the POEMS syndrome (polyneuropathy, organomegaly, endocrinopathy, monoclonal gammopathy and skin changes), in which high levels of circulating IL-6 and TNFa have been reported, and these possibly contribute to this paraneoplastic syndrome. In this variant there is unbalanced activation of osteoblasts but no special features of the myeloma cells have been reported. In rare cases such as MM with thrombocytosis, the osteomyelosclerosis may be the result of a concomitant myeloproliferative disorder. Osteosclerosis may also occur after chemo- and radiotherapy or administration of bisphosphonates.

'Myelofibrotic' MM

These are characterised by osteosclerosis, marrow fibrosis and focal megakaryocytic hyperplasia without the atypia characteristic of the cMPD. These cases must also be distinguished from Castleman's disease. However, such distinctions are not widely accepted, and their clinical usefulness has yet to be established.

Morphologic classification of MM

Many previous studies have stressed the relationship between plasma cell morphology and prognosis of MM, several morphologic classifications have recently been proposed; and prognostic cytologic features sought. The following were found to be associated with an unfavorable outcome:

1. *Plasma cell type* (Figure 29.28 and 29.32): (a) nucleolated, (b) cleaved nuclei, (c) large nuclei, (d) mitotic figures in plasma cells, (e) high PCLI.

2. *Plasma cell growth*: (a) nodularity, (b) packed marrow pattern.

3. *Plasma cell mass*: (a) percentage of plasma cells in the bone marrow.

4. *Alterations of bone and marrow*: (a) high osteoclastic index, (b) coarse fibrosis, (c) marrow atrophy, (d) myelodysplasia, (e) diffuse bone marrow lymphocytosis (and occasionally lymphoid nudules; Figure 29.33), (f) amyloidosis (Figures 29.34 and 29.35), (g) secondary neoplasia.

The spectrum of myeloma cells could be divided into type, according to the predominant plasma cell (Figures 29.28–29.32). Analogous to the malignant lymphomas, these 6 types were combined into three prognostic grades: low, intermediate and high grade malignancy (Figure 29.27).

Generally speaking, in MM the frequency of p53 point mutations is relatively low, about 10%, and is thought to be associated with the aggressive and leukemic forms of MM. We were able to confirm these observations on immunohistology (I.H.) (Figure 29.27). Wild-type and mutant p53 has been detected in 24 and 22% of myeloma patients respectively. Alterations in p53 function are also likely to influence BCL2, elevated levels of which prolong cellular survival, decrease sensitivity to cytotoxic therapy, and inhibit apoptosis.

In a prospective investigation, grading of the plasma cells proved to be the most significant prognostic parameter of all the diagnostic variables tested. There was no correlation between percentages of nucleolated plasma cells and PCLI, indicating that nucleoli in plasma cells correlate with ribosomal activity, rather than proliferative capacity or immaturity of plasma cells. In smoldering MM levels of PCLI and SB2M were low (<1% and <3 mg/l respectively) as were nucleolated plasma cells

<10% and low percentages of plasma cells in the bone marrow – minimal infiltration, interstitial growth pattern and low grade malignancy.

In contrast with CLL, in which a nodular infiltration pattern indicates an indolent course and long survival, nodularity in MM signals a progressive course, osteolytic lesions and an unfavorable prognosis, thus reflecting the intrinsic aggressivity rather than the 'stage' of the tumor.

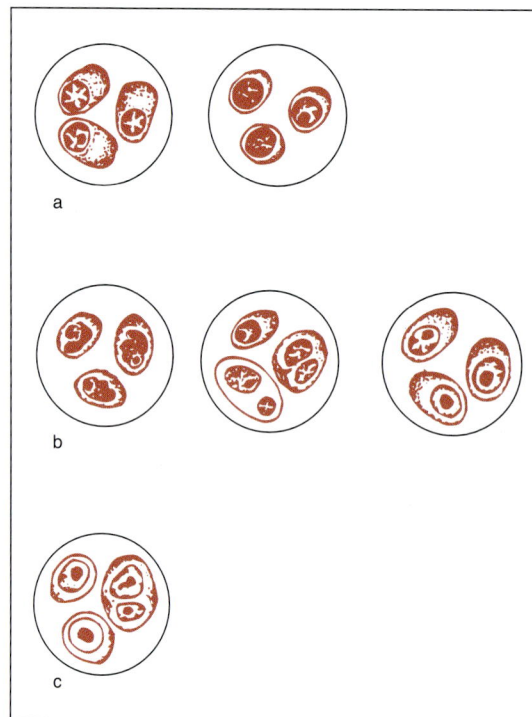

29.27 Representation of the types of plasma cells in the three histological grades of malignancy (a) low grade: Marschalko (left), small cell (right); (b) intermediate grade: cleaved (left), polymorphous (center), asynchronous (right); (c) high grade: blastic.

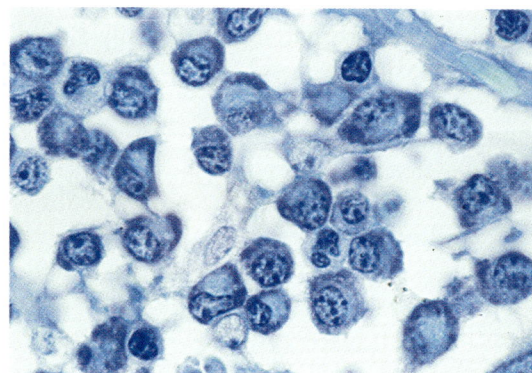

29.28 BMBS plastic, Giemsa, illustrating myeloma cell type, Marschalko, most closely resembling normal plasma cells.

29.29 (left) BMBS plastic, Giemsa, myeloma cells with irregular, cleaved nuclei.

29.30 (right) BMBS plastic, Giemsa, asynchronous type of myeloma cell – immature nucleus with mature cytoplasm.

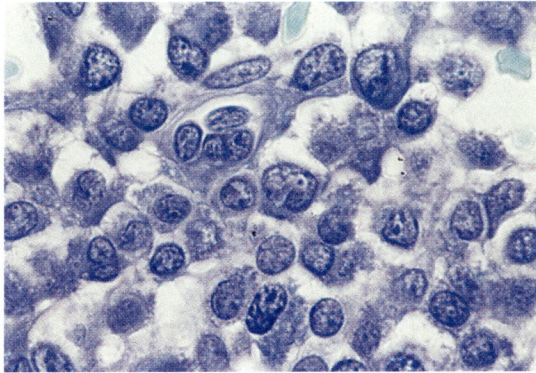

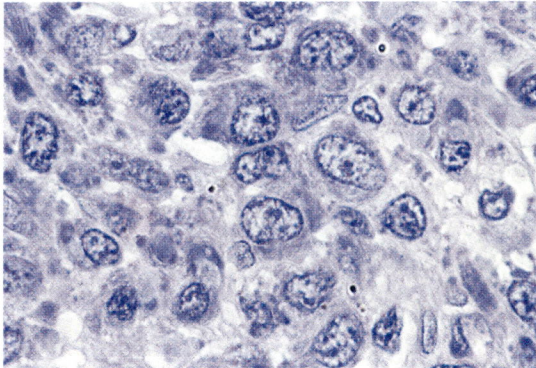

29.31 (left) BMBS plastic, Giemsa, showing polymorphous MM exhibiting a range of shapes and sizes of myeloma cells.

29.32 (right) BMBS plastic, Giemsa, MM consisting mainly of plasmablasts, large cells with immature nuclei and large nucleoli, and a high nucleo-cytoplasmic ratio.

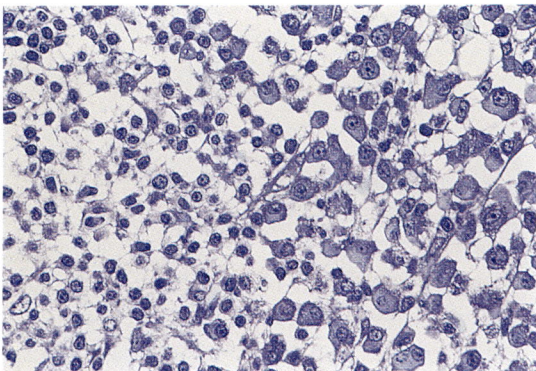

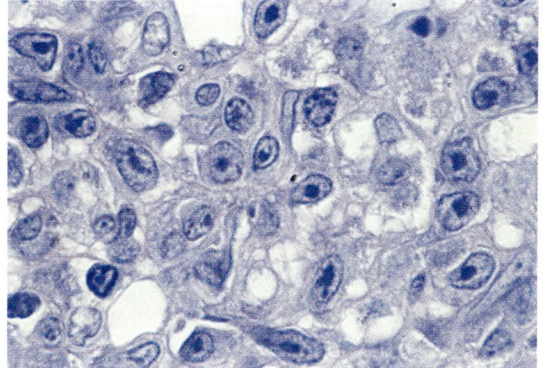

29.33 (left) BMBS plastic, Giemsa, showing lymphocytic aggregate, left and myeloma cells, right.

29.34 (right) BMBS plastic, Giemsa, MM, packed marrow type with deposition of amyloid in vascular walls.

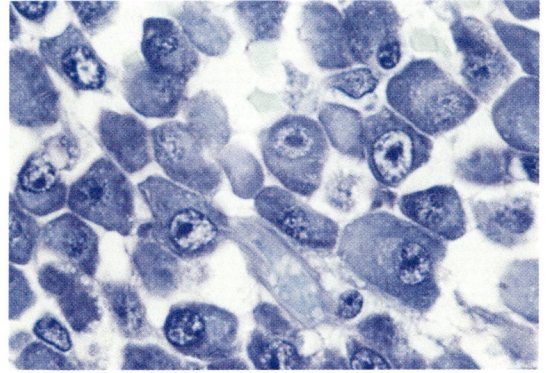

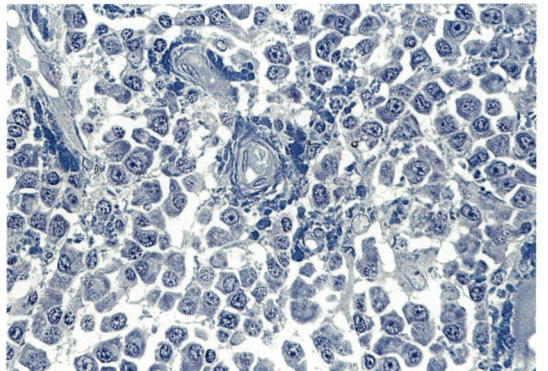

Staging of MM

Staging is required to categorise patients and to select treatment, though most patients present with systemic disease. Originally, the estimated tumor cell burden was used, more recently levels of SB2M, PCLI, the acute phase reactants C reactive protein and α1 anti-trypsin have been utilised to define two broad prognostic groups with excellent >10 years and poor 2.5 years median survivals.

The relationship between percentages of plasma cells in smears and the patients' survivals has been proposed as a factor in staging but its validity has been questioned due to the possibility of over and underestimation (as mentioned above). However, the amount of plasma cell infiltration in biopsy sections may be reliably and reproducibly estimated (if the biopsy is adequate) and utilised for histologic staging:

1. MM histologic stage I: <20 vol % plasma cells in the biopsy and a median survival of 53 months from date of first biopsy.

2. MM histologic stage II: 20–50 vol %, 25 months.

3. MM histologic stage III: >50 vol %, 15 months.

These histologic stages also correlate well with the morphologic grades; therefore histologic estimation of the plasma cell burden supplements whatever clinical staging system is used. There is also a significant correlation between histologic stage, osteoclastic index and amount of bone (Figure 29.23).

Histology in monitoring of MM

Pretreatment phase

Myeloma cell types, growth patterns and variants result from interactions between the plasma cell clones and the complex regulatory systems of the bone marrow. Features such as nodules suggestive of aggressivity and progressive disease, should be taken into consideration in planning immediate therapy including bisphosphonates, to avoid osseous complications. In contrast, patients with plasma cells of low grade malignancy, even with relatively high tumor cell burdens, may not experience rapid progression. Likewise, a minimal interstitial infiltration of mainly mature plasma cells with low levels of PCLI and biochemical parameters have an indolent course and the clinical approach of 'watch and wait' is justified. A change in rate of progression will be detected by regular follow-up investigations. An estimate of the quantity of plasma cells in the bone marrow may also be obtained by flow cytometry (Figure 29.36).

Treatment phase

Initially there is reduction of the plasma cell mass and marked edema. With attainment and maintenance of a stable plateau phase

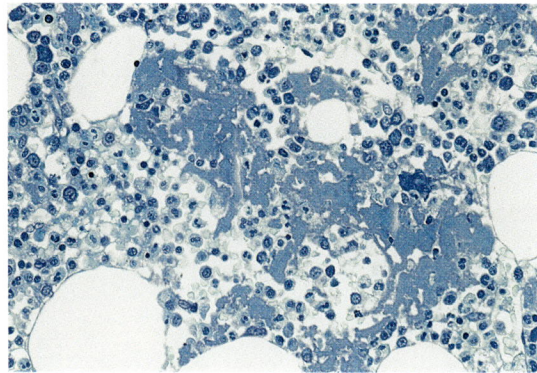

29.35 BMBS plastic, Giemsa, interstitial amyloidosis with minimal plasmacytic infiltration in a case with smoldering MM.

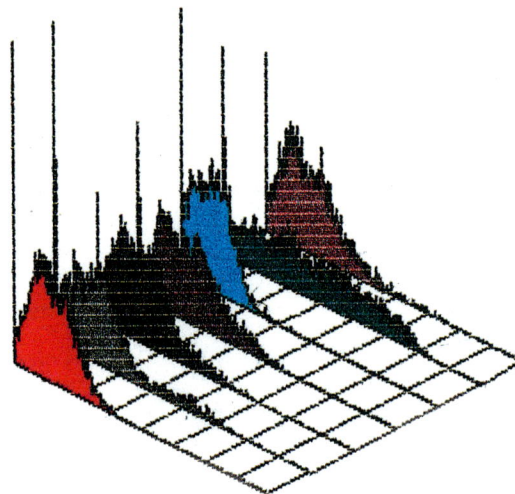

29.36 Histogram of flow cytometry of nucleated cells of bone marrow aspirate. Left to right: red, control; gray, CD5 10%; black, CD2 8%; brown, CD20 12%; blue, CD23 6%; green, CD38 51%; light brown, CD19 10%. Note CD38 plasma cells about half of all the nucleated cells present.

only a minimal residual interstitial infiltration remains. This phase may last up to 5 years or more. With successful chemotherapy plus anti-osteoclastic drugs (e.g. bisphosphonates) osteoclastic resorption is reduced while osteoblasts, osteoid seams and trabecular bone volume is increased.

Continued or maintenance chemotherapy may have cumulative toxic effects on hematopoiesis: myelodysplasia, aplasia, fibrosis. Rises in levels of SB2M, changes in plasma cell grade and development of nodularity all signal imminent relapse. Transformation to an immunoblastic lymphoma or, rarely, to an acute lymphoblastic leukemia has been described.

Refractory cytopenias, myelodysplasias, suspected amyloidosis as well as hematologic or other secondary neoplasias are all indications for taking biopsies for clarification and appropriate therapy.

Heavy chain disease

Gamma, alpha and mu chain: no specific histopathological pattern in the bone marrow has been reported. Increases in plasma cells, lymphocytes, histiocytes may be found as well as some areas of trabecular osteolyses.

Castleman's disease (Angio-follicular lymphoid hyperplasia), and the POEMS syndrome

Based on lymph node histology, two subtypes are recognised: the hyaline vascular type and the plasma cell variant characterised by sheets of plasma cells in the interfollicular regions. It is still not clear whether these are variants of the same disease process or two distinct disorders. The bone marrow lesions show lymphoid nodules, or follicle-like structures and plasmacytic infiltration, lymphocytes and lymphoplasmacytoid cells are also present. There are both localised and multicentric forms of Castleman's disease: the latter shows evidence of multisystem involvement including anemia and thrombocytopenia due to bone marrow involvement. However, in some cases even an intense bone marrow plasmacytosis may be polyclonal, so that the question arises as to whether this is part of the disease process or a reaction to it. Generalised lymphadenopathy with morphological features of the multicentric variant of Castleman's disease has also been observed in AIDS. Moreover, there appears to be a link between Castleman's disease and plasma cell dyscrasias, and several cases of the plasmacytic type of Castleman's disease have had the features of the POEMS syndrome (polyneuropathy, organomegaly, endocrinopathy, M-proteins and skin changes). However, it should be noted that most cases of the POEMS syndrome so far reported have been associated with osteosclerotic multiple myeloma. Many of these patients have plasma cell infiltrates in the osteosclerotic areas rather than a diffuse marrow involvement. The bone marrow may also show small follicular structures associated with infiltrations of plasma cells.

Immunologic characterisation of plasma cells and monoclonal gammopathy of undetermined significance (MGUS)

Monoclonality may be demonstrated by means of antibodies to heavy or light chains. Moreover, a ratio of 16 or more of one of the two light chains to the other – kappa to lambda or vice versa – indicates MM. Nevertheless, even with immunohistology it is not always possible to distinguish between MM and MGUS and follow-up studies are required. Monoclonal peripheral blood lymphocytes at a late stage of B cell differentiation are found in patients with MM, but usually not in MGUS or smoldering MM.

MGUS may occur in patients with many long-standing disorders, including infections, inflammations, tumors and cardiovascular, neurologic and renal disorders, and may regress completely with successful treatment of the underlying condition. Patients have been reported with MGUS who later developed Waldenstrom's macroglobulinemia, heavy chain disease, CLL, 1° amyloidosis and other lymphoproliferative disorders. Time from demonstration of MGUS to overt disease has varied from 6 months to 22 years. Development of MM after MGUS has been reported after intervals of 10–25 years. Myeloma cells have a characteristic pattern of antigen expression: CD38++, CD56+, CD54+ and cIg+; they have a variable expression of CD40 (which possibly suppresses apoptosis) and lack CD19, CD20, CD45 and membrane Ig.

No significant correlation has been detected between the pattern of surface markers, the M-type, the morphologic classification and clinical stage and status in MM and MGUS patients.

Check list: Multiple Myeloma

- Adequate biopsy: 30 mm excluding cortex.
- Cortical bone – reduced – porous.
- Trabecular bone – osteolyses and/or osteopenia – remodeling increased, especially focal.
- Involvement – topography, frequently uneven distribution.
- Clusters, aggregates, nodules; or interstitial infiltration, or both.
- Fibrosis, reticulin stain.
- Quantity and pattern of infiltration.
- Cytologic features of plasma cells. I.H.: LCA, kappa, lambda, CD79[a].
- Residual hematopoiesis – dysplastic features. I.H.: myeloperoxidase, Factor VIII, glycophorin. Also PAS.
- Residual fat cells.
- Vascular or interstitial amyloidosis. Check periosteal blood vessels also, Giemsa stain, methyl violet, Congo red.

- Symptomatic hyperviscosity.
- Bleeding tendency; recurrent infections, due to decreased production of normal immunoglobulin.
- Neurologic symptoms – compression of nerve roots.
- Renal insufficiency, amyloidosis and its complications.
- Monitor and follow-up by levels of immunoglobulins in blood and urine, levels of B_2 microglobulin, bone lesions.
- Preventive therapy with osteoclast inhibiting agents – osseous complications reduced.
- Clonal chromosomal characteristics
  MM
  14q+
  t(11;14)(q13;q32)
  6q−
  abnormalities of 1.

  Also reported
  del(5)(q13q32),t(6;14)(p21q32),t(8;14)
  (q24q32),t(14;18)(q32;q21),i(17)(q),17p+,
  t(9;22)(q34;q11)
  numeric abnormalities of chromosomes 7, 11, X and Y.

  Heavy chain disease
  rearrangement of 14q32
  t(9;14)(p11;q32)
  t(2;14)(p12;q32)

Monoclonal gammopathy of undetermined significance: in 40% of patients, gains of chromosome 3 have been detected, using interphase FISH. Less frequently affected are chromosomes 7, 11 and 18.

Clinical correlations

- Biochemical profile: immunoglobulins, paraprotein.
- Hypercalcemia, bone pain, fractures.
- Anemia, later neutropenia, thrombocytopenia; weakness, fatigue.
- Young adults and older age groups.

Bibliography

Abildgaard N., Bentzen S.M., Nielsen J.L., Heickendorff L. (1997) Serum markers of bone metabolism in multiple myeloma: prognostic value of the carboxy-terminal telopeptide of type I collagen (ICTP). *Br. J. Haematol.*, **96 (1)**, 103–10.

Anderson K.C., Barut B.A., Ritz J. *et al.* (1991) Monoclonal antibody-purged autologous bone marrow transplantation therapy for multiple myeloma. *Blood*, **77 (4)**, 712–20.

Bagg A., Becker P., Bezwoda W. *et al.* (1989) Circulating monotypic B-cells in multiple myeloma: association with lambda paraproteins. *Br. J. Haematol.*, **72 (2)**, 167–72.

Barlogie B. (ed) (1997) *Hematology/Oncology Clinics of North America: Multiple Myeloma*. Philadelphia: W.B. Saunders.

Barlogie B., Jagannath S., Epstein J. *et al.* (1997) Biology and therapy of multiple myeloma in 1996. *Sem in Hematol.*, **34 (1)**, 67.

Bartl R., Frisch B. (1989) Bone marrow histology in multiple myeloma: prognostic relevance of histologic characteristics. In *Haematol Rev*. Harwood.

Bartl R., Frisch B. (1993) *Biopsy of Bone in Internal Medicine*. Boston: Kluwer Academic.

Bartl R., Frisch B. (1995) Diagnostic morphology in multiple myeloma. *Curr Diagnost Pathol.*, **2**, 222–35.

Bartl R., Frisch B., Diem H. *et al.* (1989) Bone marrow histology and serum beta 2 microglonulin in multiple myeloma – a new prognostic strategy. *Eur J Haematol.* **51**, 88–98.

Bartl R., Frisch B., Diem H. *et al.* (1991) Histologic, biochemical and clinical parameters for monitoring multiple myeloma. *Cancer*, **68**, 2241–50.

Bartl R., Frisch B., Wilmanns W. (1995) Morphology of multiple myeloma. In Malpas, Bergsagel and Kyle (eds), *Myeloma*. Oxford: Oxford University Press, pp. 82–123.

Bartl R., Frisch B., Fateh-Moghadam A. *et al.* (1987) Histologic classification and staging of multiple myeloma. A retrospective and prospective study of 674 cases. *Am. J. Clin. Pathol.*, **87 (3)**, 342–55.

Bataille R., Chappard D., Marcelli C. *et al.* (1990) Osteoblast stimulation in multiple myeloma lacking lytic bone lesions. *Br J Haematol.*, **76**, 484.

Baur A., Stabler A., Bartl R. *et al.* (1996) Infiltration patterns of plasmacytomas in magnetic resonance tomography. *Rofo Fortschr Geb Rontgenstr Neuen Bildgeb Verfahr*, **164 (6)**, 457–63.

Billadeau D., Ahmann G., Greipp P., Van Ness B. (1993) The bone marrow of multiple myeloma patients contains B cell populations at different stages of differentiation that are clonally related to the malignant plasma cell. *J Exp Med.*, **178 (3)**, 1023–31.

Billadeau D., Van Ness B., Kimlinger T. *et al.* (1996) Clonal circulating cells are common in plasma cell proliferative disorders: a comparison of monoclonal gammopathy of undetermined significance, smoldering multiple myeloma, and active myeloma. *Blood*, **88 (1)**, 289–96.

Brigaudeau C., Trimoreau F., Gachard N. *et al.* (1997) Cytogenetic study of 30 patients with multiple myeloma: comparison of 3 and 6 day bone marrow cultures stimulated or not with cytokines by using a miniaturized karyotypic method. *Br J Haematol.*, **96**, 594–600.

Burger R., Wendler J., Antoni K. *et al.* (1994) Interleukin-6 production in B-cell neoplasias and Castleman's disease: evidence for an additional paracrine loop. *Ann. Hematol.* **69 (1)**, 25–31.

Buss D.H., Prichard R.W., Cooper M.R. (1988) Plasma cell dyscrasias. *Hematol/Oncol Clin N Amer.*, **2 (4)**, 603.

Buss D.H., Prichard R.W., Hartz J.W., Cooper M.R. (1987) Comparison of the usefulness of bone marrow sections and smears in diagnosis of multiple myeloma. *Hematol. Pathol.*, **1 (1)**, 35–43.

Calasanz M.J., Cigudosa J.C., Odero M.D. *et al.* (1997) Cytogenetic analysis of 280 patients with multiple myeloma and related disorders: primary breakpoints and clinical correlations. *Genes Chromosomes Cancer*, **18(2)**, 84–93.

Caligaris-Cappio F., Bergui L., Gregoretti M.G. *et al.* (1991) Role of bone marrow stromal cells in the growth of human multiple myeloma. *Blood*, **77 (12)**, 2688–93.

Carbone A., Manconi R., Sulfaro S. *et al.* (1987) Practical importance of routine paraffin-embedded bone marrow biopsy in multiple myeloma. *Tumori*, **73 (3)**, 315–19.

Cassel A., Leibovitz N., Hornstein L. *et al.* (1990) Evidence for the existence of circulating monoclonal B-lymphocytes in multiple myeloma patients. *Exp. Hematol.*, **18 (11)**, 1171–3.

Cavo M., Galieni P., Zuffa E. *et al.* (1989) Prognostic variables and clinical staging in multiple myeloma. *Blood*, **74 (5)**, 1774–80.

Chauhan D., Uchiyama H., Akbarali Y. *et al.* (1996) Multiple myeloma cell adhesion-induced interleukin-6 expression in bone marrow stromal cells involves activation of NF-kappa B. *Blood*, **87 (3)**, 1104–12.

Cook G., Dumbar M., Franklin I.M. (1997) The role of adhesion molecules in multiple myeloma. *Acta Haematol*, **97 (1–2)**, 81–9.

Corrado C., Santarelli M.T., Pavlosky S., Pizzolato M. (1989) Prognostic factors in multiple myeloma: Definition of risk groups in 410 previously untreated patients: a Grupo Argentino de Tratamiento de la Leucemia Aguda study. *J Clin Oncol*, **7 (12)**, 1839–44.

Di Benedetto G., Cataldi A., Verde A. *et al.* (1989) Gamma heavy chain disease associated with Hodgkin's disease. Clinical, pathologic, and immunologic features of one case. *Cancer*, **63 (9)**, 1804–9.

Durie B.G.M. (1991) Multiple myeloma: biology and treatment. *Oncology Today*, **3**, 15.

Epstein J., Xiao H.Q., He X.Y. (1990) Markers of multiple hematopoietic-cell lineages in multiple myeloma. *N. Engl. J. Med.*, **322 (10)**, 664–8.

Evans C.E., Galasko C.S.B., Ward C. (1989) Does myeloma secrete an osteoblast inhibiting factor? *J Bone Joint Surg.*, **71B**, 288.

Facon T., Lai J.L., Nataf E. *et al.* (1993) Improved cytogenetic analysis of bone marrow plasma cells after cytokine stimulation in multiple myeloma: a report on 46 patients. *Br J Haematol.*, **84** (4), 743–5.

Faravelli A., Ponzoni M., Zoldan M.C. *et al.* (1994) Monoclonal gammapathies: differential diagnosis with bone marrow biopsy. *Pathologica*, **86** (3), 258–66.

Feiner H.D., Bannan M., Marsh E. *et al.* (1992) Monoclonal gammopathy of undetermined significance: a morphologic and immunophenotypic study of the bone marrow. *Mod Pathol.*, **5** (4), 372–9.

Fermand J.P., Brouet J.C., Danon F., Seligmann M. (1989) Gamma heavy chain 'disease': heterogénity of the clinico-pathologic features. Report of 16 cases and review of the literature. *Medicine*, **68** (6), 321–35.

Frewin R., Henson A., Provan D. (1997) ABC of clinical haematology: haematological emergencies. *BMJ*, **314**, 1333–6.

Harster G.A., Krause J.R. (1987) Multiple myeloma in two young postpartum women. *Arch. Pathol. Lab. Med.*, **111** (1), 38–42.

Huvos A.G. (1991) Multiple myeloma, including solitary osseous myeloma. In A.G. Huvos (ed), *Bone Tumors: Diagnosis, Treatment and Prognosis*. Philadelphia: W.B. Saunders.

Jarosová M., Scudla V., Bakovsky, K. *et al.* (1996) Two cases of t(9;20) in multiple myeloma. *Cancer Genet Cytogenet*, **90** (2), 106–8.

Joshua D., Gibson J., Brown R. (1996) Myeloma: biology, prognosis and treatment. *Hematol Rev and Comm*, **9** (4), 227–50.

Kimlinger T., Witzig T.E. (1997) Expression of the hematopoietic stem cell antigen CD34 on blood and bone marrow monoclonal plasma cells from patients with multiple myeloma. *Bone Marrow Transplant.*, **19** (6), 553–6.

Klein B., Zhang X.G., Jourdan M. *et al.* (1990) Interleukin-6 is the central tumor growth factor in vitro and in vivo in multiple myeloma. *Eur. Cytokine. Netw.*, **1** (4), 193–201.

Krzyzaniak R.L., Buss D.H., Cooper M.R., Wells H.B. (1988) Marrow fibrosis and multiple myeloma. *Am. J. Clin. Pathol.*, **89** (1), 63–8.

Kurabayashi H., Miyawaki S., Murakami H. *et al.* (1989) Ultrastructure of multinucleated giant myeloma cells: report of one case. *Am. J. Hematol.*, **31** (4), 284–5.

Kyle R.A. (1987) Monoclonal gammopathy and multiple myeloma in the elderly. *Bailliere's Clinical Hematol.*, **1** (2), 533.

Kyle R.A. (1990) Multiple myeloma: an update on diagnosis and management. *Acta Oncol.*, **29**, 1.

Levo Y., Behar A.J., Blum I., Frisch B. (1987) A benign course of multicentric Castleman's disease with involvement of the spleen and bone marrow. *Eur. J. Hematol.* **39** (5), 471–4.

Ludescher C., Grunewald K., Fend F. *et al.* (1989) Osteosclerotic myeloma with polyneuropathy and hypocalcemia. *Blut*, **58** (4), 207–10.

Marmont F., Pich A., Chiusa L. *et al.* (1996) Correlation between argyrophilic nucleolar organizer region counts and labelling index in multiple myeloma. *Eur J Haematol*, **56** (1–2), 39–44.

Menke D.M., Greipp P.R., Colon-Otero G. *et al.* (1994) Bone marrow aspirate immunofluorescent and bone marrow biopsy immunoperoxidase staining of plasma cells in histologically occult plasma cell proliferative marrow disorders. *Arch Pathol Lab Med*, **118** (8), 811–14.

Merville P., Dechanet J., Desmouliere A. *et al.* (1996) Bcl-2+ tonsillar plasma cells are rescued from apoptosis by bone marrow fibroblasts. *J Exp Med.*, **183** (1), 227–36.

Molina T., Brouland J.P., Bigorgne C. *et al.* (1996) Pseudo-myelomatous plasmacytosis of the bone marrow in a multicentric Castleman's disease. *Ann Pathol*, **16** (2), 133–6.

Mundy G.R. (1990) Hypercalcemia of malignancy. In Avioli and Krane (eds), *Metabolic Bone Disease*. Philadelphia: W.B. Saunders.

Pasqualetti P., Casale R., Collacciani A. *et al.* (1990) Multiple myeloma: relationship between survival and cellular morphology. *Am J Hematol*, **33** (2), 145–7.

Pasqualetti P., Colantonio D., Casale R. (1990) Prognostic value of the ratio of bone marrow plasma cells in multiple myeloma. *Minerva Med.*, **81** (3), 129–33.

Paule B., Quillard J., Bennet P. *et al.* (1989) Morphologic heterogeneity and plasmablastic transformation in advanced plasma-cytic/plasmablastic myeloma: a study of 35 serial bone marrow biopsies in 9 patients. *Nouv Rev Fr Hematol.*, **31** (3), 203–8.

Pich A., Chiusa L., Marmont F., Navone R. (1997) Risk groups of myeloma patients by histologic pattern and proliferative activity. *Am J Surg Pathol.*, **21** (3), 339–47.

Pileri S., Poggi S., Baglioni P. *et al.* (1989) Histology and immunohistology of bone marrow biopsy in multiple myeloma. *Eur J Hematol Suppl.*, **51**, 52–9.

Pulsoni A., Bianco P., La Verde G. *et al.* (1993) Coexistent multiple myeloma and myelofibrosis. *Leukemia and Lymphoma*, **10** (4–5), 401–3.

Roy D.N., Mitra S., Biswas T.K. *et al.* (1988) Bence–Jones myeloma. *J. Indian Med. Assoc.*, **86** (3), 70–2.

Ruhlmann J., Bockisch A., Dewes W. *et al.* (1989) Bone marrow scinitgraphy and magnetic resonance tomography in plasmacytoma. *Onkologie*, **12** (1), 38–41.

Sailer M., Vykoupil K.F., Peest D. *et al.* (1995) Prognostic relevance of a histologic classification system applied in bone marrow biopsies from patients with multiple myeloma: a histopathological evaluation of biopsies from 153 untreated patients. *Eur J Haematol*, **54** (3), 137–46.

Samanta A., Hilton D., Roy S. (1990) Peripheral neuropathy, polymyalgia and arthralgia: a paraneoplastic syndrome associated with myeloma. *Clin Rheuumatol*, **9** (2), 246–8.

Schambeck C.M., Bartl R., Hochtlen-Vollmar W. *et al.* (1996) Characterization of myeloma cells by means of labeling index, bone marrow histology, and serum beta 2-microglobulin. *Am J Clin Pathol*, **106** (1), 64–8.

Schmidt U., Ruwe M., Leder L.D. (1995) Multiple myeloma with bone marrow biopsy features simulating concomitant chronic idiopathic myelofibrosis. *Nouv Rev Fr Hematol*, **37** (2), 159–63.

Singer C.R.J. (1997) ABC of clinical haematology: Multiple myeloma and related conditions. *BMJ*, **314**, 960.

Smadja N., Krulik M., Louvet C. *et al.* (1991) Similar cytogenetic abnormalities in two cases of plasma cell leukemia. *Cancer Genet. Cytogenet.*, **52** (1), 123–9.

Solé F., Woesnner S., Acin P. *et al.* (1996) Cytogenetic abnormalities in 13 patients with multiple myeloma. *Cancer Genet Cytogenet*, **86** (2), 162–4.

Stewart A.K., Freedman J., Garvey M.B. (1990) Acute leukemia evolving from

multiple myeloma and co-expressing myeloid and plasma cell antigens. *Am. J. Hematol.*, **34** (3), 210–4.

Taniwaki M., Nishida K., Ueda Y., Takashima T. (1996) Non-random chromosomal rearrangements and their implications in clinical features and outcome of multiple myeloma and plasma cell leukemia. *Leukemia and Lymphoma*, **21**, 25–30.

Tasaka T., Berenson J., Vesico R., Hirama T. *et al.* (1997) Analysis of the p^{16INK4A}, p^{15INK4B} and p^{18INK}.

Teoh G., Anderson K.C. (1997) Interaction of tumor and host cells with adhesion and extracellular matrix molecules in the development of multiple myeloma. *Hematol/Oncol Clinics of N. Amer.*, **11** (1), 27.

Thiry A., Delvenne P., Fontaine M.A., Boniver J. (1993) Comparison of bone marrow sections, smears and immunohistological staining for immunoglobulin light chains in the diagnosis of benign and malignant plasma cell proliferations. *Histopathology*, **22** (5), 423–8.

Vacca A., Di Loreto M., Ribatti D. *et al.* (1995) Bone marrow of patients with active multiple myeloma: angiogenesis and plasma cell adhesion molecules LFA-1, VLA-4, LAM-1, and CD44. *Am. J. Hematol.*, **50** (1), 9–14.

Van den Berghe H. (1989) Chromosomes in plasma-cell malignancies. *Eur. J. Hematol. Suppl.*, **51**, 47–51.

Van Riet I., De Greef C., Del Favero H. *et al.* (1994) Production of fibronectin and adherence to fibronectin by human myeloma cell lines. *Br J Haematol.*, **87** (2), 258–65.

Van Riet I., Heriman C., Lacor P. *et al.* (1989) Detection of monoclonal B lymphocytes in bone marrow and peripheral blood of multiple myeloma patients by immunoglobulin gene rearrangement studies. *Br J Haematol*, **73** (3), 289–95.

Vendrell J., Richart C., Arteaga R. *et al.* (1992) Monoclonal gammopathy as a clue to the presence of thyroid lymphoma associated with auto-immune thyroiditis. *Aust. N.Z. J. Med.*, **22** (5), 510.

Vescio R., Rosen L., Schmulbach E., Berenson J. (1996) Multiple myeloma and chronic lymphocytic leukemia. *Current Opinion in Hematol*, **3** (4), 288–96.

Yermiahu T., Peiser J., Beharroch D., Ovnat A. (1989) Aggressive behavior of carcinoma of the colon associated with nonsecreting plasma cell myeloma. A case report. *J Clin Gastroenterol*, **11** (5), 565–7.

Zukerberg L.R., Ferry J.A., Conlon M., Harris N.L. (1990) Plasma cell myeloma with cleaved, multilobulated, and monocytoid nuclei. *Am J Clin Pathol*, **93** (5), 657–61.

30 Mononuclear phagocyte and immunoregulatory effector system (M-PIRES)

General aspects

The above designation has replaced the previous more comprehensive name of 'reticuloendothelial system' as this included non-phagocytic cells, such as fibroblast and endothelial cells, and cells which did not arise from the monocyte-macrophage progenitor, which also produces the granulocytic cell line. Recent studies have provided additional support for earlier conclusions on the derivation and function of monocytes and macrophages. The bone marrow stem cells produce the committed progenitor which gives rise to the monoblast, promonocyte and monocyte in the bone marrow. The monocytes leave the bone marrow after maturation, remain only a short time in the peripheral blood and migrate out into the tissues where they become macrophages. In previous chapters, mention has been made of bone marrow macrophages – their number is increased in various conditions, such as infections by any of numerous agents; or disorders involving ineffective hematopoiesis with intramedullary cell destruction and subsequent accumulation of numerous hemosiderin-containing macrophages in the bone marrow stroma. Thus, the bone marrow produces monocytes that become macrophages in the tissues of the body, but monocytes can also become macrophages and perform their phagocytic functions in the bone marrow itself. Moreover, scavenging and phagocytosis are not their only activities: the mononuclear phagocyte produces a variety of secretions; it participates in regulation of the immune response and macrophages function as antigen-presenting cells. Activated monocytes act in concert with other cells in various biological processes, for example bone resorption. The inflammatory reactions that occur in the bone marrow, and the agents which evoke them, have been dealt with previously. It should be emphasised that epithelioid and multinucleated giant cells are all derived from the mononuclear phagocyte system.

Inherited disorders of the mononuclear phagocyte system

Storage diseases
These are the consequence of inherited enzyme deficiencies that lead to accumulation

of the substances that are incompletely catabolised in the cells of the mononuclear phagocyte system in organs such as liver, spleen and bone marrow. Many of these products are derived from lipids of the cell membrane.

Gaucher's disease (Figures 30.1–30.5)

This is due to a defective lysosomal glucosidase (glucocerebrosidase) which splits beta-glucose-cerebrosides. Mutations occur at the locus for this enzyme on chromosome 1q21. There are different levels of enzymic activity in the mononuclear phagocyte system and these in turn influence the time of appearance of the disease so that three types are recognised: infantile, juvenile and adult.

Macrophages containing cerebroside accumulate in the liver, spleen and bone marrow. Subsequently, there may be pancytopenia due to replacement of the bone marrow and increased splenic destruction. Lytic bone lesions and aseptic necrosis may lead to pathological fractures.

Within the bone marrow the aggregates of large macrophages with the typical wrinkled silk or tissue-paper appearance of Gaucher cells alternate with areas of normal hematopoietic tissue. Fat cells are decreased, macrophages in all stages of development to Gaucher cells are found in the marrow. In some cases, patches of fat cells remain and hematopoiesis is decreased in spite of the occupation of large areas of the marrow by Gaucher cells. Immunoglobulin production in Gaucher's disease is increased due to chronic stimulation of the immune system which eventually may lead to development of a lymphoproliferative disorder (e.g. MM) in both adults and children. The course of the disease is variable, and a heterozygous genotype is associated with a mild clinical course.

30.1 (left) BMBS paraffin, H&E, showing aggregate of typical Gaucher cells, left, and hematopoiesis, right.

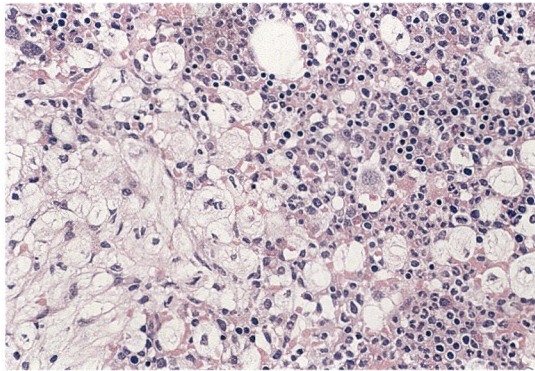

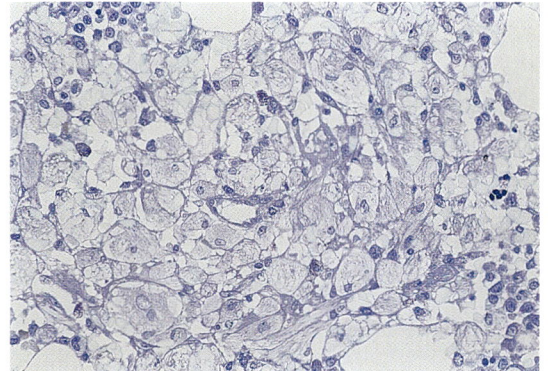

30.2 (right) BMBS plastic, Giemsa, large aggregate of Gaucher cells.

30.3 (left) BMBS paraffin, I.H., with CD68; note that the smaller Gaucher cells are more strongly positive than the larger ones.

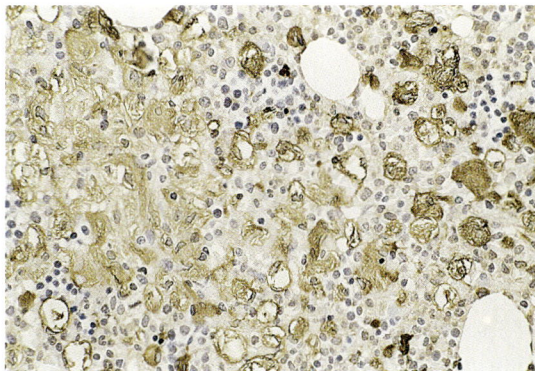

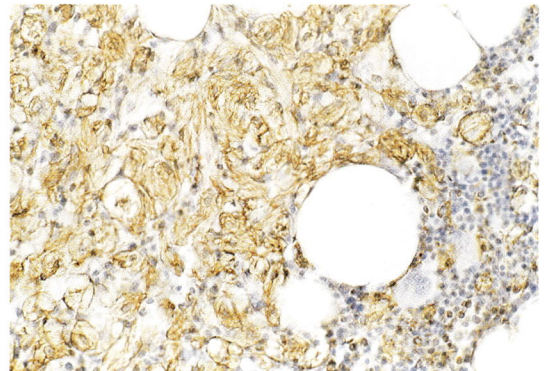

30.4 (right) BMBS paraffin, I.H., vimentin, most of the storage cells are stained.

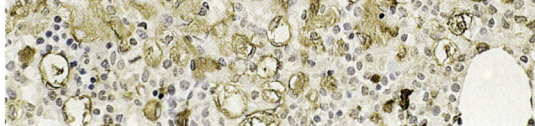

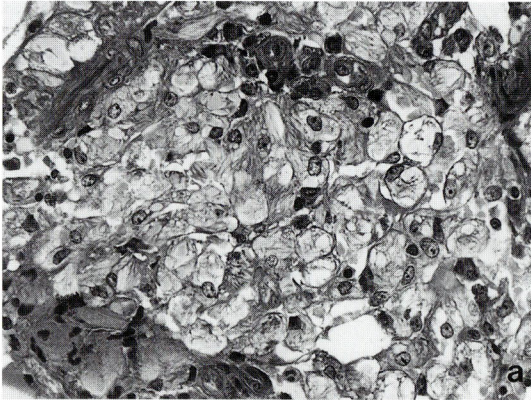

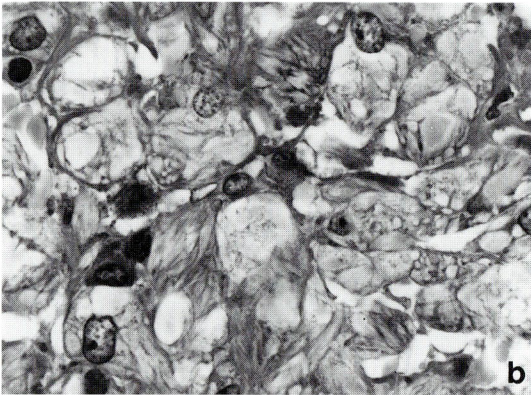

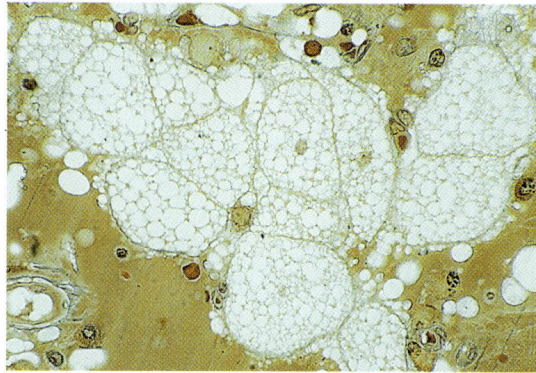

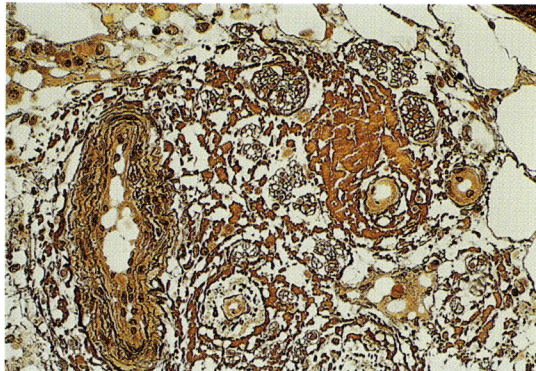

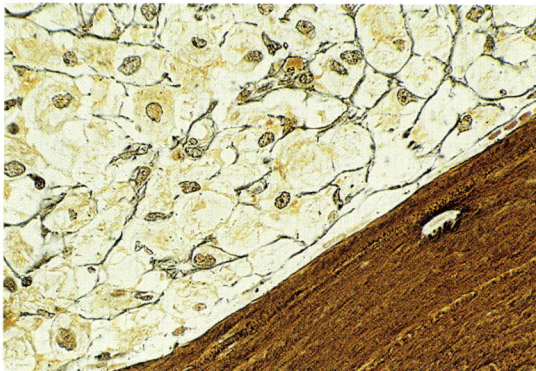

30.5a and b (left) BMBS plastic, Giemsa, M, Gaucher, the typical wrinkled tissue paper aspect of the cytoplasm of the storage cells is highlighted.

30.6 (right top) BMBS plastic, Gomori, high magnification illustrating large foamy cells, Nieman Pick.

30.7 (right bottom) BMBS plastic, macrophages in Fabry's disease.

Nieman–Pick disease (Figure 30.6)

This is also a heterogenous group of diseases. Large foamy cells with small eccentric nuclei accumulate in bone marrow. Most cases are diagnosed in infancy and childhood as the disease is rapidly fatal.

Fabry's disease (Figure 30.7)

This is due to lack of the enzyme alpha galactosidase (an inborn error of metabolism of a glycolipid), resulting in a storage disease affecting not only the mononuclear phagocyte system but also parenchymal cells of other organs. The macrophages have a foamy whorled appearance.

Farquhar's disease (lymphohistiocytosis) (Figure 30.8)

This was originally called familial hemophagocytic reticulosis; it is possibly an acute variant of the Letterer–Siwe syndrome. There is widespread histiocytosis, in some cases also involving the meninges. The disease affects

30.8 BMBS plastic, Gomori, histiocytes in Farquhar's disease.

infants and young children and is rapidly fatal.

Lipid storage disease (Figure 30.9)

In these conditions, also known as the hyperlipidemias (such as alpha-lipoprotein deficiency), macrophages containing cholesterol or cholesterol esters may be found in the bone marrow. However, in sections of the bone marrow the cholesterol is dissolved out during the histological processing, so that empty spaces are left. These macrophages are large and multiloculated. Such macrophages are also found in other conditions such as diabetes, hyperthyroidism and hypercholesterolemia. The mechanism controlling the deposition of cholesterol or its esters is not known. Cholesterol embolism from atherosclerotic plaques has been observed in the bone marrow.

Hermansky–Pudlak syndrome
(Figure 30.10)
This is one variant of oculocutaneous albinism, characterised by hypopigmentation of the skin, hair and eyes. The following features are found in the Hermansky–Pudlak variant: it is autosomal recessive; tyrosinase positive; there is an enzyme defect leading to deposition of a ceroid-lipofuchsin-like material in macrophages; there is a storage-pool defect in

platelets which causes functional disturbances and hence bleeding complications, especially in females (reproductive system) and during and after surgical interventions. The macrophages in the bone marrow are dispersed singly or in clusters among the hematopoietic cells, are large, may contain vacuoles and pigment, which is negative in stains for iron.

Sea-blue histiocytosis
Macrophages containing sea-blue-colored inclusions may be found in the bone marrow in many different conditions including thalassemias, myeloproliferative disorders, chronic granulomatous conditions and others. Whether it occurs as an independent entity has not yet been settled. The occurrence of these histiocytes in the disorders mentioned above (all with a high cellular turnover rate) may well be due to overloading of the mononuclear phagocyte system.

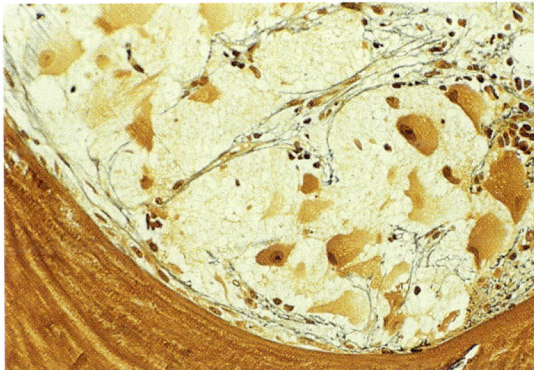

30.9 BMBS plastic, Gomori, histiocytes in lipid storage disease; note irregular nuclei.

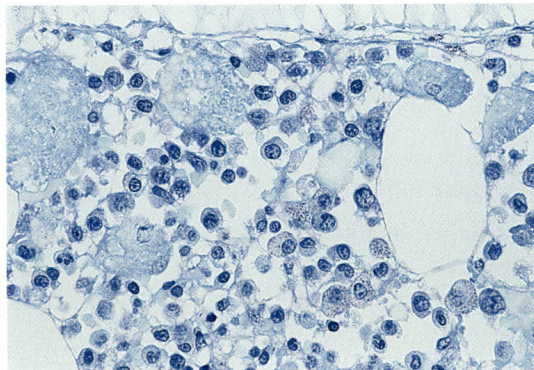

Pseudo-Gaucher (or pseudo-storage disease)
Many congenital or acquired conditions involve ineffective hematopoiesis with a consequently high turnover rate. This may lead to the development of Gaucher-like macrophages in the bone marrow, for example in CML. But the large multiple aggregates with replacement of the marrow seen in Gaucher's disease do not occur in these conditions. Conditions in which pseudo-Gaucher cells have been observed include CML, thalassemia, after intensive chemotherapy, in tumors and in other disorders with a high cellular turnover rate.

Histiocytosis X
This designation comprises eosinophilic granuloma, Hand–Schüller–Christian disease (HSC) (Figures 30.11 and 30.12), and Letterer–Siwe disease. The cause is unknown, though a disturbance of immune regulation has been postulated. This group of diseases has now been renamed Langerhans cell histiocytosis, and specific criteria established for the definitive diagnosis.

30.10 BMBS plastic, Giemsa, large, pale blue-stained macrophages, top left and right from a case of Hermansky–Pudlak syndrome.

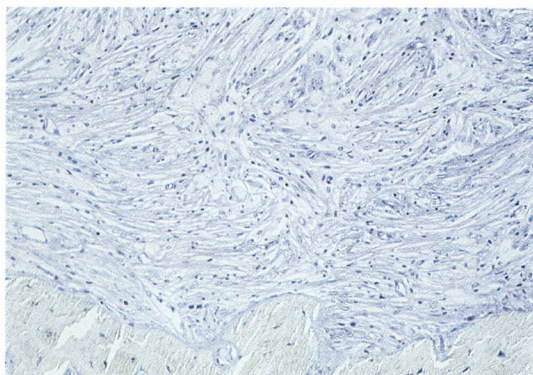

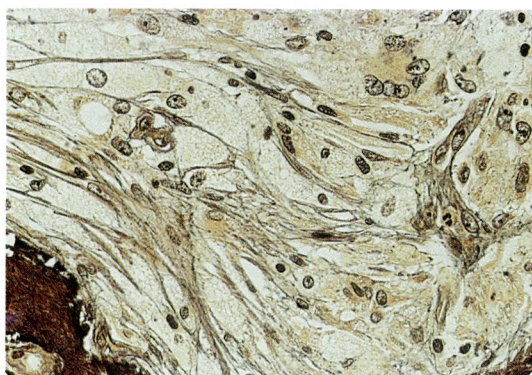

30.11 (left) BMBS plastic, Giemsa, showing histiocytes, fibroblasts and fibers replacing the bone marrow in histiocytosis X.

30.12 (right) As for Figure 30.11, Gomori illustrating extent of fibrosis.

Eosinophilic granuloma of bone

Though occurring more often in males and young people, females and any age group may be affected. The lesions may be single or multiple and consist of aggregates of macrophages and eosinophils; foam cells, giant cells and fibers may also be present. Multiple lesions indicate a chronic disorder, with generalised manifestations.

Hand–Schüller–Christian disease

This occurs mainly in children and involves the bone as well as many other organs. The lesions consist of monomorphic infiltrations of histiocytes (sometimes with cholesterol crystals), and include lymphocytes, plasma cells, eosinophils, fibroblasts and fibers. The histiocytes have irregular nuclei and abundant, well-demarcated cytoplasm.

Letterer–Siwe disease

Infiltrates similar to those described above in HSC and eosinophilic granuloma are found. The diagnoses of these variants are made on clinical grounds and not only on a purely histopathological basis.

Langerhan's cell histiocytosis in adults

Bone marrow involvement is sporadic but represents an aggressive form with an unfavorable prognosis. The extensive childhood form of the disease has a different phenotype than the adult form, which appears to be more differentiated.

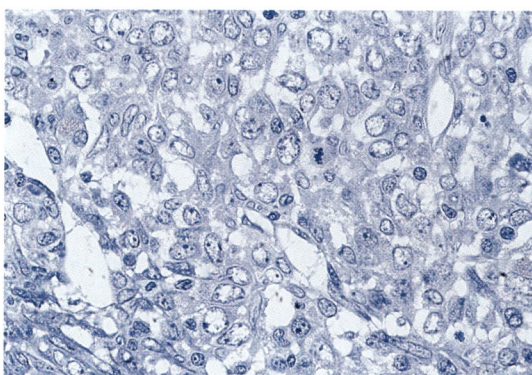

30.13 BMBS plastic, Giemsa, showing pleomorphic nuclei in cells of malignant histiocytosis.

Malignant histiocytosis (also known as histiocytic medullary reticulosis HMR) (Figure 30.13)

This is considered a malignancy of the mononuclear phagocyte system with neoplastic proliferation of histiocytes in the bone marrow, liver and spleen. The bone marrow structure is effaced, hematopoiesis and fat cells are reduced, and the histiocytes show hemophagocytosis. In early cases, small aggregates and diffusely dispersed histiocytes are found, without effacement of the normal marrow. Nevertheless, there is still some uncertainty about the etiology of the disease and the nature of the histiocytes. An association between HMR and EBV infection has been demonstrated, supporting previous suggestions that HMR may be a fatal form of infectious mononucleosis. The differential diagnosis includes viral-associated hemophagocytic syndrome (VAHS), and hemophagocytosis in other infections. Histiocytic proliferations with hemophagocytosis may accompany diseases such as lymphoproliferative disorders, especially in their terminal phases, or gastric carcinoma; sinus histiocytosis with massive lymphadenopathy; and erythrophagocytic T cell lymphoma. Increase in bone marrow histiocytes with erythrophagocytosis is also found in Kawasaki's disease.

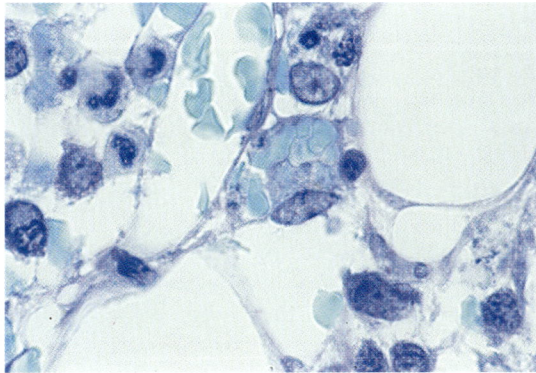

30.14 BMBS plastic, Giemsa, macrophage with engulfed erythrocytes.

Viral-associated hemophagocytic syndrome

This resembles malignant histiocytosis both clinically and histologically. There is hyperplasia of the mononuclear phagocyte system in the bone marrow with striking hemophagocytosis; multinucleated giant cells may also be present. The marrow architecture is disrupted and hematopoiesis and fat cells are decreased. The morphological distinction between the two conditions (i.e. HMR and VAHS) may be very difficult. A relationship between histiocytic medullary reticulosis and T cell lymphomas has recently been proposed (Figures 30.14 and 30.15)

Bone marrow in Acquired Immune Deficiency Syndrome (AIDS)

(Figures 30.16–30.19)

There are an estimated 22 million people worldwide with HIV infection (as of February 1997) and though potent new antiviral combination therapies have led to new optimisim

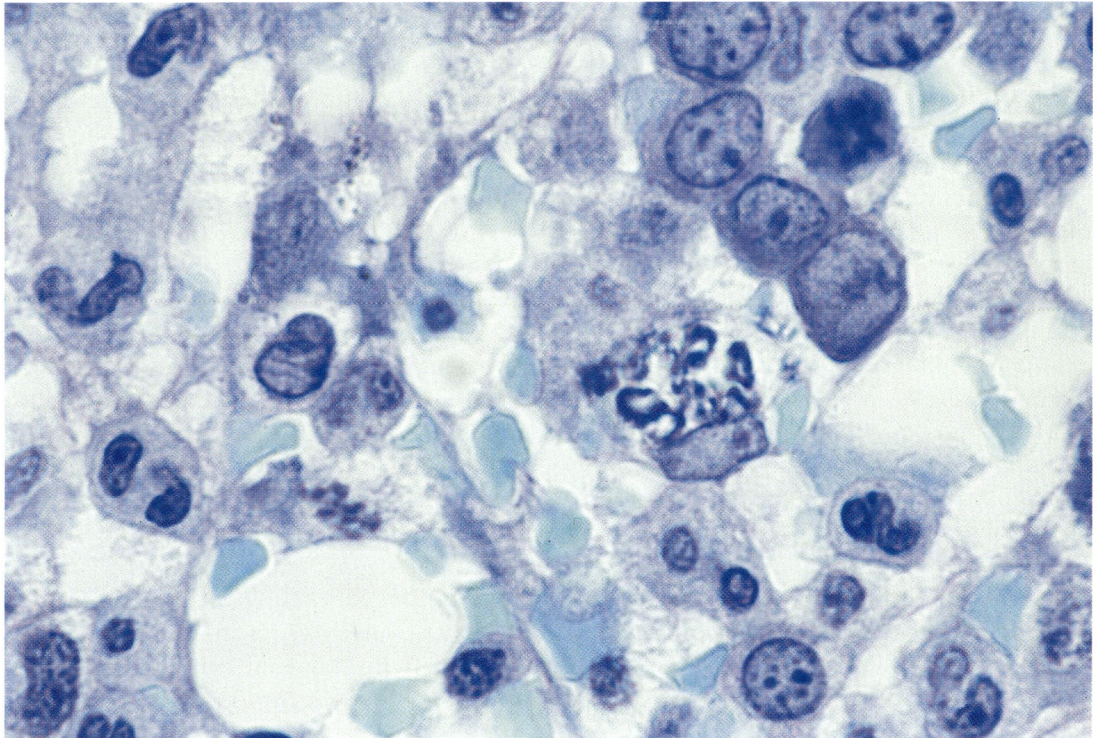

30.15 As for Figure 30.14, macrophage with cellular debris.

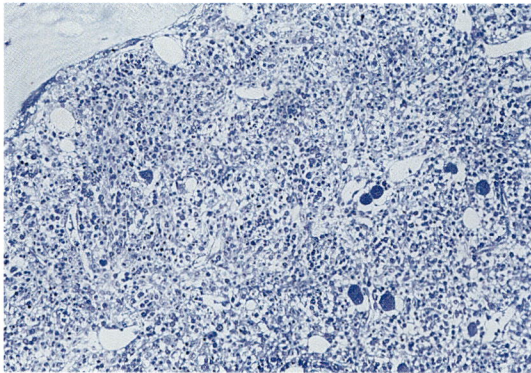

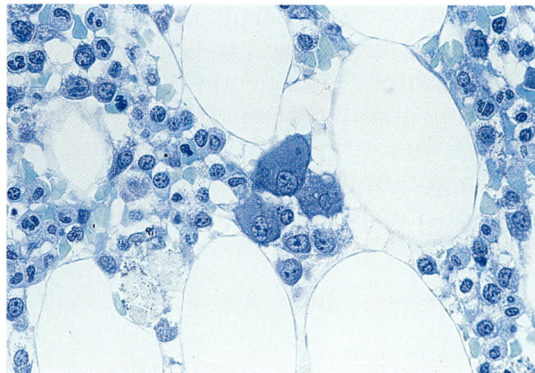

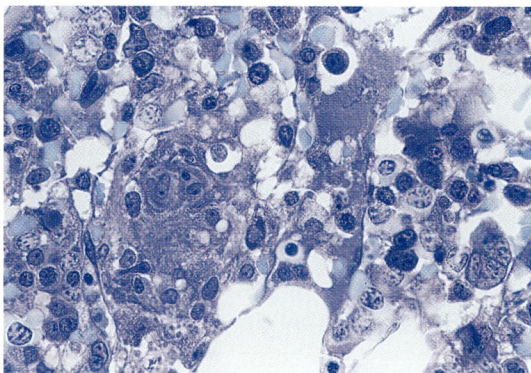

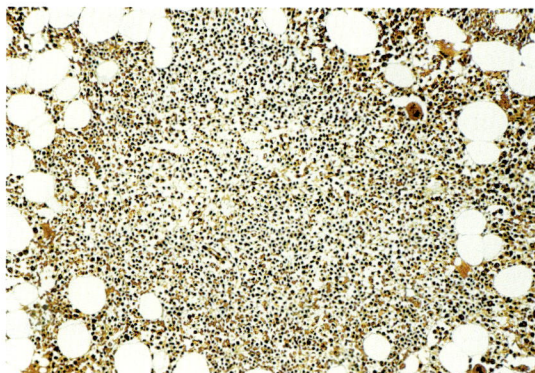

30.16–30.19 Aspects of histologic findings in biopsies of patients with AIDS. 30.16 (left) BMBS plastic, Giemsa, showing hypercellular bone marrow with disorganisation of the marrow architecture, decrease in fat cells and increase in reticular fibers. 30.17 (right) BMBS plastic, Giemsa, area from hypocellular marrow with dysplastic features; note dyserythropoiesis and small, mononuclear megakaryocytes. 30.18 (left) BMBS plastic, Giemsa, showing poorly circumscribed granuloma, lower left. 30.19 (right) BMBS plastic, Gomori, showing large lymphocytic aggregate; patient did not have lymphoma.

and opportunities for treating patients, prospects for a cure remain uncertain, and even improved treatment is unaffordable for most people infected with HIV.

Over the past few years, bone marrow histopathology in AIDS has been extensively studied. The results of even the early investigations led to the speculation that the bone marrow is a target organ in AIDS, though to date no direct evidence has been put forward to support this claim, as retroviral infection of bone marrow progenitors has not been demonstrated. AIDS virus has been detected in macrophages from brain tissue of AIDS patients with encephalopathy. Presumably these macrophages were infected at the portal of entry and migrated. Therefore, the bone marrow could become infected in a similar fashion. Since the macrophage is directly and initially involved in AIDS, it was considered appropriate to consider the bone marrow manifestations of AIDS in this section.

With the increase in the number of patients suffering from AIDS has come the recognition that AIDS patients are especially susceptible, and that disease manifestations in these patients may differ from those in the general population. This applies to a variety of infections, as well as to the development of malignant lymphomas, Kaposi's sarcoma, and other neoplasms. For example, the gastrointestinal tract, brain and heart as predominant sites for malignant lymphomas, the incidence of which has been steadily increasing in AIDS patients. Hematological abnormalities are also common in AIDS patients, who therefore frequently undergo examination of the bone marrow during investigation for cytopenias, opportunistic infections, malignancies and fever of unknown origin.

A wide spectrum of findings has been reported in the bone marrow, ranging from marked hypocellularity to normocellularity and hypercellularity with disappearance of fat cells (Table 30.1). An 'AIDS pattern' has been described, characterised by separation of fat cells by hematopoietic elements in contrast with normal marrow where small groups of fat cells are closely apposed without intervening hematopoietic elements. However, this finding was not confirmed by other workers in subsequent reports. Other features include marrow damage, areas of serous or gelatinous atrophy, or even necrosis with or without hemophagocytosis, lymphoplasmacytic aggregates, histiocytosis, plasmacytosis, eosinophilia, uni-, bi-, or trilinear myelodysplasias, 'naked' megakaryocyte nuclei, giant neutrophil and megaloblastoid erythroid elements and hypoplasias, granulomas, an increase or decrease of stainable iron, reticulin fibrosis and demonstrable organisms, especially *Mycobacterium avium intracellulare*. These have been found in granulomas which are poorly circumscribed, as well as in macrophages dispersed in the marrow,

and some of these macrophages may resemble the storage cells in Gaucher's disease. The lymphohistiocytic aggregates may be accompanied by vascular proliferations, and may be indistinguishable (by morphology alone) from bone marrow involvement by peripheral T cell lymphoma or AILD or HD. Diffuse bone marrow lymphocytosis, as well as lymphocytic aggregates, nodules and follicles, have been observed. Since both HD and malignant lymphomas may be present in the bone marrow in these patients, the findings must be distinguished from purely reactive changes. Both morphologic characteristics and immunohistologic investigations are required. The increase in the incidence of lymphomas and HD in patients with HIV infection is directly related to immunosuppression. There is presumably expansion of multiple clones of lymphocytes infected with Epstein–Barr virus; they develop into high-grade lymphomas arising at extranodal sites. These AIDS-related HD and malignant lymphomas usually have an advanced stage at presentation, and follow an aggressive course, though responsive to therapy, at least initially. The bone marrow is frequently involved. The Reed–Sternberg-like cells have an activated B cell phenotype and are EBV-LMP-1 positive, often CD30+ and CD15−.

In summary, the pathogenesis of the bone marrow findings in AIDS is undoubtedly multifactorial: (1) possibly involving direct retroviral infection of hematopoietic precursors, (2) abnormal regulation of hematopoiesis due to micro-environmental defects, (3) a variety of immune phenomena, (4) the response of the bone marrow to the infections, (5) the direct effects of the infections on the marrow (it is of interest that a case of transmission of HIV through transplantation of bone has recently been reported), and (6) effects, often adverse, of therapy of HIV on the bone marrow.

The bone marrow in the primary immunodeficiency syndromes

The diagnosis is made on the basis of the clinical findings, laboratory tests and peripheral blood examinations. A bone marrow biopsy is generally not taken.

TABLE 30.1 Bone and marrow changes in iliac crest biopsies of AIDS patients

	Percentage
Hematopoiesis	
Hypercellular	32
Hypocellular	24
Myelodysplastic	75
Stroma	
Serous atrophy	42
Plasmacytosis	72
Increased iron stores	85
Vasculitis, mast cells	35
Diffuse fibrosis	25
Lymphoid nodules (follicles)	15
Granulomas	10
Organisms	8
Bone	
Osteopenia	20
Osteosclerosis	4
Increased osseous remodeling	20

Check list: Mononuclear Phagocyte System (MPS, M-PIRE)

- Adequate biopsy; 20–30 mm after exclusion of cortex.
- Structure of cortical and cancellous bone.
- Lytic lesions?
- Active remodeling?
- Foci of involvement – patchy, complete?
- Type of mononuclear cell population. I.H.: CD68, TRAP, αI antitrypsin, lysozyme.
- Nuclear characteristics.
- Cytoplasm – amount, features, inclusions.
- Characteristics of stored material and phagocytosis, PAS, iron stain.
- Residual hematopoiesis: quantity, dysplastic features, I.H.: myeloperoxidase, Factor VIII.
- Quantity and location of fibrosis, reticulin stain. I.H.: vimentin, actin.

Clinical correlations

LCH – Langerhans Cell Histiocytosis

- Uni- or multifocal, uni- at any age, multi- in children.
- Lesions involve ribs, mandible, vertebrae, pelvis.
- Lesions asymptomatic, or pain and swelling may occur.
- Bone scans, CT, MRI – to determine number of sites.
- Association with other conditions, e.g. ML.
- Clonal chromosomal characteristics

  Gaucher disease
  the gene is at chromosome 1q21.

  Niemann–Pick disease
  the autosomal recessive gene has not yet been characterised.

  Fabry's disease
  x-linked recessive disease.

  Histiocytosis
  autosomal recessive disorder.

  Malignant histiocytosis
  t(2;5)(p23;q35)
  t(1;5)(p32;q35)
  t(5;6)(q35;p12).

Bibliography

Abe R., Akaike Y., Yokoyama A. *et al.* (1990) High incidence of 17p13 chromosomal abnormalities in malignant histiocytosis. *Cancer*, **65 (12)**, 2689–96.

Ahluwalia C., Bernstein-Singer M., Beckstead J., Brynes R.K. (1991) Kaposi's sarcoma in the bone marrow of a patient with AIDS. *Am. J. Clin. Pathol.*, **95 (4)**, 561–4.

Arkin A.M., Schein A.J. (1948) Aseptic necrosis in Gaucher's disease. *J Bone Jt Surg.*, 30A, 631.

Armstutz H.C., Carey E.J. (1966) Skeletal manifestations and treatment of Gaucher's disease. *J Bone Jt Surg.*, **48A**, 670.

Barton N.W., Brady R.O., Dambrosia J.M. (1991) Replacement therapy for inherited enzyme deficiency – macrophage-targeted glucocerebrosidase for Gaucher's disease. *N Engl J Med.*, **324**, 1464.

Baumann M.A., Pacheco J., Paul C.C. *et al.* (1988) Paroxysmal nocturnal hemoglobinuria associated with the acquired immunodeficiency syndrome. *Arch. Intern. Med.*, **148 (1)**, 212–13.

Baumgartner I., von Hochstetter A., Baumert B. *et al.* (1997) Langerhans'-cell histiocytosis in adults. *Med Pediatr Oncol.*, **28 (1)**, 9–14

Beighton P., Goldblatt J., Sacks S. (1982) Bone involvement in Gaucher's disease: a

century of delineation and research. In Desnick and Grabowski (eds), *Progress in Clinical and Biological Research*, vol. **95**. New York: Alan R. Liss, p. 107.

Bello J.L., Burgaleta C., Magallon M. *et al.* (1990) Hematological abnormalities in hemophiliac patients with human immunodeficiency virus infection. *Am J Hematol*, **33 (4)**, 230–3.

Beutler E. (1991) Gaucher's disease. *New Engl J Med.*, **325**, 1354.

Bigorgne C., Le Tourneau A., Messing B. *et al.* (1996) Sea-blue histiocyte syndrome in bone marrow secondary to toal parenteral nutrition including fat-emulsion sources: a clinicopathologic study of seven cases. *Br J Haematol*, **95** (2), 258–62.

Brizzi M.F., Porcu P., Porteri A., Pegoraro L. (1990) Hematologic abnormalities in the acquired immunodeficiency syndrome. *Hematologica*, **75** (5), 454–63.

Browett P.J., Varcoe A.R., Fraser A.G., Ellis-Pegler R.B. (1988) Disseminated tuberculosis complicated by the hemophagocytic syndrome. *Aust., N.Z. J. Med.*, **18** (1), 79–80.

Brunning R.D., Mckenna R.W. (1994) Histiocytic proliferations of the bone marrow. In *Tumors of the Bone Marrow. Atlas of Tumor Pathology*, 3rd series, fascicle 9. Washington: Armed Forces Institute of Pathology, pp. 439–55.

Callihan T.R. (1995) Langerhans' cell histiocytosis (histiocytosis X). In E.S. Jaffe (ed), *Surgical Pathology of the Lymph Nodes and Related Organs*, 2nd edn, **16**, pp. 534–59.

Candido A., Rossi P., Menichella G. *et al.* (1990) Indicative morphological myelodysplastic alterations of bone marrow in overt AIDS. *Hematologica*, **75** (4), 327–33.

Casassus P., Roulot D., Le Roux G. *et al.* (1990) Lymphomatous bone marrow necrosis in a case of AIDS. *Ann. Med. Interne.*, **141** (5), 476–8.

Castella A., Croxson T.S., Mildvan D. (1985) The bone marrow in AIDS. A histologic, hematologic and microbiologic study. *Clin Pathol.*, **84**, 425.

Chan J.K., Ng C.S., Law C.K. *et al.* (1987) Reactive hemophagocytic syndrome: a study of 7 fatal cases. *Pathology*, **19** (1), 43–50.

Chen R.L., Su I.J., Lin K.H. *et al.* (1991) Fulminant childhood hemophagocytic syndrome mimicking histiocytic medullary reticulosis. An atypical form of Epstein–Barr virus infection. *Am. J. Clin. Pathol.*, **96** (2), 171–6.

Chetty R., Biddolph S., Gatter K. (1997) An immunohistochemical analysis of Reed–

Sternberg-like cells in post-transplantation lymphoproliferative disorders: the possible pathogeneic relationship to Reed–Sternberg cells in Hodgin's disease and Reed–Sternberg-like cells in non-Hodgkin's lymphomas and reactive conditions. *Hum Pathol.*, **28** (4), 493–8.

Christensson B., Braconier J.H., Winqvist I. *et al.* (1987) Fulminant course of infectious mononucleosis with virus-associated hemophagocytic syndrome. *Scand. J. Infect. Dis.*, **19** (3), 373–9.

Ciaudo M., Doco-Lecompte T., Guettier C. *et al.* (1994) Revisited indications for bone marrow examinations in HIV-infected patients. *Eur J Haematol*, **53** (3), 168–74.

Clatch R.J., Krigman H.R., Peters M.G., Zutter M.M. (1994) Dysplastic haemopoiesis following orthotopic liver transplantation: comparison with similar changes in HIV infection and primary myelodysplasia. *Br J Haematol*, **88** (4), 685–92.

Cohn J.A. (1997) Recent advances; HIV infection – I. *BMJ*, **314**, 487–91.

Dash S., Behera K.C., Patnaik B.K. (1990) Type-II infantile form of Guacher's disease. *Indian J. Pathol. Microbiol.*, **33** (2), 190–2.

Daum G.S., Sullivan J.L., Ansell J. *et al.* (1987) Virus-associated hemophagocytic syndrome: identification of an immunoptoliferative precursor lesion. *Hum. Pathol.*, **18** (10), 1071–4.

Davis B.R., Zauli G. (1995) Effect of human immunodeficiency virus infection on haematopoiesis. *Bailleres Clin Haematol*, **8**, 113–30.

de Cremoux H., Monnet I., Fleury J., Chleq C. (1991) Histiocytic medullary reticulosis occurring with small cell lung carcinoma. *Eur. Respir. J.*, **4** (1), 122–4.

Dehner L.P. (1991) Morphologic findings in the histiocytic syndromes. *Semin Oncol.*, **18**, 8.

Delacretaz F., Perey L., Schmidt P.M. (1987) Histopathology of bone marrow in human

immunodeficiency virus infection. *Virch Arch.*, **411**, 543.

Diebold J., Tabbara W., Marche C. *et al.* (1991) Modifications de la moelle osseuse a divers stades de l'infection par VIH etudiees par biopsie medullaire chez quatre-vingt-cinq patients. *Arch Anat Cytol Pathol*, **39** (4), 137–46.

Elema J.D., Atmosoerodjo-Briggs J.E. (1984) Langerhans' cells and macrophages in eosinophilic granuloma: an enzyme-histochemical, enzyme-cytochemical, and ultrastructural study. *Cancer*, **54**, 2174.

Emilie D., Touitou R., Raphael M. *et al.* (1992) *In vivo* production of interleukin-10 by malignant cells in AIDS lymphomas. *Eur. J. Immunol.*, **22** (11), 2937–42.

Falini B., Pileri S., de Solas I. *et al.* (1990) Peripheral T-cell lymphoma associated with hemophagocytic syndrome. *Blood*, **76** (10), 434–44.

Favara B.E. (1991) Langerhans' cell histiocytosis pathobiology and pathogenesis. *Sem Oncol*, **18**, 3–7.

Frank T.S., Reed J.C., Brooks J.J. (1993) Absence of expression of c-sis and transforming growth factor-β mRNA in malignant fibrous histiocytoma. *Surg Pathol*, **5** (2), 141–50.

Frisch B., Bartl R., Goebel F.D. (1989) Bone marrow manifestations in the acquired immune deficiency syndrome (AIDS). A study of 40 patients and review of the literature. *Haematol Rev.*, **3**, 177.

Geissler R.G., Ottmann O.G., Eder M. *et al.* (1991) Effect of recombinant human transforming growth factor beta and tumor necrosis factor alpha on bone marrow progenitor cells of HIV-infected persons. *Ann. Hematol.*, **62** (5), 151–5.

Gold J.E., Schwam L., Castella A. *et al.* (1990) Malignant plasma cell tumors in human immunodeficiency virus-infected patients. *Cancer*, **66** (2), 363–8.

Goldstein D. (1996) HIV associated malignancies. *Hematol Rev and Comm*, **9** (4), 275–84.

335

Gollub H., Machill K., Sander P. (1989) Infection-associated hemophagocytic syndrome with a lethal outcome. *Dtsch. Med. Wochenschr.*, **114 (44)**, 1697–701.

Gonzalez C.L., Medeiros L.J., Braziel R.M., Jaffe, E.S. (1991) T-cell lymphoma involving subcutaneous tissue. A clinicopathologic entity commonly associated with hemophagocytic syndrome. *Am. J. Surg. Pathol.*, **15 (1)**, 17–27.

Gonzalez C.L., Jaffe E.S. (1990) The histiocytosis: clinical presentation and differential diagnosis. *Oncology*, **4**, 47–60.

Greenfield G.B. (1970) Bone changes in chronic adult Gaucher's disease. *Amer. J Roentgenol.*, **110**, 800.

Groopman J.E., Golde D.W. (1981) The histiocytic disorder: a pathophysiologic analysis. *Ann Intern Med.*, **94**, 95.

Hara T., Mizuno Y., Ueda K. *et al.* (1989) Virus-associated hemophagocytic syndrome: the diagnostic usefulness of immature histiocytes with benign features in the bone marrow. *Nippon. Ketsueki. Gakkai. Zasshi.*, **52 (4)**, 796–9.

Hassinger S.L., Schiffer C.A., Sun C.C. (1989) Acute myeloblastic leukemia with extensive erythrophagocytosis mimicking malignant histiocytosis. *Am J Clin Pathol*, **92 (5)**, 696–700.

Henry K., Costello C. (1994) HIV-associated bone marrow changes. *Curr Diagnost Pathol.*, **1**, 131–41.

Henter J.I., Elinder G., Ost A. (1991) Diagnostic guidelines for hemophagocytic lymphohistiocytosis. *Sem Oncol.*, **18**, 29–33.

Howard M.R., Kesteven P.J. (1993) Sea blue histiocytosis: a common abnormality of the bone marrow in myelodysplastic syndromes. *J Clin Pathol*, **46 (11)**, 1030–2.

Itoyama T., Sadamori N., Sasagawa I. *et al.* (1991) A T-cell neoplasia showing clinicopathologic features of malignant histiocytosis with novel chromosomal abnormalities and N-ras mutation. *Cancer*, **67 (8)**, 2103–10.

Jurlander J., Caligiuri M.A., Ruutu T. *et al.* (1996) Persistence of the AML1/ETO fusion transcript in patients treated with allogeneic bone marrow transplantation for t(8;21) leukemia. *Blood*, **88 (6)**, 2183–91.

Kaneko Y., Maseki N., Sakurai M. *et al.* (1995) Clonal and non-clonal karyotypically abnormal cells in haematophagocytic lymphohistiocytosis. *Br J Haematol*, **90 (1)**, 48–55.

Karcher D.S. (1993) Clinically unsuspected Hodgkin's disease presenting initially in the bone marrow of patients infected with the human immunodeficiency virus. *Cancer*, **71 (4)**, 1235–8.

Karcher D.S., Frost A.R. (1991) The bone marrow in human immunodeficiency virus (HIV)-related disease. Morphology and clinical correlation. *Am. J. Clin. Pathol.*, **95 (1)**, 63–71.

Keen C.E., Philip G., Parker B.C., Souhami R.L. (1990) Unusual bony lesions of histiocytosis X in a patient previously treated for Hodgkin's disease. *Pathol Res Pract.*, **186**, 519.

Kohalmi F., Strausz J., Egervary M. *et al.* (1996) Differential expression of markers in extensive and restricted Langerhans Cell Histiocytosis (LCH) *Pathol Oncol Res.*, **2 (3)**, 184–7.

Komatsu M., Katakura M., Aizawa T. *et al.* (1991) Unusual clinical presentation of malignant histiocytosis in a 70-year-old woman. *J. Intern. Med.*, **230 (1)**, 73–7.

Kosmo M.A., Mitsuyasu R.T., Sparkes R.S., Gale R.P. (1987) Trisomy 12 in Burkitt-like lymphoma associated with acquired immunodeficiency syndrome. *Cancer Genet. Cytogenet.*, **29 (2)**, 245–51.

Lee R.E. (1988) Histiocytic diseases of bone marrow. *Hematol/Oncol Clin N Amer.*, **2 (4)**, 657.

Levine A.M. (1992) Acquired immunodeficiency syndrome-related lymphoma. Response. *Blood*, **80 (11)**, 2945–46.

Levy J., Wodell R.A., August C.S., Bayever E. (1990) Adenovirus-related hemophagocytic syndrome after bone marrow transplantation. *Bone Marrow Transplant.*, **6 (5)**, 349–52.

Loy T.S., Diaz-Arias A.A., Perry M.C. (1991) Familial erythrophagocytic lympho-histiocytosis. *Sem Oncol.*, **18**, 34–8.

Mankin H.J., Doppelt S.H., Rosenberg A.E., Barranger J.A. (1990) Metabolic bone disease in patients with Gaucher's disease. In Avioli and Krane (eds), *Metabolic Bone Disease*. Philadelphia: W.B. Saunders, p. 130.

Marche C., Tabbara W., Michon C. *et al.* (1990) Bone marrow findings in HIV infection: a pathological study. *Prog. AIDS Pathol.* **2**, 51–60.

Maya M.M., Fried K., Gendel E.S. (1993) AIDS-related lymphoma: An unusual cause of omental caking. *Am. J. Roengenology*, **160 (3)**, 661.

Milam M.W., Balerdi M.J., Toney J.F. *et al.* (1990) Epitheloid angiomatosis secondary to disseminated cat scratch disease involving the bone marrow and skin in a patient with acquired immune deficiency syndrome: a case report. *Am J Med*, **88 (2)**, 180–3.

Mogilner B.M., Barak Y., Amitay M., Zlotogora J. (1990) Hyperphosphatasemia in infantile GMI gangliosidosis: possible association with microscopic bone marrow osteoblastosis. *J Pediatr.*, **117 (5)**, 758.

Mollnes T.E., Harboe M. (1996) Clinical immunology. *BMJ*, **312**, 1465–9.

Morales L.E. (1996) Gaucher's disease: a review. *Ann Pharmacother.*, **30 (4)**, 381–8.

Mroczek E.C., Weisenburger D.D., Grierson H.L. *et al.* (1987) Fatal infectious mononucleosis and virus-associated hemophagocytic syndrome. *Arch. Pathol. Lab. Med.*, **111 (6)**, 530–5.

Muller H., Weier S., Schneider M. *et al.* (1990) Comparison of HIV-associated dyshemopoiesis in myelodysplastic HIV-negative patients. *Verh. Dtsch. Ges. Pathol.*, **74**, 149–54.

Namiki T.S., Boone D.C., Meyer P.R. (1987) A comparison of bone marrow findings in patients with acquired immunodeficiency syndrome (AIDS) and AIDS related conditions. *Hematol Oncol.*, **5**, 99.

Newcom S.R. (1992) Acquired immunodeficiency syndrome-related lymphoma. *Blood*, **80 (11)**, 2944–5.

Ng C.S., Lam T.K., Chan J.K. *et al.* (1988) Juvenile chronic myeloid leukemia. A malignancy of S-100 protein-positive histiocytes. *Am. J. Clin. Pathol.*, **90 (5)**, 575–82.

Oh J., Bailin T., Fukai K. *et al.* (1996) Positional cloning of a gene for Hermansky–Pudlak syndrome, a disorder of cytoplasmic organelles. *Nat Genet*, **14 (3)**, 300–6.

Ohshima K., Kikuchi M., Eguchi F. *et al.* (1991) Virus-associated hematophagocytic syndrome with Epstein–Barr virus infection. *Virchows Arch. A. pathol. Anat. Histopathol.*, **419 (6)**, 519–22.

Paulson J.A., Marti G.E., Fink J.K. *et al.* (1989) Richter's transformation of lymphoma complicating Gaucher's disease. *Hematol. Pathol.*, **3 (2)**, 91–6.

Paxton W.A., Martin S.R., Tse D. *et al.* (1996) Relative resistance to HIV-1 infection of CD4 lymphocytes from persons who remain uninfected despite multiple high-risk sexual exposures. *Nature Med*, **2 (4)**, 412–16.

Pinckney L., Parker B.R. (1977) Myelo-sclerosis and myelofibrosis in treated histiocytosis X. *Amer J Roentgenol.*, **129**, 521.

Prego V., Glatt A.E., Roy V. *et al.* (1990) Comparative yield of blood culture for fungi and mycobacteria, liver biopsy and bone marrow biopsy in the diagnosis of fever of undetermined origin in human immuno-deficiency virus-infected patients. *Arch Intern Med*, **150 (10)**, 2204.

Prevot S., Raphael M., Fournier J.G., Diebold J. (1993) Detection by *in situ* hybridization of HIV and *c-myc* RNA in tumour cells of AIDS-related B-cell lymphomas. *Histopathology*, **22 (2)**, 151–6.

Pugh-Humphreys R.G.P. (1992) Macrophage-neoplastic cell interactions: implications for neoplastic cell growth. *FEMS Microbiol Immunol.*, **105 (5–6)**, 289–308.

Reynolds P., Saunders L.D., Layefsky M.E., Lemp G.F. (1993) The spectrum of acquired immunodeficiency syndrom (AIDS)-associated malignancies in San Francisco, 1980–1987. *Am. J. Epidemiology*, **137 (1)**, 19–30.

Rice E.O., Mifflin T.E., Sakallah S. *et al.* (1996) Gaucher disease: studies of phenotype, molecular diagnosis and treatment. *Clin Genet.*, **49 (3)**, 111–18.

Riley U.B., Crawford S., Barrett S.P., Abdalla S.H. (1995) Detection of mycobacteria in bone marrow biopsy specimens taken to investigate pyrexia of unknown origin. *J Clin Pathol*, **48 (8)**, 706–9.

Sacchi G., Zorzi F., Fiorentino M. *et al.* (1990) Bone marrow biopsy in HIV-positive patients with thrombocytopenia. Light and electron microscopy. *Pathologica*, **82 (1080)**, 371–80.

Sakarelou N., Kosmaidou Z., Mesogitis S. *et al.* (1997) Gaucher's disease (type 1) and pregancy. *Cytogenet Cell Genet.*, **77**, 137.

Sheu S.S., Chan L.P., Liao S.C. *et al.* (1994) Fabry's disease: clinical, pathologic and biochemical manifestations in two Chinese males. *Chung Hua I Hsueh Tsa Chih (Taipei)*, **54 (5)**, 368–72.

Shimada M., Kojima M., Tani G. *et al.* (1993) Rheumatoid arthritis and B cell lymphoma with pathological changes of reactive histiocytosis. *J. Clin. Pathol.*, **46 (11)**, 1064.

Thiele J., Zirbes T.K., Bertsch H.P. *et al.* (1996) AIDS-related bone marrow lesions – myelodysplastic features or predominant inflammatory-reactive changes (HIV-myelopathy)? A comparative morphometric study by immunohistochemistry with special emphasis on apoptosis and PCNA-labeling. *Anal Cell Pathol*, **11 (3)**, 141–57.

Turner M.L., Gilmour H.M., McLaren K.M. *et al.* (1993) Regressing atypical histiocytosis: report of two cases with progression to high grade T-cell non-Hodgkin's lymphoma. *Hematol. Pathol.*, **7 (1)**, 33–47.

van Furth, R. (1989) Origin and turnover of monocytes and macrophages. *Curr. Top. Pathol.*, **79**, 125–50.

Vespignani S., Sardeo G., Castronovo S. *et al.* (1991) A case of virus associated hemophagocytic syndrome and malignant histiocytosis: sometimes a difficult distinction. *Recenti. Prog. Med.*, **82 (2)**, 80–2.

Wiley E.L., Perry A., Nightingale S.D., Lawrence J. (1994) Detection of Mycobacterium avium-intracellulare complex in bone marrow specimens of patients with acquired immunodeficiency syndrome. *Am J Clin Pathol*, **101 (4)**, 446–51.

Wong K.F., Chan J.K. (1989) Foamy histiocytes in repeat marrow aspirates (letter). *Pathology*, **21 (2)**, 153–4.

Wong K.F., Chan J.K., Ng C.S. *et al.* (1991) Anaplastic large cell Ki-1 lymphoma involving bone marrow: marrow findings and association with reactive hemophagocytosis. *Am J. Hematol.*, **37 (2)**, 112–19.

Wong K.F., Hui P.K., Chan J.K. *et al.* (1991) The acute lupus hemophagocytic syndrome. *Ann. Intern. Med.*, **114 (5)**, 387–90.

Writing Group of the Histiocyte Society (1987) Histiocytosis syndromes in children. *Lancet*, **January 24**, 208–9.

31 Effects of cytotoxic therapy and bone marrow transplantation (BMT or PBSCT)

Immediate toxicity after ablative chemotherapy (and/or radiotherapy)

The nature of the changes seen after chemotherapy prior to BMT depends on the type, quantity, duration of treatment and length of the interval elapsed following ablative treatment before the transplantation. Though considerable variability has been noted, generally there is rapid and widespread degeneration and necrosis of the hematopoietic and stromal constituents: with complete effacement of the marrow architecture, dilatation and disruption of sinusoids with edema and hemorrhage, and areas of fibrinoid, eosinophilic and somewhat granular serous atrophy (Figures 31.1–31.4). Macrophages with phagocytosed cellular debris, red cells and hemosiderin as well as large fat cells, often multiloculated, appear early after chemotherapy, together with a mild transient increase in reticular fibers. Perivascular and interstitial plasma and mast cells, and some lymphocytes may be found, and there is early activation of osteoblasts. Granulomas are also observed.

Rarely, massive bone marrow necrosis may follow chemotherapy.

With less intensive chemotherapy – and of shorter duration – the changes observed are also less drastic: some reduction in hematopoiesis, increase in fat cells and macrophages and marked megaloblastoid aspect of the erythroblasts. Other cases may show myelodysplastic features reminiscent of MDS, or of aplastic anemia with 'hot spots'. A special influence of adipocytes and of endosteal lining cells on the process of bone marrow regeneration has been postulated on the basis of histological studies before and after therapy for acute leukemia.

Restitution of hematopoiesis
(Figures 31.5–31.9)

This usually starts at 7–14 days – small foci of immature cells appear and tend to occur in the paratrabecular regions, and in close association to fat cells, sometimes precursors surround the fat cells. Possibly there is some connection with restoration of the microenvironment

31.1 (left) Aspects of bone marrow toxicity. BMBS plastic, Gomori, low-power showing widespread ablation of bone marrow.

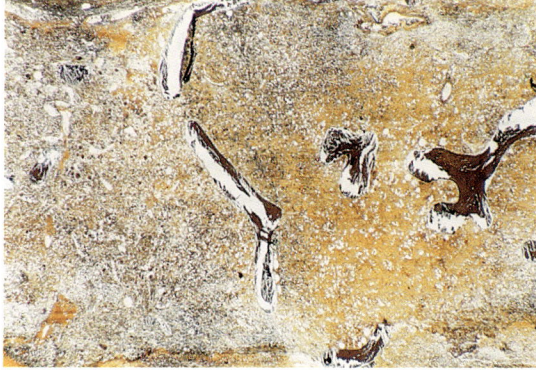

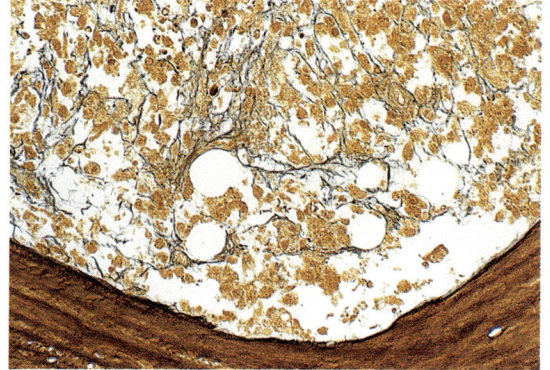

31.2 (right) BMBS plastic Gomori, necrosis of tumor cells several days after initial chemotherapy.

31.3 (left) BMBS plastic, Giemsa, showing marrow atrophy with some plasma cells and lymphocytes.

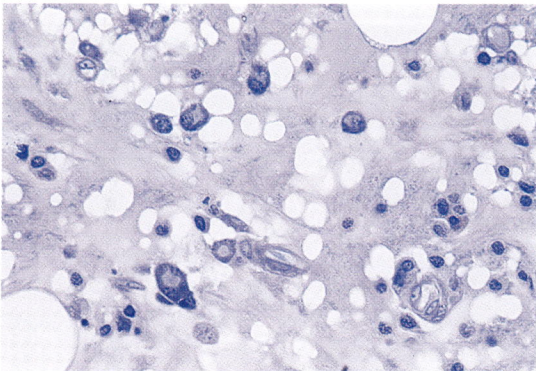

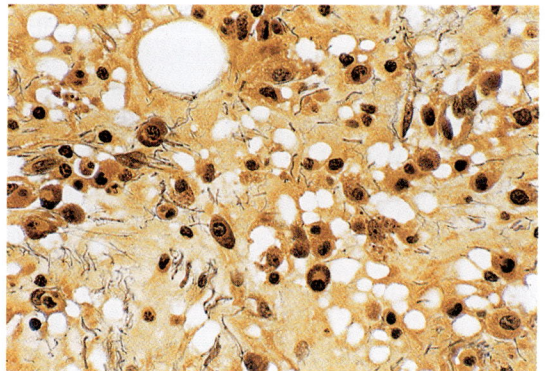

31.4 (right) BMBS paraffin, reticulin stain, necrosis of marrow and fibrosis after chemotherapy.

31.5 (left) BMBS plastic, Gomori, incipient regeneration foci of erythropoiesis, fat cells present, but stroma not yet restored.

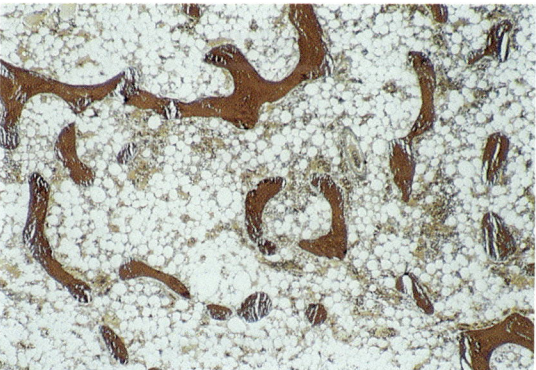

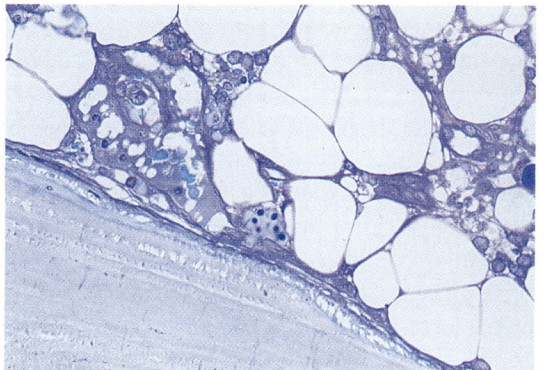

31.6 (right) BMBS plastic, Giemsa, showing small group of erythroblasts at trabecular surface.

31.7 (left) BMBS plastic, Giemsa, hematopoietic precursors, incomplete restoration of stroma with residual fibrosis.

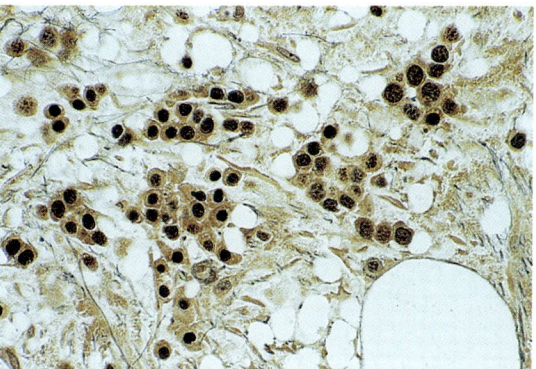

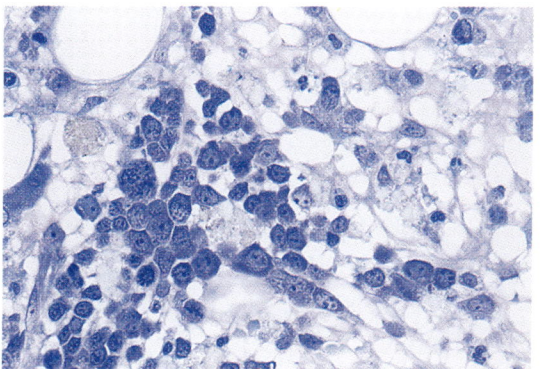

31.8 (right) BMBS plastic, Giemsa, showing progressive regeneration, large erythroid island with megaloblastoid features and maturation arrest.

required for hematopoiesis; while the para-trabecular localisation may be due to an association of hematopoietic stem cells with endosteal lining cells. Erythro- and myelopoiesis appear before megakaryopoiesis. The foci of regenerating cells gradually increase. All three cell lines show dysplastic features initially – megablastosis, maturation arrest, left shift and other changes in size and shape of nuclei. The dyserythropoiesis includes ringed sideroblasts. As regeneration proceeds, the stroma is also reconstituted, the edema and hemorrhage are absorbed, and macrophages and reticular fibers decrease. Islands and clusters of erythroid, myeloid and megakaryocytic precursors are then found throughout the marrow. Dysplastic features may persist for variable periods of time. Moreover, considerable variability in the speed and sequence of restitution of hematopoiesis has also been described when biopsies were analysed from 2 to 56 weeks from start of therapy.

Persistent effects (Figure 31.10)

In some cases, long-lasting effects have been documented especially after combined chemo- and radiotherapy or direct radiation to areas containing active hematopoietic marrow. Irreversible stem cell and stromal damage is produced and these sites remain hypo- or aplastic, as subsequently circulating peripheral blood stem cells apparently do not settle and repopulate them.

In other patients, the myelodysplasia may not resolve and leukemia eventually develops.

This occurs especially in patients who received alkylating agents or combinations of radio- and chemotherapy.

Additional manifestations

Occasionally multiple or large granulomas are seen and/or increases in macrophages and histiocytes which may indicate intercurrent infections, especially viral. The rate of regeneration and maturation of hematopoiesis may be altered so that foci and clusters of blasts, or sheets of promyelocytes, or of erythroid and megakaryocytic precursors at the same stage of maturation are found. Lymphoid cell precursors ('hematogones') may be prominent in children.

Bone (Figure 31.11)

Following ablative chemotherapy with or without radiation, effects are seen on the bone cells: estimated osteocyte viability decreased for over 4 weeks after transplantation; and further loss of osteocytes was noted subsequently. At the same time, osteoblastic activity with formation of new osteocytes began at the trabecular surface. Subsequently, osteoblastic trabecular bone remodeling may be increased – it appears to be more prominent in hypocellular bone marrows. Extensive osteoid seams may also develop, so that the picture resembles that in osteomalacia; as well as foci of osteoblastic remodeling with accompanying increase in blood vessels and fibers.

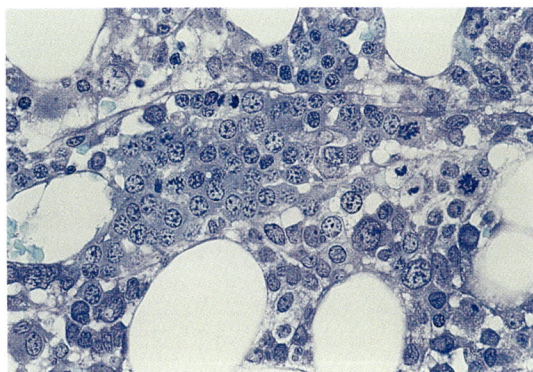

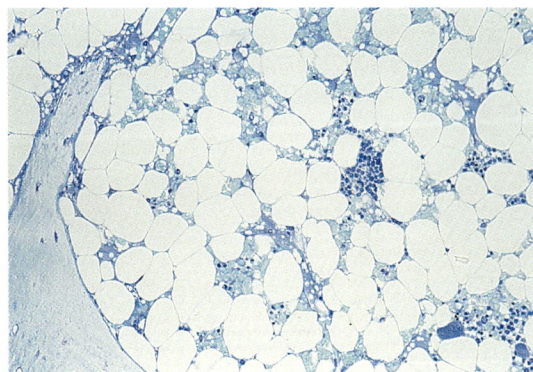

31.9 (left) BMBS plastic, Giemsa, illustrating large erythroid islands and mainly immature myeloid precursors.
31.10 (right) BMBS, plastic, Giemsa, bone marrow of patient with persistent cytopenia after aggressive chemotherapy for breast cancer. No restitution of hematopoiesis.

31.11–31.21 Examples of residual disease following chemotherapy, confirmed by immunohistology and/or flow cytometry.

31.11 BMBS, plastic, Giemsa, showing increased osteoblastic remodeling with wide osteoid seams in patient treated for ML before transplantation.

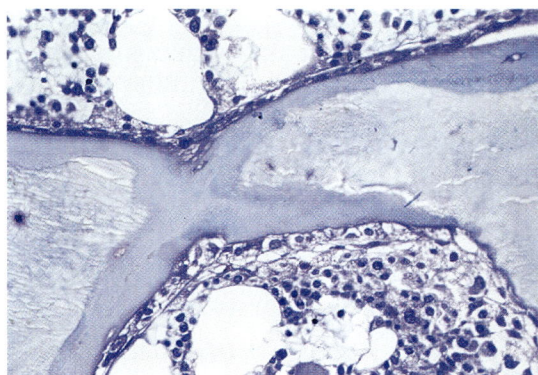

TABLE 31.1 Indications for BT and PBSCT

Lymphomas
Acute leukemias
Multiple myeloma
Hodgkin's disease
Chronic myeloid leukemia
Myelodysplasias
Aplastic anemia
Hereditary hematologic conditions
Disseminated solid tumors

Bone marrow transplantation

The aim of BMT is reconstitution of the hematopoietic system by transfer and engraftment of pluripotent (stem) cells from the patient (autologous transplant) or a suitable donor (allogeneic) transplant, after the underlying disease has been eliminated. In both cases, the cells may be obtained from the bone marrow or the peripheral blood (peripheral blood stem cell transplantation, PBSCT). BMT or PBSCT are now carried out in both hematologic and other malignancies, and non-malignant conditions (Table 31.1). However, this is not yet a routine procedure, and each patient is carefully evaluated beforehand; children as well as adults. Moreover, the late effects of

bone marrow transplantation still need to be determined in a large population, particularly the risk of new solid cancers.

The effects on the bone marrow – both hematopoiesis and stroma of the ablative chemo- and/or radiotherapy, are similar to those described above. Regeneration occurs 7–14 days after BMT and initially consists of one cell type, monotypic. Within days, however, intertrabecular colonies of all three cell types are present. There appears to be a relationship between fat cells and hematopoietic precursors as well as with other stromal elements in the re-establishment of hematopoiesis indicating its requirement for the proper microenvironment.

Delayed engraftment may be due to: a mismatched graft, a T cell depleted bone marrow, a damaged bone marrow due to previous extensive cytotoxic therapy. Administration of colony-stimulating factors may be useful in some of these patients. The myelosuppression and immune dysfunction in transplanted patients predispose them to a large variety of potentially fatal infections with both conventional and unusual organisms.

Severe bone marrow fibrosis before cytotoxic therapy and bone marrow transplantation may have an adverse effect on subsequent hematopoietic recovery. In addition, in allograft recipients, immunosuppressive therapy such as antithymocyte globulin or cyclosporin may result in reduction in lymphocytes in the bone marrow, and dysplastic features in the hematopoietic cell lines.

Failure of bone marrow transplantation – rejection and graft versus host disease (GVHD)

GVHD, which occurs within 100 days of transplantation, is called acute, and chronic if the onset is after that time. The severity of GVHD correlates with the number of donor T cells infused. One of the hallmarks of chronic GVHD is myelosuppression (Figures 31.12 and 31.13).

Declining peripheral blood cell counts (or failure to regenerate in the first instance) indicate any of the above. The bone marrow shows a decrease in cellularity, necrosis of hematopoietic and stromal elements, edema, hemorrhage, macrophages and other infiltrating cells, in particular histiocytes with foamy eosinophilic cytoplasm. Failure of bone marrow transplant engraftment could also be due to a microenvironmental defect in the recipient's marrow.

As the transplanted, regenerating marrow is more susceptible to infections (especially viral) and to drugs (including some antibodies and antiviral agents), both may also cause graft failure.

Relapse of acute leukemia in transplanted patients may be accompanied by myelodysplasia of all three cell lines.

Transplantation of other organs

Dysplastic features in hemopoietic cell lines are also found after transplantation of organs other than bone marrow; for example, liver, kidney and pancreas.

Detection of residual disease
(Figures 30.14–30.21)

Many of the sophisticated methods now available for the detection of residual and of minimal residual disease are highly sensitive, and range from >1 to 5%; for example, in certain cases one malignant cell in 100,000 or even 1,000,000 normal bone marrow aspirate cells may be identified. When foci or clusters of residual cells are found by morphology,

cytochemistry or immunologic methods, there is some doubt about their significance. Moreover, three main questions still beset the problem of residual disease:

1. The heterogeneity of the bone marrow itself and the large variations in distribution of

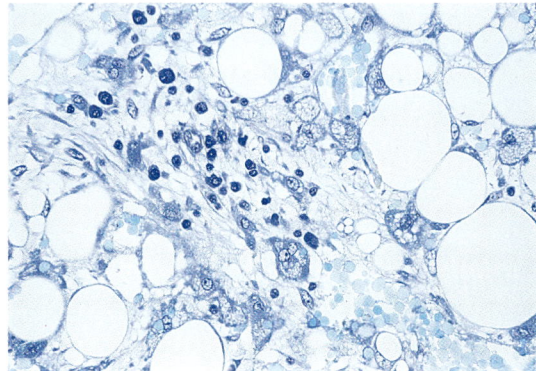

31.12 BMBS plastic, Giemsa, illustrating graft versus host disease after 3 weeks, presenting as sudden, severe pancytopenia. There was virtually no hematopoiesis, some infiltrating cells, disruption of marrow stroma and numerous macrophages.

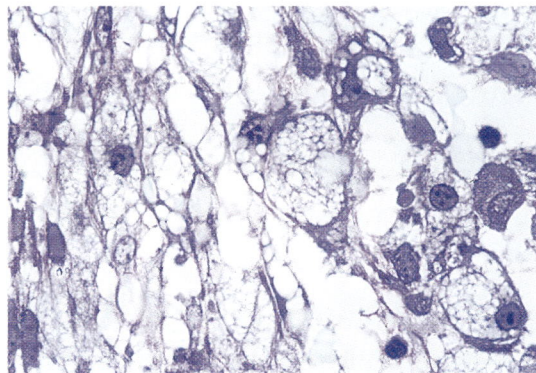

31.13 As for Figure 31.12, BMBS, showing macrophages containing hematopoietic precursors, upper left and lower right.

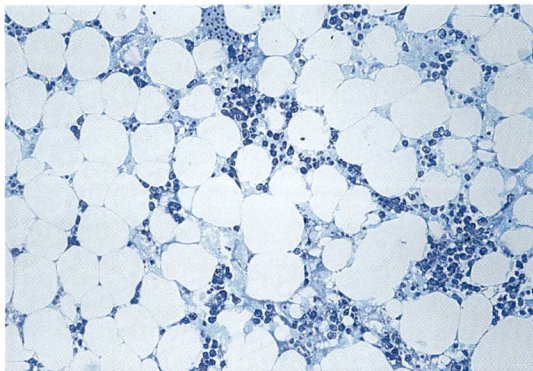

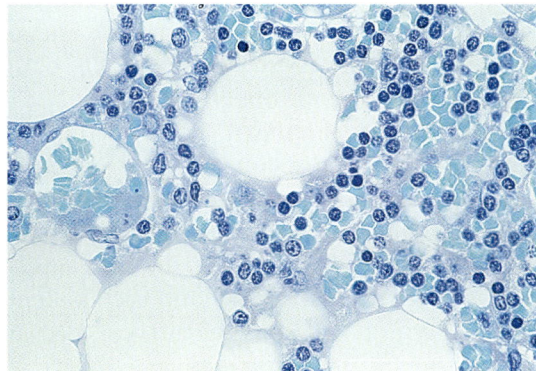

31.14 (left) BMBS plastic, Giemsa, showing residual acute leukemia.

31.15 (right) BMBS plastic, Giemsa, showing residual CLL.

31.16 (left) BMBS plastic, Giemsa, showing residual myeloma; note nucleolated cells.

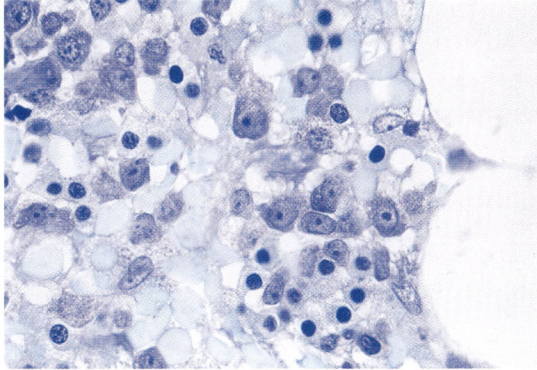

31.17 (right) BMBS plastic, Gomori, with residual nodules in atrophic marrow, after aggressive therapy of MM.

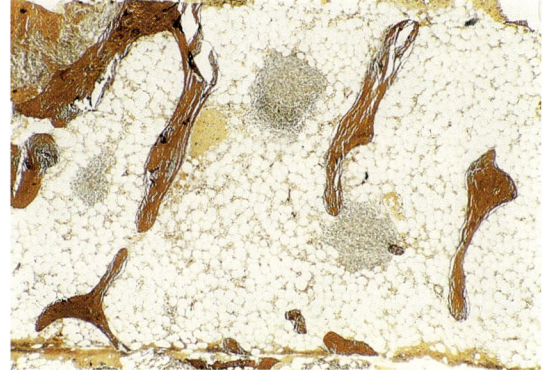

31.18 (left) BMBS paraffin, H&E, residual hairy cell infiltration after therapy.

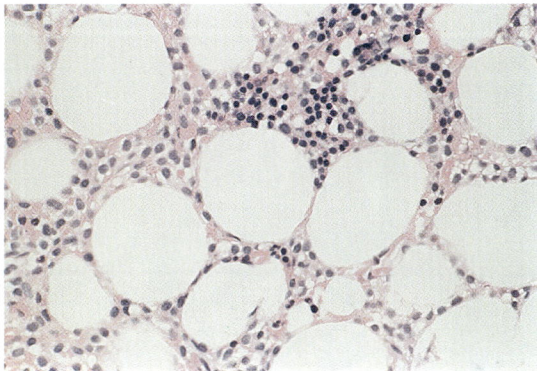

31.19 (right) BMBS paraffin, same biopsy as for Figure 31.18, stained with hairy cell antigen demarcating residual hairy cell infiltration.

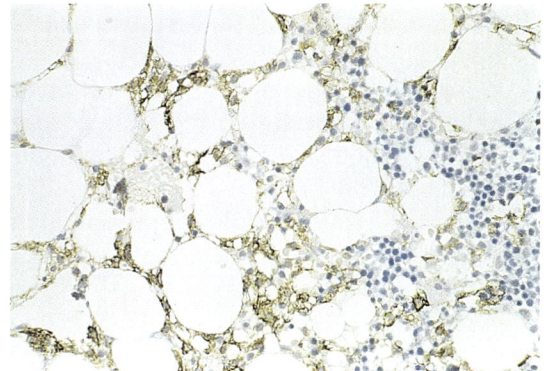

31.20 BMBS plastic, Gomori, case of prostatic cancer, post-therapy with residual metastasis.

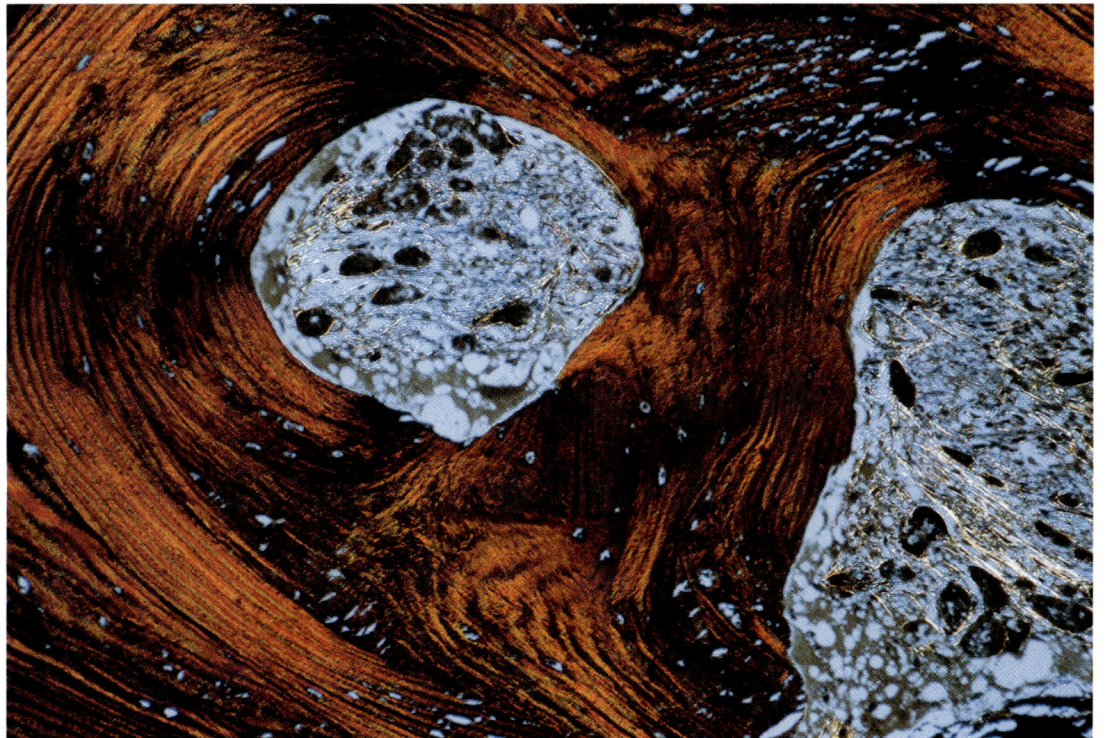

malignant cells so that the involved areas may not be sampled: for example, a focal pattern of residual involvement in APL. Residual disease may therefore be widespread and difficult, if not impossible, to evaluate quantitatively.

2. Cytotoxic therapy may interfere with the host's immune surveillance and ability to eradicate the malignant cells and prevent recurrence. For example, it is well known that patients apparently cured of breast cancer may develop distant metastases (previously unrecognised in spite of intensive investigation) 5–20 years later. Presumably the malignant cells were held in check and kept dormant by host factors, until something happened to upset the balance.

3. The clinical significance of the detection of minimal residual disease has not yet been established unequivocally. For example, minimal hairy cell infiltration may be found in patients who are in complete remission after treatment for HCL and there are conflicting reports as to its significance; likewise for some cases of AML expressing the AML7/ETO fusion transcript in complete remission, indicating that these cells were not eradicated by the cytotoxic therapy. In addition, it has been shown that in acute and chronic leukemias the detection of minimal residual disease does not necessarily predict relapse, therefore, there is a need to redefine the concept of remission. Moreover, when bone is very carefully checked in biopsies of patients treated for lymphomas, residual disease may sometimes be found in the cortex. Whether this constitutes a 'sanctuary site' or even has any practical significance is entirely unknown. Similarly, metastatic cells may also occasionally be seen in bone after the patient has received chemotherapy; but a large series would have to be examined before any conclusions could be drawn. Recurrence of a lymphoma may occur several years after chemotherapy (Figure 31.22).

Bone marrow response to cytokine therapy: effect of growth factors on bone marrow

This depends on whether single or multiple agents are given. Following granulocyte-

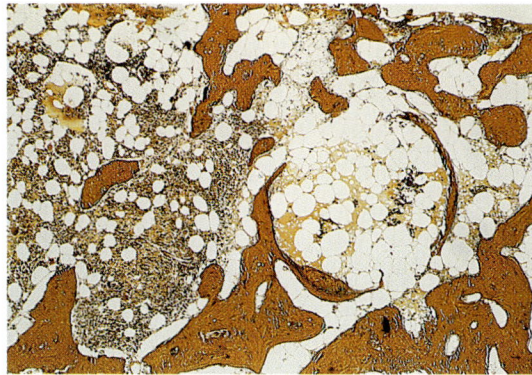

31.21 BMBS plastic, Gomori, with residual evidence of previous metastasis as shown by the osteosclerotic reaction, but no metastatic cells were found.

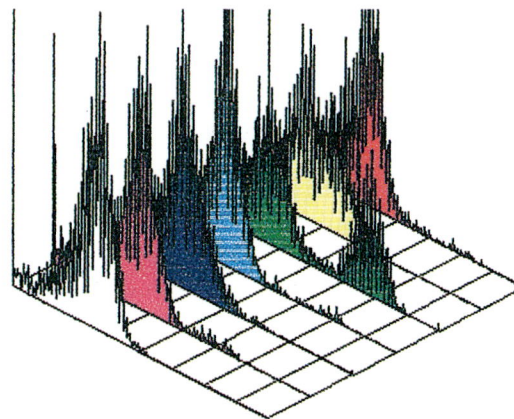

31.22 Histogram of flow cytometry of nucleated cells in bone marrow aspirate. Left to right: white, control; pink, CD4 7%; dark blue, CD8 4%; pale blue, CD2 5%; green, CD19 35%; yellow, CD20 14%; pink, CD14 9%. Case of recurrence, as shown by CD19 – 35%, and CD20 – 14%.

monocyte colony-stimulating factor, there is marked stimulation of myeloid precursors, with immature stages near the trabeculae and progressively more mature ones in the central regions; while erythropoietin administration results in stimulation of erythropoiesis. Marked megakaryocytic hyperplasia has also been observed, including atypical megakaryocytes.

Future perspectives

Transplantation of BMT and PBSCT is a rapidly developing field with constant widening of the indications, for example, to hereditary conditions in which hematopoietic stem cells may be used as vehicles for delivering missing or abnormal genes, as well as in autoimmune diseases and other disorders.

Check list: Effects of Cytotoxic Therapy and Bone Marrow Transplantation

- Adequate biopsy.
- State of cortex and trabeculae.
- Remodeling: extent and location.
- Cellularity.
- Gelatinous atrophy, necrosis, degenerating cells?
- Presence of fibrosis – distribution? Reticulin stain.
- Hematopoiesis – quantity, distribution, composition, dysplastic features.
- Presence of hot spots?
- Residual infiltration – aspect, quantity, location?
- Immunohistology: appropriate immunohistology for confirmation of residual infiltration.

Cytokines and growth factors
- Adequate biopsy.
- Cellularity.
- Atrophy – fibrosis, necrosis?
- State and quantity of erythropoiesis – myelopoiesis – megakaryopoiesis.
- Dysplastic features.
- Residual disease.

Clinical correlations

- State of patient depends on previous disease and therapy.
- Duration of interval since BMT or PBSCT.
- Allogeneic or autotransplant.
- Type of current therapy.
- Peripheral blood values.
- Clinical features of acute GVHD: dermatologic: rash, abdominal: pain and diarrhea; jaundice; may be mild or fatal.
- Chronic GVHD: skin and joint manifestations, mucosal ulcers and malabsorption, jaundice, infections, bone marrow failure.
- Therapy of GVHD – prevent progression and alleviate symptoms.

Bibliography

Aboulafia D.M., Demirer T. (1995) Fatal bone marrow necrosis following fludarabine administration in a patient with indolent lymphoma. *Leuk Lymphoma*, **19** (1–2), 181–4.

Abramson N., Castro S., Goldstein J.D. (1997) Lipid-laden macrophage infiltration of human adenocarcinoma in vivo associated with taxol and GCSF treatment. *Cancer Invest.*, **15** (1), 18–22.

Antman K.S., Griffin J.D., Elias A. *et al.* (1988) Effect of recombinant human granulocyte-macrophage colony-stimulating factor on chemotherapy-induced myelosuppression. *N. Engl. J. Med.*, **320 (14)**, 939–40.

Argiris A., Maris T., Papavasiliou G. *et al.* (1996) Radiotherapy effects on vertebral bone marrow: easily recognizable changes in T2 relaxation times. *Magn Reson Iamgining*, **14 (6)**, 633–8.

Azuno Y., Kaneko T., Nishimura M. *et al.* (1996) Donor leukocyte transfusions and discontinuation of immunosuppressants to achieve an initial remission after allogeneic bone marrow transplantation in a patient with primary refractory acute leukemia. *Bone Marrow Transplant.*, **18** (1), 257–9.

Barriga F.J., Legues M.E., Bertin P. (1996) Selective engraftment of the granulocyte compartment after allogeneic bone marrow transplantation in a patient with severe aplastic anemaia. *J Pediatr Hematol Oncol*, **18** (2), 216–7.

Bergman B.S., Lyman G.H., Ballester O.F. *et al.* (1995) Therapeutic use of granulocyte colony stimulating factor after induction chemotherapy in acute myelogenous leukemia: an analysis of clinical practice. *Hematol Rev and Comm*, **9 (3)**, 213–222.

Bertheas M.F., Fraisse J., Vasselon C. *et al.* (1988) The contribution of cytogenetics to the evaluation of residual disease in malignant hemopathies. *Pathol. Biol.*, **36 (1)**, 52–5.

Bessho M., Itoh Y., Kataumi S. *et al.* (1992) A hematological remission by clonal hematopoiesis after treatment with recombinant human granulocyte-macrophage colony-stimulating factor and erythropoietin in a patient with therapy-related myelodysplastic syndrome. *Leuk. Res.*, **16 (2)**, 123–31.

Bilgrami S., Almeida G.D., Quinn J.J. *et al.* (1994) Pancytopenia in allogeneic marrow transplant recipients: role of cytomegalovirus. *Br J Haematol.*, **87 (2)**, 357–62.

Blayney D.W., Longo D.L., Young R.C. *et al.* (1987) Decreasing risk of leukemia with prolonged follow-up after chemotherapy and radiotherapy for Hodgkin's disease. *N Engl J Med.*, **316 (12)**, 710–4.

Boque C., Pujol-Moix N., Linde M.A. *et al.* (1989) Use of monoclonal anti-actin as a megakaryocyte marker in paraffin wax embedded bone marrow biopsy specimens. *J Clin Pathol*, **42 (9)**, 982–4.

Bosserman L.D., Murray C., Takvorian T. *et al.* (1989) Mechanism of graft failure in HLA-matched and HLA-mismatched bone marrow transplant recipients. *Bone Marrow Transplant*, **4 (3)**, 239–45.

Bradstock K.F., Gottlieb D.J. (1995) Interaction of acute leukemia cells with the bone marrow microenvironment: implications for control of minimal residual disease. *Leuk Lymphoma*, **18 (1–2)**, 1–16.

Brunning R.B., McKenna R.W. (eds) (1994) Tumors of the bone marrow. In *Atlas of Tumor Pathology*, 3rd series, fascicle 9. Washington: Armed Forces Institute of Pathology, pp. 182–91.

Cabanillas F., Pathak S., Zander A. *et al.* (1987) Monosomy 21, partial duplication of chromosome 11, and structural abnormality of chromosme 1q21 in a case of lymphoma developing in a transplant recipient: characteristic abnormalities of secondary lymphoma? *Cancer Genet Cytogenet.*, **24 (1)**, 7–10.

Chopra R., Wotherspoon A.C., Blair S. *et al.* (1994) Detection and significance of bone marrow infiltration at the time of autologous bone marrow transplantation in Hodgkin's disease. *Br J Haematol*, **87 (3)**, 647–9.

Chucrallah A.E., Crow M.K., Rice L.E. *et al.* (1994) Multiple myeloma after cardiac transplantation: an unusual form of post-transplant lymphoproliferative disorder. *Hum. Pathol.*, **25 (5)**, 541–5.

Coustan-Smith E., Behm F.G., Hurwit C.A. *et al.* (1993) N-CAM (CD56) expression by CD34+ malignant myeloblasts with implications for minimal residual disease detection in acute myeloid leukemia. *Leukemia*, **7**, 853.

Cross N.C.P., Feng L., Bungey J., Goldman J.M. (1993) Minimal residual disease after bone marrow transplant for chronic myeloid leukemia detected by the polymerase chain reaction. *Leukemia and Lymphoma*, **11 (Suppl. 1)**, 39–43.

Cross N.C.P., Feng L., Chase A. *et al.* (1993) Competitive polymerase chain reaction to estimate the number of BCR-ABL transcripts, 39–43.nic myeloid leukemia patients after bone marrow transplantation. *Blood*, **82 (6)**, 1929–36.

Curtis R.E., Rowlings P.A., Deeg H.J. *et al.* (1997) Solid cancers after bone marrow transplantation. *N Engl J Med.*, **336 (13)**, 897–904.

Davey D.D., Kamat D., Lasewski M. *et al.* (1989) Epstein–Barr virus-related lymphoproliferative disorders following bone marrow transplantation: an immologic analysis. *Mod Pathol*, **2 (1)**, 27–34.

De Graaf H., Mulder N.H., Willemse P.H. *et al.* (1995) The additive effect of peripheral blood stem cells harvested with low-dose cyclophosphamide, to autologous bone marrow reinfusion on hematopoietic reconstitution after ablative chemotherapy in breast cancer patients with localized disease. *Anticancer Res*, **15 (6B)**, 2851–6.

Dietrich P.Y., Henry-Amar M. *et al.* (1994) Second primary cancers in patients continuously disease-free from Hodgkin's disease: a protective role for the spleen? *Blood*, **84 (4)**, 1209–15.

Duhrsen U., Villeval J.L., Boyd J. *et al.* (1988) Effects of recombinant human granulocyte colony-stimulating factor on hematopoietic progenitor cells in cancer patients. *Blood*, **72 (6)**, 2074–81.

Duncombe A. (1997) ABC of clinical haematology: bone marrow and stem cell transplantation. *BMJ*, **314**, 1179–92.

Duncombe A.S., Grundy J.E., Prentice H.G., Brenner M.K. (1991) IL2 activated killer cells may contribute to cytomegalovirus induced marrow hypoplasia after bone marrow transplantation. *Bone Marrow Transplant.*, **7 (2)**, 81–7.

El-Naggar A.M., Hanna I.R.A., Chanana A.D. *et al.* (1980) Bone marrow changes after localized acute and fractionated X irradiation. *Radiat Res.*, **84**, 46.

El-Rifal W., Ruutu T., Vettenranta K. *et al.* (1996) Minimal residual disease after allogeneic bone marrow transplantation for chronic myeloid leukaemia: a metaphase-FISH study. *Br J Haematol.*, **92**, 365–9.

Ellison D.J., Sharpe R.W., Robbins B.A. *et al.* (1994) Immunomorphologic analysis of bone marrow biopsies after treatment with 2-chlorodeoxyadenosine for hairy cell leukemia. *Blood*, **84 (12)**, 4310–5.

El Rifai W., Ruutu T., Elonen E. *et al.* (1997) Prognostic value of metaphase-fluorescence in situ hybridization in follow-up of patients with acute myeloid leukemia in remission. *Blood*, **89 (9)**, 3330–4.

Engel H., Goodacre A., Keyhani A. *et al.* (1997) Minimal residue disease in acute myelogenous leukaemia and myelodysplastic syndromes: a follow-up of patients in clinical remission. *Br. J. Haematol.*, **99**, 64–75.

Euvrard S., Pouteil Noble C., Kanitakis J. *et al.* (1992) Brief report: Successive occurrence of T-cell and B-cell lymphomas after renal transplantation in a patient with multiple cutaneous squamous-cell carcinomas. *New Eng. J. Med.*, **327 (27)**, 1924–26.

Falini B., Pileri S.A., Flenghi L. *et al.* (1990) Selection of a panel of monoclonal antibodies for monitoring residual disease in peripheral blood and bone marrow of interferon-treated hairy cell leukemia patients. *Br. J. Haematol.* **76 (4)**, 460–8.

Favrot M.C., Herve P. (1987) Detection of minimal malignant cell infiltration in the bone marrow of patients with solid tumors, non-Hodgkin lymphomas and leukemias. *Bone Marrow Transplant.*, **2 (2)**, 117–22.

Ferrera J.L.M., Deeg H.J. (1991) Graft-versus-host disease. *N Engl J Med.*, **324 (10)**, 667–74.

Filipovich A.H., Mathur A., Kamat D. *et al.* (1994) Lymphoproliferative disorders and other tumors complicating immuno-deficiencies. *Immunodeficiency*, **5 (2)**, 91–112.

Foucar K. (1994) Effects of therapy and transplantation and detection of minimal residual disease. In K. Foucar (ed), *Bone Marrow Pathology*. Chicago: ASCP Press, pp. 531–52.

Foucar K., Dick F.R. (1992) Interpretation of postchemotherapy and post-transplantation bone marrow specimen. *Neoplastic Hematol*, ed. D.M. Knowles, 1439–57.

Franco V., Florena A.M., Quintini G., Musso M. (1994) Bone marrow granulomas in hairy cell leukemia following 2-chlorodeoxy-adenosine therapy. *Histopathology*, **24 (3)**, 271–3.

Franklin W.A., Shpall E.J., Archer P. *et al.* (1996) Immunocytochemical detection of

breast cancer cells in marrow and peripheral blood of patients undergoing high dose chemotherapy with autologous stem cell support. *Breast Cancer Res Treat.*, **41 (4)**, 1–13.

Gale R.P., Horowitz M.M., Weiner R.S. *et al.* (1995) Impact of cytogenetic abnormalities on outcome of bone marrow transplants in acute myelogenous leukemia in first remission. *Bone Marrow Transplant.*, **16 (2)**, 203–8.

Goodrich J.M., Mori M., Gleaves C.A. *et al.* (1991) Early treatment with ganciclovir to prevent cytomegalovirus disease after allogeneic bone marrow transplantation. *N Engl J Med*, **325**, 1601–7.

Gore S.D., Kasta M.B., Goodman S.N., Civin C.I. (1990) Detection of minimal residual T cell acute lymphoblastic leukemia by flow cytometry. *J. Immunol. Methods.*, **132 (2)**, 275–86.

Gorin N.C., Coiffier B., Hayat M. *et al.* (1993) Hematopoietic recovery factor (GM-CSF) after autologous bone marrow transplantation. A randomized, double-blind, multicentric trial in 91 cases of non-Hodgkin's malignant lymphoma. *Presse Medicale*, **22 (3)**, 109–20.

Goulden N., Langlands K., Steward C. *et al.*, (1994) PCR assessment of bone marrow status in 'isolated' extramedullary relapse of childhood B-precursor acute lymphoblastic leukaemia. *Br J Haematol.*, **87 (2)**, 282–5.

Gratwohl A., Hermans J., Niederwieser D. *et al.* (1993) Bone marrow transplantation for chronic myeloid leukemia: Long-term results. *Bone Marrow Transplant.*, **12 (5)**, 509–16.

Greenberger J.S. (1991) Toxic effects on the hematopoietic microenvironment. *Exp Hematol*, **19**, 1101–9.

Harousseau J.L., Attal M. (1997) The role of autologous hematopoietic stem cell transplantation in multiple myeloma. *Sem in Hematol.*, **34 (1)**, 61–7.

Heslop H.E., Duncombe A.S., Reittie J.E. *et al.* (1991) Interleukin 2 infusion induces hemopoietic growth factors and modifies marrow regeneration after chemotherapy or autologous marrow transplantation. *Br. J. Hematol.*, **77 (2)**, 237–44.

Humblet Y., Feyens A.M., Sekhavat M. *et al.* (1989) Immunological and pharmacological removal of small cell lung cancer cells from bone marrow autografts. *Cancer Res.*, **49 (18)**, 5058–61.

Isaacs R.E. (1995) The role of cytokines in the management of patients undergoing bone marrow transplantation. *Hematol Rev and Comm*, **9 (2)**, 85–104.

Jouan H., LeDeist F., Nezelof C. (1987) Omenn's syndrome – pathologic arguments in favor of a graft versus host pathogenesis: a report of nine cases. *Hum Pathol*, **18 (11)**, 1101–8.

Kampmeier P., Spielberger R., Dickstein J. *et al.* (1994) Increased incidence of second neoplasms in patients treated with interferon alpha 2b for hairy cell leukemia: a clinicopathologic assessment. *Blood*, **83 (10)**, 2931–8.

Kobayashi S.D., Seki K., Suwa N. *et al.* (1991) The transient appearance of small blastoid cells in the marrow after bone marrow transplantation.

Kolb H.J., Schattenberg A., Goldman J.M. *et al.* (1995) Graft-versus-leukemia effect of donor lymphocyte transfusions in marrow grafted patients. *Blood*, **86 (5)**, 2041–50.

Konwalinka G., Dchirmer M., Hilbe W. *et al.* (1995) Minimal residual disease in hairy-cell leukemia after treatment with 2-chlorodeoxyadenosine. *Blood Cells Mol Dis*, **21 (2)**, 142–51.

Koppler H., Pfluger K.H., Havemann K. (1991) Hematopoietic reconstitution after high-dose chemotherapy and autologous nonfrozen bone marrow rescue. *Ann. Hematol.*, **63 (5)**, 253–8.

Kurihara K., Hill W., Burkhardt R., Kettner G., Hashimoto N. (1987) Bone marrow changes following chemotherapy for multiple myeloma – a clinicopathological study of biopsy cases. *Nippon Ketsueki Gakkai Zasshi*, **50** (4), 876–89.

Lazarus H.M., Gale R.P. (1997) Blood cell and bone marrow transplants. *Bone Marrow Transplant.*, **18** (5), 839–41.

Leitenberg D., Rappeport J.M., Smith B.R. (1994) B-cell precursor bone marrow reconstitution after bone marrow transplantation. *Am J Clin Pathol.*, **102** (2), 231–6.

Lemoli R.M., Cavo M., Fortuna A. (1996) Concomitant mobilization of plasma cells and hematopoietic progenitors into peripheral blood of patients with multiple myeloma. *J Hematother.*, **5** (4), 339–49.

Leonard R.C., Duncan L.W., Hay F.G. (1990) Immunocytological detection of residual marrow disease at clinical remission predicts metastatic relapse in small cell lung cancer. *Cancer Res.*, **50** (20), 6545–8.

Levine E.G., Bloomfield C.P. (1992) Seminars in Oncology, **19** (1), 47–84.

Locatelli F., Niemeyer C., Angelucci E. *et al.* (1997) Allogeneic bone marrow transplantation for chronic myelomonocytic leukemia in childhood: a report from the European Working Group on Myelodysplastic Syndrome in Childhood. *J Clin Oncol.*, **15** (2), 566–73.

Macedo A., Orfao A., Gonzalez M. *et al.* (1995) Immunological detection of blast cell subpopulations in acute myeloblastic leukemia at diagnosis: implications for minimal residual disease studies. *Leukemia*, **9** (6), 993–8.

Macon W.R., Tham K.T., Greer J.P., Wolff S.N. (1995) Ringed sideroblasts: a frequent observation after bone marrow transplantation. *Mod Pathol*, **8** (7), 782–5.

Mangan K.F., Mullaney M.T., Rosenfeld C.S., Shadduck R.K. (1988) In vitro evidence for disappearance of erythroid progenitor T suppressor cells following allogenic bone

marrow transplantation for severe aplastic anemia. *Blood*, **71** (1), 144–50.

Maritaz O., Combaret V., Favrot M.C. (1988) The significance of immunological analysis for the detection of residual neuroblasts in bone marrow. *Pathol Biol*, **36** (1), 21–4.

Michelson JD., Gornet M., Codd T. *et al.* (1993) Bone morphology after bone marrow transplantation for Hodgkin's and non-Hodgkin's lymphoma. *Exp Hematol*, **21** (3), 475–82.

Mouratidou M., Sotiropoulos D., Deremitzaki K. *et al.* (1993) Recurrence of acute leukemia in donor cells after bone marrow transplantation: Documentation by *in situ* DNA hydridization. *Bone Marrow Transplantation*, **12** (1), 77–80.

Negrin R.S., Kiem H.P., Schmidt-Wolf I.G. *et al.* (1991) Use of the polymerase chain reaction to monitor the effectiveness of ex vivo tumor cell purging. *Blood*, **77** (3), 654–60.

Pantel K. (1996) Detection of minimal disease in patients with solid tumors. *J Hematother.*, **5** (4), 359–67

Pekarske S.L. (1996) Bone marrow changes induced by recombinant granulocyte colony-stimulating factor resembling metastatic carcinoma: distinction with cytochemical amd immunohistochemical studies. *Am J Hematol.*, **51** (4), 332–4.

Philips G.L., Reece D.E., Lerner K.G., Connors J.M. (1990) Intensive chemotherapy and autologous peripheral blood stem cell transplantation in a patient with persistent marrow involvement with Hodgkin's disease. *Bone Marrow Transplant*, **6** (1), 45–7.

Pileri S., Sabattini E., Poggi S. *et al.* (1994) Bone marrow biopsy in hairy cell leukaemia (HCL) patients. Histological and immuno-histological analysis of 46 cases treated with different therapies. *Leuk Lymphoma*, **14** (Suppl. 1), 67–71.

Radich J. (1996) Detection of minimal residual disease in acute and chronic

leukemias. *Current Opinion in Hematol*, **3** (4), 310–14.

Randhawa P.S., Jaffe R., Demetris A.J. *et al.* (1991) The sytemic distribution of Epstein–Barr virus genomes in fatal post-transplantation lymphoproliferative disorders. An in situ hybridization study. *Am J Pathol.*, **138** (4), 1027–33.

Rosenthal N.S., Farhi D.C. (1991) Dysmegakaryopoiesis resembling acute megakaryoblastic leukemia in treated acute myeloid leukemia. *Am J Clin Pathol*, **95**, 556–69.

Rosenthal N.S., Farhi D.C. (1994) Failure to engraft after bone marrow transplantation: bone marrow morphologic findings. *Am J Clin Pathol*, **102** (6), 821–4.

Rowland P., Mirro J. Jr. (1994) Clinical applications of the hematopoietic growth factors. *Current Opinion in Hematol*, **1**, 303–9.

Salloum E., Tallini G., Levy A., Cooper D.L., Burkitt's lymphoma-leukemia in patients treated for Hodgkin's disease. *Cancer Invest*, **14** (6), 527–33.

Samoszuk M., Ravel J., Ramzi E. (1992) Epstein–Barr virus and interleukein-5 mRNA in acquired immunodeficiency syndrome-related lymphomas with eosinophilia. *Hum. Pathol.*, **23** (12), 1355–59.

Sanz M.A., Sempere A. (1996) Immuno-phenotyping of AML and MDS and detection of residual disease. *Baillière's Clin Haematol.*, **9** (1), 35–55.

Schultze J.L., Gribben J.G. (1996) Minimal residual disease in non-Hodgkin's lymphoma. *Biomed and Pharmacother*, **50**, 451–8.

Siena S., Bregni M., Brando B. *et al.* (1991) Flow cytometry for clinical estimation of circulating hematopoietic progenitors for autologous transplantation in cancer patients, **77** (2), 400–9.

Simmons P., Kaushamsky K., Torok-Storb B. (1990) Mechanisms of a cytomegalo-virus-mediated myelosuppression: perturbation of stromal cell function versus direct infection of myeloid cells. *Proc Natl Acad Sci.*, **87**, 1386–80.

Simmons P.J., Przepiorka D., Thomas E.D., Torok-Storb B. (1987) Host origin of marrow stromal cells following allogeneic bone marrow transplantation. *Nature*, **328**, 429–32.

Snover, D.C. (1989) Biopsy interpretation in bone marrow transplantation. *Pathol. Annu.*, **24 (2)**, 63–101.

Stoppa A.M., Hirn J., Blaise D. *et al.* (1990) Autologous bone marrow transplantation for B cell malignancies after in vitro purging with floating immunoheads. *Bone Marrow Transplant.*, **6 (5)**, 301–7.

Sugimoto M., Takahashi S.M., Toguchida T. *et al.* (1991) Changes in bone after high-dose irradiation: biomechanics and histomorphology. *J Bone Joint Surg.*, **73B**, 492.

Swerdlow S.H. (1997) Post-transplant lymphoproliferative disorders: a working classification. *Curr Diagnost Pathol.*, I4, 28–35.

Thaler J. Dietze O., Faber V. *et al.* (1990) Monoclonal antibody B-ly7: a sensitive marker for detection of minimal residual disease in hairy cell leukemia. *Leukemia*, **4 (3)**, 170–6.

Thorne A.C., Malbin K.F., Jain M. *et al.* (1996) Autologous bone marrow harvesting in outpatients. *J Clin Anesth.*, **8 (7)**, 551–6.

Travis L.B., Curtis R.E., Glimelius B. *et al.* (1993) Second cancers among long-term survivors of non-Hodgkin's lymphoma. *J. Nat. Cancer Inst.*, **85 (23)**, 1932–37.

van den Berg H., Kluin P.M., Vossen J.M. (1990) Early reconstitution of haematopoiesis after allogeneic bone marrow transplantation: a prospective histopathological study of bone marrow biopsy specimens. *J Clin Pathol*, **43**, 365–9.

van den Berg H., Beverstock G., Westerhof J.P., Vossen J.M. (1991) Chromosomal studies after bone marrow transplantation for leukemia in children. *Bone Marrow Transplant.*, **7 (5)**, 335–42.

van den Berg H., Kluin P.M., Zwaan F.E., Vossen J.M. (1989) Histopathology of bone marrow reconstitution after allogeneic bone marrow transplantation. *Histopathology*, **15 (4)**, 363–73.

van Gorp J., Doornewaard H., Verdonck L.F. *et al.* (1994) Post-transplant T-cell lymphoma. Report of three cases and a review of the literature. *Cancer*, **73 (12)**, 3064–72.

van Rhee F., Marks D.I., Lin F. *et al.* (1995) Quantification of residual disease in Philadelphia-positive acute lymphoblastic leukemia: comparison of blood and bone marrow. *Leukemia*, **9 (2)**, 329–35.

Vescio R.A., Han E.J., Schiller G.J. *et al.* (1996) Quantitative comparison of multiple myeloma tumor contamination in bone marrow harvest and leukapheresis autografts. *Bone Marrow Transplant.*, **18 (1)**, 103–10.

Wheaton S., Tallman M.S., Hakimian D., Peterson L. (1996) Minimal residual disease may predict bone marrow relapse in patients with hairy cell leukemia treated with 2-chlorodeoxyadenosine. *Blood*, **87 (4)**, 1556–60.

Wilkins B.S., Bostanci A.G., Ryan M.F., Jones D.B. (1993) Haematopoietic regrowth after chemotherapy for acute leukaemia: an immunohistochemical study of bone marrow trephine biopsy specimens. *J Clin Pathol*, **46 (10)**, 915–21.

Wittels B. (1980) Bone marrow biopsy changes following chemotherapy for acute leukemia. *Am J Surg Path*, **4**, 135–42.

Zaccaria A., Rosti G., Testoni N. *et al.* (1987) Chromosome studies in patients with Philadelphia chromosome-positive chronic myeloid leukemia submitted to bone marrow transplantation – results of a European Cooperative Study. *Cancer Genet. Cytogenet.*, **26 (1)**, 5–13.

Appendix: Methods

Plastic embedding

Bone biopsies are cut into two pieces and half is fixed for embedding into plastic (see below) and the other half for embedding into paraffin or for frozen sections. Small pieces may also be carefully removed for EM.

Fixation

Put the specimen into the fixative (Schaffer's solution) and leave for 4–16 h, depending on biopsy width and amount of bone.

Composition of the fixative

Methanol absolute G.R. (Merck) – 96 ml;
Glucose phosphate buffer – 4 ml;
Formol neutralised G.R. – 50 ml.
Formol is neutralised by the addition of CaCo₃ – ca.50 g/liter. The fixative can be kept in the refrigerator at 4°C.

Glucose Phosphate buffer pH 7.4

Na_2HPO_4. $2H_2O$ – 48.0 g;
KH_2PO_4 – 8.7 g;
Glucose. $1H_2O$ (mol. wt. 198.17) – 154.0 g;
Aqua dest. Ad – 5000 ml.
Sterilise by filtration through a bacterial funnel. The buffer can be kept for 3–4 weeks in the refrigerator at 4°C. The bottled, sterile and unopened buffer can be kept for longer (±5 months).

Reagents

Formaldehyde solution GR 35% – Merck no. 4003;
Methanol GR – Merck no. 6009;
$Na_2HPO_4 \cdot 2H_2O$ (di-sodium hydrogen phosphate 2-hydrate GR) – Merck no. 6580;
KH_2PO_4 (Potassium dihydrogenphosphate GR) – Merck no. 4873;
D(+)Glucose (-monohydrate) – Merck no. 8342.

Dehydration

Transfer specimen (biopsy) from fixative directly to absolute methanol (100%), change the methanol after 0.5, 1 and 2 h; dehydrate in the absolute methanol 4–6 h altogether depending on the size of the biopsy. The vial should be tightly closed during dehydration.

Embedding

The biopsy is transferred directly from 100% methanol to the fluid methyl methacrylate, in a vial with just enough of the methacrylate to cover the specimen, left for 0.5 h, the methacrylate is changed, left for 1 h and changed again. After 1 h the methacrylate is poured off and the vial filled with fresh methacrylate. The vial is tightly closed and left in a water bath or in a dish with water in an incubator overnight at ±45°C. In the morning the vial is placed in the freezer for about 0.5 h, then it is smashed and the hardened block trimmed. Sections are cut at 2 or 3 µm and are floated on hot (>70°C) water to stretch them, and are picked up on gelatin coated glass slides, blotted dry with some pressure, and left for ±30 min in the incubator at ±45°C. The sections are now ready for staining, and any of the stains routinely used in histopathology can be applied after removal of the methacrylate; for example, Giemsa, hematoxylin and eosin, toluidine blue for calcified bone and osteoid; fiber stains for reticulin and collagen, and PAS for glycoproteins.

The exact times required for optimal staining are usually determined by each laboratory individually, but it should be borne in mind that, generally speaking, thin sections require longer staining times; the procedures are the same as those given for paraffin sections in any text on histopathologic techniques, Giemsa and toluidine blue are given below as examples.

Procedure for coating glass slides

Clean glass slides are dipped into the gelatin solution, drained and dried for a few minutes at room temperature or in an incubator at 37–46°C and used to pick up the sections from the water bath.

Gelatin solution

Dissolve 6.75 g gelatin in 1500 ml distilled water at 60°C; cool to 50°C and add 58 ml 4% potassium chromium (III) sulfate solution; add several crystals of thymol and four drops of Plastoid N. The gelatin solution is stable at room temperature for about 10–14 days, and longer when kept in the refrigerator; gelatinised slides can be kept for 2 days or longer if put into boxes and kept in the refrigerator.

Removal of the methacrylate from the sections

Sections mounted on the glass slides are used. The slides are placed into benzene (Benzol).
benzene I – 20 min;
benzene II – 20 min;
then into absolute methanol – 2 min;
96% methanol – 2 min;
80% methanol – 2 min;
methanol ammonia solution – 10 min;
Aqua dest. – 10 min.
The sections are now ready for staining.

Methanol ammonia solution

70% Methanol – 100 ml;
ammonia 25% – 10 ml.

Benzol (benzene) GR – Merck no. 1783;
Methanol GR – Merck no. 6009;
Ammonia solution GR (mon 25%) – Merck no. 5432.

Giemsa stain – for cytological details

Remove the methacrylate and put the slides into distilled water for 10 min. Drain and put into Giemsa solution pH 6.7 at 50°C for 45 min; then into Giemsa solution pH 6.6 at 40°C for 25 min. Dip in distilled water and dry the slides immediately by gentle blotting with filter paper, dip into xylol, cover with a mounting medium (Entallan) and cover glass; as mentioned above, these staining times are approximate.

Phosphate buffer pH 6.7, 0.066 mol/l

0.066 mol/l Disodium hydrogen phosphate (Na_2HPO_4): 43.4 ml;
0.066 mol/l potassium dihydrogen phosphate (KH_2PO_4): 56.6 ml.

Phosphate buffer pH 6.6, 0.066 mol/l

0.066 mol/l Disodium hydrogen phosphate (Na_2HPO_4): 36 ml;
0.066 mol/l potassium dihydrogen phosphate (KH_2PO_4): 64 ml.

Giemsa pH 6.7 (prepare fresh before use)

Distilled water: 49 ml;
phosphate buffer pH 6.7: 1 ml;
Giemsa solution: 2 ml.

Giemsa solution pH 6.6

Distilled water: 49 ml;
phosphate buffer pH 6.6: 1 ml;
Giemsa solution: 2 ml.
The times for staining are calculated for 3 μm section thickness; thinner sections need more time.

Toluidine blue stain

This is used for rapid diagnostic evaluation, as well as for calcified bone and osteoid. Dissolve the methylmethacrylate as described above. Then stain in toluidine blue 0.1% in distilled water, at ca.50°C for 5–20 min, dip in water, blot gently, dry in air for 1–5 min, dip in xylol, cover with mounting medium and cover-glass.

The method for plastic embedding and immunohistology is given in Table 1.

Paraffin embedding and immunohistology

Fixation

The biopsies are fixed in 10% neutral buffered formalin for 4–6 h or overnight, depending on the size (width) of the biopsy. The biopsies are then placed in the decalcification liquid (De Cal Rapid N° HS 105 National Diagnostics, Atlanta, GA, USA) for 20 min–1 h, depending on the width of the biopsy and the estimated amount of bone present.

Then the biopsies are rinsed in distilled water for 30 min and transferred to 70%

TABLE 1 Method for plastic embedding and immunohistology

Time	Procedure
	Fixation
18 h (over night) (for biopsies of 2–3 mm diameter)	45 ml tetrahydrofuran 45 ml ethanol 96% 10 ml ethyleneglycol
	Dehydration
3 h overall, 3 changes	tetrahydrofuran 100%
	Infiltration
3 h overall, 2 changes, under vacuum	84% methylmethacrylate 14% dibutylphthalate 1% polyethylenglycol 600 0.7% benzoylperoxide, dried } A
	Polymerisation
18 h (over night)	15 ml A and 50 µl dimethyltoluidine in a waterbath in the refrigerator at 4°C, each biopsy in a small glass vial

Method developed by J. Sturm and R. Bartl.
Reagents supplied by Merck and Sigma.

methanol. The specimens can then be processed automatically in a tissue processor as any other piece of tissue for histopathologic examination. Sections for immunohistology are picked up on polylysine-coated slides, dried overnight in the incubator at 37°C and used the next day after removal of the paraffin. Antigen retrieval and antigen–antibody reactions are carried out according to the manufacturer's instructions or data-sheets. Bone biopsy sections must be checked against tissues known to react with the antibody being used, to avoid errors in interpretation. In many cases, kits are available which contain detailed instructions, and it is advisable to follow these carefully.

Frozen sections

A piece of the biopsy is immediately soaked in Histocon (cat no. 0582, Polysciences Inc., Warrington, PA, USA) at 4°C, for 2–16 h, after which it is snap-frozen in liquid nitrogen and stored at −180°C, till cut in a cryostat. For sectioning, the biopsy is mounted on a tissue-holder covered with OCT (cat. no. 4583, Raymond Lamb, London, UK) and sections are cut at 3–5 µm at −18 to −25°C, depending on the amount of adipose tissue present. The sections are mounted on albuminised slides, air-dried and kept in the refrigerator at 4°C till incubation, a section stained with H&E, or toluidine blue, or Giemsa is first examined to ascertain that sufficient marrow is present; for details, see, Frisch and Bartl (1990).

Electron microscopy

Spicules or small pieces of the biopsies are fixed in glutaraldehyde, dehydrated and embedded in resin, for example Araldite, Epon, or maraglas. Pyramids are obtained by hardening of the resin in appropriate moulds, sections are first cut at about 1 µm, stained and examined in the light microscope to select the appropriate area for cutting for EM. Thin sections are then cut, stained, e.g. by lead citrate and uranyl acetate, and examined. For details, see Rozman *et al.* (1993).

Flow cytometry (FACS)

About 3–5 ml bone marrow is aspirated and immediately placed into RPMI medium and 20% fetal calf serum containing heparin to prevent coagulation. PBS with heparin is also used. This mixture of marrow and medium can be left at room temperature, if necessary, until the next morning when the nucleated cells are first counted in a Coulter counter before separation on Ficoll-Hypaque and incubation with the appropriate antibodies, which usually are already attached to the appropriate fluorescent dye. Samples are counted in the flow cytometer and histograms obtained showing the proportions of the cells which have been labeled by the fluorescent antibodies. These procedures are now standardised and given in the texts dealing with these techniques (see Preface).

Cytogenetics: conventional and FISH

As for FACS, 3–5 ml bone marrow are taken into medium with heparin and antibiotics. If possible, cultures are set up the same day; if not, the bone marrow is left at room temperature (or in the refrigerator) till the next morning when the cells are counted and the cultures are set up. In most cases, a direct culture is prepared as well as 8, 12, 24 h or longer, depending on how many nucleated

cells the aspirate contained. Details of the methods are available in any of the many texts on this subject.

Giemsa banding is routinely used in our laboratories and the metaphase spreads are analysed on a computer screen, simultaneously with observation of the chromosomes in the microscope. Alternatively, a series of metaphases may be stored in the computer and subsequently analysed.

Fluorescent *in situ* hybridisation (FISH) may be carried out on the same slides or on additional slides or cells stored for that purpose. FISH is especially useful in cases with few or poor quality metaphases, as well as for investigation of larger numbers of cells as many interphase nuclei can be counted, and for identification of 'marker' chromosomes which cannot be identified by banding techniques.

Cytogenetic nomenclature

This is based on the results of several international conferences after each of which reports containing recommendations for a uniform system of karyotype description were published. The most recent is An International System for Human Cytogenetic Nomenclature (1995) ISCN.

Chromosomes are classified according to their size, the location of the centromere, and the banding pattern along each arm. The autosomes are numbered from 1 to 22 in descending order of length; the sex chromosomes are referred to as X and Y, female and male respectively.

Nomenclature symbols

p   short arm (above the centromere);
q   long arm (below the centromere);
+   before the chromosome indicates gain of a whole chromosome (e.g. +8, trisomy chromosome 8); after the chromosome indicates gain of part of chromosome (e.g. 14q+ added material at the end of the long arm of chromosome 14);
−   before the chromosome indicates a loss of a whole chromosome (e.g. −7, monosomy

chromosome 7); after the chromosome indicates loss of part of the chromosome (e.g. 5q–, loss of part of the long arm of chromosome 5);

? indicates uncertainty about the identity of the chromosome or band listed just after the ?

Each chromosome arm may consist of one or more regions. Each region is delimited by specific landmarks; consistent, distinct morphological features of importance in chromosome identification. A region consists of one or more bands and is defined as the area that lies between two adjacent landmarks. A band is defined as a chromosomal area that is distinguishable from adjacent segments by appearing darker or lighter by one or more banding techniques. Regions and bands are numbered consecutively from the centromere outward along each chromosome arm.

In designating any particular band, four items are therefore required:

the chromosome number, e.g. 9;

the arm symbol, e.g. p;

the region number, e.g. 2;

the band number within that region, e.g. 4;

These items are given in consecutive order without spacing or punctuation.

In the karyotype description, the first item to be recorded is the total number of chromosomes, followed by a comma. The sex chromosome constitution is given next. Thus, a normal male karyotype is written 46,XY – the normal female karyotype 46,XX.

Chromosome aberrations may be numerical or structural. The first means the loss or gain of an entire chromosome, written by placing a (–) or (+) before the chromosome in question. The second occurs as an abnormal repair process after chromosome breakage.

To specify structurally altered chromosomes, the number of the chromosome or chromosomes involved in the rearrangement is specified within parenthesis immediately following the symbol indicating the type of rearrangement. If two or more chromosomes are altered, a semicolon is used to separate their designations. If one of the rearranged chromosomes is a sex chromosome, this is listed first; otherwise the rule is that the lowest

chromosome is mentioned first. The breakpoints given in parenthesis are specified in the same order as the chromosomes involved, and a semicolon is again used to separate the breakpoints.

The karyotype designations of different clones are separated by a slant line, /. The number of cells that constitute a clone is given in square brackets, [ ], after the karyotype. For example, 47,XX,+8[5]/46,XX,del(5)(q13)[4]/45,XX,–7[3].

Structural chromosome rearrangements

Translocation (t): a break in at least two chromosomes with exchange of material; the chromosomes involved are noted in the first set of brackets and the breakpoints in the second brackets. The Ph chromosome is t(9;22)(q34;q11).

Deletion (del): loss of a chromosomal segment. Whether a deletion is interpreted as terminal or interstitial is apparent from the breakpoint designations. For example, del(5)(q13) involves the long arm and del(5)(q13q33) indicates an interstitial deletion with breakage and reunion of bands 5q13 and 5q33.

Inversion (inv): two breaks occur in the same chromosome with rotation of the intervening segment. For example, inv(3)(q21;q26).

Insertion (ins): a chromosome segment has moved to a new, interstitial position in the same or another chromosome. The chromosome in which the segment is inserted is always specified first, e.g. ins(5;3)(q14;q21q26).

Duplication (dup): presence of an extra copy of part of the chromosome. The breakpoints delineate the duplicated segment, e.g. dup(1)(q21q31).

Isochromosome (i): identical copies of one chromosome with the loss of the other arm. An isochromosome for the entire long arm of one chromosome 17, i(17)(q24).

Derivative chromosome (der): any structurally rearranged chromosome generated by an abnormality involving two or more chromosomes.

Dicentric chromosome (dic): an abnormal chromosome possessing two centromeres produced by breakage and recombination of two chromosomes, e.g. 45,XX,dec(13;15)(q22.q24).

Ring chromosome (r): produced when breaks have occurred in both the short and the long arms with subsequent fusion to form a ring structure.

Marker chromosome (mar): structurally abnormal chromosome that cannot be identified by classical cytogenetics. FISH is a powerful tool to ascertain its origins.

Complex rearrangements: all of the above anomalies can occur in association with each other.

Chromosome breakage syndromes: specific inherited defects of DNA repair mechanisms which give rise to a loosely associated group of conditions.

Homogeneously staining regions (hsr): describe the presence, but not the size, of a homogeneously staining region in a chromosome arm, segment or band.

Double minute (dmin): some chromosome aberrations usually do not appear in constitutional karyotypes because they may be lost at cell division. For example, acentric fragments are subject to random loss at cell division, e.g. 47xx +8 ldmin.

Glossary

Aberration: observable chromosome change. The term is used to describe any abnormality of chromosome number or structure.

Aneuploid: an abnormal chromosome number due either to gain or loss of chromosome.

Autosome: any chromosome other than the sex chromosome; in the human diploid cell there are 22 pairs.

Banded chromosomes: chromosomes with alternating dark and light segments due to special stains or to pretreatment of metaphase cells with enzymes before staining. Each chromosome pair has a unique pattern of bands. The most commonly used procedures are Q-, G-, C-, R- and T-banding.

Breakpoint: location of a break in a chromatid or chromosome denoted by the exact band involved.

Centromere: the primary constriction of the chromosome where the short and long arms are seen to meet. It is the region of attachment of spindle fibers. The centromere of all the chromosomes are characterised by the presence of highly repetitive sequences.

Chromatid: one of the two strands resulting from replication of the chromosome.

Chromosome: structure in the cell nucleus containing a linear thread of DNA, which transmits genetic information.

Congenital: condition present at birth; may be of genetic or environmental etiology, or a combination of both.

Clone: population derived from a single progenitor. In the cytogenetic sense, two cells with the same additional or structurally rearranged chromosome or three cells with loss or addition of the same chromosome.

Cytogenetics: microscopic study of chromosome structure and behavior during cell division.

Diploidy: normal chromosome number and normal composition of chromosomes.

Gene: unit of heredity. At the present a gene is equated with a chromosomal unit of function, for example, the sequence of DNA required to code for one polypeptide.

Genotype: the chromosome complement of a cell or individual.

Hyperdiploid: presence of additional chromosomes (modal number 47 or greater).

Hypodiploid: loss of chromosomes (resulting in a modal number of 45 or less).

Interphase: the resting phase of the cell cycle where there is no visible evidence of cell division.

Karyotype: arrangement of chromosomes according to their size and position of the centromere. A normal female karyotype is described as 46,XX and a normal male karyotype is 46,XY.

Metaphase: the phase in cell division prior to separation of the sister chromatids; the phase utilised for cytogenetic examination.

Mitosis: cell division which produces daughter cells with exactly the same chromosome constitution as the parent cell.

Monosomy: presence of only one member of a pair of chromosomes.

Mutation: a permanent heritable change (loss, gain or exchange) in the genetic material.

Probe: DNA or RNA fragment used to identify a complementary sequence (by molecular hybridisation).

Pseudodiploid: the chromosome number is diploid but there are abnormalities in the karyotype.

Sex chromosomes: the X and Y chromosomes in humans.

Trisomy: presence of three copies of a particular chromosome.

Unique specific sequences: cosmid probes are used in cancer specimens for the detection of gene amplification, such as N-myc in neuroblastoma and are particularly useful for detecting fusion events resulting from specific translocations, t(9;22) or t(15;17) for example, as well as small deletions such as del(13)(q) in retinoblastoma.

Whole chromosome painting probes: these probes enable the identification of human chromosomes in metaphase spreads and in interphase nuclei, by hybridisation to unique sequences spanning the length of the target chromosome.

Bibliography

Abrahamsen J.F., Smaaland R., Skjaerven R., Laerum O.D. (1996) Flow cytometric measurement of DNA S-phase in human bone marrow cells: correlating for peripheral blood contamination. *Eur J Haematol.*, **56** (3), 138–47.

Andrade R.E., Wick M.R., Frizzera G., Gajl-Peczalska K.J. (1986) Immunophenotyping of haematopoietic malignancies in paraffin sections. *Hum Pathol.*, **19**, 394–402.

Auld J. (1994) Immunonews, **3**, 4–5.

Bancroft J., Stevens A. (eds) (1990) *Theory and Practice of Histological Technique*, 3rd edn. New York: Churchill Livingstone.

Baron R., Vignery A., Neff L. *et al.* Processing of undecalcified bone specimens for bone histomorphometry. In R.R. Recker (ed), *Bone Histomorphometry: Techniques and Interpretations*. Boca Raton: CRC Press.

Bauer K.D., Duque R.E., Shankey T.V. (1993) *Clinical Flow Cytometry*. Bulbinse: Willams & Williams, Baltimore.

Bentley S.A., Taylor M.A., Killian D.E. *et al.* (1995) Correction of bone marrow nucleated cell counts for the presence of fat particles. *Am J Clin Pathol.*, **104** (1), 60–4.

Berman J.J., McNeill R.E. (1989) Cytologic evaluation of Papanicolaou-stained bone marrow aspirates. *Diagn Cytopathol*, **5** (4), 383–7.

Bernhards J., Weitzel B., Werner M. *et al.* (1992) A new histological embedding method by low-temperature polymerisation of methyl methacrylate allowing immuno- and enzyme histochemical studies on semi-thin sections of undecalcified bone marrow biopsies. *Histochemistry*, **98**, 145–54.

Blythe D., Hand N.M., Jackson P. *et al.* (1997) Use of methyl methacrylate resin for embedding bone marrow trephine biopsy specimens. *J Clin Pathol.*, **50** (1), 45–9.

Boque C., Pujol-Moix N., Linde M.A. *et al.* (1989) Use of monoclonal anti-actin as a megakaryocyte marker in paraffin wax embedded bone marrow biopsy specimens. *J. Clin. Pathol.*, **42** (9), 982–4.

Brigaudeau C., Gachard N., Clay D. *et al.* (1996) A 'miniaturized' method for the karyotypic analysis of bone marrow or blood samples in hematological malignancies. *Hematol Cell Ther*, **38** (3), 275–7.

Burgio V.L., Pignoloni P., Baroni C.D. (1991) Immunohistology of bone marrow: a modified method of glycolmethacrylate embedding. *Histopathology*, **18** (1), 37–43.

Cheong S.K., Lim Y.C. (1990) Frozen bone marrow trephine biopsy – a technical evaluation. *Malays. J. Pathol.*, **12** (1), 51–6.

Coignet L.J., Van de Rijke F.M., Bertheas M.F. *et al.* (1996) Automated counting of in situ hybridization dots in interphase cells of leukemia samples. *Leukemia*, **10** (6), 1065–71.

Coignet L.J.A., Schuuring E., Kibbelaar R.E. *et al.* (1996) Detection of 11q13 rearrangements in hematologic neoplasias by double-color fluorescence in situ hybridization. *Blood*, **4**, 1512–19.

Compston J.E., Vedi S., Webb A. (1985) Relationship between Toluidine Blue-stained calcification fronts and tetracycline-labeled surfaces in normal iliac crest biopsies. *Calcif. Tissue*, **37**, 32.

Connor M., Ferguson-Smith M. (1997) *Essential Medical Genetics*, 5th edn. London: Blackwell.

Crisan D., Farkas D.H. (1993) Bone marrow biopsy imprint preparations; use for molecular diagnostics in leukemias. *Ann Clin Lab Sci*, **23** (6), 407–22.

Dean P.N. (1990) Data processing. In *Flow Cytometry and Sorting*. New York: Wiley-Liss, pp. 415–44.

DeLellis R.A., Faller G.T. (1977) Cell and tissue staining methods. In S.G. Silverberg, R.A. Delellis and W.J. Frable (eds), *Principles and Practice of Surgical Pathology and Cytopathology, 3rd edn*. Edinburgh: Churchill Livingstone, pp. 43–62.

Ebener U., Hauser S., Wehner S., Kornhuber B. (1989) Retrospective marker analyses performed with blood and bone marrow smears using an immunoenzyme procedure (alkaline phosphatase-anti-alkaline phosphatase technic). *Klin. Padiatr.*, **201 (4)**, 242–6.

Erber W.N., MacLachlan, J. (1989) Use of APAAP technique on paraffin wax embedded bone marrow trephines. *J. Clin. Pathol.*, **42 (11)**, 1201–5.

Flandrin G., Daniel M-T., Crockard A. (1991) Cytochemistry in the classification of leukemias. *The Leukemic Cell*, **2**, 23–46

Frierson H.F. Jr., Linder J. (1977) Flow and image cytometry. In S.G. Silverberg, R.A. Delellis and W.J. Frable (eds), *Principles and Practice of Surgical Pathology and Cytopathology, 3rd ed*. Edinburgh: Churchill Livingstone, pp. 95–112.

Givan A.L. (ed) (1992) *Flow Cytometry: First principles* Chichester: Wiley-Liss.

Gurley A.M., Cluroe A.D., Roberts E.C. (1977) *Principles and Practice of Surgical Pathology and Cytopathology, 3rd ed*. Silverberg, S.G., Delellis R.A., Frable W.J. (eds). Churchill Livingstone, pp. 127–36.

Henry K. (1992) In Edited by K. Henry and W. St. C. Symmers, *Thymus, Lymph Nodes, Spleen and Lymphatics, 3rd edn*. Edinburgh: Churchill Livingstone.

Henry K., Costello C. (1994) HIV-associated bone marrow changes. *Curr Diag Pathol*, **1**, 131–41.

Hoffman R., Benz E.J. Jr., Shattil S.J. *et al.* (1995) *Hematology: Basic Principles and Practice*, 2nd ed. Edinburgh: Churchill Livingstone.

Huegel A., Coyle L., McNeil R., Smith A. (1995) Evaluation of interphase fluorescence in situ hybridization on direct hematological bone marrow smears. *Pathology*, **27 (1)**, 86–90.

Hyun B.H., Stevenson A.J., Hanau C.A. (1994) Fundamentals of bone marrow examination. *Hematol Oncol Clin North Am.*, **8 (4)**, 651–63.

Invernizzi R., Cazzola M., De Fazio P. *et al.* (1990) Immunocytochemical detection of ferritin in human bone marrow and peripheral blood cells using monoclonal antibodies specific for the H and L subinit. *Br. J. Hematol.*, **76 (3)**, 427–32.

Ivanyi J.L., Kiss A., Thomazy V. (1989) Histochemical observations on bone marrow biopsies embedded in glycol methacrylate (Technovit 7100). *Appl. Pathol.*, **7 (2)**, 116–21.

Kass L. (1995) Identification of normal and abnormal human megakaryocytes based on acid fast metachromasia after staining with basic black MSP. *Biotech Histochem.*, **70 (5)**, 271–4.

Keinanen M., Bloomfield C.D., Machnicki J. *et al.* (1989) Human bone marrow cytogenetics: growth factors stimulate metaphases for specific lineages. *Leukemia*, **3 (6)**, 405–12.

Kerim, S., Rege-Cambrin, G., Scaravaglio, P. *et al.* (1991) Effect of recombinant human IL-3 on the mitotic index and karyotype of hemopoietic cells. *Cancer Genet. Cytogenet.*, **55 (2)**, 235–41.

Koller U., Haas O.A., Kornmuller R. *et al.* (1989) Immunofluorescence and immunocytochemical stain methods for simultaneous cytogenetic and phenotypic characterization of mitotic cells. *Wien Klin Wochenschr.*, **101 (3)**, 111–7.

Kotylo P. (1995) Flow cytometric analysis in diagnostic hematology. In *Diagnost Haematol*. Rodak, Saunders, pp. 425–35.

Kristensen J.S. (1994) Immunophenotyping in acute leukemia, myelodysplastic syndromes and hairy cell leukemia. The use of monoclonal antibodies against myeloid differentiation antigens. *Dan. Med. Bull.*, **41 (1)**, 52–65.

Lebeau A., Muthmann H., Sendelhofert A. *et al.* (1995) Histochemistry and immuno-histochemistry on bone marrow biopsies. A rapid procedure for methyl methacrylate embedding. *Pathol Res Pract*, **191 (2)**, 121–9.

Louw I., De Beer D.P., Du Plessis M.J. (1994) Microwave histoprocessing of bone marrow trephine biopsies. *Histochem J*, **26 (6)**, 487–94.

Macera M.J., Szabo P., Verman R.S. (1989) A simple method for short-term culturing bone marrow and unstimulated blood from acute leukemias. *Leuk. Res.*, **13 (9)**, 729–34.

MacLennan K.A., Reynolds G. (1992) In K. Henry and W St C Symmers (eds), *Thymus, Lymph Nodes, Spleen and Lymphatics, 3rd edn*. Edinburgh: Churchill Livingstone.

Mason D.Y., Erber W.N. (1991) Immunocytochemical labeling of leukemia samples with monoclonal antibodies by the APAAP procedure. *The Leukemic Cell*, **2**, 196–214.

McCluggage W.G., Roddy S., Whiteside C. *et al.* (1995) Immunohistochemical staining of plastic embedded bone marrow trephine biopsy specimens after microwave heating. *J Clin Pathol*, **48 (9)**, 840–4.

Merkel D.E., Dressler L.G., McGuire W.L. (1987) Flow cytometry, cellular DNA content, and prognosis in human malignancy. *J Clin Oncol.*, **5**, 1690–703.

Mitelman F. (ed) (1995) *ISCN 1995: An International System for Human Cytogenetic Nomenclature (1995)*. Basel: Karger.

Nadji M., Morales A.R. (1977) Immunohistochemical techniques. In S.G. Silverberg, R.A. Delellis and W.J. Frable (eds), *Principles and Practice of Surgical Pathology and Cytopathology*, 3rd edn. Edinburgh: Churchill Livingstone, pp. 63–76.

Naish S.J. (ed) (1989) *Handbook of Immunochemical Staining Methods*. Carpinteria, Ca. Dako Corp.

Novak A., Kruskic M., Ludoski M., Jurukovski V. (1994) Rapid method for obtaining high-quality chromosome banding in the study of hematopietic neoplasia. *Cancer Genet Cytogenet.*, **74 (2)**, 109–14.

Pasquale D., Chikkappa G. (1995) Bone marrow biopsy imprints (touch preparations) for assessment of iron stores. *Am J Hematol*, **48 (3)**, 201–2.

Pellegrini W., Facchetti F., Marocolo D. *et al.* (1995) Assessment of cell proliferation in normal and pathological bone marrow biopsies: a study using double sequential immunophenotyping on paraffin sections. *Histopathology*, **27 (5)**, 397–405.

Robinson J.P. (ed) (1993) *Handbook of Flow Cytometry Methods*. Chichester: John Wiley.

Ruck P., Horny H.P., Greschniok A. *et al.* (1995) Nonspecific immunostaining of blast cells of acute leukemia by antibodies against nonhemopoietic antigens. *Hematol Pathol*, **9 (1)**, 49–56.

Shi S.R., Cote R.J., Taylor C.R. (1997) Antigen retrieval immunohistochemistry: past, present, and future. *J Histochem Cytochem.*, **45 (3)**, 327–43.

True L.D. (ed) (1990) *Atlas of Diagnostic Immunohistopathology*. New York: Gower Medical.

Ucci G., Danova M., Ricardi A. (1995) Optimal bone marrow samples for cell kinetic studies. *Cytometry*, **20 (3)**, 268–9.

Williams B., Allan D.J. (1996) Combonation of SCF, IL-6, IL-3, and GM-CSF increases the mitotic index in short term bone marrow cultures from acute promyelocytic leukemia (APL) patients. *Cancer Genet Cytogenet.*, **91 (1)**, 77–81.

Wolf E., Roser K., Hahn M. *et al.* (1992) Enzyme and immunohistochemistry on undecalcified bone and bone marrow biopsies after embedding in plastic: a new embedding method for routine application. *Virchows Archiv A Pathol Anat.*, **420**, 17.

Yunis J.J. (1976) High resolution of human chromosomes. *Science*, **191**, 1268–70.

Yunis J.J., Sawyer J.R., Ball D.W. (1978) The characterization of high-resolution G-banded chromosomes of man. *Chromosoma*, **67**, 293–307.

Index

Note: page numbers in *italics* refer to tables, those in **bold** refer to figures